User–Driven Healthcare and Narrative Medicine:
Utilizing Collaborative Social Networks and Technologies

Rakesh Biswas
People's College of Medical Sciences, India

Carmel M. Martin
Trinity College Dublin, Ireland

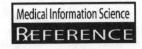
Medical Information Science
REFERENCE

MEDICAL INFORMATION SCIENCE REFERENCE

Hershey · New York

Director of Editorial Content:	Kristin Klinger
Director of Book Publications:	Julia Mosemann
Acquisitions Editor:	Lindsay Johnston
Development Editor:	Dave DeRicco
Typesetter:	Deanna Zombro and Keith Glazewski
Production Editor:	Jamie Snavely
Cover Design:	Lisa Tosheff

Published in the United States of America by
    Medical Information Science Reference (an imprint of IGI Global)
    701 E. Chocolate Avenue
    Hershey PA 17033
    Tel: 717-533-8845
    Fax: 717-533-8661
    E-mail: cust@igi-global.com
    Web site: http://www.igi-global.com

Library of Congress Cataloging-in-Publication Data

User-driven healthcare and narrative medicine : utilizing collaborative social
networks and technologies / Rakesh Biswas and Carmel Mary Martin, editors.
      p. ; cm.
  Includes bibliographical references and index.
  Summary: "This book explores various individual user-driven strategies that
assist in solving multiple clinical system problems in healthcare, using
social networking to improve their healthcare outcomes"--Provided by
publisher.
  ISBN 978-1-60960-097-6 (h/c) -- ISBN 978-1-60960-099-0 (e-ISBN) 1.
Clinical medicine--Decision making. 2. Narrative medicine. 3. Social
networks. 4. Medical informatics. 5. Consumer-driven health care. I.
Biswas, Rakesh. II. Martin, Carmel M.
  [DNLM: 1. Community Networks. 2. Decision Support Techniques. 3.
Information Systems. 4. Narration. 5. Social Support. W 26.55.I4 U84 2011]
  RC48.U86 2011
  616--dc22
                              2010019426

British Cataloguing in Publication Data
A Cataloguing in Publication record for this book is available from the British Library.

All work contributed to this book is new, previously-unpublished material. The views expressed in this book are those of the authors, but not necessarily of the publisher.

Table of Contents

Section 2

Detailed Table of Contents

Section 1

Chapter 1
Joan W. Young, Independent Researcher, USA

Young describes her engagement with the healthcare system and the insights she gained during her struggle to restore her health. She also chronicles how this life-changing event prompted her to help educate others diagnosed with similar diseases and to form an active community for sharing and expanding medical knowledge. After a synopsis of the author's medical journey in the introduction, these topics are woven into three main sections: Medical Evidence, Complementary and Alternative Treatments, and the Influence of Technology.

Chapter 2
Anirban Chaudhuri, Consultant Physician, India
Joan Young, Platelet Disorder Support Association, USA
Carmel M. Martin, Trinity College Dublin, Ireland
Joachim Sturmberg, Monash University and The University of Newcastle, Australia
Rakesh Biswas, People's College of Medicine, India

Choudhuri and colleagues introduce the reader to a world of clinical problem solving in blood disorders as presented in hematology lectures. These lectures encompass multiple perspectives, the patient, his/her relatives, healthcare students, consultant health professionals and society. This style of lecture aims to enable these key stakeholders in the health care system to utilize the continued learning derived from sharing their narratives toward attaining the goal of improved healthcare outcomes. The chapter has three narratives which are intertwined – the patient narratives of their experiences with disturbances in their blood stream, the blood system disease narratives of the medical professionals and the stream of consciousness expressed in poetry evoked by the first two narratives.

Chapter 3

Paramartha Bhattacharya, Consultant Physician, India
Amar Puri Asanga, Yoga consultant, Nepal
Rakesh Biswas, People's College of Medicine, India

Bhattacharya and colleagues present physician and patient perspectives of their gastrointestinal system problem solving experiences beginning from one anatomical end, stomodeum and continuing toward the other end proctodeum of the gastrointestinal tube. These experiences reflect user driven health care to the extent that they have been largely shared and developed over a web interface through email narratives and illustrate conversational learning in a patient centered manner.

Chapter 4

Paul Bradley, Hertfordshire Partnership NHS Foundation Trust, UK
Peter Griffin, Teacher in Further Education, UK
Ann Griffin, Caregiver and Mother, UK
Kamalika Mukherj, Hertfordshire Partnership NHS Foundation Trust, UK

In this chapter Bradley and colleagues present the narratives of some people with autistic spectrum disorders (also known as autism spectrum conditions) as well as those of their families and carers. It describes the history and development of the diagnostic concept of autistic spectrum disorders and how the clinical features impact on daily life and their families. It examines the different stages through which people progress, based on their contact with services – before diagnosis, at the time of diagnosis and their life since then. The chapter concludes with a personal account of all these stages.

Chapter 5

R. K. Goyal, NY Presbyterian Hospital, USA
M. O'Neill, NY Presbyterian Hospital, USA
N. Agostinelli, NY Presbyterian Hospital, USA
P. Wyer, Columbia University, USA

Goyal and colleagues illustrate that the care of the critically-ill patient in the acute setting, an 'everyday' occurrence in most urban emergency departments, often proceeds through the dictates of Parsonian paternalism: the Physician knows best. Through a discussion of three such 'everyday' encounters, the authors hope to complicate this notion and find a place for healthcare patient users in the decision making process.

Chapter 6

Carmel M. Martin, Trinity College Dublin, Ireland
Rakesh Biswas, People's College of Medical Sciences, India
Ankur Joshi, People's College of Medical Sciences, India
Joachim Sturmberg, Monash University and The University of Newcastle, Australia

Martin and colleagues argue the need for a paradigm shift to focus health care from a top down fragmented process driven activity to a user-driven journey of the individual whose health is at stake. Currently many person/patients express needs that are often overlooked or not understood in the health
system, and the frontline care workers express frustration in relation to care systems that prevent them
from optimizing their care delivery. They propose the Patient Journey Record System (PaJR) as a fundamental concept to transform health care so it supports and improves the experience of patients and
improves the quality of care through adaptable and interconnected information and care systems. A case
is made for placing Patient Journey Record Systems at the centre of care to which patients, caregivers,
physicians, allied health professionals and students can contribute. PaJR's become a 'discovery tool'
of new knowledge arising from different types of experiences ranging from the implicit knowledge in
narratives through to the explicit knowledge that is formalized in the published peer reviewed literature.
They show that complex adaptive systems and social constructionist theories provide a link for knowledge translation that ultimately will lead to improved health care and better personal health outcomes/
experiences.

Chapter 7

Carmel M. Martin, Trinity College Dublin, Ireland
Rakesh Biswas, People's College of Medical Sciences, India
Joachim Sturmberg, Monash University and The University of Newcastle, Australia
David Topps, Northern Ontario School of Medicine, Canada
Rachel Ellaway, Northern Ontario School of Medicine, Canada
Kevin Smith, National Digital Research Centre, Ireland

Martin and colleagues articulate key considerations for the translation of the concept of the Patient
Journey Record Systems (PaJR) into real world systems. The key concept lies in the 'discovery' of
the use of patient narratives to locate the phase of illness in a patient journey. They describe their developmental framework in the context of ambulatory care for older patients with multiple morbidity,
who are at a high risk of hospitalizations and other adverse consequences. The framework addresses
the feasibility and usability of an information technology based solution to avert adverse outcomes of
hospitalization when this is potentially avoidable by activities in primary care. Key considerations in
the PaJR knowledge systems are the design and implementation of robust expert knowledge and data
support systems. The patient, caregiver, physician and care team perspectives drive clinical usability
and functionality requirements. Experts from computer science domains in artificial intelligence, expert
systems, and decision support systems ensure the requirements for the functionality of underlying sys-

tems architecture are met. They explore this transdisciplinary perspective and ways in which coherence may be achieved among the many practitioners and expert domains involved in a developmental framework for PaJR. Finally they make a case for the implementation of PaJR systems as part of a universal move to electronic user driven health care.

Ross illustrates that the personal experience of Medicine by each physician is the product of a large number of dynamic and diverse factors: inborn talents and deficiencies, social and cultural environments, type of schooling, exposure to teachers and mentors, colleagues, family and friends, and of course, perhaps most important of all, encounters with patients. She demonstrates that many of these influences are beyond the direct control of the physician, and nearly all continue to change throughout a lifetime. Finally she concludes that out of this seemingly random and chaotic mix of influences, each physician develops his or her own highly unique, and ever evolving understanding of what it means to practice Medicine today.

Dhakal and Ross trace the learning experiences of a medical student through his career journey in medical training from two different world settings of Nepal and US. The chapter sketches the student's interactive learning with his patients through his case notes right from his medical student days in Nepal to residency in the US. The juxtaposed commentary from a senior physician provides a longer view lens through which these learning points may be considered. These case notes and narrative insights from the health professional's perspective aim to demonstrate and stimulate experiential learning in medicine, a valuable means of obtaining expertise.

Morgan illustrates the fact that doctors have unique and privileged opportunities to observe and participate in the illness narratives (stories) that patients present with. Hearing, understanding and respecting the patient narrative is as important as correctly practising the technical aspects of medical diagnosis and treatment, and yet traditionally has received much less emphasis during medical education. The stories below (which have all been altered to preserve patient confidentiality) illustrate how attention to the patient's narrative enables a richer and deeper interaction with them that enhances the therapeutic aspects of the consultation.

Das narrates the stories of patients with cardiac illnesses requiring surgery and reveals how the physician-surgeon tries to reconcile a low resource setting patient care narrative with resource demanding modern scientific medicine and the areas of disconnect that this generate. This chapter is written in three parts. The first part is a narrative of training that the author received and the development of his philosophy of medicine. The second part describes his experiences in the government health services in the State of West Bengal in India and the third describes how from a remote location in Nepal, the author was able to set up a cardiothoracic unit. The chapter narrates the problems, solutions and outcomes of surgery in these circumstances and how it was possible to overcome difficulties to offer a service to the patients which, while having many flaws, did offer treatments that would have never been possible for them to access otherwise.

O Shea explores aspects of professional blindness in the family practice setting. This exploration uses the vehicle of an exercise in practice audit, which resulted in a more meaningful level of interaction between the GP and a particular group of individuals in his practice. He illustrates that what set out as a quantitative exercise in audit inadvertently threw up valuable qualitative insights and reflections on how a family doctor had previously viewed this group of individuals in the past, and more importantly, would do so in the future. In particular, the exercise challenges the audience to look for and see the ambitions and hopes of those individuals who attend health professionals for medical care, in order to properly respect these important aspects of their humanity, and to assist health professionals in more easily rising beyond the confines unwittingly imposed and accepted by a passive acceptance of disease defined horizons and the medical model.

James illustrates a life in medical practice and emphasizes the importance of lifelong learning in medicine through sharing of lived experiences. The life narratives display the authors own observations of what he has learned and unlearned over the years. Also added are observations about his retirement project - editing and publishing abstracts of the current primary care medicine literature - that exemplifies the need for health care professionals to continue sharing life-long.

Hegde provides a personal view on learning medicine and summarizes his lessons learnt in a medical career that has made him explore medical traditions primarily to refute false dogmas that in his view continue to permeate the sciences to this day.

Chapter 15

Conroy uses the example of sex work research in Africa to ask the question "useful to whom?" In over 800 papers on sex work in Africa published over more than two decades, the focus has been on sex workers as spreaders of HIV, enriching the research community while further stigmatising the sex workers who participate in the research. In a study conducted by the author and partly run by sex workers themselves, the focus was on targeting micro-economic aid, and documenting the violent and abusive culture in which sex work is practised. The chapter illustrates the data analysis using Stata. However, it tries to place the descriptive statistics into their wider context in the research agenda, including a discussion of the ethics of research into vulnerable groups.

Chapter 16

Shanker provides a broad idea of what are the Medical Humanities (MH) and directs his readers to understand the advantages of teaching MH to medical students. He also introduces them to a selection of MH programs in developed and developing nations and explores connections between medical ethics and MH. The chapter also provides an overview of MH in the Asian context through the author's experiences with MH modules and familiarizes the reader with possible challenges and future directions for MH in developing nations.

Section 2

Chapter 17

Biswas and colleagues provide an introduction to user driven learning that initially dwells on features that are unchanged such as the role of collaborative social interactions in human learning and later move on to describe certain aspects that are evolving and helping create a learning transformation through web based technologies. The chapter is interspersed with user driven learning narrative examples taken from the authors' own experience of sharing data over the web to accumulate learning points as well as the experience of a significant population of other web based learners in discussion forums, blogs and other networking sites. This is an attempt to create a background that may help illustrate the evolution of user driven health care, which is another form of user driven learning on the web with particular reference to individual user clinical problem solving, be it initiated by patients, health professionals or other actors in a care giving collaborative network across a web interface.

Kochar explores her personal journey in teaching math and traces her path toward initiating student user driven learning strategies in math. It begins by spelling out the need for different math learning strategies and progresses to illustrate student user output which she has savored over the years. Finally it emphasizes the importance of letting go.

Garg and colleagues introduce the reader to a sample 'User driven learning environment' created in an online community with a special interest centred on trees and plants. It traces the development of an online learning community through the lived experiences and thoughts of its founding members and also includes conversational learning experiences of other users to illustrate the process of 'user driven learning' in online communities. It illustrates innovative sense making methodologies utilized by group members to create a more meaningful 'User driven learning environment' while simultaneously contributing in a positive way to create information resources at no cost along with creating awareness & scientific temper among members.

Shaefer and Dervin demonstrate the utilization of a discussion group design and analytical process informed by Sense-Making Methodology to highlight the relationship between situational aspects of online dialogue and consensus/dissensus activity. Their findings suggest that, counter to received theories advocating the privileging of user-to-user interaction within online discussion groups, both consensus and dissensus appeared to be important for robust communicative activities.

Sarbadhikari discusses examples of information needs and information-seeking behaviors of patients and students of healthcare. The role of the Internet (infrastructure), and especially the WWW (applications and content), is elucidated with respect to the concepts of online collaborative learning as applied to medical education and practice where the emphasis is on user driven healthcare.

Chapter 22

Jane Fitzpatrick, University of the West of England, UK
Willie Ako, University of Bristol, UK

Fitzpatrick and Ako examine how health care professionals can work with a range of stakeholders in designing and delivering health care focused on service user needs. It further examines how health care professionals can engage in understanding user perspectives in order to develop effective health care policies and programs. It argues that this type of approach will enable the development of effective partnerships in designing and implementing user focused approaches to healthcare.

Chapter 23

Edward Kim, Robert Wood Johnson Medical School, USA

Kim examines how descriptions of psychiatric illness may be the richest and most challenging narrative for consumers to develop because core symptoms of disease may distort perceptual and interpretative brain functions. These distortions may fragment and disrupt personal narratives of wellness, illness, and recovery. As Internet access becomes more common among all strata of societies, the use of Web-based social networking may accelerate the development of new models of recovery. Social networking may expand the consumer's understanding of their past and present through web-based shared discussions with other consumers and professionals. Online psychiatry-related activity generally falls into several categories related to information acquisition, treatment facilitation, and social networking. The tension between confidentiality and transparency, and the potential for deception due to anonymity are ethical challenges that must be addressed as Virtual Communities and social networking evolve in health care.

Chapter 24

Maartje H.J. Swennen, University Medical Centre Utrecht, The Netherlands

Swennen explores why doctors, do, and do not, incorporate high quality evidence into their routine practice. She takes us down the road to how she became more and more intrigued by all the challenges that EBM faces. In addition, she explains how she hopes to contribute to closing the gap between what is knowable using EBM methods and what we do in clinical practice.

Chapter 25

Daz Greenop, Liverpool John Moores University, UK
Sheila Glenn, Liverpool John Moores University, UK
Martin Walshaw, Liverpool Heart and Chest Hospital NHS Trust, UK
Martin Ledson, Liverpool Heart and Chest Hospital NHS Trust, UK

Greenop and colleagues explore how a group of adults with cystic fibrosis (N=40) manage and account for self-care. By focussing of the development of 'character and plot', narrative analysis illustrates how distinct patient identities may be constructed and performed as participants defend and justify their preferred self-care practices. Drawing on exemplars of 5 distinct types of storytelling an alternative user-driven taxonomy is suggested which not only recognizes a range of self-care practices but also affirms their legitimacy beyond the horizons of mainstream biomedicine.

Chapter 26

Susan Sliedrecht, Auckland Spinal Rehabilitation Unit, New Zealand
Elmarie Kotzé, University of Waikato, New Zealand

Sliedrecht and Kotze report on a qualitative research project which explored patients' experiences of counseling and which provided the impetus for changes to be incorporated in the rehabilitation and health care provided at a spinal cord rehabilitation unit in Auckland, New Zealand. It illustrate how navigating different landscapes of meaning, philosophies, ideas and practices from approaches such as the relationship-centred model and narrative medicine developed into a collaborative meaning-making partnership between the patient team and the multidisciplinary team that further shaped practices of doing reasonable hope together.

Chapter 27

Chris Peterson, La Trobe University, Australia
Evan Willis, La Trobe University, Australia

•

Peterson and Willis describe how a typical biomedical perspective on illness tends to focus on disease and its causes without considering the social world within which health and illness occur, and the way in which social forces shape these concepts and experiences. In their chapter they aim to present some narratives by patients, consumers, medical and health practitioners, and other stakeholders in blogs, discussions and forums on the Internet that examine the relevance of looking at social construction for understanding chronic illness, and at the effects of social factors on understanding illness. In addition this chapter focuses on the problems associated with illnesses that have not achieved a legitimate status according to biomedical criteria.

Chapter 28

Bjerg describes relevant dimensions of a personal life-journey support system – across health, handicaps and illness. The chapter demonstrates a new road to facilitate private logging of phenomena, a coherent and sedimenting self-narrative not only in text, picture and sound, but also through user-network-developed pictographic fonts. Inclusion of biotelemetric data and virtual body imaging as part of such support systems are considered. And questions are raised concerning the future of thus skilled chronic patients' interfacing most trusted helpers, fellow-sufferers and wider shared social platforms of Patient Journey Records.

Chapter 29

Basu and colleagues provide a review of two key concepts of online social learning (social presence and media richness) and explore how they can be implemented in the current wave of web based collaboration tools, and indicate their place in medical education. They also provide a few examplars of how educators are incorporating web based or online social tools in student learning in the context of medical education and indicate some ways to extend this approach further.

Chapter 30

Gavgani introduces a model for Information Therapy service through social networks. It discusses how health care providers including physicians, medical specialists and residents can prescribe reliable, evidence based health information to patients in a web 2.0 environment. This chapter deals with definition of Information Therapy, importance of information therapy, changes in the preference of information users about how to access right information, Web 2.0, application of Web 2.0 in rendering Information Therapy Service, and a proposal model for Information Therapy service through web 2.0.

Chapter 31

Norman begins his chapter with an emphasis on how complex problems require strategies that leverage the knowledge of diverse actors working in a coordinated manner in order to address them in a manner that is appropriate to the context. Such strategies require building relationships among groups that enable them to network in ways that have the intensity of face-to-face meetings, but also extend over time. He proceeds to describe the 'Complexity, Networks, EHealth, & Knowledge Translation Research' (CoNEKTR) model that draws upon established methods of face-to-face social engagement supported with information technology and further proscribes an approach to issue exploration, idea generation and collective action that leverages social networks for health innovation.

Vicdan aims to describe transformations in market roles and relations that reflect collaborative, connective and communal characteristics among healthcare market actors, in light of technological advances and changing consumer/marketer institutional relationships. She further exemplifies how these transformations influence current market dynamics by providing a deep understanding of web 2.0 applications in healthcare, specifically organizations that turn social networking into an enterprising virtual community in healthcare. In doing so, she seeks to explore how and why such systems develop and function, what makes patients and other actors in healthcare become a part of these systems, and how their interest and participation in these systems is maintained as they share their private health information and contribute to real-time medical research.

LaPorte and colleagues evaluate and illustrate the utility of Google Tools for assessing research communications in Global Health. Page Ranks (PR) appear to be an important tool or utility for ranking the impact pages with the logic that PR determine which pages will be seen in a search. Google Trends provide very intriguing results as with this one can assess the temporal trends in searching. Google analyses appear to be very powerful to evaluate the translation of scientific knowledge.

Chapter 34

> *Tom Axtell, National Aboriginal Health Organization, Canada*
> *Cassandra Chaulk, Nunatsiavut Health & Social Development, Canada*
> *Dianne Kinnon, National Aboriginal Health Organization, Canada*
> *Carmel M. Martin, Trinity College Dublin, Ireland*
> *Michele Wood, Nunatsiavut Health & Social Development, Canada*

Axtell and colleagues describe focus group testing in a small community in the Labrador Inuit Land Claim area of the online information system 'Community Accounts,' developed by the province of Newfoundland and Labrador. Key data users were engaged in a hands-on process to help determine what information and data would be useful in an Inuit Web directory. The purpose was to obtain a better understanding of how Inuit use statistics to better understand the broad determinants of health. Inuit continue to take further steps toward managing Inuit specific data in order to create comprehensive health policies and programs and affect decision-making.

Afterword

> *Joachim Sturmberg, Monash University and The University of Newcastle, Australia*

Sturmberg takes a conceptual rather than a technical or social perspective towards exploring user-driven health care and views user-driven health care as an emergent phenomenon in the context of a rapidly evolving web-based communication infrastructure. He highlights that knowledge has many dimensions each of which contribute unique insights to the understanding of health as a personal adaptive experiential state that needs to be distinguished from the health professional preoccupation with pathologies. Information technologies increase connectivity between people and the sharing of knowledge and experience narrows the 'gap between experts in the pathology and experts in the dis-ease' which finally may give people the power to shift the attractor of the health care system to the health needs of the people, resulting in truly people-centred health care reform.

Foreword

As doctor-driven medicine sinks into disreputable old age, user-driven medicine is the hope of the future. This transition is already taking place across the world, and doctors and other health professionals should welcome it and play a creative role in shaping it. This book is a beginning in that process: a collecting together of materials, of stories, of insights, of ways of thinking, of problems and potential solutions, from users ("patients" - a word which needs to disappear) and from health professionals. A new kind of shared health care will emerge out of the current chaos not by the imposition of a single will, but through the shaping that emerges spontaneously from the creative efforts of many individuals and many different forces. The unprecedented privilege of our time is that we can each participate in this on a global scale, and this book is one illustration of how this process can get started.

Medicine in our time has become alienated from its users, and even from its practitioners. We are all, to a varying extent, pawns in a global business which is only incidentally related to helping ill people. And yet our individual efforts are well motivated and overwhelmingly successful compared to those of previous generations. I write as a doctor who has practised for 35 years, and when I look back I can be proud of many things achieved, but also frustrated: not just by personal shortcomings, which all of us have, but by the restraints of systems we all have to work in and which could be far more effective and creative than they ever seem capable of becoming. It is to liberation of this creativity, of organic development through shared aims between users and professionals, that this book is directed.

Doctors for the main part lead crowded and emotionally demanding lives. I am told that when doctors go on narrative medicine courses and are asked to write stories from their lives, the commonest subject is the patient they killed (or blame themselves for killing). By contrast, the weekly medical magazines which are sent to general practitioners throughout the UK always include columns about silly things that patients do and say and the ways they find to annoy us. Between confessional anguish and shared world-weariness, we manage to survive and protect ourselves. This may be necessary, but we need to move well beyond it. If personal continuous care by doctors for individual sick people is to be transformed into user-driven health care, delivered by genuinely integrated health professional teams. There is a need to share values as well as effective systems of operation.

For doctors, to be "user-driven" means an increase in the vulnerability which we already find so stressful. It means opening up to the demands of people with physical and mental problems, whether or not these bear any relation to the diagnostic categories that appear in medical school courses and textbooks. It means that the traditional defence mechanisms of doctors - ranging from carefully limited consulting times to shared rote-learning from "expert" lecturers - need to be replaced by far more open and interactive forms of shared communication and learning with sick individuals, or users.

I find this model of user-driven medicine quite frightening. I don't know if I have the required mental flexibility or the right repertoire of skills. It may be that nobody has, but that these will simply develop as we open up to new ways of helping users in need of our services. They are almost always be in a position of disadvantage in relation to us - they will be ill, or worried, or distressed, and may lack the resources to assess what they need - just as we often do, the moment we become sick. We can fall back on our usual defensive armoury, including emblems of authority like the white coat, ways of speaking which are more elevated and technical than the patient can follow, the ordering of batteries of investigations, etc, for which they may respond with a seeming gratitude which reinforces our bad habits. We can really listen to their needs and adopt a much wider repertoire of genuine empathy and help. It is our failure to do this that drives patients so often to seek "complementary" therapies with a proven lack of physical benefit. We need to widen the debate about these forms of user-professional interaction, both remote and face-to-face. Both users and health professionals have hurdles of vulnerability to overcome before they can align themselves more closely.

Medicine only became effective when it ceased to be based on transmitted authority and aligned itself with science, which is a truth-seeking activity. The "truth" of medicine was sought first of all in the physical realities of how the body functions and how disease arises, and it continues to be sought this way, with spectacular success. Most people go into medicine with the idea of putting this success into practice, and actually succeed to the extent of doing much more good than harm throughout their working lives. Additionally we now seek "truth" by constantly assessing that balance of good versus harm in the wide range of scientifically plausible treatments that we use. This has come to be called evidence-based medicine. We discover that many treatments which have a good basis in scientific logic do not in fact benefit the majority of people. We also discover the frayed edges of seemingly objective truth as we struggle for precise definitions of such conditions as "heart failure" or "major depression", and then look at outcomes from interventions in populations which bear little resemblance to the patients who most often come to see us.

User-driven health care must include the aligning of our understanding of the truth with that of the patient. By this I do not mean trying to explain the full science of every situation as we understand it. On the contrary, it means recognising that our understanding of the situation is usually critically dependent on what the user can tell us, and our management is always aimed at making the user better, not simply at discovering or ruling out disease. We want to know above all what the person before us is experiencing and how this affects them. This concordance of understanding can then lead to a concordance of aims. Without such concordance, we can act as effective technicians in certain circumstances, but we can never provide any deeper help to a person facing the distress of illness, loss or death. Without it we cannot begin to develop a research agenda that deals with real causes of distress, rather than the things that are convenient or lucrative to write papers about.

If we limit ourselves to the technical, the user will be free to leave us and seek a different practitioner, perhaps non-medical, and we are thus relieved of further responsibility. If this is the future of "user-driven" health care, then I want no part in it. It is not that I am opposed to the principle of free choice among users - far from it - but rather that I believe that such a take-it-or-leave-it system degrades health professionals and exploits sick people, and ultimately makes health care unaffordable for those who need it most. To me, an encounter between a sick person and a professional involves an assumption of responsibility, above all the responsibility of understanding and helping.

We will know when we have arrived at a proper model of user-driven medicine when there is a free dialogue between patient experience and evidence-based medicine. Above all we will know it when every person (user) in the world has access to health professionals whom they can trust to listen to them and help them, and a health system which will provide them with the best available care. If only a small percentage of health professionals in the world united behind this aim, it could be realised within the lifetime of most of us.

Richard Lehman
Oxford University, UK
7th March 2010

Richard Lehman *is a Senior Research Fellow in the Department of Primary Care at Oxford University. He is perhaps best known for his individual weekly reviews of the principal general medical journals, maintained for the last 12 years and posted worldwide by the Centre for Evidence Based Medicine and on the BMJ website. His clinical interests are wide and in 2006 he was responsible for the first book on Palliative Care for Heart Failure. Following retirement this year from clinical practice R has been acting as medical adviser to the Health Experiences Research Group at Oxford and their groundbreaking website of patient interviews covering 70 clinical areas on www.healthtalkonline.org. His current main interest is in combining qualitative and quantitative research methods to identify patient-important outcome measures, especially in chronic illnesses as exemplified by type 2 diabetes.*

CONVERSATIONS

Physician, Ireland:
Strongly agree with the need to discontinue the use of the word 'patient,' but the word 'user' does also have some fairly significant negative and pejorative connotations. Could we simply refer to 'people centred,' 'people,' and 'individuals,' or even 'individualised.'
In this profound re orientation of our personal practices in healing and caring, it is important we do not throw out any babies with the bathwater. As with any revolution, overtly political or merely within the infinities of the mind, it is important to retain carefully the good of the older while bringing on the new. As a younger Doctor, I was vividly taught by Dr. Manne Berber, a Dublin based Jewish Family Doctor, the art of positive unconditional regard when in the presence of any individual consulting me professionally. At the core of this manouvre was the effective ability to ruthlessly exclude any other concern or distraction other than the issues of importance for this individual at this moment in time. Thus taught, it has informed many of my own consultations, and though it originates from well within the twentieth century, it is well deserving of a place in the twenty first.

Editors:
Just to add to our official perspective (also detailed on our journal web page) on the term "user":
The term "user" includes health professionals as well as patients and anyone who uses the web with a user name. These "users" generate an information flow that "drives" the system's workflow (hence the choice of the term "driven"). "User driven healthcare" aims at improved healthcare through clinical problem solving utilizing concerted experiential learning in conversations between multiple users and

stakeholders, primarily patients, health professionals, and other actors in a care giving collaborative network across a Web interface.

User driven health care is actually Patient/People centred but it is as much about health professionals as much as it is about patients.

Physician, Dublin, Ireland:

I think 'we' know what we mean by the word 'user,' which is fine. Its a practical and utilitarian term. It is strictly accurate. But all of this still does not make it the best choice as a successor to the word 'patient.' This is, I believe, because it has negative connotations as in 'bloody users,' friendly user,' and even 'user friendly,' which in itself is nowadays more often used ironically and sarcastically than in its original sense where it started off life as part of the marketing jargon of peddlers of computer consumables...

Anyway, I'll get over it!!

Editors:

Yes it is not a successor to the word patient because there is a 'patient user' as well as a 'health professional user.' I guess as of now it is a successor to the word 'humans' perhaps.

Asst Prof, Marketing, Eastern Kentucky University, USA:

It was important for me to learn about the thoughts or feelings of a physician about user-generated healthcare, since physicians now become more conscious of their expertise and of course become vulnerable with shared decision-making and active involvement from patients. Quick question though, at the very end, the author talks about a free dialogue between patient experience and evidence based medicine? What does he exactly mean by free? Also, is there a clear cut between patient experience and evidence based medicine?

Dr Lehman, Oxford, UK:

What I mean is that in future research questions should be generated by users on the basis of their experiences and answered by the methods of EBM, and that people generally should be much better informed of how medical decisions are made, how evidence is generated, and what the shortcomings are.

Epidemiologist and Associate Professor, Dublin, Ireland:

Quoting from Dr Lehman, "Medicine in our time has become alienated from its users, and even from its practitioners"

This equates medicine with Medicine - I would see the alienation of users from Medicine as indexed by the huge profitability of alternative medicine(s). The demand on behalf of users to define their own problems (rather than the typical Doctor retort of "Let me be the judge of that") and to decide on their own treatment has led to an explosion of spending on medicine outside the professional sphere of Medicine.

Quoting from Dr Lehman, "Medicine only became effective when it ceased to be based on transmitted authority and aligned itself with science, which is a truth-seeking activity"

Yes but...

Yes but the whole enterprise of scientific medicine has been hijacked by the vast commercial interest involved. The ten highest earning companies in the Fortune 500 are ALL pharma companies. And furthermore, these ten companies together earn more than the other 490 companies put together. At these high stakes, of course the dice are loaded.

Psychology Researcher, Copenhagen, Denmark
Quoting from Dr Lehman, "We want to know above all what the person before us is experiencing and how this affects them. This concordance of understanding can then lead to a concordance of aims."

But a preliminary concordance of understanding between doctor and patient necessary to develop a research agenda that deals with the real causes of distress may –at least in chronic cases- have to involve an assumption of patient responsibility as an empiricist.
The focus on the brief (and expensive) face-to-face encounters between patient and doctor (and patients' on the spot recollection and condensed narrative of selected distresses) tends to distract from the data resources available through long-term involvement of the patient in documentation.

To reach a free dialogue between patient experience and evidence based medicine, patients - in an age where the 200 dollars laptop is globally available- must be provided free tools to collect their own evidences of what they - when they are not before us - have been experiencing, and how this has and now affects them around the clock and along the weeks, months and years, before , between and after their encounters with health-providers.
"An abundance of unrealised potential that is waiting to be unleashed"...yes indeed. And this is also a question of acknowledging the more or less global access to Internet 2.0, and creating a user-driven approach to the presence and future of medicine.

Sociologist, Liverpool, UK:
I can't really comment on the vulnerabilities experienced by practitioners but as a regular user of healthcare and a social scientist, however, I am concerned with other 'vulnerabilities'. Indeed, my main concern is with what goes on 'outside' the medical encounter: the lived experience of patients, the barriers (and resources) they must daily negotiate within wider structures of inequality.

Patients are not just disadvantaged because of illness and loss but also because of the alienation they experience when encountering health professionals. The institutions of medicine are, like it or not, constructed and designed by a privileged few for the (greater) benefit of a privileged few and utilized most 'effectively' by such. My concern then is that it is the latter who become the focus of user-driven healthcare and, consequently, health inequalities may become even more pronounced. These are also the same people who have generally enjoyed the unprecedented 'successes' of medicine in the past – which is easily evidenced today in, for example, in the enduring (and unacceptable) differences in rates of mortality and morbidity both within and between different societies across the globe.

This not, of course, to take anything away from the achievements of medicine but, clearly, as the author of the foreword intimates there remains an abundance of unrealized potential that is waiting to be unleashed.

It is a connected point but I do wonder, also, if we all understand the term 'user' (the best term we have, I think). Does it designate anyone who comes into contact with a health professional, only those who have a health 'condition' (which could include all of us) or those undergoing some kind of 'treatment'? I think Rakesh uses the term (in this book and elsewhere) in relation to all 'stakeholders' whereas the author of the foreward seems to confine it (as I generally do) to 'patients' as opposed to health professionals (paras 1&5) or practitioners (para 2) or doctors (para 4). I wonder if this may cause some confusion to readers.

Like much of the emerging debates in 'user-driven healthcare' we need to get beyond semantics and listen to what 'users' actually say and do not just in medical encounters but in everyday life for the latter is the real 'test' of what drives them. User-driven healthcare can I hope contribute to the on-going dialogue that is needed to address these issues (and others) but we must never lose sight of the multiple disadvantages experienced by many and we cannot presume to speak on their behalf.

Preface

We welcome you to review a journey that began long back, perhaps when you were born, perhaps when you first became aware of an entity that you identified as yourself, your body.

Welcome to a reconsideration of this bodily voyage of learning that permeates our cognitive being each day that we live, a voyage that ends only in death (some would say even death is a temporary ending). Our book is about making sense of this journey that most of us as humans have been fortunate to have begun.

We begin this book with a focus on individual narrative descriptions of learning journeys in healthcare students/professionals, patients, their relatives and to break the tedium of an anthropocentric healthcare focus, even math and botany enthusiasts.

Most of these journeys document individual concrete experiences, their reflective observations, abstract conceptualizations and particular instances of their active experimentation.

For today's learner about health be it as patient or professional, new horizons are opening. New options for sharing the journey with others are emerging. With patient-professional access to Internet the world of "Health 2.0" empowers them to dive into a wealth of information on the diagnoses and therapy offered and received.

And not least: to join networks, relevant for particular diagnoses, locate other patients or professionals, with comparable problems, and exchange subjective narratives of personal patient or professional journeys through personal bloggings. This is the new – and global – noosphere: the soil, from which user-driven healthcare grows (K. Bjerg, personal communication, 2010).

It makes a difference if we conceive of patient journey in the sense of the narrow patient journey concept or in the sense of the wider patient journey concept of an individual explorer, whose life-journey earlier or later turns into travelling through pains and problems, encounters with medicine men, passage through admissions, tolls to be paid, - or not afforded -waiting times to be endured, encampment in more or less friendly healthcare institutions, undergoing tortures and sufferings, deprivations and starvations , uncertainties of outcomes, demands of endurance, and potential return to a continuation of previous life voyage, more or less radical change of life-course, or terminal more or less affordable more or less palliative terminal care (K. Bjerg, personal communication, 2010).

From the individual we move on to the collective and focus on learning trends gleaned from online search engines.

We may commiserate upon the ways technologies and gadgets are intruding into our lives, so widely necessary and adopted, making all of us dependant and vulnerable to the whims of engineers, commercial markets and administrations.

New kinds of vulnerabilities are growing upon the human species, not least as our pursuits and their waste is going to thread the ecosystem we share with other species.

Yet one of the prime reasons humans are likely to be device dependent for good is that they have always felt the need to be connected optimally and the new media (albeit device dependent) does inspire a feeling of connectivity that seems phenomenal in comparison to our recent past and that shows no signs of reducing for the moment.

This book is about a kind of human learning, which has always existed as a social process that currently seems to have been augmented in this new media driven wave of connectivity. This book explores how humans make faster learning associations utilizing the new social spider that cuts across barriers of time and space and traps learning in its web of persistent conversations, intersecting life trajectories and lived experiences displayed in flowing narrative.

We have built upon this framework of conversational learning by introducing conversations between readers after quite a few chapters and we hope it stimulates some readers who may even prefer to read the conversations prior to reading the chapters.

Finally all our work in this book of bringing together insights from hitherto undocumented perspectives from all stakeholders in healthcare will evolve further in the "International Journal of User Driven Health Care," that has been launched recently with the Information Resources Management Association IRMA to accommodate the enthusiasm of authors and readers that overflowed while preparing this book. It can be accessed from the IGI global web site and we hope to continue this journey with our audience through their active participation in the journal and invite their fresh perspectives and continued feedback.

Rakesh Biswas, People's College of Medical Sciences, India

Carmel M. Martin, Northern Ontario School of Medicine, Canada

April 2010

Acknowledgment

To all care seekers and caregivers who inspired us to work for this book.

   To all our authors, reviewers and editorial staff without whom this book wouldn't have seen the light of day.

Rakesh Biswas, People's College of Medical Sciences, India

Carmel M. Martin, Northern Ontario School of Medicine, Canada

Section 1

Chapter 1
A Healing Journey with a Thousand Echoes

Joan W. Young
Independent Researcher, USA

ABSTRACT

In this personal account, the author describes her engagement with the healthcare system and the insights she gained during her struggle to restore her health. It also chronicles how this life-changing event prompted her to help educate others diagnosed with similar diseases and to form an active community for sharing and expanding medical knowledge. After a synopsis of the author's medical journey in the Introduction, these topics are woven into three main sections: Medical Evidence, Complementary and Alternative Treatments, and the Influence of Technology.

INTRODUCTION

Like many patients, I thought life was going along fine. Sure, my job wasn't very fulfilling, but it did pay well. I was worried about my two daughters who had graduated from college and were trying to find their way in life, not unlike many young adults. I was living with "Paul" and that relationship was alright, but not great. I was eating the standard American diet along with a daily dose of chocolate and way-too-frequent french fries, had redecorated a few rooms in the winter with insufficient ventilation, cleaned my

home with the volatile products one finds on the supermarket shelves, and had sprayed some plants with pesticides. I was oblivious to the increasing toxicity of my lifestyle. That is until I caught what seemed like the flu, after getting chilled on vacation during the July 4 holiday in 1992, and my physical resilience gave way to a disease I couldn't ignore, although I tried.

After that vacation, I had trouble getting out of bed and just collapsed after work, thinking the fatigue and lack of vitality would go away with rest. The bruises that mysteriously appeared on my arms were odd but would go away too, I thought. I became more suspicious when I bumped my thigh on the edge of my bed and noticed a black and

DOI: 10.4018/978-1-60960-097-6.ch001

blue mark the size of a grapefruit. I became more alarmed when I bit my tongue and it didn't stop bleeding for what seemed like way too long. The little things I tried to get back to normal, resting, traveling to San Francisco to breathe the bay air, eating more vegetables, were not helping. It was then that I decided to go to a doctor.

I wasn't anxious to have a deep involvement with the medical profession. In my late twenties I had my thyroid removed when the lumps in that gland were found to be cold nodules with a small amount of papillary cancer. In my late thirties I had what might have been a seizure, partly due to poor regulation of my Synthroid dose, replacing the functions of my missing thyroid. The Dilantin prescribed for the seizure made it difficult for me to concentrate or do my computer job and I was included in the corporate down-sizing. It took me years after discontinuing that medication, plus some experiments with vitamins and diet, to feel myself again and rebuild my career, in time for the flu and bruises to consume my life.

The hematologist I consulted told me I probably had idiopathic thrombocytopenic purpura, ITP. He wrote it on a piece of paper since there was no possibility of my remembering those strange words. He explained that my body was attacking my platelets as it would attack a virus or bacteria. ITP was in the same autoimmune category as multiple sclerosis or lupus, diseases I had at least heard of. And, like those diseases, there was no definitive cause, although sometimes the low platelets were linked to various environmental toxins.

Since I didn't have many platelets (6×10^9/L, or 6,000/mL) my blood would have difficulty clotting and there were insufficient platelets to plug up the holes in my veins and arteries. All this made logical sense given my symptoms. I was glad to have an explanation I understood.

When I questioned the prognosis, he said the disease was fatal in a small percent of cases, but most times it could be managed with treatments. However, when he talked about the treatment options I recoiled. The first choice was prednisone,

and I knew from a girlfriend who had taken the drug for her asthma that it could change your personality in addition to other unwelcome side effects. After he mentioned the usual second-line treatment, a splenectomy, I was disheartened. I'd already lost my adenoids and tonsils as a child and my thyroid as a young adult, and the loss of each of these may have solved some problems but certainly caused others. I wasn't anxious to lose another organ, especially one that was healthy.

I finally did agree to the prednisone, despite the difficult side effects, since it seemed to be the usual first-line recommendation for treating ITP from what I read on the Internet, and a splenectomy was certainly lower on my list of preferences. However, the prednisone barely raised my platelet count and caused more than the usual share of problems.

I didn't know it at the time, but this was only the beginning of a series of treatments, including several courses of IVIg (immunoglobulin G), a splenectomy, additional rounds of prednisone, colchicine, Danocrine, vincristine, and a Prosorba A column that resulted in another series of treatments to manage the side effects that included possible damage to my digestive system, a suspected seizure, tachycardia, a possible heart attack, and a near-death experience. I was a walking pill box.

Unfortunately, despite everyone's best efforts, none of the treatments succeeded in keeping my platelet count much above 5,000/mL for more than a few weeks and their cumulative destruction left me bald and so weak I could barely walk up stairs. From my diagnosis in August, 1992 to February, 1993, I spent 51 days in the hospital, was on short-term disability from my job, and felt I had no life.

As the treatments my hematologist recommended continued to fail and the side effects mounted I began to look outside of the medical mainstream. If I wanted to live to see the children my daughters wanted and be able to ski again, I clearly needed to change course. I had consulted a naturopath with mixed success when attempting to recover from Dilantin, so I knew something about that option and decided to pursue it again.

The first naturopath I consulted wasn't very helpful and seemed downright nasty. However, the second one suggested some diet changes and supplements that helped stabilize my energy and platelet count, albeit at a low level. That is until I caught the flu in February, my counts plummeted, and I was hospitalized again.

Encouraged by the diet and supplement success, I continued to look for healing options and found many. My psychologist gave me an inspirational diet book and helped me become more assertive. A Reiki practitioner/nurse helped balance my energy and became my wellness coach. A macrobiotic counselor and dietician created an individualized, healing diet. A medical intuitive suggested behavioral changes. An Ayurvedic physician prescribed herbs and gave me a nine-page list of exercise, meditation, and other suggestions. I also reduced the toxins in my environment and began to heal lifelong patterns of self-deprecation.

With these interventions I was able to stay out of the hospital, return to my job, and regain a normal platelet count by June, 1993. Needless to say, I was thrilled.

I had no doubt that the healing path I pursued was responsible for my recovery. One by one, for convenience or cost, I had discontinued the diet, energy treatments, or herbs, and with each absence experienced a minor relapse. When I saw my platelets go down and even small bruises appear I panicked and immediately resumed the discontinued practice. Each time, with my renewed commitment to my healing routine, my platelet count rose again. The end result was a sustained, normal platelet count, an improvement in my overall health, an increased spiritual awareness, and a greater appreciation of the gift of life.

My recovery, from a platelet count hovering near zero to one stabilized for years in the normal range, was dramatic. I thought doctors specializing in ITP would want to know what I had done and perhaps use that knowledge to help their patients.

This was very naïve. Of the two top ITP doctors I told, one was not confident I was telling the truth, although I had all my medical records, and the other was interested, but dismissive.

Discouraged, I could have just stopped there and kept my story to myself. But I knew that others had struggled with the treatments and side effects just as I did, and would want to regain their life, just as I had. When I was dealing with the disease I would have been extremely grateful if someone had told me about the things that I eventually learned, so I decided to bypass the medical community that seemed to only put up roadblocks and go directly to the patients. It was 1997 and the Internet was just beginning to grow. Since I had spent many years as a computer programmer and systems analyst and was not afraid of technology, I decided to create a Web site.

I researched Web software, taught myself Front Page, then wrote and published a small Web site that included my story, other information about ITP, and a discussion group. It would just have a few visitors, I thought, and I would go back to my computer job. I was very wrong.

In just a few months the site attracted people from many countries, hungry for more information about ITP and anxious to meet others who were struggling with similar problems. I worked nights and weekends to update the site, answer e-mails, and determine how to fund the growing enterprise.

The mission of the site was to help others and it seemed like a non-profit organization was the best fit, one where people could donate their time and money for a worthy cause. In 1998 I founded the Platelet Disorder Support Association (PDSA) and my life hasn't been the same since.

PDSA grew from a few hundred contacts to tens of thousands in 130 countries. Through the years I have answered thousands of e-mails and talked to hundreds of patients about their problems, giving me a unique perspective on the disease and the patients who deal with it. What I noticed were communication and treatment threads, many consistent with my experience with ITP, despite differences in age, gender, background, or country.

The subsequent sections of this chapter highlight some of the recurring themes in my own experience that are mirrored by the messages from others.

THE PHYSICIAN/PATIENT COMMUNICATION GAP

I thought the high blood pressure, generalized anger, puffy face, and loss of muscle tone were the worst side effects I would get from the 60 mg of prednisone on my 130-pound frame, but they were only the beginning. When I took a dose one morning at home, after not taking any the day before at my hematologist's suggestion, my head began to spin, I collapsed on the bed, and my partner, "Paul", called an ambulance to take me to a hospital where I was diagnosed with a seizure.

The doctor in the emergency room suggested Dilantin, which I refused, remembering the years I spent recovering from the side effects of that drug, and admitted me to the hospital for tests and to monitor my condition.

The neurologist assigned to my case came into my room daily, first with a simple statement, then more forceful suggestions to take Depakote, another seizure medication. Each time I refused the medication she became angrier, finally threatening to report my unmedicated seizure condition to the state of New Jersey where the authorities would revoke my driver's license. She knew I lived in suburbia and a life without a car would be debilitating.

It was not clear to me that I had a seizure since the incident was clearly precipitated by the medication, my EEG was normal, I was not confused or incontinent when I gained consciousness, and "Paul" was the only witness to the incident. Nevertheless, her diagnosis was firm and I was not doing what she said.

In time, I did take the seizure medication to keep my driver's license and because I became frightened when I felt some strange crackling in my head. My neurologist also assured me that Depakote wouldn't harm my bone marrow and any diminished intellectual capacity would be minor and reverse.

A few days after starting the medication, I could feel my brain power fade. This was confirmed when I couldn't play a computer Scrabble game that had helped me overcome the tedium of the hospital. My complaints were dismissed as trivial. Only a game, she said. It wasn't only a game to me; it was the same type of reasoning I used in my job. It was then I wondered if I would be able to function at work, even if I could return to the office.

After I was discharged from the hospital, during a follow-up office visit, I complained again about my inability to reason. This time the neurologist said that mental capacity usually returns after the medication is discontinued. "Usually" was not the term she had used prior to my taking the drug.

I felt deceived and stuck with a medication that could possibly reduce my platelet count, as I later learned, just as I was trying to raise it, and was taking part of my reasoning ability with it. That was the last time I talked to her and subsequently switched to another neurologist and another medication.

My first neurologist was not the only physician I encountered who had the "take it or I'll…." attitude. As I learned more, I was not surprised. The whole literature on the "compliant patient" reinforces the notion that the doctor is in charge and obviously knows best. The very term "compliance" signals a difference in the balance of power between the patient and the doctor, implying that the patient is less than the doctor, follows orders, perhaps blindly or under duress. With this attitude, no wonder there is a problem with compliance.

I'm sure some doctors who are pressed for time, have thoughts of a malpractice suit, or are thinking back to the years spent in medical school and the high price their knowledge commands, feel it is much easier and faster to just tell the patient what he or she needs and apply whatever strong-arm pressure to get their way. The doctor may firmly believe that s/he knows best and that if only the patient would listen and just do what they say, the patient would understand.

This attitude doesn't work for many patients. It certainly didn't work for me. There were just too many times in my life when I was harmed by a doctor's suggestion, self-serving or not, based on the best evidence at the time, or not.

Yes, there are some who want their doctor to just tell them what to do, and there are some who believe that the doctor always knows best. I'm glad when that scenario works. But in time, when one of the suggestions fails, both the patient and doctor are left with a possible intractable communication void and the seeds of blame and distrust.

It took me a long time and much help from my psychologist to learn to deal with the many doctors in my life, and it wasn't always easy or successful. During my bout with ITP I was obviously compromised physically and emotionally, both from the disease and the treatments, and that made communication more difficult for both of us. At times one of my doctors prescribed anti-anxiety medication. I refused that since I felt it was just designed to make me more complacent, and yes, compliant.

I was an older, close-to-50, female when I was diagnosed with ITP. Most of my doctors were male, about my age or younger. In time I realized that age and gender were sometimes playing a role in our communication. At one point, when I wanted to leave the hospital but felt I was being coerced into staying, I asked my younger brother to attend a hospital discharge meeting. That sufficiently changed the dynamics and I was able to go home.

Medicine, like most well-paying professions in the United States, is dominated by men. I noticed some of the same behavior in the hospital as in my corporate experience. At the large company where I worked when I became ill, the male management

bonded over joint interests in sports, their golf handicap, stock prices, and protected their friends during corporate upheavals. The few women who made it to the upper echelons seemed to spend years toughening their hides and demeanor to fit into the culture. I saw the same type of behavior, a tough and game-playing attitude, by some of the female doctors I encountered. It was as if they had to take on dominant male characteristics in order to succeed.

This male-dominant stance was only one of the complicating factors in my medical care. My treatments were expensive and I was fortunate to have good insurance coverage and a full salary from my short-term disability job status. But my financial situation also made it easier for both me and the doctors to request more tests and approve more treatments, sometimes to my detriment. In the United States, with the ease of malpractice litigation, the high cost of treatments, the variable ability to pay, and the complexities of insurance coverage, determining the best treatment approach is a high-wire balancing act. However, I believe a patient-centric approach and open, honest communication help ease the decisions and the consequences. Fortunately I encountered some doctors who knew how to keep a patient focus within the difficult system, who I felt were more interested in helping me heal than protecting their buddies, showing off their knowledge, or wrestling control. I valued their input, their honesty, and their ability to understand the true nature of what I was trying to convey. Their help was invaluable and their presence a true blessing.

Like my recovery, I thought I was alone in sometimes having difficulties communicating with my doctors, but I was wrong about that, too. After talking to hundreds of patients, I noted a recurrent theme to many of the calls: a disconnect between the patients' intuition and desires, what they felt or wanted, and what they were hearing from their doctor. It didn't matter if they were talking about a splenectomy, prednisone, or another approach to treating their disease, the subtext was the same: a difference between what their doctor told them and an instinctual feeling that the doctor's suggestion was not right for them. They were emotionally stuck between society's message, the one that taught them to always listen to their doctor, and the message from their gut.

After listening to the patient, I often agreed with their assessment based on my knowledge of ITP, the usual treatments for the disease, or communication that can foster healing. I often replied with a suggestion for a second medical opinion, sent copies of research that supported their case, or just listened and empathized.

I certainly wasn't in a position to direct their care and didn't attempt to do that. I could, however, provide information that I hoped would lead to a good decision, give them permission to take themselves and their thoughts seriously, and advocate sharing their feelings with their doctors.

Just as patients complain about their doctors, I know that doctors sometimes complain about their patients. Perhaps this is just human nature and as unavoidable as the complaints of even the most loving married couple.

In many ways I feel the best doctor/patient communication is like a marriage, one that is based on respect, open communication, honesty, sharing unique viewpoints, and arriving at decisions based on joint input. When the respect and care are gone, as in some marriages, the best thing people can do for themselves is discontinue the relationship.

Patient communication comes down to one word, 'love', not in the romantic sense but in a deep caring for a shared positive outcome.

MEDICAL EVIDENCE

I didn't want to have my spleen removed from the very beginning. My spleen was perfectly fine, doing its job removing antibody-coated platelets from my blood. My first hematologist ignored my concerns and tried to schedule the requisite im-

munizations within a month of my diagnosis. His replacement was more understanding and it wasn't until I became refractory to the IVIg treatments and felt the other treatment options would be more damaging and less successful, that I agreed to the operation. My hematologist told me the surgery sometimes failed, but that the success rate was 85%. Pretty good odds, I thought.

After the very risky surgery, given my platelet count of 2,000/mL my platelet count did rise to 180,000/mL only to plummet three weeks later, while I still had staples holding together the ten-inch gash on my left side. I was angry about the needless loss, demoralized about another failed treatment, and even more frightened about my future.

Years later I learned that the odds for splenectomy success are 66% overall for a five to ten year boost in platelet counts (Kojouri 2004) and I've heard at least one doctor suggest that even that percent is too high because it takes into account those people who may have recovered if their splenectomy was postponed until a year after diagnosis. For those over 40, the response curve and the chances for success dip dramatically (Fabris 2001). The 85% success rate was true, if you only considered the platelet count as the patient left the operating table and disregarded the fact that splenectomies often fail later, as mine did.

I don't know if my hematologist purposely failed to communicate the fine points of the literature or if he honestly didn't know them since he had many disease states to follow and some of the more accurate assessments of splenectomy success were published after 1992, when my splenectomy decision was made. I do know when I learned about the actual success rate for splenectomies, I was angry, felt deceived, and had a growing mistrust of what my doctors told me.

While there is no way to know if I would have made a different decision with better information, I continue to mourn my lost spleen. I also share my knowledge of the splenectomy success rates with anyone who calls or writes concerning the operation. There are many.

At least once per week PDSA receives a phone call or e-mail that goes: "My doctor wants me to have a splenectomy and I don't want to. What else can I do?" The staff always assures the caller that they have lots of company in that difficult decision, sends them the best research papers on the subject, and makes sure that those over 40 know that their odds are different than the younger patients. They also point them to a comprehensive list of treatments for the disease. At least we can provide people with better information than I had.

I'd always known that science was a slow process, subject to reversals in recommendations. I felt lucky when I was told I escaped the newer research suggesting radiation for my thyroid papillary cancer diagnosis. However it wasn't until I immersed myself in research literature that I discovered more of the beauty and the flaws of basing medical decisions on scientific evidence.

Certainly information is better than guesswork, but many patients are as naïve as I was and are not aware of the bias in some of the published evidence. I've seen first hand just how expensive and difficult it is to get something published. I know of results that would have been shared if someone had the money and time to write the article. I've also witnessed data that was not highlighted because they didn't fit with what the biotech company sponsor wanted to feature. Researchers have sometimes shared their dreams with me, ideas that could advance medical knowledge, and mourned that they had no funds to pursue them. These situations are probably well-known to anyone who has participated in medical research for more than a few months, but most patients I know are not aware of the publishing and funding hurdles, and sometimes the compromises, that go into the making of medical evidence. For patients, the message is usually black and white: when published evidence exists, it is sacrosanct; when published evidence does not exist, there is nothing. The reality is so much more nuanced.

Some of the most interesting post-splenectomy research, the work indicating that splenectomized people have a higher ratio of microparticles and are more susceptible to dementia (Ahn 2002) and blood clots (Fontana 2008), was done by a research group with private funding, led by someone who didn't have to worry about locating a sponsor for the research, and who wasn't worried that he was going against some mainstream thinking. He mentioned to me that he had more difficulty finding a publisher for his initial splenectomy/microparticle research than any other work he had done. I figured that was because it was clearly counter to the pro-splenectomy findings dominating the articles and conversations on splenectomies at the time.

Much like the climate debate where there are scientists who feel strongly about whether the planet is getting warmer or not, the splenectomy issue has its supporters and detractors. I heard one clinician who sees many ITP patients mention that he hasn't recommended a splenectomy in years and know of another who feels it is a choice that should be suggested soon after diagnosis for almost everyone with ITP.

Science, at its best, is a deep, objective, open inquiry, without personal or financial bias. But add the views of the investigator, funding sources, reviewers, and prevailing wisdom and it is less than the perfect system that it is held up to be.

When doctors tell their patients about treatment research and medical evidence, it is important that they communicate their imperfect knowledge of the entire scope of research on a particular subject, the funding source of the research they are mentioning, and any personal bias. I also hope they encourage the patient to do his or her own research on a topic.

Looking back on my recovery after I went into remission, I felt at a disadvantage knowing so little about ITP compared to my doctors. I was lucky to live near a medical school, but it was time-consuming to locate the articles and difficult to understand their content. There was little patient information about ITP and the lay literature for other medical subjects disappointed me, with content I thought was overly simplistic and sometimes self-serving, depending on the source. So when I founded PDSA I decided to use a different patient communication model, one that would follow the latest research and make it accessible, but not dilute it, a model that would give the patients access to the same information their doctors had. This philosophy led to my attending medical conferences, subscribing to journals, visiting the National Library of Medicine, and developing a comprehensive Web site and other patient publications.

With the increased availability of on-line journal articles, medical conference presentations, CME offerings, along with PDSA publications, I sometimes hear from patients who feel they know as much as their doctors about ITP. Since hematologists have many diseases to follow, often concentrate on malignant conditions, and usually see only a few ITP patients per year, this is a possible scenario.

Some doctors welcome the additional patient knowledge; others are intimidated by it. Hopefully, there will be an increase in physicians who value and encourage a well-educated patient. There is no way to predict what will happen to any particular patient, even with the best evidence-based medicine, so additional transparency and additional information are sure to foster better medical decisions.

COMPLEMENTARY AND ALTERNATIVE TREATMENTS

I was sitting in a chair, tissue in hand, across from "Dr. Bolton," my psychologist, explaining through my tears that my platelet count was still at a dangerous level despite the splenectomy, another round of IVIg, and now a high dose of Danocrine. All my hematologist's best efforts were failing and I felt stuck, hopeless, and terrified that a brain bleed would bring an abrupt end to my life.

"Dr. Bolton" was been very sympathetic and tried to separate the aspects of my depression that I could address from those that were exacerbated by the treatments, since it seemed like most of the prescribed medications I was taking had 'depression' listed as one of their side effects. At each appointment she encouraged me to do something to take charge of my health…to not be a victim of the treatments, the physicians, or the disease. Since victim-hood was a very comfortable response for me, we were dealing with a fundamental behavioral change in addition to a medical cure.

At one session she gave me a relaxation tape, at another a deep breathing exercise. At this appointment she asked me if I had ever considered changing my diet to help me heal. I had already eliminated the junk food from my diet and was eating more vegetables, I replied, but that did not answer her question. She wanted to know whether I considered using what I ate to heal my disease. It was not something that had entered my mind.

To help me understand the possibilities of diet, "Dr. Bolton" handed me a copy of *Recovery from Cancer* by Elaine Nussbaum. I took the book, went home, started to read, and didn't stop until I had finished the story. Elaine had a severe case of uterine cancer. In the process of being treated she lost her hair, was confined to a wheelchair, and had blood counts that were dangerously low. After she went on a macrobiotic diet, received shiatsu treatments, and improved other aspects of her lifestyle she regained her health. It was a fascinating healing story and I was hooked.

I bought a book on macrobiotics, at the core a whole-foods, non-dairy, mostly vegetarian diet. The big difference in this diet approach from others I knew was that it considered the energetic properties of food, not just the vitamin and mineral content or the protein or carbohydrate classification. From an energetic view, some food is very expansive and, like refined sugar, can make you giddy or a bit vacant. Some food, like meat, is very contractive and fosters a tightness or possibly anger. The macrobiotic food philosophy, simplistically, is to eat in the middle, not too contractive or too expensive, and to fine-tune the balance depending on the body's condition. Since my blood was literally escaping from my body, an obviously expansive problem, eating more contractive foods could counteract this tendency. The diet's promise was to help heal my ITP, center my body, calm my mind, and still my soul. That was just what I needed.

I figured if Elaine Nussbaum could help cure her cancer with a diet, surely eating differently might help me. I also didn't think it would hurt to eliminate refined sugar, meat, dairy products, and processed food, as well as add large amounts of fresh vegetables, beans, and whole grains to my meals. The naturopaths I had visited suggested my diet go in that direction, so embracing macrobiotic philosophy was a step, not a wholesale difference from what others recommended.

I embraced the new diet adventure, tried many new foods, learned a very different way of meal planning and cooking, and even scheduled a personal counseling session with Ms. Nussbaum. I was rewarded with welcomed weight loss, lowered cholesterol, and more energy. To my disappointment, my platelets didn't make a fast leap upward when I changed my diet, but they did seem more stable and on a positive trend. I decided to keep the diet on my list and continue looking for other things to try.

I was lucky to have a disease where the progress was easily measured by a simple platelet count and by looking at my bruises. So when something failed I knew it fairly rapidly and could discontinue the practice. And when something helped, even a little bit, and there were no difficult side effects, I kept that on my list of things to do and continued my search. I just had to think back to the horrors of prednisone, the failed splenectomy, and losing my hair from the vincristine to keep me motivated. My philosophy was to try one thing at a time, weigh the potential benefits and risks, and monitor my progress closely.

When my intuition, the experts, and the available information agreed, especially if there was little downside risk to an approach, I knew I was following a good path. The macrobiotic diet philosophy also piqued my interest in other healing modalities whose purpose was to keep the energy (chi, ki, prana) vibrant and flowing in my body and environment. It is an ancient, time-honored approach to healing with a thousand-plus years of clinical practice to prove its value.

In time I added other complementary healing practices that took an energetic view of the body (Reiki, shiatsu, herbs and meditation from Ayurvedic medicine) one by one, and addressed other, less-than-healthy aspects of my life. All the effort led to a normal platelet count, stopping my seizure medication, and eliminating the Tenormin I'd been taking for my tachycardia. The shift in focus that began with the macrobiotic diet initiated a change in the way I dealt with the disease and ultimately, I believe, my recovery.

With my combination of diet changes, energy therapy, herbs, and meditation I thought I had found a singular cure for the disease. That was not the case. Almost immediately after I founded PDSA I heard from many people who discovered things outside of the medical mainstream they claimed helped resolve their ITP.

These enterprising patients, many working with alternative practitioners, discovered a variety of antioxidants, supplements, diets, energy treatments, and herbs that helped raise their platelet count either temporarily or for many years. Until PDSA, they could only communicate their success with their family or their doctor, if they felt comfortable doing that. Now, they had a central place to share their experiences and someone who would listen. What PDSA found was a whole world of cures hidden from collective sight.

Some doctors were interested in knowing about this type of success, but often the stories were dismissed. It wasn't long before PDSA's acceptance of alternative successes was criticized by a major biotech company, a large professional medical organization, and some noted hematologists. This was in contrast to the patients who called and often asked if there was something they could do, eat, try, that did not make them fat and crazy, among other major corticosteroid complaints, remove a healthy organ, deplete their immune system, or keep them out of work for days tied to an infusion bottle.

In order to help determine what things had been most helpful for ITP, in 2001 we did a survey in conjunction with a noted hematologist. Close to 1,000 people replied, a record for a rare disease. The top answer, prayer and positive thinking (Survey 2001), was not easily tested and unfortunately, we didn't have the time or funding to pursue other approaches.

In our survey we did learn that 52% of the respondents used some form of complementary medicine and about one-third of them didn't tell their doctors about it. It is obviously important for patients to communicate all the things they are doing to manage their illness outside of the office and without their doctor's suggestion, whether or not the communication is met with acceptance. It is also important for the doctor to ask.

Since my return to health and PDSA began publishing healing stories, we did hear about some research on the interplay of diet and ITP. Dr. Alan Lazarus searched the literature and found one study linking a calorie-restricted diet in mice to improvement in their platelet count (Mitzutani 1994). When Dr. James Zehnder began researching the link between ITP and oxidative stress, possibly exacerbated by diet, he found only one prior study (Polat 2002). His lab confirmed the link in children (Zhang 2009). Their research continues. When Dr. James George's lab did a meta-analysis of all the splenectomy studies they found 135 papers with a sufficient number of patients that met their analysis criteria (Kojouri 2004). I can only imagine how the treatment of ITP would differ if there were 137 serious studies on diet and only one or two on splenectomy.

Unlike the study of diet and ITP, there has been significant research in linking diet to the prognosis of other diseases. There has also been a greater focus on empowering people to take charge of their health as illustrated by the *Expert Patients Programme* in the United Kingdom and the current emphasis on dietary education and legislation in the United States. With the increasing number of hospitals and clinics that have an integrated and complementary medical program, it is clear that a more comprehensive view of healing is gaining traction.

Viewing the body as both an energetic and biologic entity can lead to powerful synergy. I lived that theory and I believe I am alive today because of it. And I am not alone. So, I think it is time to halt the competitive stance, stop the name calling, balance the funding and research, choose a combination of interventions for each patient based on the best prospects for potential help versus potential harm, monitor progress, and adjust accordingly.

PDSA will continue to provide information on a wide range of interventions, encourage patients to share both their failures and their successes, monitor and promote research, and foster an open dialog with the physicians who treat ITP patients. And I will continue to follow the diet and other practices that were so instrumental in renewing my health and have served me so well to this day.

I am indebted to "Dr. Bolton" and the other practitioners who introduced me to the many healing tools. While sometimes my diet, energy treatments, and other lifestyle changes set me apart, they are a small price to pay for regaining my health and teaching me so much about life.

THE INFLUENCE OF TECHNOLOGY

After my diagnosis and my hematologist suggested prednisone I turned on my computer to discover what I could about ITP. This was 1992 and I found only a few articles on Compuserve and Medline about the disease and possible treatments. My research confirmed what I'd heard about prednisone and listed even more side effects. I also found a reference to IVIg, another treatment for ITP. "Oh, you found out about that?" my hematologist replied with some surprise in his voice when I told him. By his quizzical look and startled response it was clear that a patient who did computer research was something new to him.

By the time I created an ITP Web site in 1997, patients looking for information on cyberspace were no longer an oddity. I'd already met some likeminded people on an AOL forum, so when someone suggested I place a discussion group on the Web site, I readily agreed.

At first I answered all the questions, but it wasn't long before that part of the Web site became a large social network, growing monthly as more people found it. Some bookmarked that part of the site and visited daily since if often provided the only contact they had with others with the disease.

For those who found us, the Internet, and the personal connections made, changed their lives. This connection was not limited to the United States. Soon after PDSA was formed we received a check from someone in the United Arab Emirates because we helped his daughter who lived in California and I was able to give physician recommendations to patients in Bangladesh and the Maldives. I talked to a patient in Singapore and found a volunteer in Australia to assist with the Web site.

Our reach became quite apparent when a young woman from Tashkent, Uzbekistan, visited our office near Washington, DC, to share her appreciation for the information we provided, thanking us for the name of a hematologist in London who helped her, and hoping we could assist her with the paperwork involved in seeing a noted hematologist in New York she found through our Web site.

First, from an upstairs bedroom, and later from an office, PDSA touched the world of ITP and made it smaller. We fostered friendships, provided information, and created a patient community that didn't exist, and couldn't exist, without the Internet. Through this loose international patient collaboration, we shared success stories, the latest research experiences, and served as a pool of resources for research studies. In just a relatively few years, the patients with ITP have access to as much information as their physicians and can be a true partner in their care.

Cyberspace continues to evolve and so does PDSA. Our discussion group now keeps company with Facebook, MySpace, and Buzz. Instead of one or two Web sites describing the disease and treatments there are many. When I was diagnosed I had a problem finding information. The problem for patients now is sorting through all the information they find. Organizations like PDSA, whose mission is to gather data from many areas, to be a central repository and trusted source for patients, can assist, but are not the total answer for the information overload. I don't know what is, but I'm sure that someone will find a creative solution. Technology is fluid, advances at lightning speed, and today's capabilities were not imagined just a few years ago. Despite the flux, some things are certain: technology will continue its breakneck pace, the world will get smaller, patients will continue sharing, and there is no going back.

REFERENCES

Ahn, Y. S., Horstman, L. L., Jy, W., Jimenez, J. J., & Bowen, B. (2002). Vascular dementia in patients with immune thrombocytopenic purpura. *Thrombosis Research*, *107*(6), 337–344. doi:10.1016/S0049-3848(02)00337-7

Fabris, F., Tassan, T., Ramon, R., Carraro, G., Randi, M. L., & Luzzatto, G. (2001). Age as the major predictive factor of long-term response to splenectomy in immune thrombocytopenic purpura. *British Journal of Haematology*, *112*, 637–640. doi:10.1046/j.1365-2141.2001.02615.x

Fontana, V., Jy, W., Ahn, E. R., Dudkiewicz, P., Horstman, L. L., Duncan, R., & Ahn, Y. S. (2008). Increased procoagulant cell-derived microparticles (C-MP) in splenectomized patients with ITP. *Thrombosis Research, 122*(5), 599–603. doi:10.1016/j.thromres.2007.12.022

Kojouri, K., Vesely, S. K., Terrell, D. R., & George, J. N. (2004). Splenectomy for adult patients with idiopathic thrombocytopenic purpura: a systematic review to assess long-term platelet count responses, prediction of response, and surgical complications. *Blood, 104*(9), 2623–2634. doi:10.1182/blood-2004-03-1168

Mizutani, H., Engelman, R. W., Kurata, Y., Ikehara, S., & Good, R. A. (1994). Energy restriction prevents and reverses immune thrombocytopenic purpura (ITP) and increases life span of ITP-prone (NZW x BXSB) F1 mice. *The Journal of Nutrition, 124*(10), 2016–2023.

Polat, G., Tamer, L., Tanriverdi, K., Gürkan, E., Baslamisli, F., & Atik, U. (n.d.). Levels of Malondialdehyde, Glutathione and Ascorbic Acid in Idiopathic Thromboctytopoenic Purpura. *East African Medical Journal, 79*(8), 446-449.

Survey of Non-traditional Treatments of ITP. (2001). *Survey of Non-traditional Treatments of ITP*. Retrieved from http://www.pdsa.org/about-itp/surveys/item/113.html

Zhang, B., Shen, L., Jeng, M., Jones, C., Wong, W., Engleman, E., & Zehnder, J. (2009). Increased VNN1/PPARG Gene Expression Ratio Is Correlated with Developing Chronic ITP and Oxidative Stress Exposure to PBMC in Vitro. *Blood, 114*(22), 368.

APPENDIX A

Chapter 1 Conversations

Internist US

This is a great story, well-told, of a patient's perspective on illness, and her amazingly constructive and thoughtful response to it.

Timely and particularly important are the points made about patient 'compliance', age and gender effects in the doctor-patient relationship, and what makes a good doctor-patient relationship.

Lecturer Sociology, UK

It is a minor criticism but I felt that at times the style was a little too 'academic'. While I agree with the thrust of the author's argument, it is least convincing when attempting to critique medical research which we all know is motivated by personal ambition, etc, but this does not necessarily negate its validity – in randomized controlled trials RCTs at least. The problem, of course, is that this knowledge does not always translate into the real lives of people living in the real world very well.

Cardiac Surgeon and Clinical Stem Cell researcher, Malaysia

Joan Young is a patient of ITP who has in an excellent patient narrative detailed her experiences with the disease and its treatment. She has clearly brought out the feelings of a patient who feels that the physicians who handled her condition(s) did not, first, tell her all the options and clearly inform her about the pros and cons; second often proposed cures that were worse than the disease and third assumed an attitude that was that of a patron client relationship and resented any inputs from the patient regarding her illness.

It is easy to sympathize with her in her predicament as we are all too familiar with treatments that are prescribed with confidence, cost a huge amount, often cause severe morbidities and are later found to be of no particular use. I can think of the Vineberg operation for ischemic heart disease, colectomies for all sorts of "nervous disorders" and so on. During the nineties, cardiologists were using (and discarding) intracoronary devices as fast as the manufacturers could make them.

However while it is true that doctors do not know everything, it is also true that in the vast majority of cases they do know more than the patient about the disease condition that the patient is suffering from. There are a large number of studies testifying to horrendous consequences of so called alternative therapy. In our practice in India where homeopathy is common and every third person has set himself up as a homeopathic practitioner, it is very common too find cases of oesophageal carcinoma and distal limb ischemia treated until the disease is incurable or even beyond palliation by such practitioners. However just as these incidents do not nullify the entire gamut of alternative medicine, so similar successes which are often poorly documented should not be allowed to dominate the discourse about treatment of disease.

I must hasten to say that this does not preclude the very important points that have been raised. It is common to find physicians either contemptuously dismissing, or getting angry with patients who ask questions. I am sure that I have been guilty of this myself. It is important to point out that patients are better informed and demand a discussion rather than a didactic session when they visit their doctors. However again, we must not throw the baby of scientific evidence out with the bathwater of prejudices. This road can only lead to disaster!

It should be compulsory reading for young doctors and those in training as it can be an eye opener to how patients view physicians and what are the defects in our attitude and training while dealing with what are literally life and death questions.

Prof Medicine, India

The chapter reminded me that my original engagement and present obsession with "User Driven Healthcare" was initiated after having been inspired by the author's earlier blog that led me to use it for a power point lecture on ITP.

Like all mainstream physicians (I guess I still am one) I too was slightly uncomfortable with alternative healing approaches but then putting all approaches in a level playing field subjecting them equally to rational scrutiny has made me warm up to it (as I hope other mainstream physicians would/ should). My apprehension about the alternative healing part is chiefly because a large audience of this book is likely to be mainstream physicians and medical students. I personally feel (as much as my formal medical training allows) that it was the power of positive thinking that helped you and the alternative rituals were a vehicle to harness your positive thinking. In fact if you may allow me to put forward alternative possibilities as to how it worked I would say that you received from your alternative care givers what mainstream physicians could have given you but didn't: non paternalistic listening, touch and empathy.

I respect your opinion, but disagree with the statement about the benefit of the alternatives being due to positive thinking and non-paternalistic listening, touch, and empathy. It is true that the alternative practitioners were generally more attentive. However, this was not always the case. One of my alternative practitioners was very curt and directive, and several of my traditional doctors were very empathetic.

After my platelets reached the normal range, I stopped taking the herbs, expanded my diet, and discontinued energy therapy. I made these changes individually, and each time I stopped an intervention my platelets dipped. When I reintroduced the treatment, my platelets rose again. My understanding is that this type of challenge is used and accepted in verifying the efficacy of treatments. JY

APPENDIX B

Chapter Conversational Learning Exercises

Learning points:
- Important insights can be derived from a patients' perspective on illness, especially if their response to it is constructive and thoughtful.
- Patients can be left with a feeling that the physicians who handle their condition(s) do not, first, tell them all the options and clearly inform them about the pros and cons; second often propose cures that are worse than the disease and third assume an attitude that is of a patron client relationship and resent any inputs from the patient regarding their illness.
- Medical research may be motivated by personal ambition, etc, but this may not necessarily negate its validity – even in the case of randomized controlled studies, the present gold standard of clinical research.

- Knowledge gained from randomized controlled trials may not always translate into the real lives of people living in the real world very well. This may require that medical research is supplemented by greater detail about lived experiences of patients
- Patient perspectives may be compulsory reading for health professionals as they can reveal how patients view physicians and the defects in our attitude and training, while dealing with what are often life and death questions.
- Mainstream physicians may be uncomfortable with alternative healing approaches. Putting all approaches in a level playing field and subjecting them equally to rational scrutiny is desirable.
- Alternative caregivers may be more trained in giving what mainstream physicians can also provide but very often choose not to namely, non-paternalistic listening, touch, and empathy. This hints at encouraging mainstream medical education system to incorporate these into the curriculum in a more contextual manner.
- There is the possibility that interventions outside of the medical mainstream may lead to improved health.

Points for further exploration and search (in subsequent chapters):

- What is the magnitude of chronic illness in the community and what resources can one access to study in detail the patient's perspective and lived experiences from chronic illnesses?
- How may health professionals utilize sense-making approaches to make better shared decisions with their patients in a healthcare environment that is likely to be fraught with diagnostic uncertainty?
- Does evidence based on average patient data, which occupies most of our present day information databases, fulfill the needs of individual patient-centered healthcare? Amidst current unprecedented expansion in medical information, do we still not have the types of information required to allow us to tailor optimal care for a given individual patient?
- For each and every individual patient who suffers, is it possible to electronically document her/his clinical encounter with a provision to share it with the entire social network that supports her/his healthcare, such that it serves as a valuable learning resource that may improve the quality of medical decisions?
- Do patients gain from Web-based forums and online portfolios that enable them to anonymously share their individual disease problems with a wider network of similar patients as well as interested healthcare professionals?
- Can Web-based interactions serve as an opportunity for health professionals to find interesting patients in their specialties with detailed illness experiences with whom they have a high likelihood of maintaining a persistent informational continuity conducive to lifelong medical learning?

Chapter 2
Hematology:
The River Within

Anirban Chaudhuri
Consultant Physician, India

Joan Young
Platelet Disorder Support Association, USA

Carmel M. Martin
Trinity College Dublin, Ireland

Joachim Sturmberg
Monash University and The University of Newcastle, Australia

Rakesh Biswas
People's College of Medicine, India

ABSTRACT

This chapter introduces the reader to a world of clinical problem solving in blood disorders as presented in hematology lectures. These lectures encompass multiple perspectives, the patient, his/her relatives, healthcare students, consultant health professionals and society. This style of lecture aims to enable these key stakeholders in the health care system to utilize the continued learning derived from sharing their narratives toward attaining the goal of improved healthcare outcomes. The chapter has three narratives which are intertwined – the patient narratives of their experiences with disturbances in their blood stream, the blood system disease narratives of the medical professionals and the stream of consciousness expressed in poetry evoked by the first two narratives.

INTRODUCTION

"I am all impatience to be off...I dream of rocky cliffs that border this river, the endless bendings and turnings, the lakes and sloughs along its length, *little riverside towns and villages, fishing boats, freighters, new faces, squatters, bottomland folks, birds, animals, trees, and wild fruit. But, most of all, I dream of great freedoms to come where the living is quiet, where the struggle to survive is less."*
River Journey by Clarence Jonk Published by Minnesota Historical Society Press, 2003

DOI: 10.4018/978-1-60960-097-6.ch002

This chapter on blood disorders begins from a very simple biological perspective with a human context that may be relevant to a person trying to understand and cope with his/her blood disorder or a student of health sciences beginning his or her journey into the topic of hematology. The material presented in this chapter was originally developed by author RB to remove the tedium of his Medicine lecture classes. RB began introducing his students to the patients' world, through their personal narratives, that otherwise remain unexplored in conventional approaches to disease in mainstream medical texts.

Although RB initially utilized his own experience of narrative encounters with patients he found that the Internet was a treasure house of rich narratives, written to share, thus waiting to be understood from a health professional learner's perspective. Although RB found the length and detail of patients' experiences sometimes quite difficult being unnecessarily lengthy and somewhat dense, he realized that once these narratives were adequately explored and relevant portions selected for quoting and discussion, they could serve as powerful learning material, particularly to hold student interest. (Biswas 2009)

This chapter reads as if RB was giving his lecture. That is, this is the lecturer's narrative journey through the river of blood with learner/reader. The poetry around the river metaphor has been inserted to remind readers of the many layers of meaning we humans attach to rivers, both those inside of us and in the world around us. The narrative snippets have been taken from Web-based discussion forums, articles, and blogs to illustrate non-linear narrative with the usual linear lecture session.

Questions about Blood at an Elementary Level

The following questions are invariably asked by medical learners ranging from students to those with medical conditions.

- What does blood look like under a microscope?
- What are the cellular elements of blood?
- How does the river of blood run?
- How and why does the river of blood fail sometimes?

Discovering the River through Human Conversations in the Context of the Illness Experience

A patient's experience of disorders of the blood system can be a powerful introduction towards an understanding of the anatomical and functional constituents of blood – red blood cells, white blood cells and platelets:

a) Red Blood Cell Narrative:
"I was extremely involved at my high school, as well as in the community, and I thought my exhaustion was due to being so busy all the time.

It wasn't until around exam time that I began to think maybe there really was something wrong. I had difficulty breathing (thought it was asthma) and horrible chest pains (I just tried to ignore them).

Eventually, my doctor received my blood test results and told me that I had severe anemia and the RBCs in my blood looked smaller and pale." (Kittenwithawhip 2005)

b) White Blood Cell Crisis:
"In the summer of 1991, just after my 37th birthday, I began feeling an unshakable fatigue and a persistent pain in my left side.

Like most people, I had had episodes of hypochondria -- could that headache be a brain tumor? -- But I had always been in generally robust health.

By October, I was worried enough to see my physician for a long-overdue physical.

"You seem fine," he told me, "but let's do some blood tests just to be sure."

The next day, the phone call came that divided my life into everything before that moment and everything after.

My doctor told me that my white-blood-cell count was way too high -- close to 75,000 per cubic meter of blood, compared with the norm of 5,000." (Landro 1996)

c) Platelets:

"In a few weeks I noticed some black and blue marks on my arm and panicked when I didn't stop bleeding from a small cut.

My days became a struggle to continue life as I once knew it and understand why my body was betraying me.

After a short stint in the hospital for tests, the diagnosis was confirmed… The hematologist wrote it down so I could remember what it stood for.

My count was 6,000, a severe case, potentially fatal. I didn't know what a platelet was." (Young 1997)

Having a blood disorder is a real and personal experience. Yet our understanding of the blood system mirrors our human development and is intimately linked to our evolving construction of our place in the order of things. Blood has developed from a mysterious life giving liquid to an understandable and manageable component of the body.

"The story of blood is one of metamorphosis, of a liquid that became symbolically transformed as society learned how to deconstruct and manage it." http://www.djspooky.com/articles/kutculture.html

In contrast, knowledge about blood developed over time can be presented 'objectively', devoid of the context of patient experiences.

RED BLOOD CELL DISORDERS

Bypassing the marsh and low-country swamps
We meander through
I see antlers in the distance
"Savannah River Meander" by BlessedOne
http://www.gspoetry.com/savannah-river-mean-der-sonnet-poems-346516.html

In this chapter we shall just focus here on RBC disorders leading to anemia and ignore polycythemias.

Now we must try to match a functional diagnosis to our patient histories.

In the RBC narrative we find that the patient has anemia which was reported to be associated with smaller and paler RBCs in her peripheral blood

Figure 1. Slide: Objective knowledge about the formation and development of blood cells

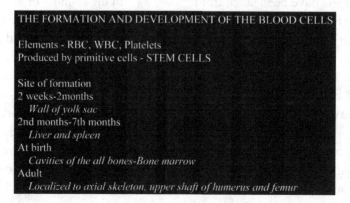

Figure 2. Slide: Conditions related to a functional deficiency in RBC production

Conditions of functional deficiency in RBC production:
1. **Marrow production defects (Hypoproliferative)**
Iron deficiency
Marrow Damage: Infiltration, Fibrosis, Aplasia
Decreased Stimulation: Renal disease, Inflammation, Metabolic disease
2. **Defects in RBC maturation (Ineffective erythropoiesis)**
Cytoplasmic defects: Iron deficiency, Thalassemia, Sideroblastic anemia
Nuclear defects: Folic acid deficiency, Vitamin B12 deficiency, Drug toxicity,
Refractory anemia
3. **Decreased RBC survival:**
Blood loss, Hemolysis, Metabolic defect, Membrane Abnormality,
Hemoglobinopathy, AI disease

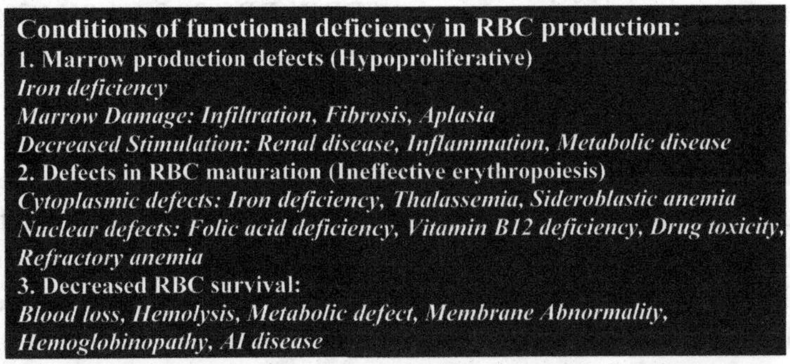

Figure 3. Blood work results of the patient in the RBC narrative

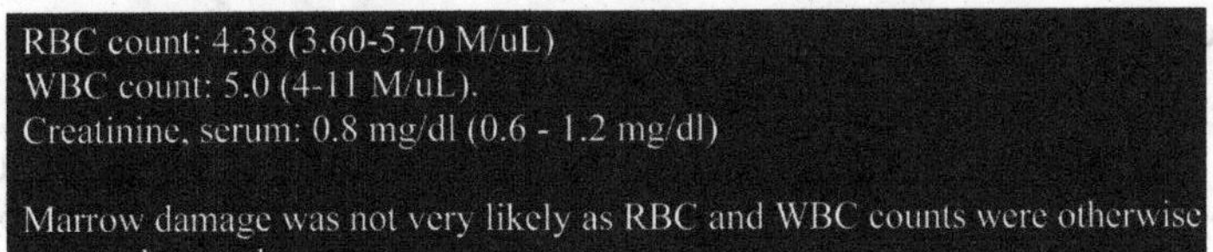

RBC count: 4.38 (3.60-5.70 M/uL)
WBC count: 5.0 (4-11 M/uL).
Creatinine, serum: 0.8 mg/dl (0.6 - 1.2 mg/dl)

Marrow damage was not very likely as RBC and WBC counts were otherwise reported normal.

smear and for this she needs further tests to find out among which of the previously summarized causes of anemia she was likely to fit into.

Some more information on her counts and relevant biochemical parameters were obtained.

Drink again this river that is the taker of pain, the giver of beauty; In these cool waves what can be lost, Only the sorry cost of the thing, not the thing itself; Gone is the fever, but not the river-melted, frozen pride; The tranquil tide runs never the warmer, never the colder; Immerse the dream, dip the song into the stream.
-William Wordsworth

If we again look at our list of causes, it could still be a marrow production defect but then further down the list in the subcategory of marrow production defects, renal causes were unlikely as her renal functions were normal. It could be a pure red cell aplasia of the marrrow but we would not consider that at the beginning for its rarity. She didn't seem to have any sign of chronic inflammation anywhere else in her body and nor did she appear to have a metabolic disease.

Small and pale RBCs, or to use their medical term, microcytic hypochromic, are characteristic of iron deficiency anemia but may be also seen in hemoglobin disorders like thallasemias, chronic inflammation, or sideroblastic anemias. The smaller and paler appearance obviously was indicative of an RBC maturation defect. Again, to be associated with causes other than iron deficiency like vitamin deficiencies of B12 and folate, we could have expected RBCs to look larger in size, which was also not the case here. Hemolysis or destruction of RBCs would have given rise to distortions in the RBC shape (poikilocytosis) and size (anisocytosis).

May the river flow without end, meandering through pastoral valleys, past temples and castles, through the miasmal and mysterious swamps; Down into a desert of red rock, blue mesas, domes and pinnacles, and down again into a deep ancient unknown charm...Where something strange and more beautiful than your deepest dreams, waits for you beyond the next turning.
- Edward Abbey

So from this preliminary appearance of the blood under the microscope, iron deficiency appeared the most likely culprit.

Most of the iron in the body is located on the hemoglobin molecules of red blood cells. When red blood cells reach a certain age, they are degraded and engulfed by specialized scavenging macrophages. These cells internalize the iron-containing hemoglobin, degrade it, put the iron onto transferrin molecules, and then export the transferrin-iron complexes back out into the blood. Most of the iron used for blood cell production comes from this cycle of hemoglobin recycling.

All cells use some iron, and must get it from the circulating blood. Since iron is tightly bound to transferrin, cells throughout the body have receptors for transferrin-iron complexes on their surfaces. These receptors engulf and internalize both the protein and the iron attached to it. Once inside, the cell transfers the iron to ferritin, the internal iron storage molecule. (Human iron metabolism 2009)

There's a dreamy river flowing
Down the street from my house
I walk down there after work
But I paddle my way home
Spencer Breau (10/12/74 / San Diego)
http://www.poemhunter.com/poem/dreamy-river/

Managing Iron Deficiency Anaemia

RBC narrative related by a patient (Lotsawalls 2009)

"So I had my levels checked last week at the doctors. Called today, my iron levels are terrible.

Ferritin less than 1 (22-291 ng/mL)
Iron 11 (35-160 ug/dL)
Transferrin Sat % is 2 (15-55%)
TIBC 449 (228-428 ug/dL)
TIBC Unsat 438 (92-365 ug/dL)
HGB 6.7 (11.5-15.0 g/dL)

Hematocrit 27.0 (34.0-46.0%)
RDW, RBC 20.3 (11.9-14.3%) (What is this?)
Red Blood Cell Count 4.38 (3.60-5.70 M/uL)
MCV 62 (80-100 fL)
Platelet Count 363 (140-400 K/uL)

My doctor just said to start taking iron supplements and recheck in a month. I told her I was concerned, as my diet is not seemingly deficient in iron (I eat some meat, not a lot, snack on almonds, cereal is always high in iron, etc). I have a normal diet. She seems to think that it could be caused by my somewhat heavy clotting during menstruation, and most people have trouble maintaining their iron levels by just diet alone.

Does this sound right to you? My ferritin level freaked me out...less than 1???

Anyone share numbers like this, and is your doctor only having you take iron pills?

Thanks for sharing any info you have!" (Lotsawalls 2009)

All this material has been posted by the patient utilizing an anonymous user name, Lotsawalls, onto an online discussion forum. All humans need to understand what is happening to them and need help from whoever may have the knowledge (either through formal training or by their experience of having gone through the same). (Sturmberg, et al. 2010)

Summarized Background Knowledge Created Over Time

To answer some of the queries of Lotsawalls, a health professional would definitely delve into his or her own background knowledge which is supposed to get updated with evidence base medical (EBM) guidelines.

Quality of Evidence

The serum markers of iron deficiency are low ferritin, low iron and raised total iron binding capacity. Serum ferritin is the most powerful test

Figure 4. Side: The levels of evidence in a particular EBM paradigm (ref)

> The quality of evidence for recommendations based on guidelines is as follows:
> - Grade A Based on meta-analysis or large randomized controlled studies
> - Grade B Based on good evidence from small or nonrandomized studies
> - Grade C Based on specialist opinion

for iron deficiency (Gr A Evidence). The cut-off level of ferritin which is diagnostic varies between 12–15 µmg/L. (Guidelines for the management of iron deficiency anemia, British Society of Gastroenterology 2005)

Also to answer Lotsawall's query on RDW one could just use plain background knowledge supplemented by wikipedia:

The red blood cell distribution width, or RDW, is a measure of the variation of red blood cell (RBC) width that is reported as part of a standard complete blood count. Usually red blood cells are a standard size of about 6-8µm. Certain disorders, however, cause a significant variation in cell size. Higher RDW values indicate greater variation in size. Normal reference range in human red blood cells is 11 - 15%. Iron deficiency anemia initially presents with a varied size distribution of red blood cells, and as such shows an increased RDW. (Red blood cell distribution width 2009) www.wikipedia.com

Interestingly within 2 hours another lady with an anonymous user name of Flowergirl responds mentioning a similar experience in her past.

"My Hb was 8.5 and I had a 2 ferritin, I can't imagine the symptoms that you must be having. My Primary Care Physician told me that at a 7 they would transfuse me.

Another alternative is to have IV iron infusion, but it is not without risk either.

I only took iron tabs orally to get my numbers up, your Hb should respond within 30-45 days. It took me two months to get from a 8.5 to 12.9 with ferris sulfate, but it almost killed my guts. Then I wasn't able to take iron for a while and I dropped again because I was still having periods with no ferritin. It takes up to a year to fill the ferritin through the oral route. I think that your doctor should do more for you." (Flowergirl 2009)

Text Book and Evidence Based Medical Literature on Iron Therapy in Iron Deficiency Anemia

Iron therapy should be continued for about 2 months after correction of the anemia and its etiological cause in order to replenish body stores of iron. Ferrous sulfate is the most common and cheapest form of iron utilized. Tablets contain 50-60 mg of iron salt. Other ferrous salts are used and may cause less intestinal discomfort because they contain a smaller dose of iron (25-50 mg).

Carbonyl iron (Feosol) is sometimes used as a substitute for ferrous sulfate. Has a slower release of iron and is more expensive than ferrous sulfate. Slower release affords the agent greater safety if ingested by children. On an mg basis, it is 70% as efficacious as ferrous sulfate. Claims are made that there is less gastrointestinal toxicity, prompting use when ferrous salts are producing intestinal symptoms and in patients with peptic ulcers and gastritis. Tablets are available containing 45 mg and 60 mg of iron. (Conrad 2006)

There's a dreamy river flowing
On every street corner in the world
And if that young moon is in the sky
She'll wink at you and let you pass by
Spencer Breau
(10/12/74 / San Diego)
http://www.poemhunter.com/poem/dreamy-river/

The EBM literature addresses further Flowergirl's concerns:

Parenteral iron may be used when there is intolerance or noncompliance with oral preparations. (Guidelines for the management of iron deficiency anemia, British Society of Gastroenterology 2005)

Does this mean that it is not a recommended substitute to achieve a quicker effect on very low hemoglobin?

A previous EBM guideline is more categorical that the rise in hemoglobin is no quicker than with oral preparations. It also adds that the hemoglobin concentration should rise by 2 g/dl after 3–4 weeks. Failure to do so is usually due to poor compliance, misdiagnosis, continued blood loss, or mal-absorption. (Goddard 2000)

Flowergirl's statement about the risks of IV iron therapy contradicts the EBM guidelines:

Intravenous iron sucrose, when given according to the manufacturers' instructions, is reasonably well tolerated (35% of patients have mild side effects) with a low incidence of serious adverse reactions (0.03–0.04%). Bolus intravenous dosing of iron sucrose (200mg iron) over 10 minutes is licensed and more convenient than a two-hour infusion. Intravenous iron dextran can replenish iron and haemoglobin levels in a single infusion but serious reactions can occur (0.6–0.7%) and there have been fatalities associated with infusion. (Guidelines for the management of iron deficiency anemia, British Society of Gastroenterology 2005)

About Flowergirl's concerns on the need for transfusion the EBM literature mentions:

Blood transfusions should be reserved for patients with, or at risk of, cardiovascular instability due to their degree of anemia (C). Transfusions should aim to restore hemoglobin to a safe level, but not necessarily normal values. Iron treatment should follow transfusion to replenish stores.

Another post from our patient *Lotsawalls* after 2 days: *Just released from hospital*

"Just got released from the hospital....felt somewhat dizzy Sat evening so went to the ER. The nurse showed some concern that my doctor wasn't taking my 6.7 Hb (12-16 normal) number more seriously. She said I looked quite pale. Doctor said 6.7 wasn't too much of a concern, as I seem to be compensating well with heart rate, oxygen level, etc and didn't feel the need to do anything more. I waited for my labs to come back, and then the action started...

Doctor came back in and said he needed to transfuse me, since my Hb had dropped to a 5.1 (from 6.7) since last week. I didn't want to get the blood, but he said I had a 50% chance of a heart attack or stroke so I had to do it. They gave me 3 units, which brought my Hb up to 8.1.

Home tonight with referral to OBGYN as they still think it's menstrual related. Thanks again Flowergirl for your feedback, it helped me to take this a little more seriously than my doctor was!" (Lotsawalls 2009)

To this *Flowergirl* agreed that it was the next logical step after showing the appropriate concern for what *Lotsawalls* had gone through.

The river, the life giver...Forever the Circles charge, I have coursed through our Mother's veins; now hear my sorrow and pain, in thy river's rush, the pain...
-Percy Bysse Shelley

At this point the discussion is joined by a new member who had a possibly similar nature of illness experience:

"Wow...you have really been through it! I hope you get some answers from the OB/GYN. My internist put me on the birth control pill that runs for three months, so I only have one (minimal) period at the end of each quarter, basically. I've read on here, however, that those with severe anemia should be put on something to prevent menstrual bleeding."

Another two days later Lotsawalls finds herself again in the ER due to palpitations but is again thankfully found to have no significant cardiac problems and is released, This episode had a profound effect on her.

"That being said, I did get some good news... my HG was up to 10! A jump from the 8 it was after my blood transfusion.

In the last 2 weeks, I've dealt with a melanoma scare with my husband (benign, praise God), the funeral of a dear friend who died of cancer, my admission to the hospital fiasco, and now an ambulance trip! I'm sure viewing life a little differently now. I can't seem to snuggle my kids enough!

Take care all. Here's hoping for an uneventful weekend!" (Lotsawalls 2009)

Misty River
So peaceful
No one is around but me
With my fishing boat
Aldo Kraas
(July 15 1964 / Sao Paulo Brazil)
http://www.poemhunter.com/poem/misty-river/

The chapter of iron deficiency anemia may end for a particular patient with the end of an ordeal but for a health professional and other patients who continue to sustain interest, the learning continues to grow every day with more conversations from patients with similar narratives and yet dissimilar settings and outcomes.

WHITE BLOOD CELL DISORDERS

While preparing for a lecture class on a specific topic related to blood disorders author RB came across a very interesting narrative by a journalist and life-threatening illness survivor, Laura Landro, who has also popularized the term "well informed patient." RB prepared a PowerPoint lecture interspersed with text book headings and EBM notes for the benefit of his students. Following are extracts from the lecture which have heavily quoted Ms Landro.

"In the summer of 1991, just after my 37th birthday, I began feeling an unshakable fatigue and a persistent pain in my left side.

Like most people, I had had episodes of hypochondria -- could that headache be a brain tumor? -- But I had always been in generally robust health.

By October, I was worried enough to see my physician for a long-overdue physical.

"You seem fine," he told me, "but let's do some blood tests just to be sure."

The next day, the phone call came that divided my life into everything before that moment and everything after.

My doctor told me that my white-blood-cell count was way too high -- close to 75,000 per cubic meter of blood, compared with the norm of 5,000." (Landro 1996)

Her clinical features are highly suggestive of chronic myeloblastic leukemia. The clinical manifestations of CML are insidious and are often discovered incidentally when an elevated WBC count is revealed by a routine blood count or when an enlarged spleen is revealed during a general physical examination.

Most patients are diagnosed while still in the chronic phase. The diagnosis shakes the foundations of one's existence.

"At first, I despaired.

Under Darwin's survival-of-the-fittest theory, I brooded, I was a flawed specimen not meant to last.

Terror soon followed. My own mortality, something I hadn't ever seriously considered, was staring me in the face.

The first thing I learned was that my disease was in an early stage.

My hematologist put me on a drug, hydroxyurea that gave me back some of my energy by

Figure 5. Slide Chronic Myeloblastic Leukemia phases

Chronic Myeloblastic Leukemia (CML)
There are three clinical phases
1) Initial chronic phase
2) Accelerated phase
3) Blast crisis

helping stem the flood of white blood cells my defective bone marrow was pumping into my bloodstream.

That enabled me to continue working full time and to travel thousands of miles to visit hospitals with transplant centers." (Landro 1996)

Myelo-suppressive therapy, was formerly the mainstay of treatment to convert a patient with CML from an uncontrolled initial presentation to one with hematologic remission and normalization of the physical examination and laboratory findings.

Hydroxyurea (Hydrea), an inhibitor of deoxynucleotide synthesis, is the most common myelosuppressive agent used to achieve hematologic remission. The initial blood cell count is monitored every 2-4 weeks, and the dose is adjusted depending on the WBC and platelet counts.

"I continued to plan for the future as though cancer would be only a brief interruption.

The man I had been living with for two years, a lawyer, had provided great help and support.

We decided to get married the following March. Knowing that the therapy I would eventually undergo would leave me infertile, we entered the in vitro fertilization program at … University Medical Center…

After I endured a month of hormone injections, we produced nine embryos that were frozen in cryopreservation vaults.

Searching for the cause of my disease was pointless. With leukemia, family history plays no significant part.

I hadn't been exposed to nuclear radiation or petrochemicals like benzene, two carcinogens linked to leukemia.

As an infant, I had lived in a town crisscrossed by high-tension electrical wires, but there is no proof this has anything to do with the disease." (Landro 1996)

It is characterized by a cytogenetic aberration consisting of a reciprocal translocation between the long arms of chromosomes 22 and 9; t (9; 22). The translocation results in a shortened chromosome 22, an observation first described by Nowell and Hungerford and subsequently termed the Philadelphia (Ph) chromosome after the city of discovery.

This translocation relocates an oncogene called *abl* from the long arm of chromosome 9 to the long arm of chromosome 22 in the *BCR* region.

A new approach to treatment of this disease is to directly inhibit the molecular cause of the disease…using a protein-tyrosine kinase inhibitor that inhibits the bcr-abl tyrosine kinase. Tyrosine kinase inhibitor (TKI) therapy has significantly changed the treatment paradigm for patients with chronic myeloid leukemia (CML). The first generation inhibitor, imatinib, has demonstrated remarkable efficacy in most chronic-phase patients. Disease progression remains a significant risk for the first 2 to 3 years of TKI therapy, but the risk falls significantly thereafter. Early recognition of each individual's risk of progression may facilitate a customized approach to TKI therapy. (White 2009)

Figure 6. Slide profile of CML

CML accounts for 20% of all leukemias affecting adults.

Increased incidence was reported among individuals exposed to radiation in Nagasaki and Hiroshima after the dropping of the atomic bomb.

The presence of BCR/ABL rearrangement is the hallmark of CML. CML is an acquired abnormality that involves the hematopoietic stem cell.

We call upon the river, the water that rims the earth, horizon to horizon; That flows in our rivers and streams, teach us and show us the way.
-David Zwich

Gratwohl and co-workers (1993) conducted a retrospective analysis on data collected by the European Bone Marrow Transplantation Group since 1979. A total of 1480 BMTs for CML were done between 1979 and 1990. Of these, 1082 patients were transplanted in first chronic phase, 88 in a subsequent chronic phase, 251 in accelerated phase and 59 in blast crisis. For these four patient groups, leukemia-free survival at 5 years was 39%, 22%, 22% and 0%, respectively.

This long-term analysis allowed a few conclusions: (i) patients with CML in blastic transformation should not be considered routine candidates for BMT; (ii) BMT should be carried out as soon after diagnosis as possible if an HLA-identical sibling is available; and (iii) age, donor/recipient sex combination, time span from diagnosis to transplant and initial disease status influence outcome. (Gratwohl 1993)

"From everything I was reading, the only hope for a cure was a bone-marrow transplant from a matched donor, ideally a sibling.

I have two brothers, and we quickly arranged tests to determine whether either could provide the lifesaving marrow I needed. We had always been close, but it turns out my brothers and I were even closer than we thought.

By an immense stroke of luck -- and luck should never be played down in medicine -- both brothers were identical matches to me. I had juggled my normal life and my illness for eight months now, seeing friends, going to parties, seeing movies, and traveling for business.

Planning my wedding had been a fun distraction.

On July 14, the pre-transplant conditioning began.

The first chemotherapy drug, Cytoxan, was pumped into me through the catheter.

I also swallowed daily doses of five giant gelatin capsules, each containing five tiny pills of the other chemo drug, busulfan. I was instantly nauseated, and sometimes threw them right up.

I was awakened one night by the blare of a fire alarm.

It turned out to be a piercing ringing in my own ears, brought on by a drug

I focused all of my energy on getting through each day."

The river that runs, runs water; the river that breeds a son and a daughter; The river that runs, Runs waves...who will sail?
- Lord Byron

"But on one of my worst days, I told my mother that I understood why people asked for assisted suicides.

If things were never going to get any better than this, life wasn't worth living.

Even then, however, things were starting to turn around.

I was slowly growing stronger. My white-blood-cell counts, which had been blasted to zero, were returning to normal.

My immune system was recovering. In early September, I was released from the hospital.

The first year was a slow process of resuming normal life, watching for my hair to start growing (it finally did)...

... and working to regain my strength and muscle tone.

My ovaries no longer functioned, and I would be on hormone-replacement therapy for the rest of my life.

Over the next three years, my tests for leukemia remained negative.

I wasn't out of the woods, but I was thrilled to be alive.

The smallest things made me happy -- enjoying a fine restaurant meal, looking in the mirror and recognizing the person reflected in it etc.

There were difficult times; my marriage ended in divorce, and we agreed not to use our frozen embryos.

But while most of my friends were traumatized as they turned 40, I was thankful to get there." (Landro 1996)

The needs of both the patient and the clinician for connection and meaning in their lives are possibly met through a transpersonal dimension of medical care that may be recognized in occasional moments during medical encounters. These moments are often marked by a physiologic reaction, such as gooseflesh or a chill; by an immediacy of awareness of the patient's situation (as if experiencing it from inside the patient's world); by a sense of being part of a larger whole; and by a lingering feeling of joy, peacefulness, or awe. Such moments seem to be therapeutic for the patient and the clinician alike. (Matthews 1993).

"My doctor tells me that my risk of getting the disease now is no greater than for the general population, I take nothing for granted.

Let's just say so far, so good." (Landro 1996)

Laura Landro is an editor and award-winning writer for the Wall Street Journal. In 1991, Laura was diagnosed with chronic myelogenous leukemia. Over the course of the months and years that followed, she used her training as a reporter to obtain critical information about the disease affecting her, improving her ability to interact with her doctors and eventually emerging as a survivor. Laura won the National Print Journalism Award from the Leukemia Society of America for her WSJ article, "A Survivor's Tale," and is the author of Survivor: Taking Control of Your Fight Against Cancer; she remains an outspoken advocate of patient empowerment through education. (Family Medicine Net Guide 2004)

PLATELET DISORDERS

"It all started in the summer of 1992 when I returned from a long 4th of July weekend in Quebec City, Canada. It was cool and rainy there. I ate too many gravy coated french fries, drove home in damp clothes, and caught what I thought was the flu.

It didn't respond to my usual cure of lying on the sofa and watching four rented videos.

In a few weeks I noticed some black and blue marks on my arm and panicked when I didn't stop bleeding from a small cut.

My days became a struggle to continue life as I once knew it and understand why my body was betraying me." (Young 1997)

In this passage which begins an individual clinical encounter with an audience (us) we notice that the initial queries generated even by a patient are always something like:

- Where is the problem? (a physician's morphologic diagnosis):
- Why the problem (a physician's etiologic diagnosis) and this is is mostly answered by *pathophysiologic rationale* that patient's are not expected to know (and may not understand even through internet searches).

Figure 7. Slide of treatment goals of CML

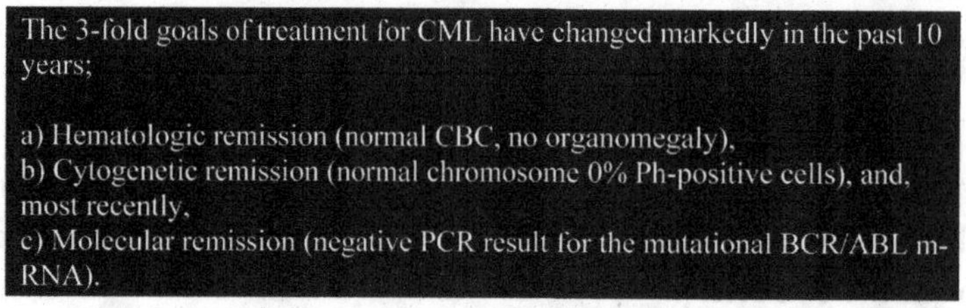

The 3-fold goals of treatment for CML have changed markedly in the past 10 years;

a) Hematologic remission (normal CBC, no organomegaly),
b) Cytogenetic remission (normal chromosome 0% Ph-positive cells), and, most recently,
c) Molecular remission (negative PCR result for the mutational BCR/ABL m-RNA).

Figure 8. Slide

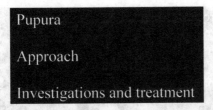

However this is what physician's are expected to know as a result of their training (and improve on with experience). The most basic of these is the knowledge of anatomy that takes time to change unlike empirical evidence in medicine that has proven to have a very short shelf life.

A physician by virtue of this basic knowledge of macro and microanatomy is able to quickly grasp other information that keeps adding to his lifelong day-to-day learning in medicine. (Biswas 2008)

A basic science question is at this point posed to the students who have had to pass their basic sciences before coming to attend this medicine lecture:

What are the mechanisms of hemostasis?

Diseases affecting the smaller blood vessels & platelets produce the clinical picture of purpura.

"After a short stint in the hospital for tests, the diagnosis was confirmed…

The hematologist wrote it down so I could remember what it stood for.

My count was 6,000, a severe case, potentially fatal. I didn't know what a platelet was." (Young 1997)

Little scientific evidence is available about the accuracy or reliability of tests for ITP. The largely clinical diagnosis of ITP, which is made by confirming the presence of isolated thrombocytopenia and by excluding concurrent causes of thrombocytopenia, is best accomplished with a history, physical examination, complete blood count, and examination of the peripheral blood smear. Clinicians sometimes do additional tests, including those to rule out other causes of thrombocytopenia (such as HIV infection, thyroid disorders, and systemic lupus erythematosus); bone marrow examination; imaging studies; and tests for immunoglobulins, platelet antibodies,

Figure 9.

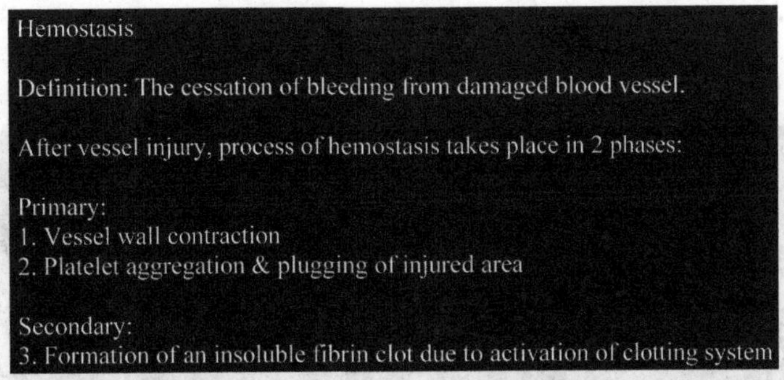

Hemostasis

Definition: The cessation of bleeding from damaged blood vessel.

After vessel injury, process of hemostasis takes place in 2 phases:

Primary:
1. Vessel wall contraction
2. Platelet aggregation & plugging of injured area

Secondary:
3. Formation of an insoluble fibrin clot due to activation of clotting system

Figure 10.

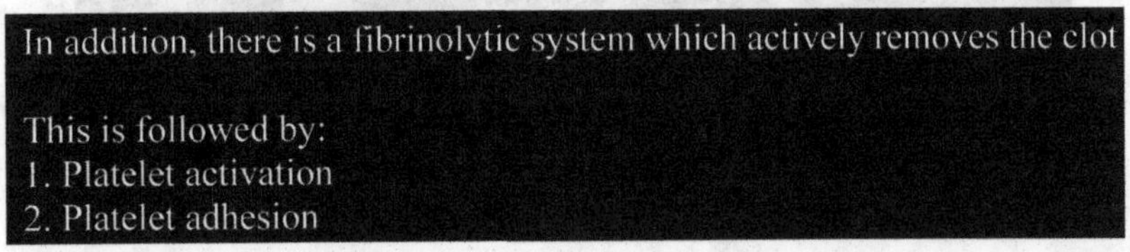

In addition, there is a fibrinolytic system which actively removes the clot

This is followed by:
1. Platelet activation
2. Platelet adhesion

Figure 11.

Haemorrhagic diseases

Can result from abnormalities of:
1. Blood vessels
2. Platelets
3. Clotting systems

Figure 12.

Diseases of clotting system

Congenital
(Hemophilia, von-Willebrand's disease)

Acquired
Deficiency of Vitamin K dependent clotting factors

Severe liver disease, anticoagulant therapy;

Hypofibrinogenemia –DIC, destruction of liver

Figure 13.

Thrombocytopenia

Causes

Impaired production:
    Marrow aplasia,
    Leukemia
    Infiltration
    Megaloblastic anemia
    Myeloma
    Myelofibrosis

Exessive destruction:
    ITP

Secondary Immune:
    SLE,CLL,viruses, Drugs eg. heparin

Sequestration:
    Hypersplenism

Dilutional:
    Massive transfusion

Other:
    DIC
    TTP

and lupus anticoagulant, but data on the predictive value or effectiveness of these tests in the typical patient are lacking. (American Society of Hematology ITP Practice Guideline Panel 1997)

Most physicians elect to not treat patients unless their platelet count is below 50,000/L or bleeding manifestations are present.

Figure 14.

Idiopathic thrombocytopenic purpura (ITP):

May occur following a respiratory or gastrointestinal viral infection

Clinical features

In children often presents 2-3 weeks after viral illness with sudden onset purpura & sometimes oral or nasal bleeding

Acute ITP

Acute, self limiting

In adults usually affects females; maybe associated with other AI disorders like SLE, Thyroid disease, AIHA ; CLL, Tumours, after infections

Chronic ITP

Course is chronic with remissions & relapses

Figure 15.

Clinical effects with different levels of Platelet Counts	
Platelet Count	Clinical defects
500,000-1,00,000	None
100,000-50,000	Moderate hemorrhage after injury
50,000-20,000	Purpura may occur, hemorrhage after injury
<20,000	Purpura common with spontaneous hemorrhage

Figure 16.

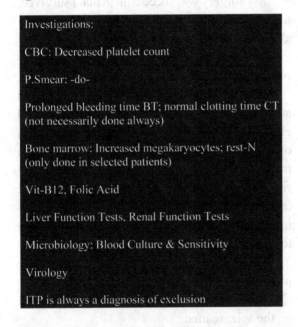

Investigations:

CBC: Decreased platelet count

P.Smear: -do-

Prolonged bleeding time BT; normal clotting time CT (not necessarily done always)

Bone marrow: Increased megakaryocytes; rest-N (only done in selected patients)

Vit-B12, Folic Acid

Liver Function Tests, Renal Function Tests

Microbiology: Blood Culture & Sensitivity

Virology

ITP is always a diagnosis of exclusion

A course of steroid therapy is often administered upon the initial diagnosis in an effort to induce a sustained remission. (Thiagarajan 2009)

"The hematologist suggested prednisone, the drug of choice. I was wary of the side effects, but this seemed to be the best option.

For three weeks I endured the brain fog, sleepless nights, and anxiety, hoping the drug would be a quick fix. It wasn't."

There was only a slight rise in my platelet count, then a fall. He then suggested IVIg." (Young 1997)

"As I was reducing the quantity of prednisone and had my first Intravenous Immunoglobulin (IVIg) treatment my body began to reel.

After a walk my blood pressure rose to an alarming level and I had chest pains.

The next day I collapsed and had a seizure.

In the many hours of the day that I lay prone, I tried to counteract the stupor of the seizure meds by doing crossword puzzles and to think about my ITP and solve that puzzle too.

My platelet count slowly went down.

The next round of IVIg was less successful in raising my counts.

Figure 17.

TREATMENT

First line:

Oral Prednisolone 60 mg/d for 4-6weeks; then tapered over a few weeks
Inravenous Immunolglobulin (IV Ig): where rapid rise required
Anti-D

The round after that had almost no effect." (Young 1997)

Next we enter the zone of *empirical evidence* that tells us what intervention to choose for our patient at hand utilizing population based data from collective experimentation. (Biswas 2008)

In general, only 15-25% of patients on steroids are expected to have lasting remission;

The remainders have disease characterized by frequent relapses and remissions.

"Splenectomy and a large number of drugs have been used as second-line therapy with variable success. Physicians are required to make individual judgments about the nature of second-line treatment based on bleeding history, comorbidities, patient expectations, and compliance.

The main goal of second-line therapy is to attain a sustained increase of the platelet count that is considered hemostatic for the individual patient. Available treatment modalities have quite different mechanisms of action and can be broadly categorized into those that are given only once (or for only one course) and are intended to induce long-term remission (splenectomy, rituximab and those that need continued or chronic administration of corticosteroids, immunosuppressive agents and thrombopoietin receptor agonists)." (Provan 2010)

"I agreed to have my spleen removed, hoping again for a quick fix and to put an end to the endless round of doctor appointments, hospitalizations and the constant fear of bumping my head and dying.

Before I left for the hospital I placed my will on my dresser." (Young 1997)

Splenectomy is effective because it removes the major site of destruction and the major source of antiplatelet antibody synthesis.

Before splenectomy, patients receive a prophylactic polyvalent pneumococcal, meningococcal C conjugate, and H influenzae b (Hib) vaccines at least 4 weeks before (preferably) or 2 weeks after splenectomy and revaccinated according to the country specific recommendations (Provan 2010)

Even if complete remission is not achieved, the platelet count will be higher after splenectomy. (Thiagarajan 2009)

"My surgery was successful in that I survived, my spleen was removed and the wound eventually healed.

However, it was not successful in raising my platelet count." (Young 1997)

Failure to respond to splenectomy has been attributed to platelet clearance in the liver and elsewhere (Cines 2007). Approximately 10-20% of patients who undergo splenectomy remain thrombocytopenic and continue to have a bleeding risk that requires continued treatment. Both steroid therapy and splenectomy are considered failures in these patients, and the patients are challenging to treat. (Thiagarajan 2009)

"Three weeks after the surgery I had as few platelets as before the operation.

Now I was without a spleen, bruised, and still on the seizure meds.

It was now Christmas and my family and I wondered if it would be our last together." (Young 1997)

A number of other second line treatments have been proposed for splenectomy and steroid failures.

Figure 18.

Second line therapies:

1) Elective Splenectomy : Chronic ITP patients who fail to maintain normal platelet count after a course of prednisolone are eligible for it. (Thiagarajan 2009)

Figure 19.

> Second line therapies (continued from figure 20):
>
> High dose corticosteroids (iv)
> High dose iv Ig
> Rituximab
> TPO receptor agonists
> Danazol, colchicine
> Vinca alkaloids
> Immunosuppresive drugs: Azathioprin, Cyclosporine, Dapsone

Most of them are not based on placebo-controlled studies, and evaluating the efficacy of these treatments in a disease associated with spontaneous remissions and relapse is difficult. (Thiagarajan 2009)

"My hematologist recommended Danazol… No luck…Colchicine failed too.

We even tried another course of IVIg hoping that my body would respond to it differently now that I didn't have a spleen.

It responded differently alright. I was hospitalized following one of the treatments for a nosebleed that didn't stop." (Young 1997)

The antigenic target in most patients appears to be the platelet glycoprotein IIb/IIIa complex.

Platelets with antibodies on their surface are trapped in the spleen, where they are efficiently removed by splenic macrophages.

The mechanism of origin of these antibodies is not known. (Thiagarajan 2009)

Since Joan's illness in 1992, the knowledge around ITP has continued to evolve. There have been newer concepts in pathogenesis such as "same antibodies that mediate platelet destruction also mediate impaired platelet production by damaging megakaryocytes and/or blocking their ability to release pro-platelets." (Cines, Bussel, Liebman et al 2009). Newer treatment options have been found that may be recommended differently for people with secondary causes of ITP such that when the underlying condition is treated, the platelets may go up. H-pylori is a striking example of this. (Stasi 2009). ITP is now immune thrombocytopenia;

the "i" is no longer "idiopathic" and "purpura" is no longer part of the name. (Rodeghiero 2009)

"I went to an ITP specialist in …and he berated my local hematologist for not putting me in the hospital.

I reluctantly agreed to a course of vincristine (chemotherapy) followed by a series of Prosorba-A blood cleansing treatments. They sneaked in more of the dreaded prednisone.

I returned to work at the end of March 1993, part time, wearing a wig, on the day that my short-term disability insurance ended."

The song of the river ends not at her banks but in the hearts of those who have loved her...
Anirban Chaudhuri

CONCLUSION

This chapter tries to highlight the power of personal experience and its role in enhancing the engagement of the learner. Not only are people's stories transferring factual information, they more importantly highlight the limitations of the textbook knowledge in particular. The "failure of the textbook" is common enough to warrant a discourse about the limitations of knowledge as much as a discourse about the impact of success and failure in medical care on the individual. We believe that this format of teaching promotes deeper insight in the learner and instills a sense of "always being humble" as a health professional.

REFERENCES

American Society of Hematology ITP Practice Guideline Panel. (1997). Diagnosis and Treatment of Idiopathic Thrombocytopenic Purpura. *Recommendations of the American Society of Hematology, 126*(4), 319–326.

Besa, C. E., & Woermann, U. (2009, February 6). *Chronic Myelogenous Leukemia. E Medicine (Medscape).* Retrieved June 16, 2009 from http://emedicine.medscape.com/article/199425-overview

Biswas, R., Martin, C., Sturmberg, J., Shankar, R., & Umakanth, S., Shanker, & Kasthuri A. S. (2008). User driven health care - Answering multidimensional information needs in individual patients utilizing post EBM approaches: A conceptual model. *Journal of Evaluation in Clinical Practice, 14,* 742–749. doi:10.1111/j.1365-2753.2008.00998.x

Biswas, R., Umakanth, S., Shetty, M., Hande, M., & Nagra, J. S. (2009). Problem based self-directed life long participatory learning in medical educators and their audience: Reflective lessons learnt from a lecture series. In Geinare, P. F. (Ed.), *Trends in continuing education.* New York: Nova Science Publishers.

Cines, D. B. (2007). Pumping out platelets. *Blood, 113*(11), 4591–4592. doi:10.1182/blood-2007-03-079483

Cines, D. B., Bussel, J. B., & Liebman, H. A. (2009). The ITP syndrome: pathogenic and clinical diversity. *Blood, 113,* 6511–6521. doi:10.1182/blood-2009-01-129155

Conrad, M. E. (2006, October). *Iron Deficiency Anemia: Treatment & Medication. E Medicine (Medscape).* Retrieved June 16 2009 from http://emedicine.medscape.com/article/202333-treatment

Family Medicine Net Guide (2004, February). Empowered! Taking Control of Your Health with the Web: advice from a survivor: a talk with Laura Landro. *Family Medicine Net Guide, 2*(1).

Flflowergirl. Ferritin less than 1? Forum post (2009, January). *Anemia message board, In HealthBoards Message Boards.* Retrieved June 15, 2009, from http://www.healthboards.com/boards/showthread.php?t=666920&highlight=lotsawalls&page=5

Goddard, A. F., McIntyre, A. S., & Scott, B. B. (2000, December). Guidelines for the management of iron deficiency anaemia. *British Society of Gastroenterology, 47*(6), 872. Retrieved June 15, 2009 from http://www.pubmedcentral.nih.gov/articlerender.fcgi?artid=1766761

Gratwohl, A., Hermans, J., & Niederwieser, D. (1993). Bone marrow transplantation for chronic myeloid leukemia: Long term results. Chronic Leukemia Working Party of the European Group for Bone Marrow Transplantation. *Bone Marrow Transplantation, 12*(5), 509–516.

Guidelines for the management of iron deficiency anaemia (2005). *British Society of Gastroenterology.* Retrieved June 15, 2009, from http://www.bsg.org.uk/pdf_word_docs/iron_def.pdf

Human iron metabolism (2009). *Wikipedia, the free encyclopedia.* Retrieved June 15, 2009, from http://en.wikipedia.org/wiki/Human_iron_metabolism

Kittenwithawhip. My anemia story.... Forum post (2005, August). *Anemia message board, In HealthBoards Message Boards.* Retrieved June 15, 2009, from http://www.healthboards.com/boards/showthread.php?t=310085&highlight=kittenwithawhip

Landro, L. A. (1996, October). Survivor's Tale: How a Wall Street Journal reporter confronted a potentially fatal cancer head-on. *The Wall Street Journal, Health & Medicine (A Special Report): Essay*. Retrieved June 7, 2009, fromhttp://leukemia.acor.org/storydir/landro.html

Lotsawalls. Ferritin less than 1? Forum post (2009, Jan). Anemia message board, In *HealthBoards Message Boards*. Retrieved June 15, 2009, from http://www.healthboards.com/boards/showthread.php?t=666920&highlight=lotsawalls&page=5

Matthews, D. A., Suchman, A. L., & Branch, W. T. (1993). Making "connexions": enhancing the therapeutic potential of patient-clinician relationships. *Annals of Internal Medicine, 118*, 973–977.

Provan, D., Stasi, R., & Newland, A. C. (2010). International consensus report on the investigation and management of primary immune thrombocytopenia. *Blood, 115*, 168–186. doi:10.1182/blood-2009-06-225565

Red blood cell distribution width (2009). *Wikipedia, the free encyclopedia*. Retrieved June 15, 2009 from http://en.wikipedia.org/wiki/Red_blood_cell_distribution_width

Rodeghiero, F., Stasi, R., & Gernsheimer, T. (2009). Standardization of terminology, definitions and outcome criteria in immune thrombocytopenic purpura of adults and children: report from an international working group. *Blood, 113*, 2386–2393. doi:10.1182/blood-2008-07-162503

Stasi, R., Sarpatwari, A., & Sega, J. B. (2009). Effects of eradication of Helicobacter pylori infection in patients with immune thrombocytopenic purpura: a systematic review. *Blood, 113*, 1231–1240. doi:10.1182/blood-2008-07-167155

Sturmberg, J. P., Martin, C. M., & Moes, M. (2010). (in press). Health at the Centre of Health Systems Reform - How Philosophy Can Inform Policy. *Perspectives in Biology and Medicine*.

Thiagarajan, P. (2009). *Platelet disorders, E-medicine (Medscape)*. Retrieved June 16 2009 from http://emedicine.medscape.com/article/201722-treatment

White, D. L., & Hughes, T. P. (2009, April). Predicting the response of CML patients to tyrosine kinase inhibitor therapy. *Current Hematologic Malignancy Reports, 4*(2), 59–65. doi:10.1007/s11899-009-0009-2

Young, J. (1997). *ITP personal stories: Success story. Platelet disorder support association*. Retrieved April 7, 2010 from http://www.pdsa.org/join-the-community/personal-stories/item/129-success-story.html.

Chapter 3
Stomodeum to Proctodeum:
Email Narratives on Clinical Problem Solving in Gastroenterology

Paramartha Bhattacharya
Consultant Physician, India

Amar Puri Asanga
Yoga consultant, Nepal

Rakesh Biswas
People's College of Medical Sciences, India

ABSTRACT

This chapter contains physician and patient perspectives of their gastrointestinal system problem solving experiences beginning from one anatomical end, stomodeum and continuing toward the other end proctodeum of the gastrointestinal tube. These experiences reflect user driven health care to the extent that they have been largely shared and developed over a web interface through email narratives and illustrate conversational learning in a patient centered manner.

INTRODUCTION

We take for granted the pleasure of being able to enjoy our food – with our eyes, our smell and our taste, and we take for granted to digest, to absorb the sustaining substances from our food, and to pass the leftovers on average once a day. However this is not the case for everyone all of the time, and it is not always easy to know the reasons for this. In this chapter we "travel" down the at times "rocky road" of the "pipe of our digestive tract". We explore the personal perspectives of the patient

as well as the doctor's struggles to understand the "troubles of the gut". These reflections extend on experiences shared in various ways in the past.

By the third week, endodermal cells have migrated around the inside of the blastocyst, completing a pouch called the yolk sac. The primitive gut, composed entirely of endoderm, develops early in the fourth week when the dorsal part of the yolk sac incorporates into the embryo during the process of folding. The gastrointestinal tract develops from modifications of the primitive gut that forms a continuous elongated tube from the future mouth (a depression called the stomodeum or oral pit that is not part of the foregut but an

DOI: 10.4018/978-1-60960-097-6.ch003

invagination of ectoderm that will become the oral cavity) to the future anus (the proctodeum or anal pit is an invagination of surface epidermal ectoderm that develops in the hindgut and develops into the anus). (Neas 2003)

In planning this chapter the narrative nature of medical knowledge is acknowledged. These include the medical story, the patient story, the notes, and the test results. And these are all interpreted in the light of previous stories within medicine - the anecdotes, the scientific literature, and stories of previous patients that seem similar. (Nicholas & Gillett, 1997)

Some of these experiences have been published before and after having obtained permission from the primary publishers we have reproduced them with appropriate referencing and citations to avoid copyright issues.

We begin our journey from the stomodeum with a window seat to our past experiences alongside our patients. These experiences have over the years gradually receded into the background and yet require continued documentation and sharing to reach further insights be it personal or collective.

Stomodeum: The Journey Begins

Sometime around April 2002 author RB saw this patient in his clinic in a teaching hospital in Nepal and posted the patient's picture along with the clinical query on to the www.jiscmail.ac.uk/lists/evidence-based-health list serv.

She is a yoga teacher on a strict vegetarian diet and has taken all possible vitamins and essential nutrients available along with various antibiotic creams (partly self medication). What are the possible causes and what further line of management would benefit the patient? Rakesh Biswas, Asst Prof, Pokhara, Nepal

Searching for Evidence

A dermatology referral was made immediately after the physician's consultation and she cor-

Figure 1. A middle aged white lady has persistent angular cheilitis and stomatitis since the last 4 months

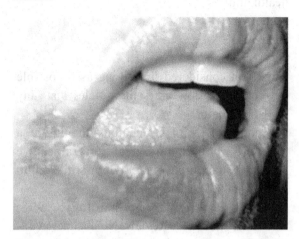

rectly made a reasonable assumption with a few differential diagnoses although the exact source of the problem remained elusive. There was no verbal contact between the dermatologist and the physician at this point of time and the physician remained unaware of her differential diagnosis. The physician formulated clinical query was then dispatched to the evidence based mailing list and following are a few of the various suggestions to our query from and outside the evidence based health mailing list

Consider Lip licking, Iron deficiency, Recurrent Herpes simplex infection (5-15 episodes per year),Syphilis, Candidiasis and other fungal infections, Vit B1 deficiency (Not corrected by oral- as first manifestatin of malabsorption syndrome or as the only manifestation. Give a therapeutic trial of Injectable Vit B.)Bechet's, Pemphigus, Dental causes: Can be related to overclosure of the mouth leading to stagnant areas in the corners of the mouth and infection. Until the problem is sorted out (for instance by making new dentures at an appropriate occluso-vertical dimension) the cause will not be removed and symptoms will persist or recur.

The transcript below can also be accessed at http://www.jiscmail.ac.uk/lists/evidence-based-health.html

Response 1

Dear Sir:

Have you considered lip licking as a possible cause? Below are some articles that may be of help.

1. Epidemiology of eczematous cheilitis at a tertiary dermatological referral centre in Singapore.Contact Dermatitis. 2000 Dec;43(6):322-6.
2. Senile lip licking.Dermatology. 1995; 191(4):339-40. Review. No abstract available.
3. Factitious lip crusting Arch Dermatol. 1981 Jun;117(6):338-40.

Anne Nichols, CRNP
Nurse Practitioner
Widener University
Chester, PA

Response 2

Hello Rakesh,

I have two questions.

First, Do the nutritional supplements the patient is taking contain Iron?

Secondly, does she have any anemia (microcytic vs. macrocytic)?

Sandeep, Physician, US

Response 3

Dear Rakesh,

Have you done a VDRL?

Regards,

Rout

Response 4

Angular stomatitis and cheilitis have these etiologies and causes as differential diagnosis-

Recurrent Herpes simplex infection (5-15 episodes per year)

Candidiasis and other fungal infections

Vit B1 deficiency (Not corrected by oral - as first manifestatin of malabsorption syndrome or as the only manifestation. Give a therapeutic trial of Injectable Vit B.)

Bechet's, Pemphigus (Both can be proved by lip biopsy)

Anurag Bharadwaj
Associate Professor of Medicine
Melaka- Manipal Medical College
Jalan Batu Hampar, Bukit Baru, 75150 Melaka
Malaysia

Response 5

Dear Rakesh,

Thank you for the data.I would consider Inflammatory Bowel Disease. I have seen pts of IBD present with persistent Apthous Ulcers. Also investigate for Syphilis and HIV.

Best wishes,

Pratap J Philip, Physician, Australia

Response 6

Dear Rakesh,

What about a fungal infection? I had someone very like this recently who responded beautifully to clotrimazole cream. Let me know what you think.

Janette, Physician, UK

Response 7

I am a dentist and regularly although not frequently see patients with both symptomatic and asymptomatic angular cheilitis (stomatitis). It may be useful to refer the patient to a dental practitioner or oral medicine specialist. Angular chelitis can be related to overclosure of the mouth leading to stagnant areas in the corners of the mouth and infection. Until the problem is sorted out (for instance by making new dentures at an appropriate occluso-vertical dimension) the cause will not be removed and symptoms will persist or

recur. Also infective agents needn't always
be bacterial (staph, strep or mixed) but may
be candidal. Miconazole can be useful.
Hope this helps
Nicola

Nicola P T Innes
GDP/ CSO Research Training Fellow University
of Dundee
nptinnes@hotmail.com

Evidence into Practice

Thanks everybody,
I shall consider a therapeutic trial of anti-fungal
cream after getting a dental evaluation and if
in the negative taking a scraping for fungal
hyphae and a blood for VDRL although it will
need a forbidding pre test counseling. If the
patient doesn't respond to this initial treatment, I may go ahead with a lip biopsy after
a repeat consultation with the dematologist.

Rakesh Biswas, Asst Prof, Medicine,
Manipal Teaching Hospital, Pokhara
Pin-33701, Nepal

Outcome

Then suddenly an email from the patient herself:
(see Box 1)

Box 1.

----- Original Message -rakesh7biswas@yahoo.com>
Sent: Monday, April 22, 2002 7:38 AM
Subject: mouth
Hello, dear Rakesh,
I just want to tell you, that my spot at the angle of the mouth has gone almost totally. As soon as Monica said, it had something to do with inside the mouth, I remembered that I didn't use mouthwash in Kathmandu. As you know in Kathmandu, the spot was so much better. So I stopped immediately using this tea-tree oil in my mouthwash and also changed the toothpaste and it has gone. Please be so kind to tell Monica, that tea tree oil was the cause of this disease and that I'm happy to be rid of it now.
Monica is our dermatologist to whom I had referred our patient immediately after I took the photo of her angular cheilitis. She did suspect contact dermatitis and enquired whether the patient was using any particular brand of new toothpaste or mouth wash. At that time our patient couldn't recall any but then… she did recall it later.

Searching Further

We did a search on tea tree oil and came across
some interesting information. Tea tree oil is a
complex chemical substance made up of almost 50
compounds. The oil is distilled from the leaves of
the *Melaleuca alternifolia* plant, native to swampy
areas of New South Wales; As early as 1933 the
British Medical Journal carried a report stating
that [tea tree] oil was a powerful disinfectant,
non-poisonous and non-irritant. Since then it
has been recommended for a variety of ailments
such as acne, arthritis, athlete's foot, boils and
abscesses, bronchitis, bruises, burns and sunburn,
candida, chilblains, colds, cold sores, corns, cuts
and abrasions, cystitis, dental plaque, dermatitis/
eczema, fungal infections, fever/flu, genital herpes, head lice, herpes, insect bites, muscular aches
and pains, respiratory tract infections, vaginal
infections, varicose veins, warts, to strengthen
the immune system(and the list is increasing
everyday).(Teatree 2002)

However the essential oil also contains turpen-
tines (limonene, alpha-pinene, phellandrene) that
are potentially allergenic. In a recent review of 14
patients who were patch tested because of eczema
to used products containing tea tree oil, 7 were
confirmed to have allergic contact dermatitis due to
tea tree oil of which two also exhibited a delayed
type IV hypersensitivity towards fragrance-mix
or colophony suggesting the possibility of cross
reaction. (Fritz 2001)

These patients used creams, hair products and essential oils containing Melaleuca alternifolia for cosmetic reasons and to treat skin affections. They were patch tested from a standard panel of allergens, topical emulgators, perfumes, plants, topical medications, metal, gloves, topical disinfectants and preservatives, dental products and rubber derivatives. Products containing Melaleuca alternifolia were tested concentrated or diluted. The safety, efficacy of tea tree oil has been reviewed elsewhere in detail. (Carson 2001)

Soul Search

Our patient presented with a persistent angular cheilitis and stomatitis and there is a definite cause and effect relationship considering the temporal course of events linked to her mouth wash usage and the development and subsequent subsidence of her ailment. Mouthwash usage is associated with cheilitis as per standard textbook descriptions. (Burton 1993)

Patch testing may have been more corroborative in a definitive sense but as evidenced on the patient's email she's quite convinced that it was her mouthwash with the tea tree oil and further testing may not be feasible(now that she's rid of the problem).

We found most of the suggestions in a standard textbook of dermatology. Syphilis has been described as a cause of macrocheilitis. We didn't find Bechet's as a cause for cheilitis although connective tissue disorders like systemic lupus can cause a severe form of cheilitis with erosions and even hemorrhagic crusts. (Burton 1993)

The six major obstacles encountered when attempting to answer doctors' questions with evidence recently identified were: the excessive time required to find information, difficulty modifying the original question, which was often vague and open to interpretation, difficulty selecting an optimal strategy to search for information, failure of a seemingly appropriate resource to cover the topic, uncertainty about how to know when all the relevant evidence has been found so that the search can stop, and inadequate synthesis of multiple bits of evidence into a clinically useful statement.(Ely 2002)

In our instance the time required to find information was shortened by the evidence based network although its final relevance is debatable. The search strategy was well defined although limited in its scope. There are a lot of helpful people on the net who are keen to solve an interesting puzzle although it may be simple laziness on the part of the person posing the clinical query, who seeks an easier solution from a wider resource instead of pouring through textbooks him/herself (which may still be the initial appropriate resource). It may have been difficult to reach a conclusion on part of the physician alone if the dermatologist hadn't intervened and the patient hadn't recalled a useful clue. The above experience has been published and reproduced here with permission (Biswas 2003)

Our next stop is slightly down below in the food pipe that one is likely to enter after clearing the stomodeum and the oral cavity. (Biswas 2002)

The Burning Food Pipe: Journey Continues

A 30 year old yoga teacher from Pokhara, Nepal, presented to us with severe prolonged heart burn and sour eructations(intermittent reflux symptoms) for 2 years not responding to Proton Pump Inhibitors and with no marked abnormality on available investigations like Upper Gastro Intestinal (UGI) endoscopy with biopsy and barium swallow. There was however a patulous lower esophageal sphincter along with a hiatus hernia noted on UGI endoscopy although there were no erosions due to reflux.

He also reported having noticed exacerbation of his symptoms particularly after Shirsasana (a yoga asana (or posture) in which the body is completely inverted, and held upright supported by the forearms, while the crown of the head rests lightly on the floor).

As to the etiology of this troublesome reflux, he recalled having had to master Kunjal kriya and also demonstrate it a number of times daily to his students.

Kunjal kriya is a special technique involving induced reverse peristalsis following intake of a large volume of water. It is supposed to have cleansing properties and it claims to throw fermented waste out of the stomach and prevents auto-poisoning of the body. It is also recommended for bronchial asthma by yogic schools…even during attacks! (Swami 1981)

Repeated induced reverse peristalsis in the form of Kunjal kriya is likely to have been responsible for the persistent esophageal reflux in this yoga teacher, since his symptoms were much better after having given up Kunjal kriya and Shirshasana (headstand) for a few months initially (but recurred again). Heartburn and acid regurgitation have a high specificity (89 and 95% respectively) for the presence of gastroesophageal reflux disease. (Parkman 1995)

This was published in 2002 and author RB is still in touch with him at 2010. Unfortunately his reflux symptoms continued to persist for the most part in the form of heart burns in spite of the proton pump inhibitors.

RB mailed his patient's problem to one of his long term colleagues working as a gastroenterology faculty in US on advice regarding further available interventions (this was somewhere around 2005):

Hi J, I have a patient-a yoga teacher who has been having reflux like burning particularly as a result of a particular yogic kriya of reverse peristalsis he demonstrated to his students for quite a few years.
I wonder if he would benefit by the Stretta procedure. He has more of a burning epigastric pain but no remarkable endoscopic findings

other than a patulous LES. Could it be that his pain is because of a neural damage to the LES although it hasn't produced much mucosal changes?
Could the Stretta benefit him by burning the raw nerve endings that are generating his pain? R

Hi R,
The benefits of either stretta or enteryx -so far as evidence based approach is concerned- is essentially short lived and most patient benefit has been decreased PPI usage and decreased GERD related QUALI. No study till date has shown long term benefit and for all practical purposes these are used in patients who do not want to use PPI or have quality of life related issues.
My approach would have been to do a manometry and Ph study on him while on PPI (*proton pump inhibitors like omeprazole etc-authors*) and depending on the result consider sending him if he does have an incompetent LES for fundoplication either laparoscopic or convention depending on the local expertise. Nobody knows the cause of GERD symptoms in patients on PPI and compliant-- non-erosive reflux or NERD may be reason but only way to prove that is with esophageal impedence studies--you must be believer in that school of thought to accept that rationale.
I don't know if this helps you or may be adds to the confusion. Let me know of any other info that I can provide. J

A mail from the patient somewhere in 2006:

Dear R,
Recently I have been looking for the place to have laparoscopic fundoplication through internet. I could not find any in Kathmandu but I found a Apollo Hospital in Delhi and I made some queries to them, since lifestyle changing and medical treatment didn't work

I am thinking to make this operation sooner or later, may be on January or February.

Do you think there maybe any such center in Kathmandu? Delhi is far away for me and also sounds very costly $2000/- for all the treatment. If this would be in Manipal it would so easy for me to do it.

Here are the answers from that hospital

Where is the hospital located? *New delhi, india*
Is that price for Indians or Westerners? *For all we dont make any distinctions*
How much in economy ward? *About 20% less*
Is that Laparoscopic Fundoplication ? YES
How big incision you make and how long it takes to recover? *5 small incisions of 1/4 to 1/2 inches*
Who is the surgeon?
How long does this operation take? 2 hours
How do you make decision whether I need this operation or not? *Going by the summary you have sent, you should benefit from the surgery*

Our patient decided not to get operated at that time.

Another mail from him recently in 2009:

Dear R,

You know my heartburn is still there, never got better.

One of my German doctor friends has suggested raising dose of Omeprazole or pantoprazole?

Follow up mail: Dear R,

I finished 40 capsules of omeprazole, maximum I had 2 capsules a day. My German friend says that it could be the quality of medicine, so he is sending me omeprazole from Germany, I will try that with 2 capsules and if symptoms remain same as it was I will try 3 and 4. Nowadays symptom is same more or less, even after such a long time of omeprazole.

Jan 13, 2010
Dear R,

I booked an airplane ticket to Delhi for 17 of January, 2010. I am going to Apollo hospital. You may have more idea about hospitals in Delhi. Please advice which one is good to go to have check up. First I will get ph monitoring done along with a biopsy of the LES (lower esophageal sphincter).

With regards

Jan 18, 2010
Dear R,

I went to sir Gangaram hospital today and they are doing ph monitoring and biopsy tomorrow. Let's see the result. Dr. was fine but had to wait so long. I will let you know about results. With best regards

Jan 20, 2010
Dear R,

Yesterday I went through the awful Ph monitoring tests and today again another endoscopy. Here I am attaching reports of them, tomorrow Dr. has called me, seems that he will insist for operation.

I would like to hear from you before I do this. If we come we will let you know. With regards

PS attached file are my reports of ph monitoring and endoscopy. (Figures 2 and 3)

Jan 20, 2010
Thanks A, for sending these. There is definite evidence of significant reflux and you also have developed erosions since the last endoscopy I remember doing on you 8 years back which didn't reveal this at that time.

I feel you would respond better to surgery although the evidence suggests that some patients still may need to continue on antireflux medications like omeprazole etc inspite of the surgery.

Figure 2. Esophageal Ph monitoring results

pH analysis results - Channel: pH-1

pH acid results

	Total
Duration	23:54 hh:mm
Duration	100.0 %
Total reflux time (pH <=4.0)	1204.4 min
Total reflux time (pH <=4.0)	84.0 %
Nr of reflux periods	69
Nr of long reflux periods >5 min.	19
Longest reflux	291.6 min

DeMeester scoring results (Score according to DeMeester normal values)
DeMeester score: 156.59 (14.72 is upper limit of 95.0 percentile of normal)

Adult scoring results

	Patient	Normal		
Total reflux time	84.0	< 4.2		► 20 Total %
Nr of reflux periods	69.3	< 50.0		100 in 24 hours
Nr of long reflux periods >5 min.	19.1	< 4.0		20 in 24 hours
Longest reflux	291.6	< 9.2		► 60 min

No Boix-Ochoa scoring results calculated. Patient is too old.

No Infant scoring results calculated. Patient is too old.

Figure 3. Erosions at lower end of esophagus

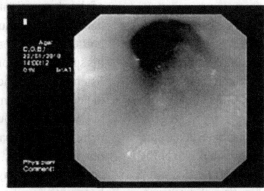

GASTRO-DUODENOSCOPY REPORT

Findings

Erosions seen at lower end of esophagus. Large hiatus hernia present. GE Junction is at 30cm.

Fundus, body, and antrum of stomach are normal

Duodenal bulb is normal
Second part of duodenum is normal

Conclusions
GERD WITH LARGE HIATUS HERNIA

I feel you have no option but to try out surgery and let us hope for the best.

Regards,

R

A got operated and here is the last conversation R had with him:

Dear R,

I am back home already 3 weeks, I was just about to email you today because since I didn't find much change they asked me to take Tablet Libotryp before bed and 40 mg of pantoprazol. I couldn't find Tablet libotryp in any medical shop here in Nepal, what is it?

I am still suffering, but may be little bit less, I still can't say.

Burping is fully stopped, so there shouldn't be reflux now but why is there pain? I still don't understand. Doctors there said that it is because of previous erosion and will take 4 to 6 weeks.

Thanks for your concern.

With best regards

A

Hi A,

Great to hear from you.

Hope you recover from the pain. I agree it may be due to the erosions. Sometimes frayed nerve endings due to the reflux could cause the persistent pain.

Hopefully now that the reflux has been taken care of the pain shall subside gradually over the next one year.

Libotryp is actually a combination of amiltryptline (the tablet Tryptomer that you used to take earlier for the same chronic pain) and Chlordiazepoxide or Librium (which is an anxiety reducing agent).

You can take them separately if the combination is not available there.

Further down we enter the stomach and then sail through the small and large intestines and considering the length of this tube there are quite a few stories to relate:

Intestines: An Outbreak

This is an unusual story related by a boy helping out with managing an outbreak of diarrhea in a rural hospital in Bengal, India along with author PB. This boy was a patient's relative as well as an enthusiastic college student volunteering his services with perhaps an altruistic motive.

"Of course, you should have given him lots of water to drink", the Doctor kept on harping in the same monotonous tone.

I was still perplexed. So long we had known if a child vomits so much he should not be given water to drink, rather it should be put in his blood as 'saline'. We also knew that when a baby vomits the baby should be denied water. But the Doctor seems to change all our beliefs!!

Standing in the ward of a overcrowded hospital of rural Bengal amongst a ghastly sight of scores of diarrhea patients sometimes we were joining hands with the nurses in fixing the saline drip bottles, sometimes helping the sole doctor with his sphygmomanometer but all the while we were listening to the clichés of health information that the doctor or the nurses were telling us.

We were a group of young boys and we were helping diarrhea patients to the hospitals, enjoying our philanthropic work to the society. We could understand as days were advancing, we were becoming familiar with the norms and systems of the hospital and the clichés of the doctor but we could understand that anxiety was mounting every day as evident by the growing wrinkles on the doctors forehead.

Then one day, probably our 5th day in the hospital, Doctor PB called us to his office in the evening and explained there was an outbreak of epidemic of diarrhoeal diseases in our neighboring block (block-II)and the doctor feared that now the disease was spreading in our block as well.

Doctor P explained that in this (Figure 4) graph series-I (blue) was the total admitted patients; series-II (red) pts. From block-I; series-III (yellow) pts.from block-II. Initially during the outbreak when the total admission was small the yellow band was big and the pts were from the neighboring block. As the outbreak progressed, the blue band increased in size the yellow band was bigger than the red counterpart.

Doctor P told us that it was necessary to cut down the source from which the epidemic was spreading to arrest the onslaught rather then providing curative care. He wanted us to go back to the villages and work door to door spreading the sermons of healthy living and preventing indispensable water which we drink or wash with every day getting contaminated or soiled.

So we went back to the community and started some health habits:

- We segregated open wells and deep tube wells as sources of drinking water and got them disinfected by health workers. Washing was prohibited near sources of drinking water.

- Ponds were used for washing and the cooking utensils were again made to wash with well water.
- Diarrhea affected individuals were encouraged to drink plenty of water and ORS.
- Daily extensive cleaning of sick houses were prioritized.
- We also used to keep good liaison with the hospital.

The two charts above were, of course, compiled later but showed how correct the doctor was when he predicted that the diarrhoeal epidemic started in block–II and then gradually spread to block–I.

In this graph (Figure 5) it was evident that there was a sudden surge of patients between 27.10 & 29.10 which certainly marks the beginning of the epidemic. This was more substantiated from the next graph (Figure 6)which shows the no. of in-hospital *admissions* and no. of in-hospital patient *load* had a parallel trend when suddenly on 26.10 the inpatient trend fell despite the rise in admissions. This was because this was the point when the in-patient admission of diarrheal cases suddenly peaked in excess of general admissions. The further trend shows again parallel trends till 22.11 when again a pattern similar to the one on 26.10 was noted which marked the discharge of

Figure 4. Shows bar graph depicting total admissions (BLUE) and the split showing pts. From block-I (red) and those from block –II (yellow)

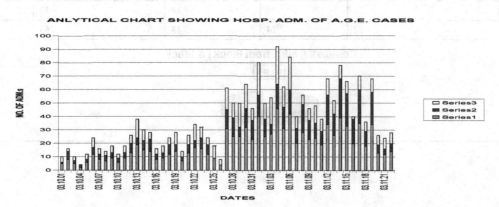

Table 1. Shows hospital admissions in October with block wise analysis

Date	No. Of Admission	Block-I	Block-Ii	Total Pt.S @12 Mn	Death
	Analytical Report Of Hosp. Admissions In Hpur R.Hospital.				
.10.01	5	1	4	48	1
.10.02	8	6	2	44	
.10.03	5	2	3	44	1
.10.04	2	2	0	35	
.10.05	6	2	4	37	
.10.06	12	5	7	46	
.10.07	8	4	4	40	
.10.08	7	4	3	32	
.10.09	9	4	5	38	
.10.10	6	3	3	32	
.10.11	9	4	5	32	
.10.12	13	7	6	40	1
.10.13	19	5	14	47	
.10.14	15	7	8	45	
.10.15	14	9	5	56	
.10.16	8	4	4	45	
.10.17	9	4	5	37	
.10.18	12	7	5	53	1
.10.19	14	5	9	46	
.10.20	7	3	4	39	
.10.21	13	6	7	47	
.10.22	17	5	12	44	
.10.23	16	8	8	54	
.10.24	12	7	5	55	
.10.25	9	0	9	39	
.10.26	4	0	4	33	
.10.27	31	14	16	40	1
.10.28	25	14	11	67	
.10.29	25	7	18	58	1
.10.30	32	14	18	63	

Comparing adm. from Block I & Block

□ 1 ■ 2

1
43%

2
57%

Table 2. Shows hospital admissions in November with block wise analysis

No. Of Admission	Block-I	Block-Ii	Total Pt.S @12 Mn	Death	
.11.01	40	16	24	80	
.11.02	25	13	12	60	
.11.03	27	7	20	67	
.11.04	46	18	28	87	
.11.05	31	16	15	64	
.11.06	42	18	24	82	
.11.07	20	11	9	64	
.11.08	28	21	7	55	
.11.09	23	14	9	52	1
.11.10	24	11	13	57	
.11.11	19	10	9	62	
.11.12	34	22	12	66	
11.13	26	16	10	62	
.11.14	39	29	10	79	
.11.15	33	24	9	86	
.11.16	20	18	2	71	1
.11.17	35	25	10	70	
.11.18	18	11	7	57	1
.11.19	34	24	10	62	
.11.20	13	6	7	49	
.11.21	12	4	8	37	
.11.22	14	6	8	34	
		340	263		

Comparing Adm. from Block I & BlockII

□1 ■2

2
44%

1
56%

diarrhea cases and admissions of general cases in excess of diarrheal cases again. This trend occurred as the diarrheal cases were in such excess so as to flood the isolation ward onto general pts. Hence the period between 26.10–22.11 is designated as the period of epidemic.

Though reports and experiences of previous years suggest a similar trend of upsurge of diarrhoeal disease after the rains details analysis re-vealed that this years' occurrence was clearly "in excess of" what was expected.

Physician's reflections: (PB)

1. That there was a definite outbreak of infec-tive diarrheal diseases over the months of Oct and Nov in the blocks Block I & II,. As is evident from the data the no. of in-hospital *admissions* and no. of in-hospital patient

Figure 5. Total hosp admission trend between 1ˢᵗ Oct and 22ⁿᵈ Nov

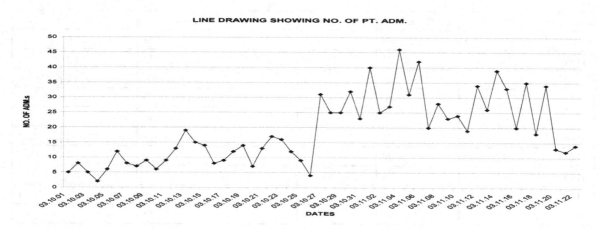

Figure 6. Shows a trend of total inpatient cases @12midnight compared with total no. of admissions

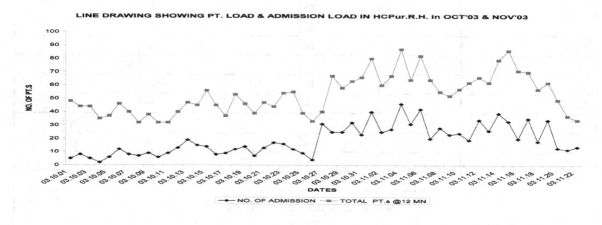

Figure 7. Shows the Year wise trend of A.G.E. case admissions in Hcpur Hosp over three years

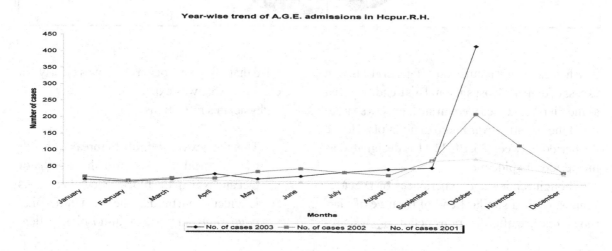

load had a parallel trend when suddenly on 26.10 the inpatient trend fell despite the rise in admissions. This was because this was the point when the in-patient admission of diarrheal cases suddenly peaked in excess of general admissions. The further trend shows again parallel trends till 22.11 when again a pattern similar to the one on 26.10 was noted which marked the discharge of diarrhea cases and admissions of general cases in excess of diarrheal cases again. This trend occurred as the diarrheal cases were in such excess so as to flood the isolation ward onto general pts. Hence the period between 26.10–22.11 is designated as the period of epidemic.

2. Such outbreak is in line with similar trends over the past year.

3. That this outbreak occurred almost within a week of heavy downpours in the second week of October. It may be stressed that in the year of study significant downpour was not seen early in rainy season.

4. Outbreak initially occurred in the villages of Block - II block and gradually spread to Block-I, as the pie diagram should suggest. And in Block I, as is evident from the sketch map, the trend of the disease was more in areas where there was no metalled road connection. I'd like to stress on this fact. It is again a fact that metalled roads do not connect most of the areas of Block II either. Here people have to use mostly muddy roads, which after the showers are slimy are excellent culture for bacteria that cause diarrhoeal disease. The aptness of this hypothesis may be confirmed by bacteriological studies.

This investigation of an intestinal diarrhea outbreak was supported by the enthusiasm of patient relatives and enthusiastic college students volunteering to help out a physician single handedly managing an epidemic in a remote village. This illustrates the power of community participation in health care and when done over the web documentation and sharing of such a multiple stakeholder partnership at a local village level is likely to instigate much needed global participation even toward managing a remote rural epidemic.

The Irritable Bowel: When the Journey is A Stop and Go Affair

The above was an experience in documenting an epidemic of acute diarrhea and what a primary care physician is more likely to see throughout his/her life is an interesting sequel that is being recognized increasingly. Results of injury to the intestinal neurons include an immediate acceleration of transit (Gwee 1995) and development of rectal hypersensitivity. Small intestinal permeability is also increased in virtually all individuals, however in those who develop post infectious irritable bowel, this abnormality persists for years (Spiller 2000).

Here is a description and discussion of a patient of irritable bowel by author RB in a recently published novel (Biswas 2009):

He was a very meticulous man and was by profession an anthropologist-teacher. His abdomen at that point of time while I was in school oblivious of my future medical career was gradually putting on a paunch. It was not however his paunch that bothered him, it was gas. However it was not the coming out of gas that seemed to bother him. It was the not coming out part that was most worrisome.

He used to feel miserable about his intermittent abdominal bloating, producing a diffuse pain. Very often he would express his anguish by percussing various parts of his abdomen, even while moving around with his daily activities until it became a habit. He even developed a philosophy of happiness which stated that all cause of human misery lay in the abdomen. If only abdominal organs functioned well, everything would be perfectly alright in this world. Surprisingly he grew out of it although it took him years and I no longer find him percussing his own abdomen.

I went on to meet similar people in my human trouble shooting career. At first I used to attribute them to protozoan infestations like Giardia or Entamoeba so very endemic in our part of the world but gradually realized that most often no cause could be detected. There were so many criteria to identify the irritable bowel and most of these problem patients would satisfy quite a few. The treatment was however dismal as the cause wasn't clear. It was a disturbance of bowel movement alright but then why should the bowel move so mischievously at times? A typical scenario was the bowel moving in alternate contraction and relaxations and suddenly at one point of time stopping randomly followed by distension of that halted segment until the human carrying the bowel winced in pain.

Mercifully it would pass off after some time, the distended colonic gas coming out silently or otherwise and you'd find a relieved expression on his face. Another way it would present was an urge to defecate at times especially when the subject was engaged in some kind of work, tedious and boring but important nevertheless. However what would come out could hardly be called fecal matter rather than that which was normally present on the surface of the colonic mucus membrane, 'mucus.' Each time one passed stools one felt there was more to pass, a sensation termed tenesmus that was possibly due to colonic spasm. Eighty of hundred patients in my outpatient clinic with abdominal pain going on for a very long time could be classified into this pattern.

It was not just the lower bowel whose movement was at fault but even the upper bowel along with the stomach would refuse to budge at times. This produced an upper abdominal epigastric discomfort frequently labeled dyspepsia. June would put in flexible telescopes with lighted lens into these mischievous bowels either from above or below to look for anything that could be treated but no it was something to do with the electrical wiring of their slow moving pipes that wouldn't

move because of frequent current failures. There was no way she could have their wiring replaced.

PROCTODEUM:

A Painful Ending: When The Last Station Breaks Down

The nature of anal sinus and anal intramuscular glands is well known, but their origin is still discussed. In the past years a surprising new theory about the invagination of the proctodeum into the hindgut was put forward. Anal intramuscular glands should be the anatomic correlate of anal fistulas.(Klosterhalfen 1991)

An anal fistula is an inflammatory tract between the anal canal and skin. Most anal fistulas originate in anal crypts, which become infected with abscess formation. When the abscess is opened or ruptures, a fistula is formed. (Legall 2009)

Consider this next series of email communications with a patient:

Dear R,
Should I bug you about a suspected fistula problem I am having for about a month? I have looked at all the info I can get from the net, but still.....
L.

Ok, here is the story.

I had a small lump that appeared a little more than a month ago. I thought it was just another casual thing that happens once in a year or so and goes away a day or two later. But this thing grew and one day I had a fever. I went to our doctor, first day he gave metrogyl, combiflam and gaspaz and asked me to come back a day later. Second day, he continued with antibiotics (I think it was Levoflaxin) and supporting pills (including some painkillers like paracetamol). I was a little concerned that he was not doing any thorough examination and giving me all these pills. He also asked me to sit on hot water sometimes.

Anyway, the lump burst, some discharge (pus) came out and a week later the lump subsided- there was occasional itch. I did not go back to the doc. But the lump did not die down. Also, I was surprised at the diagnosis that it is a fistula because though it was close to the anus, it was not quite on it, it was a bit away from it. Then about a week ago, I started feeling uncomfortable that It had not gone away. A friend here advised that I take Sporidex (cephalexin)and use fusidine ointment. So I have been taking Sporidex 375 mg twice a day and using fusidine, but not much change.

Any suggestions? In the mean time I think the lump (now small) burst again and there is more discharge and I also feel a little pain.

Perhaps with age, I am just getting more worried about all this.

Actually there is a real worry that if things get worse, it will effect my work.

L.

Hi L,

I am surprised the doctor didn't examine you!

It does sound like an ischiorectal abscess to me now with a possible fistula festering. You need to be examined proper.

I guess you need to show a surgeon (although I don't think you will need to go under the knife in case that puts you off).

Do let me know what happens.

R

Thank you so much R.

I am in a difficult situation - I cannot afford to spend a lot of money, so I do not want to go to Apollo hospital.

It is difficult to explain to someone why as a IIIT professor, I whine about money. Unfortunately, our campus physician is not able to help me. How do you get in touch with Dr L S, any phone number or email address?

I will try to look up myself.

I am planning to inquire about the Ayurved person who comes to campus.

We have two allopathy practitioners, one ayurved and one homeopathy

practioners appointed for part time visit.

L.

The name L S is familiar. Does she sing classical western vocal (like in operas)? I may have heard her once.

L.

Dear L,

I am sure she's not a classical vocalist.

I suddenly realized I have other contacts in Hyderabad. There is a medical college there where I know a few people and I shall send you a mobile number in the next email that should be able to provide you with a good surgeon's number.

Everyone will be suitably impressed by your IIIT background so you needn't worry.

But if I were you I would get myself examined for the abscess.

Warmest regards

Dear R,

I met the Ayurveda doctor in our campus. She has given me some medicines; Let me try these for a few days. The good thing is that she seemed to understand the problem immediately and she has allowed me to continue with the antibiotic if I want to. She said that I do not need surgery if this can be treated well.

Thank you for the number of Dr Reddy. I will get in touch with him soon some time. A major problem is that I am located at an end of the city from where all major medical centers are at least half an hour's drive away.

L.

Dear R,

I have finally called the contact you gave. If it is not much bother for you, it will really be helpful if you can tell him that I cannot afford high rates.

He said he is not a doctor himself but he works in an organization where doctors work.

He also said that he will look into where I can get better treatment.

I have kept the problem under control, but it has not disappeared. The discomfort is less; in fact other than a nagging worry, I do not have much.

I have been taking the Ayurvedic medicine, and washing the boil with sterilized cotton regularly. So it is under control, but has not disappeared. Both the allopathic and ayurvedic doctors say it is a fistula, but no examination other than naked eye from a distance has been used for this inference.

L

I went to a surgeon finally. The surgeon did a rectal examination. He says that there is no emergency but there is no alternative to surgery. The problem is he says it will take 6-8 weeks to heal. I am attaching his diagnosis.

L.

Good to hear that.

However you seem to have forgotten the attachment.

Attachment fixed now. I am in a fix.

I definitely do not want surgery, but I guess I do not have much of a choice.

The surgeon said it will take 6-8 weeks for recovery - this has shaken me. I am alone and I do not want to depend on people.

The doctors at Hyderabad Nursing Home were nice, but there was only room with (luckily)

an Indian style toilet that was also meant to be a urinal, all this makes me suspicious of quality of hygiene in their OT.

My institute has a contract with a nearby nursing home called Pr Hospital that I do not like. But it may be cheaper for me especially because I do not have any insurance coverage. And the Ayurvedic doctor said I should give them another 10 days.

Incidentally, is this problem a common problem- I mean do a lot of people have fistula or its only a few like me?

L.

Another email later from RB on Jun 17th 2009

Interestingly I have had a patient today who has come all the way from Coochbihar, West Bengal to get her fistula in ano operated. Her father knew me as a physician in Bangalore and they had managed to keep in touch even through my Malaysia days and now I finally got to see them here in Bhopal again.

What have you decided on the fistula now?

As for the commonality of the condition there is an interesting discussion between three patients who have had a fistulectomy at this site: http://www.healthboards.com/boards/showthread.php?t=331865&highlight t=fistula+in+ano

Do let me know how it goes.

Dear R,

I am in no condition to go for surgery.

I have been worried about it and quite frustrated with the situation.

I have kept it under control. I find the lump irritable after walking in the sun or after long drives.

Otherwise it is rather dormant. May be the Ayurvedic medicine is working. There has not been any discharge for quite some time (if it has been, I have not noticed it). I am told by some people they had a complete recovery using a homeopathic medicine. I know that there is no scientific basis for homeopathy but something goes inside and God knows if it is all placebo or whatever, and I am considering seriously to try it out for a few months. Let me see what the Ayurvedic medicine does for some time.

Incidentally, there is a possibility that I may go to US for a two day meeting in July. Is it right to worry about the possibility of fistula flaring up after long sitting in airplanes?

My problem with surgery is manifold. As you know, I have had stomach problems ever since early childhood. What if I have a similar problem after a few years? Will there be another surgery? How much can you keep chopping?

Right now, four weeks complete rest is impossible. Thanks for keeping me in mind.

L

Hi L,

At the moment even my patient who had come here to get operated for her fistula in ano all the way from Bengal has deferred her operation especially after I related the scary post op stories on the site that I had also sent you a link to (perhaps it was difficult for you to follow that site and their unreliable patient diatribes laced with country slang I guess was a put off...). However their stories although scary do have a happy ending in general albeit most of them seem to have required more than one surgery.

Yes I guess you could hang on with it as long as it is dormant and doesn't release its train of pus or blood too often.

Dear R,

I know you have been a kind friend and have put up with rather unfriendly brief replies from me. I did look at the link you sent and it did add to my depression and I agree that they kind of implied if not happy an ok ending. I am also assured that you have asked me

to hang on. In a way it is good to have it because it has compelled to me to stop drinking completely and even reduce caffeine intake. I actually feel much healthier. The Ayurvedic medicine seems to be more like a purgative with healthy stool formation. It may be inhibiting growth of bacteria and that may be one way of keeping the monster under control. I am relatively much more confident now as compared to how I felt a month ago. I have stopped using sterilized cotton wash that I was doing 2-3 times a day. All I do is use oil and take the herbal medicine.

Anyway, it is a good experience dealing with this crisis though I feel it is unfair how I seem to keep moving from one to another crisis all the time.

Thanks again,

L

Last email on the progress of the problem:

The lump has now reduced in size. The discomfort level is insignificant. But I am not yet confident that it will not flare up again.

Today someone helped me by typing and I completed the first draft of a short story.

I am going to work on it and send it for publication.

L.

CONCLUSION

As these email narrative journeys through the gastrointestinal tract illustrate, many complaints have diffuse etiologies, are difficult to explain, and result in troublesome experiences for their sufferers. Gastrointestinal problems as experienced by physician-trouble-shooters have been discussed above along with illustrations of how the discussion could be developed over a web interface through a user driven email narrative. Along with this other instances of multiple stake holder narratives relating problems cropping throughout the gastrointestinal tract in epidemics and remaining as endemic problems have been discussed. This re-affirmation of medicine as more than scientific knowledge and technical skill is part of the contemporary move towards more training in medical humanities. If this inspires further reading into gastrointestinal problem solving we shall consider having achieved our goal.

REFERENCES

Biswas, R., (2001, January). Irritable Bowel syndrome in the tropics: a possible culprit. *Journal of Indian academy of clinical medicine (letter)*, 2(1-2).

Biswas, R. (2009). *The Conscious Notebook*. New York: Nova Science Publishers.

Biswas, R., & Dalal, M. (2003, May). A yoga teacher with persistent cheilitis. *Intl Jl Clin Pract (UK)*, 57(4), 340–342.

Biswas, R., Paul, A., & Shetty, K. J. (2002, November). A yoga teacher with persistent reflux symptoms. *Intl Jl Clin Pract (UK)*, 56, 9.

Burton, J. L. (1993). The Lips. In: Rook, Wilkinson, Ebling (eds), *Textbook of dermatology*. Oxford, UK: Blackwell Scientific publications.

Carson, C. F. (2001, August). Riley TV. Safety, efficacy and provenance of tea tree (Melaleuca alternifolia) oil. *Contact Dermatitis*, 45(2), 65–67. doi:10.1034/j.1600-0536.2001.045002065.x

Ely, J. W., & Osheroff, J. A. (2002). Obstacles to answering doctors' questions about patient care with evidence: qualitative study. *BMJ (Clinical Research Ed.)*, 324, 710. doi:10.1136/bmj.324.7339.710

Fritz, T. M., Burg, G., & Krasovec, M. (2001). Allergic contact dermatitis to cosmetics containing Melaleuca alternifolia (tea tree oil)]. *Annales de Dermatologie et de Venereologie*, 128(2), 123–126.

Gwee, K. A., Leong, Y. L., Graham, C., McKendrick, M. W., Collins, S. M., & Walters, S. J.The role of psychological and biological factors in postinfective gutdysfunction. *Gut*, 44(3), 400–406. doi:10.1136/gut.44.3.400

Hoge, C. W., Shlim, D. R., & Rajah, R. (1993). Epidemiology of diarrhoel illness associated with coccidian like organism among travellers and foreign residents in Nepal. *Lancet*, 341, 1175. doi:10.1016/0140-6736(93)91002-4

Klosterhalfen, B., Offner, F., Vogel, P., & Kirckpatrick, C. J. (1991). Anatomic nature and surgical significance of anal sinus and anal intramuscular glands. Retreieved from http://www.springerlink.com/content/t4rv02umj00h6q77

Legall, I. (2009). *Anal Fistulas and Fissures E medicine*. Retrieved Oct 25, 2009, from http://emedicine.medscape.com/article/776150-overview

Neas, J. F. (2003). Digestive System Development in Embryology Atlas. Upper Saddle River, NJ: Pearson Education Inc Nhieu, J. T., Nin, F., Fleury-Feith, J., Chaumette, M. T., Schaeffer, A., & Bretagne, S. Identification of intracellular stages of Cyclospora species by light microscopy of thick sections using hematoxylin. *Human Pathology*, (10): 1107–1109.

Nicholas, B., & Gillett, G. (1997). Doctors' stories, patients' stories: a narrative approach to teaching medical ethics. *Journal of Medical Ethics*, 23(5), 295–299. doi:10.1136/jme.23.5.295

Parkman, H. P., & Cohen, S. (1995). Heartburn, regurgitation, odynophagia, chest pain and dysphagia. In Haubrich, W. S., Schaffner, F., & Berk, J. E. (Eds.), *Bockus Gastroenterology* (5th ed., pp. 30–40). Philadelphia: WB Saunders company.

Spiller, R. C., Jenkins, D., Thornley, J. P., Hebden, J. M., Wright, T., & Skinner, M. (2000). Increased rectal mucosal enteroendocrine cells, T lymphocytes, and increased gut permeability following acute Campylobacter enteritis and in post-dysenteric irritable bowel syndrome. *Gut, 47*(6), 804–811. doi:10.1136/gut.47.6.804

Swami, S. S. (1981). Hathayoga (Kunjal kriya). In Swami, S. S. (Ed.), *A systematic course in the ancient tantric techniques of Yoga and Kriya, Bihar school of Yoga* (pp. 205–214).

Teatree Oil. (n.d.). *Teatree Oil Information*. Retrieved April 2002, from http://www.teatree.co.uk/cuttings.html.

Chapter 4

Physician and Patient Perspectives:
Autistic Spectrum Disorders

Paul Bradley
Hertfordshire Partnership NHS Foundation Trust, UK

Peter Griffin
Teacher in Further Education, UK

Ann Griffin
Caregiver and Mother, UK

Kamalika Mukherj
Hertfordshire Partnership NHS Foundation Trust, UK

ABSTRACT

This chapter presents the narratives of some people with autistic spectrum disorders (also known as autism spectrum conditions) as well as those of their families and carers. It describes the history and development of the diagnostic concept of autistic spectrum disorders and how the clinical features impact on daily life and their families. It examines the different stages through which people progress, based on their contact with services – before diagnosis, at the time of diagnosis and their life since then. The chapter concludes with a personal account of all these stages.

INTRODUCTION

Autism is a disorder which profoundly effects how people communicate. Although it is often associated with intellectual disability and occasionally occurs as a part of other clinical syndromes, features often exist in people with average or above average intelligence. It is important that health professionals are able to recognise and understand this group, regardless of their discipline, in order to provide high quality care. Recent estimates put the prevalence as high as 1% amongst children and young people; this is explored further later in the chapter.

In recent years there has been more widespread awareness of the characteristic features leading to more appropriate support being offered. In the

DOI: 10.4018/978-1-60960-097-6.ch004

past some people would have been mistreated by services believing they had a mental illness like schizophrenia. Many people would have passed undetected, forming their own coping strategies seeming to society eccentric or unusual. Whilst the diagnoses are made on the basis of deficits in some areas, there are also strengths and abilities which people are able to build on.

In this chapter we will present the narratives of some people with autistic spectrum disorders (also known as autism spectrum conditions) as well as those of their families and carers. We will see how some of the clinical features impact on people's lives and include their advice on how health professionals could support them. We will look at the different stages through which people progress, based on their contact with services – before diagnosis, at the time of diagnosis and then their life since then.

PERSONAL EXPERIENCES OF AUTISM

The autistic spectrum disorders (ASDs) are classified as pervasive developmental disorders. These are conditions with an onset in early childhood and are profoundly linked to the person's experience of life in every respect. The classical features of impairments in social communication, interaction and imagination often mark children out as different to others. For children, different is quickly termed strange, weird or odd. These children then can be subject to social exclusion, compounding the difficulties they may experience.

The clinical features of autism and related disorders are well documented, but there is no substitute for the perspective of people with these disorders and their families. There are now several novels and autobiographies written about and by people with ASDs, e.g. The Curious Incident of the Dog in the Night-Time by Mark Haddon and Reflections: Me and Planet Weirdo by P. Hughes.

Another book, Autism and the Myth of the Person Alone by Douglas Biklen, features heavily the words of people with ASDs.

A qualitative study of life with high-functioning autism (Hurlbutt and Chalmers, 2002) featured the experiences of three individuals as told to researchers over the course of nine months through interviews and written material. Data was analysed by coding 150 main ideas into 29 clusters then collapsing these down to seven categories. Core themes emerged which were equally supported throughout the study. The participants wished to be "considered experts in the field of autism and to be consulted on issues related to autism. They are proud to have autism".

Other research has focussed on particular stages of life. Parenting a child with an ASD has come under great scrutiny. A grounded theory study (Lasser and Corley, 2008) involved 20 parents of children with Asperger's Disorder in the USA. They reported the phenomenon of "constructing normalcy" emerged as important for many parents. In other words, this is the struggle to establish a shared understanding of what is normal for their children. They also review some of the literature around particular challenges in parenting a child with an ASD:

- Diagnostic process
  - Waiting, loss of "idealised" child, relief
- Parental perceptions of uneven development
  - Advancement followed by loss of skills leading to confusion
- Channelling the child's strengths
  - Importance of identifying them and building upon them
- Ambiguity of future outcomes
  - Difficulty knowing how much support a child will need in the future

THE EVOLUTION OF THE TERM AUTISTIC SPECTRUM DISORDER

The term "autism" was coined by Eugen Bleuler (1857-1939), a Swiss psychiatrist, in the first definition of schizophrenia. This word was explained as a narcissistic self-interest; in other words, the tendency to be pre-occupied by oneself with a disregard for others. It is worth noting that although the term was used descriptively for people with schizophrenia, autistic spectrum disorders share little else with that diagnosis.

In 1944, Hans Asperger published a case series of children in whom he identified a recurring pattern of behaviours and abilities he described as autistic psychopathy. This research was published obscurely in a German journal, remaining largely unheard of until the 1980s.

The term psychopath has gained a variety of lay and medical meanings, but essentially means little more than a disorder of the mind. These children tended to be less aware of the feelings of others and acted without regard for them. This is more formally described as a lack of empathy. This could include aggression, especially when their needs and wishes were not recognised or addressed. They also had intense absorption in their areas of special interest, could not form relationships easily and held one sided conversations.

The first modern definition of autism as it is now known was published by Leo Kanner. This has come to be known as classical, infantile, childhood or Kanner's autism. He placed a greater emphasis on the social impairments, i.e. the deficits, than on the disturbed behaviour, i.e. the consequence. This was an important step towards the understanding of these conditions and the recognition that it could be managed positively.

However, given the origins of the term, it is not hard to see how misinterpretations were made through many years of the twentieth century. Prior to the widespread use of antipsychotic medication and the trend for social inclusion, people with schizophrenia were considered to have a poor prognosis and were largely confined to institutions away from the general population. Psychopath became a term synonymous with murderer; an association which people with autism did not benefit from.

In the mid- 20th century the prevailing view of autism was derived from psychoanalytic thinking, viewing it as a form of psychotic defence. Some early studies found a link between a more distant style of parenting and autistic features. This was dubbed the "refrigerator mother" theory and may have been the most damaging development for all involved. Parents were made to feel guilty and responsible for the natural history of the condition due to premature assumptions about cause and effect.

In 1981, Lorna Wing, then a researcher at the Institute of Psychiatry in London published an important paper, coining the term Asperger's Syndrome (AS), having come across Hans Asperger's previous case descriptions. Wing and Gould also published an important paper about the epidemiology of autism. They found that in a London borough as many as 15 /10,000 children had the impairments of social interaction, communication and imagination (which they referred to as the 'triad' of impairments), together with a repetitive stereotyped pattern of activities. Although these children did not fit into the full picture of early childhood autism (or typical autism) as described by Kanner they were identified as being within a broader autism spectrum.

By the end of the 20th century a view of classical autism, Asperger's syndrome, atypical autism and high functioning autism as parts of a spectrum had formed; the autistic spectrum disorders.

The awareness of autistic spectrum disorders, their early recognition and diagnosis is on the increase. A review of the literature on autism prevalence (Fombonne, 2003) suggested a figure between 30 and 60 / 10,000 of the population meet diagnostic criteria.

A survey by the Office of National Statistics of the mental health of children and young people in Great Britain carried out in 2004 found a prevalence of 0.9% for autism spectrum disorders. (Green et al, 2005).

In 2006 Baird and her colleagues published a report of a prevalence study (SNAP) which surveyed a population of children aged 9-10 years in the South Thames region in the U.K. The results showed a prevalence of 38.9 in 10,000 for childhood autism, and 77.2 in 10,000 for other autism spectrum disorders, giving an overall figure of 116 in 10,000 for all autism spectrum disorders. The authors concluded that services in health, education, and social care needed to recognise the needs of children with some form of ASD, who constitute 1% of the child population.

LIFE BEFORE DIAGNOSIS

Children with autistic spectrum disorders can have a wide range of abilities and deficits. Those who present early with a clear developmental delay, especially with a delay in language or behavioural disorders, are likely to be diagnosed early, but increasing numbers of adults are identifying autistic features in themselves. Here we present an example of life before diagnosis from the co-author of the chapter Peter, whose story we will hear in full later.

"I knew that I was different as I was constantly going for tests for different things so I was aware that other people thought there were issues When I first went to university I didn't have my diagnosis and it was my first time living away from home. I enjoyed myself, living with no responsibilities. If I didn't want to go to lectures I didn't. This university didn't understand my specific needs and support was not structured and only concentrated on the academic side rather than the social side."
- Peter Griffin

Peter recognised that there was a significant difference between others and himself. He was able to identify his academic strengths but also recognised his difficulties in relating to people. This kind of insight is the first step in developing ways to cope with the demands of life as part of a society.

Social interaction is a skill most people can take for granted, at least at a basic level. The ability to recognise a facial expression or tone of voice allows far more information to be conveyed than through words alone. One of the challenging aspects for a young person with autism is trying to learn these nuances consciously and for those around them to be aware that subtleties of communication may not be effective.

Put in a situation where people seem to be speaking a different language and are unwilling or unable to interact with you, it is understandable that people sometimes choose an imaginary world. However, this is often misinterpreted as evidence that people with autism do not wish to socialise. It is becoming clearer that, at least until such patterns are ingrained, many people appreciate the presence and thoughtful interaction of others although they may find it very hard to express.

"I don't need friends but do enjoy being with people I like. I like it when people are forthright with me, when they tell me that I am being inappropriate or talk too much it helps me to learn the right social etiquette"
- Peter Griffin

This demonstrates the difficulties in social communication that many people with autistic spectrum disorders experience. Language delay is the main discriminating factor between Asperger Syndrome (when it is absent) and high-functioning autism (when it is present). Even when verbal expression does develop there can be a stilted quality to its use, perhaps because of how it is learnt differently. Understanding of metaphors and figures of speech, such as "raining cats and dogs" or "bull in a china shop" can present a particular difficulty when interpreted literally.

There is sometimes a marked difference between the abilities of a person to communicate their needs and the lack of ability to engage in a two-way process of communication. This reciprocity is what gives communication the potential for a social function; we do not simply tell each other what we need but we talk for the sake of talking. For those who understand the unwritten rules of conversation this can be a great pleasure, but it can seem very daunting if the rules are not easily acquired.

COMMUNICATION OF DIAGNOSIS

There are complexities in how a diagnosis is reached and challenges maybe encountered in how this communicated. The contrast between different people's lived experience of these events can inform us how important it is to consider each person individually. It will not be possible to say "all people with autism should be told about it in this way."

It is important to be aware of the stigma of mental health diagnoses and they should never be used pejoratively or without regard for confidentiality. However, this should not be an obstacle to discussing them with the patient or their immediate carers since it can be a relief for people to understand themselves and to be understood.

Some people on the autistic spectrum are able to identify features in their own personality and behaviour that they recognise as different. The educated patient can sometimes be a challenge to the "authority" of a doctor or other health professional. The current trend is firmly away from paternalism, where a patient is told what the doctor believes they should hear, towards a collaborative approach. The patient and doctor are on an even footing and work together to advance their shared knowledge. Each person is an individual, so once again it is true to say that no single approach will suit everyone. The clinical features, their impact on behaviour and the environment will emphasise one aspect over another in every case.

LIVING WITH A DIAGNOSIS

There are now a wide range of organisations in the state, voluntary and private sector that provide support to people with autistic spectrum disorders. This can range from information about the diagnoses to full time residential care, depending on the needs and wishes of those involved. In this section we will discuss the experiences of people who are receiving services and those who through choice or lack of local provision are not.

For some people their autism is associated with intellectual disability. The more severe the disability the greater the level of support they are likely to require. Historically, these are the people who would have been managed in secure wards in long-stay institutions, poorly understood and poorly treated. Many of the challenging behaviours encountered in the care of people with severe intellectual disability are related to autistic traits. Once recognised, life with the diagnosis of autism can be vastly improved with a reduction in self-injurious behaviour and aggression which permits a lower level of security and more social integration.

There is much variation in support that people can receive and also how much they can benefit with the right opportunities. Although Asperger Syndrome is defined by the absence of a delay in language, there may be difficulties with its use in some cases. Visual communication tools can be highly effective in supporting people across the autistic spectrum. Visual timetables allow people to understand sequences of events. These can be created using diagrams or photographs of the person doing an activity for those who think in a more concrete way and may find it difficult to equate a diagram with themselves.

Communication passports are developed with the support of speech and language therapists and feature a thorough study of the effective ways to communicate with people. These are useful for a range of people, but especially for those on the autistic spectrum. Another common tool is the object of reference where a particular item is associated with an activity. For example, being shown a pair of walking shoes may indicate that the person will go out for walk.

PETER'S STORY

Peter is a 29 year old man with Asperger syndrome. He was diagnosed in 1999 at the age of 19 years. He gained a Masters Degree in Astrophysics at the University of Hertfordshire. He is currently working five days a week as a teaching assistant in a college of further education, supporting students with autism, learning disabilities and physical disabilities. He will undertake his teacher training from September 2010. He lives in the family home with his parents and younger brother who also has Asperger syndrome. This is his story, illustrating vividly many of the points made earlier in the chapter.

When I first went to university I enjoyed myself, living away from home with no responsibilities. If I didn't want to go to lectures I didn't. I didn't have a diagnosis and the university didn't understand my specific needs; support was not structured and only concentrated on the academic side rather than the social side. I knew that I was different as I was constantly going for tests for different things so I was aware that other people thought there were issues.

Diagnosis changed my perspective on life; I have changed quite a bit since then and have a better insight. With AS you don't always know something is wrong but other people see you differently. I have a very poor memory of what I was like. Diagnosis has made my life easier but I can't define in what way as I have no recollection of what I was like before. Diagnosis has led me to a

better insight but it is very subtle in the way it has changed me but the problems I had I still have.

Since diagnosis I have achieved a Masters Degree in Astrophysics once I had some focussed and structured support. The difference at the University of Hertfordshire was that I felt supported on the social side by university staff and of course, I had that support from my family. This combination worked well for me.

Without the right kind of support from the disability unit at the University of Hertfordshire I would not have achieved my degree. I don't want people to do things for me; I want people to work with me as that will help me to improve. My mentor at university gave me support but challenged me to do things for myself. I recognise that I will always need someone with me as I don't always see things as a problem and others will. I can't always see solutions to problems.

I left university in 2005 and wasn't sure what I wanted to do. It took me a while to realise that I would have liked to do a PhD but by this time it was too late. I went through a difficult time then; I had no job and did not know what I wanted to do. I play on computers because I enjoy doing this and there was nothing else I wanted to do. There was no service there to support me to find out what I could do.

I was still learning about myself, still trying to build up my understanding of myself and work out who I was in the world. All the things I have experienced have increased my knowledge of myself.

I worked at a big supermarket for many years, just one day a week. I didn't enjoy working; there were many things that made it difficult for me. The difference at university was that my mentors learnt about AS, they were friendly faces that I could go to and they had a built up a relationship that meant I could trust them and that was really important.

Now, I have good support at work which means I don't stagnate. I need to be challenged to do things I wouldn't normally do. I try very hard not to say no but will explain that I am not sure about something. Before, I would have just said no. I will try things, especially things that won't commit me to something.

The National Autistic Society has helped by getting me involved in things they are doing. It has made me think about my disability, teaching it means you can understand it more. I have had support from my social worker and psychiatrist; sometimes just knowing that someone cares helps.

I don't need friends but do enjoy being with people I like. I like it when people are forthright with me, when they tell me that I am being inappropriate or talk too much it helps me to learn the right social etiquette.

I would always have wanted and valued the diagnosis. It has had a significant impact on my life. My family accepted me anyway; just saw me as a bit eccentric.

THE IMPACT OF DIAGNOSIS ON PEOPLE ON THE AUTISM SPECTRUM

Peter asked some of his peers to comments on aspects of their experience of diagnosis and support with their autistic spectrum disorders. Two responded, giving detailed information about themselves which is presented below. Their names have been changed to maintain their anonymity.

Martin, an 18 year old male diagnosed with High Functioning Autism at age of six felt he was different to other people in the way he thought and spoke. He felt a huge relief at knowing why he was different to others. In his words "didn't feel like such a freak or outcast" when he was told of his diagnosis when he was a little older and able to understand.

Russell, a 26 year old male said that before diagnosis he used to say or do things that he regretted afterwards and wished people could delete those things from their memories. He felt that these things made him different and he wanted

people to like him and not bully him. He found it very frustrating. He was diagnosed with Asperger syndrome and OCD at 13 years of age. He felt angry when he was given his diagnosis and wanted to know who gave it to him. He didn't want and still doesn't want to be different. It has taken him a long time to understand his AS. He still does things that he regrets but with the knowledge of his AS he tries harder to fit in.

Both young men were asked if the diagnosis changed them for better or worse. Russell said for better but very slowly. Martin felt that it helped him for the better; that it gave him a clearer understanding of himself when he knew what social and mental weaknesses and gifts he had due to his condition. Neither would have preferred not to have a diagnosis. Russell felt angry to be told he was different.

Often it is thought that a diagnosis will bring services and support. Martin said he had a lot of support from teachers, psychiatrists and psychologists as well as books and other media sources. He feels this has helped him to develop and evolve as a person. Russell said that the support he received at school made him different and brought attention to him which he did not like. He has learnt that he needs help with the flat he is living in and with getting a job but not much has happened over the last two and a half years, in fact, if anything things have got worse.

The two young men were also asked if the diagnosis meant that people understood them and their needs better. Martin said that those who knew of his diagnosis did. He said "a lot of the time, people understanding you is the ability to communicate clearly how you feel and what you're thinking". Russell said "People only understand me if they understand AS. They are finding out stuff as they go along. It's frustrating." His answer reflects the views of many young people on the autism spectrum that they are often the people trying to teach those people who are providing services to them.

They were asked what positive experience in terms of diagnosis or support they had experienced. Martin was clear that it was that people (parents) cared and never gave up. Russell said that he hadn't had a positive experience outside of his family. They recognised his AS and asked for a diagnosis and found out information to help him and them.

Both also had negative experiences. Martin said the negative experiences could have been avoided by having some clear thinking strategies of how to get around certain situations. A better understanding of certain difficult situations could have been outlined more often to ASD pupils. Russell feels that you shouldn't have to ask for a diagnosis, it should be a right. People who provide adult support need to be trained to understand AS and "what it's like to be me".

Martin is still living in the family home and about to start at University on a music programme. Russell has not worked for five years and is living on his own in a flat heavily supported by his mother and sister.

MANY PERSPECTIVES BROUGHT TOGETHER

Ann, Peter's mother, summarises the perspectives of these three young men and adds her own experience:

This is not a large sample, however, from these stories and from people who contact a local support group helpline it is clear that diagnosis is extremely important. There is a belief that with diagnosis come services, support and understanding. What is clear is that most of the support comes from family carers who struggle to balance the needs of other children with working to ensure the financial stability of the family. It is often the family carers and the person with ASD who end up teaching those who are supposed to be offering services. Peter's youngest brother is also on the spectrum and when we received his diagnosis we were told to go away and find out a bit more about autism. This at a time when we were reeling from the diagnosis and feeling bereaved, our aspirations for our son had changed in that second that the diagnosis was made. This is not an uncommon experience for families. If I could change anything it would be that a diagnosis is followed up with information about what ASD means, how it impacts on lives but also about the positive nature of ASD. Given the right support early people with autism can offer a unique insight into life, they have a lot to offer us but if we get it wrong in terms of understanding them and the services they are offered we can cause them a lot of harm that can be irretrievable for them and their families.

CONCLUSION

Through this chapter we have heard the experiences of many people with an autistic spectrum disorder. Through our personal and professional lives we are all likely to meet people on this spectrum and it is rewarding to be able to gain an understanding of their perspective. We have focussed on three main areas orientated around diagnosis – before, during and after. The wide range of strengths and impairments means that despite the known features of the disorders, each person must be seen as an individual.

LEARNING POINTS

- Autistic spectrum disorders affect social communication, interaction and imagination
- People with these conditions may not be known to psychiatric services, nor be in need of them
- Awareness of their perspectives can allow all healthcare practitioners to support such people appropriately

REFERENCES

Attwood, T. (1998). *Asperger syndrome: a guide for parents and professionals*. London: Jessica Kingsley Publishers.

Autism Research Centre. (n.d.). *Autism Research Centre*. Retrieved from http://www.autismre-searchcentre.com/

Baird, G., Simonoff, E., & Pickles, A. (2006). Prevalence of disorders of the autism spectrum in a population cohort of children in South Thames: the Special Needs and Autism Project (SNAP). *Lancet, 368*, 210–215. doi:10.1016/S0140-6736(06)69041-7

Baron-Cohen, S. (2003). *The Essential Difference*. New York: Basic Books.

Baron-Cohen, S., Scott, F., Allison, C., Williams, J., Bolton, P., Matthews, F., & Brayne, C. (n.d.). Prevalence of autism-spectrum conditions: UK school-based population study. *British Journal of Psychiatry, 194*, 500-509.

Barron-Cohen, S. (2008). *Autism and Asperger Syndrome: the facts*. New York: Oxford University Press.

Biklen, D. (2005). *Autism and the Myth of the Person Alone*. New York: NYU Press.

Fombonne, E. (2003). Epidemiological Surveys of Autism and Other Pervasive Developmental Disorders: An Update. *Journal of Autism and Developmental Disorders, 33*(4). doi:10.1023/A:1025054610557

Gillberg, C. (1998). Asperger syndrome and High functioning autism, *BJPsych*

Gillberg, I., & Gillberg, C. (1989). Asperger Syndrome: Some Epidemiological Considerations. A Research Note. *Journal of Child Psychology and Psychiatry, and Allied Disciplines, 30*(4), 631–638. doi:10.1111/j.1469-7610.1989.tb00275.x

Glennon, T. (2001). The stress of the university experience for students with Asperger syndrome. Work: Journal of Prevention. *Assessment & Rehabilitation, 17*(3), 183–190.

Green, H., McGinnity, A., Meltzer, H., Ford, T., & Goodman, R. (2005). *Mental health of children and young people in Great Britain, A survey carried out by the Office for National Statistics on behalf of the Department of Health and the Scottish Executive*. London: Palgrave Macmillan.

Haddon, M. (2005). *The Curious Incident of the Dog in the Night-Time*. New York: Doubleday.

Hughes, P. (2008). *Reflections: Me and Planet Weirdo*. London: Chipmunkapublishing.

Hurlbutt, K., & Chalmers, L. (2002). Adults with Autism Speak Out: Perceptions of Their Life Experiences. *Focus on Autism and Other Developmental Disabilities, 17*(2), 103–111. doi:10.1177/10883576020170020501

Lasser, J., & Corley, K. (2008). Constructing normalcy: a qualitative study of parenting children with Asperger's Disorder. *Educational Psychology in Practice, 24*(4), 335–346. doi:10.1080/02667360802488773

National Autistic Society. (n.d.). *National Autistic Society*. Retrieved from http://www.nas.org.uk/

Wing, L., & Gould, J. (1979). Severe impairments of social interaction and associated abnormalities in children: epidemiology & classification. *Journal of Autism and Developmental Disorders, 9*(1), 11–29. doi:10.1007/BF01531288

Chapter 5
Critical Illness and the Emergency Room

R. K. Goyal
NY Presbyterian Hospital, USA

M. O'Neill
NY Presbyterian Hospital, USA

N. Agostinelli
NY Presbyterian Hospital, USA

P. Wyer
Columbia University, USA

ABSTRACT

The care of the critically-ill patient in the acute setting, an 'everyday' occurrence in most urban emergency departments, often proceeds through the dictates of Parsonian paternalism: the Physician knows best. But through a discussion of three such 'everyday' encounters, we hope to complicate this notion and find a place for healthcare users in the decision making process while developing a language and analytic basis for thinking seriously about the clinical dyad and the construction of knowledge in relationship economies. Finally, we discuss the escalation and de-escalation (terms derived from the military industrial complex) of care as it relates to medical futility.

INTRODUCTION

Unlike most medical problems that trade in years or decades, critical illnesses manifest themselves in the short span of hours or days. From a knife wound to the left chest cavity of a young man to an amniotic fluid embolus in a thirty-six week gravid expectant mother to a large hemorrhagic stroke in a hypertensive older woman returning home from her grandchild's first ballet recital, critical illness is not limited by demography, pathophysiology or organ system. While in clinical practice it is often apparent to even the most neophyte practitioner, critical illness avoids easy definition and like the fog at dawn escapes a unifying grip. Faced with critically ill patients, physicians unconsciously fall back on time-worn forms of 'evidence' like intuition, anecdote, animal and cell-based research, common sense and personal bias. While

DOI: 10.4018/978-1-60960-097-6.ch005

there is a burgeoning literature on critical illness and clinical evidence that is most developed in the ongoing research on sepsis and septic shock (Jones et al, 2008), many physicians taking care of critically ill patients perceive an impossibly wide chasm between everyday practice and the availability of results from clinical research (Marik, 2001). In addition to the lack of a clear definition, critical illness seems to resist clinical research in its perceived and real time constraints, as attested by concepts like the golden hour, for the lack of time is thought to be a barrier both to the production of new clinical knowledge and to the search for existing literature. Because of the critically ill patient's liminal position, often hovering at the limits of mortality, practitioners may grasp for and apply unproven or experimental treatment strategies. And finally, these very sick patients are thought to be voiceless, treated more appropriately as physiologic bodes than as still sentient human beings. Through this chapter, we hope to complicate these notions and find a possible place for evidence-based medicine, especially as recently re-theorized by the critical intervention of narrative medicine (Charon, 2006), in the critically ill clinical dyad and in the co-construction of knowledge.

From its inception, Evidence Based Medicine purported to be a clinical decision and practice model that unified three variously defined arenas of criteria for informing clinical decision-making. One iteration of these criteria specified: clinical expertise, research evidence and patient preferences and values (Haynes, Sackett, Gray, Cook, Guyatt, 1996). But of these three, EBM has focused almost exclusively on the second: the development of the positivist and empiricist methodologies that underlie clinical research evidence, especially as it pertains to highly sophisticated statistical analyses and tools, to the near neglect of the other two foundational pillars, doctors and patients (Silva & Wyer, 2009). Clinical expertise was assumed to encompass all of the experiences that constitute the formation of expert knowledge: an

education in the pathophysiologic basis of disease followed by a period of post-graduate training and the accumulation of experiential knowledge that could seamlessly be stitched into rich patterned tapestries. While patient values and preferences were seen as merely transparent—ask and ye shall receive. Neither the complexities of cognitive development nor the ontological vagaries of what it means to be a sick patient confronted by impossible choices received the theoretical and practical study needed to pursue the original mandate: the unification of clinical expertise, research evidence and patient preferences and values. A recent reworking of EBM, entitled narrative-evidence based medicine, attempts to correct some of these imbalances (Goyal et al, 2008). By treating the medical encounter as a truly iterative and relational event, at the same time as connecting care assessment and decisions to relevant clinical evidence, NEBM bridges the gap between the general and the particular, between the population and the patient and localizes knowledge production and the process of decision making squarely in the dyadic space co-created by the physician and the patient.

The care of the critically-ill patient in the acute setting, an 'everyday' occurrence in most urban emergency departments, often proceeds through the dictates of Parsonian paternalism: the Physician knows best (Parsons, 1951). In the 1950s, Talcott Parsons published the most extensive sociological analysis of the practice of medicine yet extant. For Parsons, the legitimation of the 'sick role' was predicated upon passivity: the understanding that the patient's sickness is not something that he or she is in control of, not something that he or she can will away, but rather something that incapacitates him and removes him from social obligation. For Parsons, within the social system, an obligation was placed on the sick patient to seek out and submit to medical care: "The obverse of the physician's obligation to be guided by the welfare of the patient is the latter's obligation 'to do his part' to the best of his ability" (Parsons,

1951, 438). In Parsons' model, the helplessness of passivity was coupled with a second negation, the lack of knowledge: "the patient has a need for technical services because he doesn't—nor do his lay associates, family members, etc.—'know' what is the matter or what to do about it, nor does he control the necessary facilities" (Parsons, 1951, 439). Not only is the patient unable institutionally to help him or herself because of the technical expansion of medicine, she does not even possess the rudimentary knowledge of what is wrong. The extremely influential Parsonian model has been critiqued by more patient or user-friendly models: patient-centeredness (May & Mead, 1999), shared-decision making (Charles, Gafni & Whelan, 1997), relationship centered care and the biopsychosocial model (Engel, 1977). But most of these counter-narratives are premised on the slow unfolding of chronic illness. Even as staunch an anti-Parsonian as the medical sociologist David Rier ("I'd often joke with my medical sociology students that much of the course could be called 'Talcott Parsons and Why he was Wrong'"), in his own moving self-portrait or auto-illness narrative suggests that Parsonian paternalism might in fact be appropriate in acute care settings: "[M]y illness provoked me to reassess the critique of Parsons I had been teaching only weeks before. For, despite my deep commitment to disclosure, negotiation and patient participation, the reactionary truth is that I was too sick to know certain details of my case, too weak to be a partner in decision making" (Rier, 2001, 73, 75). Rier describes a transfer of decision making that might not be categorized as simply paternalistic; when such a transfer reflects a mutuality of perception, preference and action, it may rather reflect a tacit acceptance of shared interests.

While the direct, volitional role of the patient may, of necessity, be limited in the acute care setting, for effective application of evidence based medicine that is in harmony with clinical expertise, research evidence and patient preferences and values, the patient must be revivified in the acute setting, not just as a body but as a speaking subject. In the following chapter, we hope to offer three case scenarios that may touch upon aspects of narrative and EBM in the critically ill patient. In the first case, we will look at the clinical and narrative evidence for inviting patients' families to watch cardiac resuscitations in the emergency room and interrogate what we want to call user trust in abstract systems and expert knowledge as it relates to Erving Goffman's distinction between the 'front stage' and 'backstage' performances that mark professionalism (Goffman, 1990). At stake here is the question of 'trust' in institutional practices and the nature of the information upon which that trust is based. In our second case, the usage of thrombolytics and prolonged CPR in cardiac arrest, we will attend to the discrepancies between high-stakes illnesses that demand 'heroic' measures and the lack of evidence for such treatments. How can we reconcile the individual needs of the critically ill dying patient in front of us with conflicting evidence derived from population-based studies? Finally, we will consider the escalation and de-escalation (terms derived from the military industrial complex) of care as it relates to end of life care.

CASE ONE

It began as a very busy day in the Emergency Department, and only became more so as the day progressed. There was an acute stroke in one room, a patient with a traumatic intracranial bleed going to the Surgical ICU in another, and it was midday, the busiest period in the ED, when the paramedics dropped our patient off. The triage nurse asked me to see the patient sooner than later, and so I entered the room reading the chart: the chief complaint was 'syncope' but her vital signs (heart rate, blood pressure, respiratory rate and temperature) were stable. I may have groaned (internally, if not audibly). In our Emergency Department, we must see this presentation at least fifty times per week, and, almost always, the patients leave the hospital without a clear understanding of the cause of their fainting spell.

Hour One: The patient was young by today's standards, 62, well-dressed, slightly overweight but with no obvious stigmata of chronic disease. She had only a small abrasion on her face from the fall, but the triage nurse was right, she did not look well. She was breathing both quickly and shallowly, and was moving around in the stretcher unable to get comfortable.

She could not or would not answer my questions, and I became increasingly more frustrated—I needed information, a complaint, an account of the day's events, some symptom to begin and direct my medical work up. Despite repeated efforts, I could not get the information I needed, and I became concerned that to spend more time in the room would compromise the care of my other patients (my acute stroke had converted into a bleed, and I needed to reassess that patient immediately). I quickly examined the patient, ordered an intravenous line and basic tests including blood work and EKG, and left to attend to my other patients.

Soon after leaving however, I was called back in by another of our nurses. The patient appeared to have become "toxic" which is a general way of stating that she seemed to be worsening. Her breathing was even more shallow and her mental status seemed to have deteriorated to the point of practical unresponsiveness. I proceeded to paralyze and intubate her. The intubation went well, and I let out a sigh of relief. In the ED, intubating a patient usually affords us a great degree of control over a disease process and also buys us time. I felt as though we had taken a step on the road to recovery.

Hour two: Almost immediately after the intubation, however, the patient's blood pressure dropped. I thought the hypotension might be due to a sedative, which was discontinued. We gave intravenous fluids, waited for the blood pressure (BP) to improve, but it did not. We repeated automatic BPs, did manual BPs, changed cuffs—her pressure remained low. None of it made sense, so I placed an arterial line: her pressure WAS dangerously low. This was not good.

I reassessed the patient. While reexamining her, I found a mass-like density in her abdomen—it seemed like it was new, though I knew the exam on an overweight patient who was intubated was very unreliable. We needed a CT scan—but we HAD to fix her blood pressure first.

Hour Three: I placed a central line to measure central venous pressures and to give vasoactive medications. I started the patient on dopamine. I felt quite confident that this would fix the problem. There was no response in her blood pressure. I increased the dopamine to maximum dose and added a second agent, norepinephrine. No response. I increased the rate of infusion of both vasoactive medications--two pressors at full dose, and still no response.

This was the point at which I started to realize how bad it might get in the next few hours...I had no idea of what to try next. And the patient was too young to die. I remember thinking this over and over. She was roughly the same age as my own mother, and with every turn my own mother's health kept flashing into my mind as it does here today.

One of the nurses's had put in a phone call to the patient's private physician who now arrived and gave us additional history which was disappointing (from a diagnostic perspective): She had been a perfectly healthy person with no prodrome of illness; she took care of herself, in fact, she had never really been ill. Later, we learned she had left her apartment merely to go shopping.

Around this time the patient's son and his wife arrived (I never found out who called them) and they looked completely lost, as if they had walked through the door of their house and somehow ended up in the hospital waiting room. I'm not sure they recognized her at first. Yesterday she was just "mom", mom whom they'd known for so long, decades, but today, intubated on a ventilator, with four intravenous pumps running, mostly unconscious, mostly naked, arms restrained, facial wounds untended, blood pooling on the floor, all with the wreckage of a resuscitation strewn throughout the room. They were dumbfounded; but then almost in unison, they started to ask what had happened. They wanted to know, they needed to know, exactly what had happened. We stepped out of the room together. We had no answers, I told them. The uncertainty only increased their distress.

Hour four: More fluids, more pressors, all with very little response. We called a surgical consult who saw the patient and agreed, we needed a CT scan; the Medical ICU became involved.

The two family members, very amicable, soft spoken, so understanding, were becoming increasingly concerned. They were remarkably polite and patient. I can see their faces. I engaged in a regular dance—kicking them out of the room for further examinations or procedures or for candid conversations of the case with consultants and with the patient's private physician followed by invitations back in to the room. Each time with the same refrain, "We just don't know what is wrong with her." I think they sensed we were growing increasingly hopeless but I don't think I ever told them that. I kept thinking to myself, "She's too young to die..." and, perhaps, also thinking "Mom's too young to die." Around this time, a second son arrived with a younger brother. They seemed better prepared to deal with her condition,

but fell speechless upon seeing her. We stepped out again. And again, I could give no answers.

Hour five: Fluids pouring in, pressors still at the highest doses, and with our patient still hypotensive, we mobilized the vent, the drips, the a-line and literally ran our unstable patient to the CT scan where we discovered a mass had grown into her renal vasculature and had caused massive internal bleeding into her abdomen.

Hour six: I placed a large gauge central catheter in the patient's groin and we activated our massive transfusion protocol. We grabbed our rapid infuser and began to infuse blood products as fast as we could—less than two minutes per unit. We mobilized the surgeons to prepare the Operating Room.

And then we did what now seems like a terrible thing. We told the patient's family that we were going to stabilize her and operate. They were so relieved that we finally had it figured out, and that we had a plan. A tumor. An operation. It was that simple and the mood was a little lifted. They were hopeful.

But just as the blood products improved her circulation, massive reperfusion injury began to occur. The patient's cardiac rhythm became abnormal, due presumably to ischemia and metabolic disarray.

Hour seven: Intermittently over the next hour, we performed Cardio Pulmonary Resuscitation (CPR) on the patient with multiple rounds of chest compressions and defibrillatory shocks. On the monitor, I could see her cardiac function deteriorating. But this time, we didn't kick her family out. They wanted to stay. Even as the CPR continued, many of us in the room seemed to know it would be over soon. When we finally stopped, we looked at each of the sons, and then pronounced her dead.

While I walked away from the bedside, I knew I hadn't walked away from the case. I spoke to the patient's personal physician a few weeks later and she stressed how important it was to the family members that they were present during the final part of the resuscitation; they felt like they were there with their mother, at the end, helping her, guiding her. They felt more connected with her passing.

Over the last few years, a growing movement in the ICU and Emergency department literature, called 'family member presence during resuscitation (FMPDR)' has begun to emerge and coalesce. Envisioned as an expansion of the healthcare model, practitioners, with the aid and direct input of family members and patients, have noticed the need to involve family in the actual practice of acute care. While EBM has recognized the importance of patient values and beliefs in decision-making, we are only now realizing that these values and beliefs may include family members. The individual, especially in times of crisis, is not marked by the strict and sharp lines drawn by the interdiction of the coloring book, but alters often to include objects and even other people: the hegemony of the individual as ending strictly at the space of the body is overthrown by a more encompassing vision of personhood.

Driven mostly by anecdote and bias, family member presence is subject to local winds. The published literature attests to benefits for some, and detriments for others. Staff members, physicians, patients, family members can all seem to be found that have either benefitted or suffered by being witness to events during a resuscitation. Some argue for closure and support while others for trauma and logistical nightmares. In his classic study of self-presence in social institutions, *The Presence of Self in Everyday Life,* the sociologist Erving Goffman distinguishes between 'front stage' and 'backstage' practices in the setting of a social situation using the metaphor of the theater or stagecraft. The front stage is what the audience (in our case, the family members) sees—it must be convincing and creditable fulfilling the dictates, mores and conventions of a social code. The stern but sensible doctor in his white coat, calm, cool and collected. The backstage is where the 'actors' are present but the audience is not—it is where the 'actors' can typically step out of character without fear of disrupting the performance. It is an area of freedom. The chaos and noise of central line kits being opened and packaging thrown on the floor, the whir and noise of machines, the doctor's curse when a needle hits an unintended artery, the gallows humor, the sweat on the brow. Trust in social institutions typically depends upon the careful separation between front stage and backstage. How could the audience believe the performance if they saw the actors conning their lines in a state of panic minutes before a performance? But family member presence during resuscitation suggests exactly this kind of upheaval. Perhaps this blind trust in institutions might be replaced by a reasoned, thoughtful perspective.

In recent years, there have been an increasing number of studies designed to determine how family members would feel at being present during resuscitations, whether their presence altered outcomes and how the staff reacted to their presence (Redley, Botti & Duke, 2006). Generally, when patients' families were surveyed, the majority of them preferred to be present during resuscitation efforts (Doyle, 1987). While most of these surveys were retrospective, at least one prospective, randomized study of family response to resuscitation suggested that family members were not traumatized by the resuscitation and gained some measure of comfort by being present (Robinson, Mackenzie-Ross, Campbell-Hewson, Egleston, Prevost, 1998). When patients who had survived resuscitation were surveyed in a qualitative manner they also seemed to favor the presence of family members: they reported feeling safer, less afraid and more at ease when their family members were present (Eichhorn et al, 2001); they also believed that the family members could act as their advocate and that physicians would be reminded by the presence of family members of the patient's personhood. In a not completely unexpected discordance, healthcare practitioners take the opposite view. A 2002 survey of critical care practitioners, including physicians and nurses, found that the overwhelming majority of them would not want patients' family members to be allowed during resuscitation (McClenathan, Torrington, & Uyehara, 2002). Part of the divergence probably lies in the "actors'" preference for maintaining the distinction between front stage and backstage. However, medical practice is not exactly like the stage (the operating theater, notwithstanding). The performance, if we can call it one, is ongoing. There is always an audience member—the patient—and there are always real, meaningful outcomes. Family member presence preserves the continuity of lives in the face of professional and technological disruptions.

CASE TWO

Our patient arrived at 11:06 AM. Unlike most patients who come to the Emergency Department in cardiac arrest, he was not brought in by an ambulance or by a paramedic. He walked in.

He arrived at triage exactly 1 minute earlier, 11:05am. In triage, he was present with his friend who notified the nurse that he had not been feeling quite up to par all morning. As a personal chauffer, he began his day around 9am. He did not quite feel like his usual self, and his wife urged him to seek medical attention. He initially refused, not impressed with what he was experiencing. An hour or so later, he spoke with his wife again. Though he expressed that he was feeling better, she still wished he would at least go to the Emergency Room to be evaluated. Approximately 20 minutes prior to his arrival to the Emergency Department he began having left-sided chest pain and numbness and tingling in his left arm. His co-worker, who was with him, noted that he became quite diaphoretic and pale. At this time, she personally

drove him to our ER. In triage, grasped his left arm with his right hand and stuttered "It's getting worse". These were the last words he uttered before becoming unresponsive.

For us, his medical team, this was another case of cardiac arrest. But it was different. Different in that patients rarely present to us as a witnessed arrest. More often they arrive via ambulance and have received a significant deal of pre-hospital care. They are usually already intubated, have already received defibrillatory shocks, have already received Advanced Cardiac Life Support care. In essence, they have already been 'down', been 'worked on' for a significant amount of time. Their mortality is increased by the time they reach us simply secondary to the amount of time that their vital organs have not been adequately perfused. What perhaps is most important in a case of cardiac arrest is time to CPR and when indicated, time to delivery of first shock.

Our patient arrived at the resuscitation bay unresponsive. He was placed on a cardiac monitor immediately and was noted to be in Ventricular Fibrillation. His first defibrillatory shock was delivered at 11:06am, and he had received his third by 11:10am. Advanced Cardiac Life Support algorithms were begun. The cardiac team and cardiac catheterization lab were activated and arrived shortly afterwards to assist in his care. He received multiple doses of epinephrine, anti-arrhythmics and a total of eight shocks. Forty minutes later, his cardiac rhythm was still Ventricular Fibrillation, and he was not responding to any of our efforts. Furthermore, he still had no pulse and no blood pressure. He was not stable enough to be transferred to the catheterization lab for definitive therapy of what we thought must have been a large myocardial infarction. The decision was made, amongst Emergency Physicians and the Cardiac team, at forty-five minutes post-arrest to deliver intravenous thrombolytics. CPR and ACLS continued concurrently. In the next few minutes the patient's blood pressure appeared to have stabilized. He regained a pulse. Given this, he was rushed to the catheterization lab.

During cardiac catheterization, he was noted to have a 100% occlusion of his Right Coronary Artery. He re-arrested twice during the procedure. He was shocked two additional times. The clot was removed with an Angiojet. As he had severe damage to his myocardium and was in cardiogenic shock, an Intra-Aortic Balloon Pump as well as a pacemaker were placed. He was transferred to the Cardiac Care Unit and his grave prognosis was delivered to his family who awaited his arrival.

Over the next few days his family sat vigil by his bedside, despite continued news of the severity of his condition by the cardiac team. If he did survive the insult to his cardiovascular system, would he even be functional? Would he have any intact neurologic capabilities? Would he be normal? Would he be himself? They seemed to understand as did everyone else that being unresponsive for over forty-five minutes in the Emergency Room was not a good clinical predictor of a happy outcome.

Yet over the next few days he began to wake up. He was responding not only to painful stimuli, but to his family. He woke up to such a degree that on day four of his hospital stay he requested extubation by writing on a piece of paper. He was weaned off all vasoactive medications.

I and some of the other members of the initial Emergency Department team were following his progress, through computer notes and updates. When we learned how well he was recovering, we decided to visit him in the Cardiac Care Unit. I think I'm safe in assuming we were all simply glad he was alive and doing well. We were not prepared for what we saw in his room on hospital day 8.

As the three of us entered the room, two physicians and a nurse, our patient (I still call him 'ours') was sitting erect in a chair by his bedside. His family was present. He took note of us and immediately began to cry. He said "Are you guys from the ER? You saved me. You saved my life". His wife began crying and said "He's been waiting for you. He's been wanting to come down to the ER ever since he woke up." We were all crying at this point. Tears and thanks continued for at least 30 minutes. This is one of the few cases of cardiac arrest that I've seen to have such a positive outcome. Throughout our training and work, we are accustomed to treat and deal with the cases we're presented. We're trained to deal with negative outcomes. In fact, we're often inured to the bad outcomes, almost numb to them. By our nature we have to continue on to the next case. Often times we wonder if any of what we're doing has any sort of positive effect. Seeing our patient not only alive that day, but fully talking, crying in the arms of his wife, left me speechless.

Current evidence-based studies show that mortality with prolonged arrest is high. It's questionable at best if administering thrombolytics this late in the process would be recommended by any academic authority. Further, rescue catheterization following thrombolytic administration is an option in only a few circumstances. The evidence that supports guidelines that we follow and practice daily shows we should have not done what we did. It also implies that our patient should not have lived. Yet by our nature as ER physicians we strive to preserve life and deliver last-ditch efforts. What remains is a husband and father who couldn't be more thankful with his second chance at life, a wife who still has her life-partner, and a teenage daughter and son who still have their father. Often we are left with negative outcomes despite our best efforts; in a certain number of cases however our clinical acumen, knowledge of medicine, and sheer dumb luck deliver otherwise.

tPA or tissue plasminogen activator is a naturally occurring serine protease found on endotheial cells that catalyzes the conversion of plasminogen to plasmin, the enzyme responsible for breaking down blood clots. A powerful compound, tPA, has been advocated and successfully used for clot lysis in pulmonary embolus, myocardial infarction and stroke (NINDS, 1995; FTT, 1994; Dong, Hao, Yue,, Wu, & Liu, 2009). But in part because of its serious side effect profile, life-threatening hemorrhages, the exact indications for tPA have been controversial. In fact, there is high grade evidence that tPA in the setting of cardiac arrest has no effect on mortality in a large population of pre-hospital patients (Bottiger et al, 2008). What was then the evidence-based role for giving this patient, tPA? Ultimately, all population evidence, when applied to a singular patient requires an inference—how well do the effects reported in a particular population trial reflect the results I would expect in my patient before me? Additionally, for every treatment, physicians and patients have to weight risks and benefits. What we think we know is that this patient had no chance of meaningful survival before the tPA was given. Therefore we assume the risks were low, we were not going to hurt him with our treatment, and the potential benefit, very high. In such high stakes settings, some researchers advocate the use of the 'N of 1' study design concept. In such a case, a single patient is the entire trial. The characteristics of interest are measured before a therapy is given, during therapy, and after the therapy is withdrawn. In our case, the first two circumstances are easy to measure, but without the last, which is impossible here, causality is difficult to adjudicate. The more unlikely the patient's expected recovery without the treatment, the more certain you might be that the recovery was then due to that treatment. It remains unclear if prolonged and effective CPR was the key to his recovery or the administration of thrombolytics. In this critically ill patient, swerving from the existing population based evidence may have saved his life.

CASE THREE

The patient and her husband were rushed in from the waiting room by the triage nurse. We hurriedly made our way to the bedside. She was dressed in slightly ill-fitting sweatpants and a sweatshirt (though it was late August) and her hair was disorderly. What immediately struck us was how fast she was breathing. Her husband somewhat disjointedly relayed that she was a double lung transplant recipient. She had developed severe post-partum pulmonary hypertension about a year and a half ago, after delivering their twin daughters (who were both well and at home with their grandmother). Having received the transplant six months previously, she had since then spent more time in the hospital than outside of it. As if to reinforce this point, we learned that she had only been discharged yesterday after a two-week course of antibiotics to fight a chronic lung infection following another intensive care stay. She and her husband were driving to the mall today, when the patient seemed to have an anxiety attack. She suffered from anxiety attacks and was on around the clock benzodiazepines. "She started breathing fast and said that she couldn't breathe. I stopped the car by the side of the road but couldn't calm her down." "It just wasn't Jennifer!" he kept repeating. "She's not like this. She's strong." Her respiratory rate was now in the thirties and her heart rate was in the one hundred thirties. We couldn't seem to get an accurate blood pressure reading. When we asked her how she was feeling, in short staccato sentences, she told us that she couldn't catch her breath. I asked a nurse to get paralytic medications, intubation supplies and a central venous catheter line kit. I also asked the patient's husband to step outside for a moment. "What do you want us to do?" I asked him. "What do you mean?" he almost screamed. "I mean, she is very sick, and we can do some things that may prolong her life, but I really don't know for how long." I went back in and tried to talk to her—she was losing ground fast and wasn't able to focus on my questions. Her breathing was getting more shallow. As I sterilized and prepared her right groin for the central line, her husband began to talk. "You're very sick," he said to her. "I'm tired" she replied. "We've had so many discussions with our doctor about what to do and we've kept on fighting but I'm tired too," he said to me. "I don't know what to do. It's not Jennifer. I don't want her to be in pain. I can't see her like this." The triage nurse had, in the meantime, called her primary transplant doctor, who now arrived at the bedside. She saw the patient's husband and they touched hands. As I was about to place my sterile gloves on for the procedure, her doctor motioned me outside of the curtain. The three of us stepped out. "What do you want to do?" she asked the husband almost in exact echo of my previous question. "I don't know." "We've talked about this before but I think she's getting worse now." "We have two kids at home and I can't do this anymore. It's not Jennifer." They looked at each other and in turn, looked at me. Her doctor just said, "OK. Let's make her comfortable." We removed the intubation equipment and the central line kit; we started slow intravenous hydration and low dose morphine and ordered her a private room on one of our wards. We sat with her, all of us. Nothing else needed to be said.

End of life care and decision-making has received much warranted attention in the last few decades. The ethical concerns with such care have traditionally focused on what is known as either patient autonomy or self-interest. When patients lose decisional capacity, these same principles require that we recollect patient's prior wishes and make decisions in accord with those wishes. *What would he or she have wanted?* However, autonomy as the central tenet in post-enlightenment western society may not be as sacrosanct as it has seemed. How can we really expect patients to make choices about futures and possibilities of which they can have no clear picture, image or understanding. Some models of patient-centeredness, shared-decision making and even EBM argue that we should put the known information before a patient and allow them to chose one of several options as if the choice were as simple as the one between carrot soup or tomato florentine. We ask patients to fill out living wills and advanced directives, we enact laws like the patient self-determination act, but in so doing, we

are asking our patients to imagine and project the impossible: their non-being. We want to protect patients from greedy corporate bottom-lines or from being appropriated by competing interests. We want to save physicians and family members the difficult choices. But a person is not an isolated individual, 'an island.' People are threads in an inter-related weave of relationships and time. The point in the illness at which a decision is made is only one point in a non-linear life. Autonomy as the bedrock principle of biomedical ethics may not be as unassailable as initially presumed (Bluhm, 2009). Interests of family, interests of personal physicians, the particular moment in its relation to all the other past and possible future moments must be considered as end-of-life decisions are made. Which patients will and which ones won't benefit from aggressive measures in critical situations is unclear and an area where meaningful research should be focused. We all knew, not in a way, perhaps, that we could clearly explain, but in a tacit manner, that our patient would not benefit in a significant way from excess interventions. Tacit knowledge, as described by Michael Polanyi, is an awareness of local contexts, prior observations, patterns and emotions that cannot always be vocalized but have an experimental and real relation to objective truths (Polyani, 1967). Our unspoken communication and commitment engineered the outcome.

The preceding three cases and their subsequent discussions were meant to suggest an expanded notion of evidence as it pertained to acute and critical illness. By considering the limits and possibilities of population-based research and an enlarged notion of patient values and concerns that come to encompass families and futures, we hoped to complicate the expected uses and abuses of EBM in critical care. Narrative considerations allowed us to broaden our notion of what constitutes evidence and to attend to details that might be missed if the subject of our practice was merely the science of bodies.

REFERENCES

Bluhm, R. (2009). Evidence-Based Medicine and Patient Autonomy. *International Journal of Feminist Approaches to Bioethics, 2*(2), 134–151. doi:10.2979/FAB.2009.2.2.134

Bottiger, B. W., Hans-Richard, A., Chamberlain, D. A., Blukhmki, E., Belmans, A., & Sanays, T. (2008). Thrombolysis during Resuscitation for Out-of-Hospital Cardiac Arrest. *The New England Journal of Medicine, 359*, 2651–2662. doi:10.1056/NEJMoa070570

Charles, C., Gafni, A., & Whelan, T. (1997). Shared Decision-making in the Medical Encounter: What does it Mean? (Or it Takes at Least Two to Tango*). Social Science & Medicine, 47*, 681–692. doi:10.1016/S0277-9536(96)00221-3

Charon, R. (2006). *Narrative Medicine: Honoring the stories of Illness*. New York: Oxford University Press.

Dong, B. R., Hao, Q., Yue, J., Wu, T., & Liu, G. J. (2009). Thrombolytic Therapy for Pulmonary Embolus. *Cochrane Database of Systematic Reviews, 3*.

Doyle, C. J., Post, H., Burney, R. E., Maino, J., Keefe, M., & Rhee, K. J. (1987). Family Participating During Resuscitation: an Option. *Annals of Emergency Medicine, 16*(6), 673–675. doi:10.1016/S0196-0644(87)80069-0

Eichhorn, D. J., Myers, T. A., Guzzetta, C. E., Clark, A. P., Klein, J. D., Taliaferro, E., & Calvin, A. O. (2001). Family Presence during Invasive Procedures and Resuscitation: Hearing the Voice of the Patient. *The American Journal of Nursing, 101*, 48–55.

Engel, G. L. (1977). The Need for a new Medical Model: a Challenge for Biomedicine. *Science, 196*, 129–136. doi:10.1126/science.847460

Fibrinolytic Therapists Trialists' (FTT) Collaborative Group. (1994). Indications for Fibrinolytic Therapy in Suspected Acute Myocardial Infarction: Collaborative Overview of early Mortality and Morbidity results from all Randomized Trials of more than 1000 patients. *Lancet, 343*, 311–322.

Goffman, E. (1990). *The Presentation of Self in everyday Life*. New York: Penguin Books.

Goyal, R. K., Charon, R., Lekas, H. M., Fullilove, M. T., Devlin, M. J., Falzon, L., & Wyer, P. C. (2008). A Local Habitation and a name: How Narrative Evidence-based Medicine Transforms the Translational Research Paradigm. *Journal of Evaluation in Clinical Practice, 14*(5), 732–741. doi:10.1111/j.1365-2753.2008.01077.x

Haynes, R. B., Sackett, D. L., Gray, J. R., Cook, D. C., & Guyatt, G. H. (1996). Transferring evidence from research into practice: 1. The role of clinical care research evidence in clinical decisions [Editorial]. *American College of Physicians Journal Club, 125*, A14–A16.

Jones, A. E., Brown, M. D., Trzeciak, S., Shapiro, N. I., Garrett, J. S., Heffner, A. C., & Kline, J. A. (2008). The effect of a quantitative resuscitation strategy on mortality in patients with sepsis: a meta-analysis. *Critical Care Medicine, 36*(10), 2734–2739. doi:10.1097/CCM.0b013e318186f839

Marik, P. E. (2001). *Handbook of Evidence Based Critical Care*. New York: Springer.

May, C., & Mead, N. (1999). Patient-centeredness: A History . In Dowrick, C., & Frith, L. (Eds.), *General Practice and Ethics: Uncertainty and Responsibility* (pp. 76–90). London: Routledge.

McClenathan, B. M., Torrington, K. G., & Uyehara, F. T. (2002). Cardiopulmonary Resuscitation: A Survey of US and International Critical Care Professionals. *Chest, 122*, 2204–2211. doi:10.1378/chest.122.6.2204

Parsons, T. (1951). *The Social System*. Glencove, New York: The Free Press.

Polyani, M. (1967). *The Tacit Dimension*. Chicago: Chicago University.

Redley, B., Botti, M., & Duke, M. (2006). Family Member Presence during Resuscitation in the Emergency Department: an Australian Perspective. *Emergency Medicine Australasia, 16*, 295–308.

Rier, D. A. (2001). The Missing Voice of the Critically Ill: a Medical Sociologist's First-Person Account. *Sociology of Health & Illness, 22*(1), 68–93. doi:10.1111/1467-9566.00192

Robinson, S. M., Mackenzie-Ross, S., Campbell-Hewson, G. L., Egleston, C. V., & Prevost, A. T. (1998). Psychological Effect of Witnessed Resuscitation on Bereaved Relatives. *Lancet, 352*, 614–617. doi:10.1016/S0140-6736(97)12179-1

Silva, S. A., & Wyer, P. C. (2009). Where Is The Wisdom? II. Evidence-Based Medicine and The Epistemological Crisis in Clinical Medicine. Exposition and Commentary on Djulbegovic, B., Guyatt, G.H. & Ashcroft, R.E. (2009) *Cancer Control, 16*, 158-168. *Journal of Evaluation in Clinical Practice, 15*, 899–906. doi:10.1111/j.1365-2753.2009.01324.x

The National Institute of Neurological Disorders and Stroke rt-PA Stroke study group. (1995). Tissue Plaminogen Activator for Acute Ischemic Stroke. *New England Journal of Medicine, 333*(24), 1581-1588.

Chapter 6
Patient Journey Record Systems (PaJR):
The Development of a Conceptual Framework for a Patient Journey System

Carmel M. Martin
Trinity College Dublin, Ireland

Rakesh Biswas
People's College of Medical Sciences, India

Ankur Joshi
People's College of Medical Sciences, India

Joachim Sturmberg
Monash University and The University of Newcastle, Australia

ABSTRACT

This chapter argues the need for a paradigm shift to focus health care from a top down fragmented process driven activity to a user-driven journey of the individual whose health is at stake. Currently many persons/users express needs that are often overlooked or not understood in the health system, and the frontline care workers express frustration in relation to care systems that prevent them from optimizing their care delivery. We argue that complex adaptive systems and social constructionist theories provide a link for knowledge translation that ultimately will lead to improved health care and better personal health outcomes/experiences. We propose the Patient Journey Record System (PaJR) as a conceptual framework to transform health care so that it supports and improves the experience of patients and improves the quality of care through adaptable and interconnected provider information and care systems. Information technology, social networking and digital democracy are proposed as major solutions to the need to put the patient and their journey at the centre of health and health care with real time shaping of care to this end. Placing PaJR at the centre of care would enable patients, caregivers, physicians, nurses, allied health professionals and students to contribute to improving care. PaJR should become a

DOI: 10.4018/978-1-60960-097-6.ch006

'discovery tool' of new knowledge arising from different types of experiences ranging from the implicit knowledge in narratives through to the explicit knowledge that is formalized in the published peer reviewed literature and translated into clinical knowledge.

Referring to the patient's journey is a very appropriate start. Travellers have always needed help. How far must I travel? What route must I take? Are there signposts along the way? Is there a map, or must I find my way from landmark to landmark? Is there someone to act as a guide, or must I act as pilot and navigator, and who is in charge? Will it hurt if I 'bump' into something on this journey? What happens upon arrival - will I be a complete stranger in a strange land? http://stanford.wellsphere.com/general-medicine-article/the-patient-s-journey/503163 Posted Nov 18 2008 12:17am

THE PATIENT'S JOURNEY

The patient journey concept has been an emergent phenomenon building on the notion of patient centeredness over the past 15-20 years. It has emerged from the dynamics of balancing the biomedical model with the biopsychosocial model, and balancing the acute care models with chronic care and community oriented patient centred models (Figure 1) (C. M. Martin, 2007). The patient journey concept recognizes that people make journeys through different stages of health and illness, through different parts of the health care systems associated with different emotional and physical experiences (C. M. Martin & Sturmberg,

Figure 1. Archetypal patient journeys underpinning the patient journey record system (PaJR)

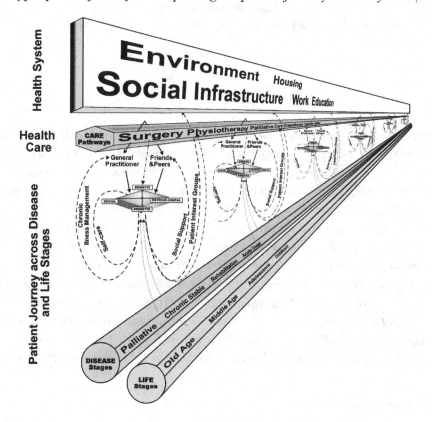

2006; Sturmberg & Martin, 2006). The individual patient journey is shaped by the systems in which they live, which are strongly influenced by the social and non-social determinants of health. A range of compelling evidence from Canada and other countries indicates that the social and economic circumstances of individuals and groups influence their health status and mortality as much as or more than health care. These circumstances affect the success rate of interventions to change personal health behaviour, such as smoking and diet, or of improved outcomes of chronic disease management. Addressing health inequities is strongly associated with the improvement of health care outcomes (Martin CM & Kaufman T, 2008).

This patient journey takes place in a western system where there is universal access to general practice and comprehensive health care. The patient journey starts from birth and early life and ends in death. The journey of the individual is through all stages of life, from wellness and risk to disease and illness. The personal nature of this unique individual journey encompasses biological, psychological, social domains of experience.

Individual journeys occur with support and interdependent relationships within their intimate family networks, their social networks of peers, friends and colleagues. Self care and the work of managing health and illness increasingly takes place with informational and disease management support from chronic disease management programs. Patients are increasingly connected through patient interest groups, blogs and other social networking sites. Individuals are located within their social network, their culture, their social and economic infrastructure. Such systems are complex and often unpredictable, thus narratives are often the best way for individual and relevant others to make sense of their journey.

The general practitioner and the primary care team have a longitudinal journey with their patient through phases of health and illness and stages of care including health promotion and prevention, risk management, diagnosis, treatment, self-management and self-care. Such care pathways pass through different care sectors from primary and community care to secondary and tertiary hospital based care. In this system continuity of care is based on relationships, information and connected management strategies. Community, secondary and tertiary care providers have episodic and sometimes long term care relationships. Doctors and care providers can increasingly network and learn from each other's experiences through traditional continuing medical education, but boosted by the immediacy of social networking.

Medical education increasingly needs to address the shift to a patient journey framework incorporating constituents of the patient journey system and needs to activate two domains of learning -cognitive and affective. Cognitive skills and competencies 'facts' are the traditional medical skills incorporating the process of comprehension, application, analysis, synthesis and evaluation. Skills to address the affective domains 'feelings and fears' of the patient journey remain highly important skills that need to be acquired by medical learners of all ages.

Social and economic circumstances of individuals and groups influence their health status and mortality as much as or more than personal health care. These circumstances influence personal health behaviour, such as smoking and diet, improved outcomes of acute and chronic disease management. Practitioners work in health services which involve education, employment, the economic, legal, welfare and political systems over time.

The theoretical framework for this chapter is based on a number of different theories including social constructionism, structuration and complex adaptive systems theory (Félix-Bortolotti, 2009; Martin CM & Peterson C, 2008). Social constructionism is a discipline within sociology that is based on sociological theories of knowledge that consider how social phenomena develop in relation to social contexts. A major focus is to uncover the ways in which individuals and groups participate in the creation of their perceived social reality. It involves looking at the ways social phenomena are created, institutionalized, and made into traditions. A socially constructed reality is one that is seen as an ongoing, dynamic process. It is reproduced by people acting on their interpretations and their knowledge, which according to 'weak' constructivists concerns subjective constructions related to objective realities (Martin CM & Peterson C, 2008). Complex adaptive systems theories have emerged from physics, mathematics and the natural sciences and permeated the organizational literature accompany the sociological streams of knowledge theory. They reflect the non-linear interdependent dynamic reality of actors and agents which are continually adapting to feedback (Félix-Bortolotti, 2009; C. M. Martin & Sturmberg, 2009).

The methodology for this chapter draws on the work of Walker and Hurt (1990). Walker and Hurt affirm that scientific and technical written communications are produced on a continuum between the two extremes of formal and informal communications (Walker & Hurt, 1990). They characterized *informal* communications as immediate fluid information; disseminator selected and interactive. Examples would include blogs, the informal and grey literature. Formal communications are characterized as public, permanently stored and typically retrievable, relatively "old" information that is primarily user selected and non-interactive. This form of information can be found in the formal peer reviewed literature, although the boundaries are increasingly becoming blurred with a proliferation of authoritative blogs and online publishing of less formal and or open access journals. In this chapter we incorporate the use of blogged narratives together with a scoping of the peer reviewed literature. Narrative and auto/biographical approaches from within the social sciences associated with post-modernism are employed in order to reflect on how social actors conceptualise the ways in which they make sense of, and re-present, the

social world (Sikes, 2007). We, as the 'actors' in health care - patients, clinicians and informatics experts - present our personal and patient narratives in order to understand the importance of the patient journey and the systems that support these journeys. A scoping of the published literature on the patient journey was conducted using 'patient journey' 'patient journey narrative' as the key search term on Pub Med, EMBASE, CINAHL and Google. The 231 journal articles identified were then filtered with additional terms: experience, audit, quality improvement, system design and information technology as the key search terms.

THE JOURNEYS

The chapter charts many patient centred journeys in health care in order to explore the key leverage points and constraints by which to improve patient health and quality of life. First. we consider the major focus of all health journeys - the patient experience as they pass through phases of illness and disease and stages of care. Second, we reflect on the doctor –patient, doctor-doctor and doctor-student experiences of the patient journey through their illnesses and the health care journey and the constraints and enabling landscapes they encounter as they try to provide high quality services. This gestalt of different experiences is, in fact, the result of interactions among diverse agents. Here, learning take place to reduce or increase agent adaptability and self organization, attending not only to structures, but also to processes and functions of complex systems (Jordon, Lanham, Anderson, & Jr, 2010).

The Patient's Journey

The complexity of issues facing people with chronic illness can be both demanding and demoralizing. Chronic illness care requires a response to broad physical, psychological and environmental issues including difficult social situations.

Bob the black country Brummie www.midtids. blogspot.com Saturday, 21 November 2009:

A couple of days ago I was taken to A&E at Sandwell by paramedic. This was the result of a "funny turn" a medical term when they can't establish what caused it. I accidently tried head butting our kitchen floor from a standing position. When they mentioned funny turn I thought I better get on stage quick before it wears off. I digress. I possibly fainted but when I was lying on my side on the floor I noticed the bottom edge of our sink unit and thought, "that is starting to break up". The misses quick as a flash dials all the nines then her mate from down the road. It wasn't long before I was on a trolley in A&E then relatively quickly transferred to Medical Assessment Unit where I was kept overnight for observation. It was early hours of the morning when I got a bed so I was very tired. I was awakened every hour with a bright light shining in my eyes followed by blood pressure, pulse, temp ect. I had difficulty getting back to sleep and this routine continued all night. Come the morning I was, well; knackered. I don't want to go into the gory details except to point out the good bits and unfortunately the bad bits. The good bits; they did a very thorough job of checking me out. They were straight and honest throughout even when the news was not particularly good. The not so good bits. In the morning they took away my bed and never found me another. I was there all day with nowhere to lie down. It is essential I stretch out during the day. Although I asked for a bed and told them why they never took me seriously. So by late afternoon I was in pain and really stressed out. I felt abandoned and neglected. It wasn't until the wife started to make a fuss that action started. The ward does not have adequate washing facilities and I did not have the motivation or strength at that time to shower (http://midtids.blogspot.com/2009/11/patients-journey.html).

Bob describes his sense of feeling 'in pain, and alone and powerless' in a big machine. Health and illness are unique personal experiences in the presence as well as in the absence of identifiable pathologies. Individuals navigate their unique personal health and illness journeys through periods of health and disease - journeys defined both by personal narratives and the data traces they leave within healthcare environments (such as family practices or hospitals). Despite decades of patient-centred research and education, people still suffer from neglect by the health care machinery. While a range of literature refers to the patient journey and there are multiple dimensions of the journeys across all sectors of health care and conditions. Complex systems theory supports the notion that it is possible to identify user driven interventions and system learning adaptive processes along the journey that can improve patient experiences and quality of care.(Leykum et al., 2007)

The journey is as much about the social and cultural experience as the physical symptoms and medical problem (Martin CM & Peterson C, 2008). General practitioners can become frustrated by the treatment of their patients in that 'system'. Providing care for chronic illness and multidimensional conditions requires whole person comprehensive care, which address the social nature of care as well as interventions that are focused on disease. Unintended consequences of health system changes such as 'contracting out' services can be a devaluing little regard for the relationships between people and their families and those who deliver care.

Carmel Martin, General Practitioner has recently worked in several countries:

Recently, while conducting regular primary care out-of-hours weekend work in a particular country where the work is contacted out to private companies, my experience with older sicker patients was punctuated by frequent urgent relative requests for visits and telephone calls with concerns about their relatives' decline. Such concerns on the week-end were delivered to a safety net service to identify and refer urgent care needs to secondary care and stabilize other needs. Some calls were misplaced when family visited older relatives who had been in deteriorating health during the week and had either not sought help or their help seeking had delivered 'weak signals' which had not been picked up. Whether these weak cries for help were based on physical disease deterioration, psychosocial or environmental contexts, the only recourses on the weekend were: maintenance strategies (of medication adjustment and psychosocial band-aid solutions); secondary care referral and admission; or long waits in Accident and Emergency Departments.

People who are ill often are unwilling to seek help and are embarrassed by an impression that they *'have been bad'* and they have not adhered to medical or health promotion advice, which have landed them in this situation. However, there is the problem of guilt or frustration at always having to seek help and 'bothering people' (C. Martin, 1998).

Annette, an Australian patient:

But now I can see, had I have taken more care earlier, it maybe wouldn't be as bad as it is... but ....it always feels like you are bothering people.

Heather, an Australian patient:

I guess they (patients who are labeled as "chronically ill") have got connotations of always being at the doctor and being a pain in the arse.

A coping strategy adopted by many older or chronically ill people is not to disclose the full extent of their pain and suffering to avoid dependency and stigmatization. This leads to delayed help seeking, and emergency admissions or visits to the emergency department (M. Martin, Hin, &

O'Neill, 2004). A patient journey record system that allows people with chronic illness to seek health advice early using an IT system that monitors and feeds back their unique status would at least, in theory, improve patient access to more timely and less bothersome help seeking.

Conversely, some patients become *'professional patients'* and live their illness thriving on the attention or developing excessive anxiety or dependency on the health system.

As Dr J says - *they live their illness* (C. Martin, 1998). Australian general practitioner and co-author, Joachim Sturmberg sees that modern technology and a patient journey record system would assist some of the people who have trouble living with illness.

Joachim Sturmberg – Australian General Practitioner:

Bill is 88 years old, lives in a hostel, and volunteers on a daily basis at the nursing home where his wife was cared for until her death 15 years ago. Bill has many health problems. The one of greatest concern to him is his shortness of breath and increasing tiredness. Bill has severe ischaemic cardiomyopathy as well as COPD, and his medication management is making him dizzy to the point of falling. Bill reduced his diuretic medications as he could not cope with having to rush to the toilet all the time, and he found that leaving the pills away made him less dizzy, but over a few days his shortness of breath became more prominent, and his legs were swelling up above his knees. Bill is well aware of his condition, and he understands the limitations of his management. He agreed to record his awakening weight, and adjust his diuretic medications, and this 'trick' is helping him to maintain a workable balance between maintaining an acceptable control of his heart failure and his desire to stay engaged with his work in the nursing home. How nice would it be to receive daily information about his physical parameters and his subjective wellbeing and being able to tweak his management whenever needed early, rather than having to see him in the surgery with a major deterioration in his health?

Social Support

John – son of Gladys, aged 82, a lady with pneumonia – in a phone call to Carmel Martin while working in the Out-of-Hours Service:

I am so concerned about my mother. I live 60 miles away and visit my mother on Sunday nights. I just feel that she needs more attention during the week and when I saw her (this) weekend, I felt she had been let down. The doctor came and went and just gave her some antibiotics, but she isn't at all well. I feel that she should have been treated earlier. I wish I could be more involved in her care during the week. At the weekend it is an OOH home visit which may take as long as 8 hours to be provided.

Social support can be simply defined as the availability of people on whom patients feel that they can depend. Currently, social support theory recognises both structural and functional elements of interpersonal relationships and social assets that contribute to the provision of support. Structural elements include the size, density, flexibility and adequacy of an individual's network of intimates, friends, colleagues and experts. Social embeddedness describes the degree and type of bonding (such as trust) between participants. Functional elements are the actual supportive acts received (and provided) and people's perceptions of their quality. Functions of support cover emotional, practical, informational, appraisal and companionship domains in human interactions. In practice, these functions are often difficult to separate and usually highly inter-correlated (House and Kahn 1985). Social support models link social, psychological and physiological levels of functioning. Health is determined by the balance between social, psychological and physiological stress and the host vulnerability or resistance (assets or resources).(C. M. Martin, 1998).

Improving Care

The literature reviewed identifies a whole world of patient journeys with a considerable focus on patient narratives on their experiences with exhortations for physicians, health care providers and health systems to refocus on such experiences as central to care (Chapple, Ziebland, & McPherson, 2004; Lapsley & Groves, 2004; Pope C, Ziebland S, Mays N, & 1999, 1999).

Educators are exhorted to improve clinical education to sensitize students to the nature of the patient journey. (Clare & Bullock, 2003; Farquhar et al., 2005; Graves, Shue, & Arnold, 2002; Maughan, Finlay, & Webster, 2001; McLeod, 2003; Muir, 2007; Powell-Tuck, 2009; Sturmberg, Reid, & Khadra, 2001; Sturmberg, Reid, & Khadra, 2002; Vegni, Mauri, & Moja, 2005; Wales, 2005, 2008)

What are we teaching our medical students? By BeamOn on 7/15/2009 4:00 PM:

The training of the young doctor has been subject to much change in recent decades. Flexner's day is done - although if you set up a medical course now and promised to excel in Basic Sciences, then you would be very very revolutionary, if a little reactionary! Still, we try to stuff the knowledge in, as much as we had to, but thankfully we are a little more aware of the patient journey and experience. We particularly like to get our students to see the other side.

Another perspective on the shift to a patient journey record systems approach is described by Joshi from the Indian sub continent. He makes the case that approaches beyond current cognitive skills of diagnosis to address context and affect should be adopted as edifying tools for medical students.

Ankur Joshi:

Often during the rendition and depiction of knowledge allied with medical sciences we emphasize on 'what' and 'how' rather than unrevealing the 'why' ………. as this 'why' always beckons to the neurons of our brains and creates an enduring, immortal affinity to the subject.

"When he set out, he did not know where he was going,

When he got there he did not know where he was,

When he returned, he did not know where he had been" (Columbus School)

Teacher should not be visualized only as a human resource input, to act as a source of information & to transmit this information to learners but should be seen as a system specialist to plan, steer & implement a formal and informal educational process. He should more be in a facilitator role rather than to act as active guide.. The success of educational system & teacher as system specialist may be measured by output specification (effectiveness of the process to achieve the desired outcome), efficiency (cost, time & resource spent) & openness of education system (sensitiveness to external stimulus & environment). These three parameters may be achieved by the formal and informal incorporation of patients narratives, pathways adopted by him/her during the illness phase and psycho-socio-demographic consideration while on treatment in the curriculum. This approach may transform the bare lecture into text-book plus eccentricity.

Incorporation of constituents of patient journey system may kindle two domains of learning - cognitive and affective.

Cognitive Domains – This domain is related with innate & inherent capacity of human race to develop intellectual skills in response to internal & external stimuli. This encompasses the process to acquire, recall and recognize knowledge and skills of the student. These domains can be further divided into knowledge (ability to recall & retrieve), comprehension (ability to visualize a idea with its fullest meaning), application (ability to used in real time scenario by using knowledge & comprehension), analysis (fragmentation of a central idea into a meaningful & interpretable finding), synthesis (ability to coherent & unified several themes/sub themes to unison) & evaluation (ability to judge the reliability, reproducibility, efficiency, effectiveness utilities & merits of a established criteria). PaJR does catalyze and facilitate the process of comprehension, application, analysis, synthesis and evaluation

Affective Domains – This taxonomic domain deals with the interpersonal relationship or communication skills and describes the learning task associated with change in attitude, interest, values & development of appreciation. In short it is associated with receiving, responding & internalization of an objective. Taxonomically it can be further categorized into receiving (consciousness to aware a idea & willing to receive it), responding (getting satisfaction by responding owe to receiving), valuing (internalization of the idea and preferential commitment to percolate it), organization (development of sound conceptual framework of learning in coherent and acceptable fashion and acting upon it) and characterization by a value complex (amalgamation of the value with philosophy to transform it into a consistent behavioral characteristics). PaJRs may light up the process of valuing, organizing and ultimately in the formation of characterization of value complex.

The learner's performance is a complex outcome of current flowing through various integrated and internalized circuits of these domains. Contemplation and introspection of these domains facilitates the learning process by encouraging the learners to think, resulting in the acquisition of knowledge, skills and attitude and PaJR undoubtedly does provide an opportunity to do so.

Despite many years and many publications across a whole range of physical and mental conditions, and quality improvements activities, patient experiences of their journey remain lonely, poorly heeded and frequently mismanaged (Alarcon & Leetz, 1998; Andrew & Whyte, 2004; Barnard, Hollingum, & Hartfiel, 2006; Baron, 2009; "Battling back from childhood sexual abuse and surviving the journey," 1998; Binkley, 1999; Blondal & Halldorsdottir, 2009; Bond et al., 2009; Centers, 2001; Curry & Stone, 1991; Graves, et al., 2002; Griffin & Fentiman, 2002; Hall, 2005; Harmel, 1986; James, Hess, Kretzing, & Stabile, 2007; Jenkins, 2006; Kelly et al., 2003; Kerfoot, 1998; Kiteley & Vaitekunas, 2006; Kobayashi, 1997; Maughan, et al., 2001; Mayor, 2006; McGrath et al., 2008; McNicholl, Dunne, Garvey, Sharkey, & Bradley, 2006; Meadows, Lackner, & Belic, 1997; Muir, 2007; Peterson, 2006; Powell-Tuck, 2009; Richardson, Casey, & Hider, 2007; Rigaux, 2005; Rockwood, Wallack, & Tallis, 2003; Storli, Lindseth, & Asplund, 2008; Thorne et al., 2009; Vegni, et al., 2005; Ventegodt, Andersen, & Merrick, 2003; Venter & Hannan, 2009; Wray & Maynard, 2008). The key message from the literature is the ongoing need to refocus and redesign care around the patient and his/her journey across all sectors of health care for long term and acute conditions.

Information technology, social networking and digital democracy is proposed as a major solution to the need to put the patient and their journey at the centre of health and health care with real time shaping of care to this end.

Social media on the Internet are empowering, engaging, and educating health care consumers and providers. While consumers use social media -- including social networks, personal blogging, wikis, video-sharing, and other formats -- for

emotional support, they also heavily rely on them to manage health conditions. The Internet has evolved from the information-retrieval of "Web 1.0" to "Web 2.0," which allows people who are not necessarily technologically savvy to generate and share content. The collective wisdom harnessed by social media can yield insights well beyond the knowledge of any single patient or physician. The outcome of this development is "Health 2.0" -- a new movement that challenges the notion that health care happens only between a single patient and doctor in an exam room. The Web is becoming a platform for convening people with shared concerns and creating health information that is more relevant to consumers. Social networks, ranging from MySpace to specific disease-oriented sites, are proliferating so rapidly that new services are already under development to help health consumers navigate through the networks. Jane Sarasohn-Kahn, The Wisdom of Patients: Health Care Meets Online Social Media- CHCF.org Posted Nov 18 2008 12:13am

Social networking - that is groups of people interacting in a dynamic system though the use of digital technology - is a way forward to promote knowledge and relationship management. Social networking is increasingly utilized in health care, comprising a range of strategies and practices used to identify, create, represent, distribute, and enable shared knowledge, either embodied in individuals experiences or embedded in formal knowledge systems or current practice (Eysenbach, 2008). Groups of individual patients, medical students and health professionals share the patient's need to increasingly interact with and seek knowledge and solutions offered by others in the network. A web based user driven social network would relax central control and make local adaptation and strategic health workers feel more engaged in the project such that it is truly user driven (Biswas et al., 2008).

Rakesh Biswas – an Indian hospital physician's perspective – promoting social networking and e-logging solutions to lack of continuity in relationships and information and care management.

We need an information system that can seamlessly integrate different types of information to meet diverse user group needs around the patient journey.

Present day e-health systems encourage increasing automation through human computer interaction whereas health and healing require human to human interaction that simply needs to be augmented by computers. This importance of human to human interaction and its augmentation by technology is illustrated below with a single day hospital ward scenario from a hospital physician consultant's e-diary (Note that care giver logs are often just telegraphic information):

1) Relooked Bed 11 ... student's request. 50 year old Male, Nephrotic syndrome with diabetes mellitus, with his diabetic foot dripping pus on the bed. No dressing since yesterday? Blood sugar values?

2) Bed 10 60 yr Male, collapsed suddenly, cirrhosis with end stage, didn't want to resuscitate but had to for protocol as we had missed out on the DNR earlier. Students had an exercise.

Another note a month later:

This was a month back I think...can't be sure... time flies so fast on the daily ward rounds. Most of my E-logs remain unutilized. In fact I first started making e-logs on my PDA chiefly to identify my information needs as a physician before I gradually started realizing even patients had similar needs and we all need to have integral solutions.

Relevance of daily E logs to solve individual patient/health professional user needs:

I had seen the diabetic man in bed 11 earlier on his morning consultation rounds but he realized

that this patient's blood sugar control had been overlooked only after a medical student requested him to have another re-look. He made a point in his mind to inform this to his junior colleague, the medical officer who would remain in the wards (also at the same time making the telegraphic note about the patient in bed 11 in his personal diary). Suddenly, at that point in time, the patient in bed 10 collapsed and he had to participate in his CPR that was emotionally and physically draining and he was relieved to escape to the outpatient department (OPD) for the day.

Ideas about Shaping an Ideal Future System Based Upon A Patient Journey Record Concept
Rakesh Biswas - Communicating valuable individual patient data – the future:

If this data were on a web portal (a kind of virtual hospital filing system) as soon as the physician entered it into his personal digital assistant (PDA), the data would have matched with his other colleague's data for the day regarding this particular patient. His junior colleague (Medical Officer/ Senior Resident) doing just a file review on his PDA would have noticed the note and acted on the diabetic man's blood sugar if it was high. Controlling it better may have benefited the wound more than the systemic antibiotics that he was already on (and which had doubtful local benefit although again it is an issue that may be debated). This technology offering a convenient local solution to improving hospital communication among in-house health professionals is evolving at present in many hospitals.

Medical Students as a Vital Force in E Learning and Improvement of Patient Care

The government generally thinks that it spends too much money in Undergraduate Medical training perhaps as these student doctors appar-

ently do not serve while they learn. However it is the medical student who has the time to listen in detail to their chosen individual patient (they do not have to see and are not responsible for all the ward patients unlike their overworked houseman/resident seniors). Medical student logs on their individual patients can be a vital source of detailed narrative data on individual patients which their consultant might often enjoy reading and also benefit from daily. The medical student who pulled the consultant to the bedside may as well have entered his thoughts about his patient on his PDA-elog that would have automatically been reviewed by the consultant or his Medical officer (Senior resident).

Continuity of information, management and relationships among physicians are key elements to support physicians doing their work to support the individual patient journey. The ideal system does not exist and the previous two narratives reflect the everyday challenges of delivering care in everyday circumstances. Why the patient journey as described by patients is consistently less than ideal, is the constant need to improve systems of care through which patients needs to journey.

KevinMD blog US:

As for patients, be aware of the difficulties physicians face when trying to talk to one another. Know your medications and medical history when seeing a new specialist or receiving care in the emergency room. Ensure that any new treatment recommendations are appropriately communicated with your primary care physician. Our health care system has plenty of room for improvement. Simply making it easier for medical providers to talk to both patients and each other would represent a significant step in the right direction.

We have been working very hard at defining and developing a much better "Patient Journey" through our practice. The whole team have been involved, as we have very much taken on board

your philosophy that the patient is like a "baton in a relay race" and that every player in the team has a responsibility to avoid "dropping the baton" by delivering fabulous personal service – a smile, eye contact, genuine interest and appreciation – all that stuff.

We organised an initial training session to discuss our views. We set aside the time to attend a day's training on "The Patient Journey" and we then came back to the practice and made a big effort to implement the ideas and revisit them at periodic team meetings. However, we do tend to keep slipping back into our old habits – we are busy most days and there just sometimes doesn't seem enough time. Most of the staff are now mildly complaining that they have forgotten the key elements of the journey and we seem to be losing the enthusiasm. I don't want this to be yet another initiative that got lost in the rush. Any hints? The top 10 tips for a Patient Journey Champion http:// www.coachbarrow.com/blog/customer-service/ the-top-10-tips-for-a-patient-journey-champion/ (date not supplied)

Medical social networking sites are flourishing (Eysenbach, 2008) and shape learning about how to care for patients in their medical journeys.

Physician use of social networking has rapidly increased in parallel with patient networking. For example, Sermo is the largest online physician community in the US. It's where practicing US physicians—spanning 68 specialties and all 50 states—collaborate on difficult cases and exchange observations about drugs, devices and clinical issues. And find potentially life-saving insights that have yet to be announced by conventional media sources. Sermo is a real-time meeting place where physicians get help with everything from patient care to practice management. They've described it as "therapeutic," a "virtual water cooler" and "vital to my everyday practice." Physicians on Sermo rank their colleagues for the value of their postings and the quality of their answers to posted questions. Highly ranked community members are turned to for respected answers and advice. (http://www.sermo.com/about/introductionaccessed21/2/2010)

Health and Social networks and systems addressing the determinants of health are significant influences on the patient journey. Thus networking would build on existing and successful collective enterprises to deliver after-hours care, improve quality and safety of individual disease management, and link with public health initiatives to extend toward implementing strategies that address the factors contributing to the genesis and evolution of disease and health outcomes (Martin CM & Kaufman T, 2008). In a well-functioning system, well-being may be enhanced by social interventions to counteract the determinants of health. The latter definitively calls for political will on the part of all agents for effective intersectorial collaboration and coordination. This is about people, multiple levels of services, and allocation of resources by the means of organizations and policymaking decisions. It is about caring for and about people in need of a wide range of services. This includes the notion of population health in the global sense of the term – clients, that is, patients who are receiving the care in order to restore or to maintain their health status, as well as the needs of direct care service providers, that is, a multidisciplinary group of health professionals in the community (Félix-Bortolotti, 2009).

THE PATIENT JOURNEY RECORD (PAJR) CONCEPTUAL FRAMEWORK

Through an iterative process of immersion and crystallization, the team developed the concept of the Patient Journey Record System as an overarching concept that requires greater explicit attention in the future to move beyond a current narrow focus on disease management.

Conceptual Framework for Developing Patient Journey Systems from the User Perspective

To enable a better understanding of the patient's health and illness experience over the trajectory of his or her chronic disease, we propose the development of the Patient Journey Record (PaJR) system. The *PaJR* will enable the development of systems to directly shape care by integrating:

1. personal narratives of the inner health/illness experiences
2. health care narratives of disease and treatment - narratives of the individual, their family and caregivers and health professional narratives
3. the personal and other narratives of life trajectory of school, work, and social support and networks, including the determinants of health (C. M. Martin, 1998).

Personal Narratives

Health is a dynamic interplay of different components and can be understood as a balance between the biological, the psychological and social viewed hrough personal sense-making narratives. As patients make their way through the health care system, they traverse their personal journeys and narratives with their health practitioners and other professionals as well as that of fellow patients they encounter along the way.

Sensemaking is the ability or attempt to understand and clear situations. More exactly, sensemaking is the process of creating situational awareness and understanding in situations of high complexity or uncertainty in order to make decisions. It is "a motivated, continuous effort to understand connections or disconnections and disjunctions (which can be with and among people, places, and events) in order to anticipate their trajectories and act effectively" (Klein, Moon, & Hoffman., 2006). By far the most common form of sensemaking is the informal and formal use of narratives. "The narrative provides meaning, context and perspective for the patient's predicament. It defines how, why and in what way he or she is ill. It offers, in short, a possibility of understanding which cannot be arrived at by any other means" (T. Greenhalgh & B, 1998).

Narratives of Care

The patient's narrative is not the only part of the sensemaking process as doctors; nurses and other clinical and non-clinical participants also have their own narratives. Bringing them together allows participants to better understand what is happening to them and others, what it means to them and in doing so bridges both cultural and professional barriers (T. Greenhalgh, 2002). Sensemaking in the cognitive domains is central skill of medical decision-making in diagnosis, treatment and management. Patient centered care (often summarized as facts, fears and feelings) also required an affective component – this domain deals with the interpersonal relationship or communication skills and describes the learning task associated with change in attitude, interest, values & development of appreciation.

Narratives of Systems in Which We Operate

At the core of the system is an understanding of local population health determinants and inequities of health outcomes, as well as local primary care demands for services. With the developments in information technology, the horizontal interconnecting of local providers is realistic and feasible; such interconnecting is essential to collectively address local needs rather than, as at present, individuals and groups working in local organizational silos. Networking builds on existing and successful collective enterprises. Thus systems and care need to be provided by interconnected practitioners, providers or agents 'at work' in their different practice settings or sectors bringing with them, their own set of individual and professional values (Félix-Bortolotti, 2009). This networking would expand existing and successful collective enterprises to deliver after-hours care, improve quality and safety of individual disease management, and link with public health initiatives to extend toward implementing strategies that address the factors contributing to the genesis and evolution of disease and health outcomes (Martin CM & Kaufman T, 2008).

Evidence is emerging of the successes of social networking in providing peer and informational support in an interactive user driven environment (Brownstein, Brownstein, Williams, Wicks, & Heywood, 2009). Evidence is also emerging about care at home through telehealth or other information technology modalities to support those who need ongoing health care as they journey through more unstable and complex phases of illness (Darkins et al., 2008). In relation to health applications, there has been a broad adoption of Web 2.0 technologies and approaches in the form of professional and personal use of electronic health records - EHR and PHR (see glossary for discussion of terms). The use of Web 2.0 technologies and/or semantic web and virtual reality approaches can enable social networking and health learning within and between these user groups and clinical carers (Eysenbach, 2008). These developments are based on a wide range of research and research and practice disciplines, and are beyond the scope of the majority of clinicians who are beginning to engage, and thus a operational framework is an important starting point. In addition, we argue that there is immediate need for a frame of reference in order to design patient journey systems for individually tailored care that can address unmet needs in current and future health and e health systems, building on existing knowledge in areas such as chronic disease management (Dorr et al., 2007).

CONCLUSION

Individuals traverse their unique disease and illness pathways through life stages, health systems, and external social and physical environments. There are potentially numerous care relationships, predictable and unpredictable, with positive and negative influences through which the patient must navigate. This is particularly the case for people experiencing phases of illness instability whose decline into hospital admissions could be prevented by timely interventions. Patient journeys take place in systems and these systems need research, education and ongoing designing. A PaJR system is proposed to provide a conceptual framework to purview ongoing activities to ensure patient-centredness in health systems. All in all there is a very strong case for a paradigm shift to placing the patient journey at the centre of knowledge generation and when translated could substantially improve health care systems. *Patient Journey Record Systems* as proposed, would encompass many existing developments in information technology supporting self care and ambulatory care, and to act as a frame of reference for future developments of technology and shift to a systems based approach to health care.

REFERENCES

Alarcon, R. D., & Leetz, K. L. (1998). Cultural intersections in the psychotherapy of borderline personality disorder. *American Journal of Psychotherapy, 52*(2), 176–190.

Andrew, J., & Whyte, F. (2004). The experiences of district nurses caring for people receiving palliative chemotherapy. *International Journal of Palliative Nursing, 10*(3), 110–118, discussion 118.

Barnard, A., Hollingum, C., & Hartfiel, B. (2006). Going on a journey: understanding palliative care nursing. *International Journal of Palliative Nursing, 12*(1), 6–12.

Baron, S. (2009). Evaluating the patient journey approach to ensure health care is centred on patients. *Nursing Times, 105*(22), 20–23.

Battling back from childhood sexual abuse and surviving the journey. (1998). *J Psychosoc Nurs Ment Health Serv, 36*(12), 13-17.

Binkley, L. (1999). Caring for renal patients during loss and bereavement. *EDTNA/ERCA Journal (English Ed.), 25*(2), 45–48.

Biswas, R., Maniam, J., Lee, E. W., Gopal, P., Umakanth, S., & Dahiya, S. (2008). User-driven health care: answering multidimensional information needs in individual patients utilizing post-EBM approaches: an operational model. *Journal of Evaluation in Clinical Practice, 14*(5), 750–760. doi:10.1111/j.1365-2753.2008.00997.x

Blondal, K., & Halldorsdottir, S. (2009). The challenge of caring for patients in pain: from the nurse's perspective. *Journal of Clinical Nursing, 18*(20), 2897–2906. doi:10.1111/j.1365-2702.2009.02794.x

Bond, A., Jones, A., Haynes, R., Tam, M., Denton, E., & Ballantyne, M. (2009). Tackling climate change close to home: mobile breast screening as a model. *Journal of Health Services Research & Policy, 14*(3), 165–167. doi:10.1258/jhsrp.2009.008154

Brownstein, C. A., Brownstein, J. S., Williams, D. S., Wicks, P., & Heywood, J. A. (2009). The power of social networking in medicine. *Nature Biotechnology, 27*(10), 888–890. doi:10.1038/nbt1009-888

Centers, L. C. (2001). Beyond denial and despair: ALS and our heroic potential for hope. *Journal of Palliative Care, 17*(4), 259–264.

Chapple, A., Ziebland, S., & McPherson, A. (2004). Stigma, shame, and blame experienced by patients with lung cancer: qualitative study. *BMJ (Clinical Research Ed.), 328*(7454), 1470. doi:10.1136/bmj.38111.639734.7C

Clare, C., & Bullock, I. (2003). Door to needle times bulls' eye or just bull? The effect of reducing door to needle times on the appropriate administration of thrombolysis: implications and recommendations. *European Journal of Cardiovascular Nursing, 2*(1), 39–45. doi:10.1016/S1474-5151(03)00005-7

Curry, L. C., & Stone, J. G. (1991). The grief process: a preparation for death. *Clinical Nurse Specialist CNS, 5*(1), 17–22. doi:10.1097/00002800-199100510-00007

Darkins, A., Ryan, P., Kobb, R., Foster, L., Edmonson, E., & Wakefield, B. (2008). Care Coordination/Home Telehealth: the systematic implementation of health informatics, home telehealth, and disease management to support the care of veteran patients with chronic conditions. *Telemedicine Journal and e-Health, 14*(10), 1118–1126. doi:10.1089/tmj.2008.0021

Dorr, D., Bonner, L. M., Cohen, A. N., Shoai, R. S., Perrin, R., & Chaney, E. (2007). Informatics Systems to Promote Improved Care for Chronic Illness: A Literature Review. *Journal of the American Medical Informatics Association, 14*(2), 156–163. doi:10.1197/jamia.M2255

Eysenbach, G. (2008). Medicine 2.0: Social Networking, Collaboration, Participation, Apomediation, and Openness. *Journal of Medical Internet Research, 10*(3), 22. doi:10.2196/jmir.1030

Farquhar, M. C., Barclay, S. I., Earl, H., Grande, G. E., Emery, J., & Crawford, R. A. (2005). Barriers to effective communication across the primary/secondary interface: examples from the ovarian cancer patient journey (a qualitative study). *European Journal of Cancer Care, 14*(4), 359–366. doi:10.1111/j.1365-2354.2005.00596.x

Félix-Bortolotti, M. (2009). Part 1 - Unravelling primary health care conceptual predicaments through the lenses of complexity: A position paper for progressive transformation. *Journal of Evaluation in Clinical Practice, 15*(5). doi:10.1111/j.1365-2753.2009.01274.x

Graves, D. L., Shue, C. K., & Arnold, L. (2002). The role of spirituality in patient care: incorporating spirituality training into medical school curriculum. *Academic Medicine, 77*(11), 1167. doi:10.1097/00001888-200211000-00035

Greenhalgh, T., & B, H. (1998). *Why Study Narrative? Narrative Based Medicine: dialogue and discourse in medical practice.*: BMJ Books.

Greenhalgh, T. (2002). Intuition and evidence--uneasy bedfellows? *The British Journal of General Practice, 52*(478), 395–400.

Griffin, I. S., & Fentiman, M. (2002). 17. Psychosocial problems following a diagnosis of breast cancer. *International Journal of Clinical Practice, 56*(9), 672–675.

Hall, B. (2005). Wound care for burn patients in acute rehabilitation settings. *Rehabilitation Nursing, 30*(3), 114–119.

Harmel, M. H. (1986). Monitoring, past, present, future. A personal journey. *International Journal of Clinical Monitoring and Computing, 3*(2), 147–153. doi:10.1007/BF01880768

James, D., Hess, S., Kretzing, J. E. Jr, & Stabile, M. E. (2007). Showing "what right looks like"-- how to improve performance through a paradigm shift around implementation thinking. *Journal of Healthcare Information Management, 21*(1), 54–61.

Jenkins, J. (2006). Survivorship: finding a new balance. *Seminars in Oncology Nursing, 22*(2), 117–125. doi:10.1016/j.soncn.2006.01.007

Jordon, M., Lanham, H. J., Anderson, R. A., & Jr, R. R. M. (2010). Implications of complex adaptive systems theory for interpreting research about health care organizations. *Forum on Systems and Complexity in Health Care in Journal of Evaluation in Clinical Practice, 16*(1), 228–231.

Kelly, M. J., Lloyd, T. D., Marshall, D., Garcea, G., Sutton, C. D., & Beach, M. (2003). A snapshot of MDT working and patient mapping in the UK colorectal cancer centres in 2002. *Colorectal Disease, 5*(6), 577–581. doi:10.1046/j.1463-1318.2003.00531.x

Kerfoot, K. (1998). Management is taught, leadership is learned. *Nursing Economics, 16*(3), 144–145.

Kiteley, C., & Vaitekunas, D. (2006). Leaving our imprints: an exploration into the nurse-patient relationship. *Canadian Oncology Nursing Journal, 16*(3), 180–190.

Klein, G., Moon, B., & Hoffman, R. R. (2006). Making Sense of Sensemaking 1: Alternative Perspectives. *IEEE Intelligent Systems, 21*(2), 70–73. doi:10.1109/MIS.2006.75

Kobayashi, J. S. (1997). The evolution of adjustment issues in HIV/AIDS. *Bulletin of the Menninger Clinic, 61*(2), 146–188.

Lapsley, P., & Groves, T. (2004). The patient's journey: travelling through life with a chronic illness. *BMJ (Clinical Research Ed.), 329*(7466), 582–583. doi:10.1136/bmj.329.7466.582

Leykum, L., Pugh, J., Lawrence, V., Parchman, M., Noel, P., & Cornell, J. (2007). Organizational interventions employing principles of complexity science have improved outcomes for patients with Type II diabetes. *Implementation Science; IS, 2*(1), 28. doi:10.1186/1748-5908-2-28

Martin, C. (1998). The care of chronic illness in general practice.

Martin, C. M. (1998). *The Care of Chronic Illness in General Practice. PhD Thesis.* Australian National University, Canberra.

Martin, C. M. (2007). Chronic disease and illness care: Adding principles of family medicine to address ongoing health system redesign. *Canadian Family Physician Medecin de Famille Canadien, 53*(12), 2086–2091.

Martin, C. M., & Kaufman, T. (2008). (in press). Do physicians have the responsibility to address health inequalities? Going beyond Primary Care to deliver Primary Health Care in our own communities . *Canadian Family Physician Medecin de Famille Canadien.*

Martin, C. M., & Peterson, C. (2008). (in press). The social construction of chronicity:- A key to understanding chronic care transformations. *Journal of Evaluation in Clinical Practice.*

Martin, C. M., & Sturmberg, J. P. (2006). Rethinking general practice – Part 2: Strategies for the future: Patient-centred responsive primary health care and the leadership challenges. *Asia Pacific Journal of Family Medicine, 5*(3).

Martin, C. M., & Sturmberg, J. P. (2009). Perturbing ongoing conversations about systems and complexity in health services and systems. *Journal of Evaluation in Clinical Practice, 15*(3), 549–552. doi:10.1111/j.1365-2753.2009.01164.x

Martin, M., Hin, P., & O'Neill, D. (2004). Acute medical take or subacute-on-chronic medical take? *Irish Medical Journal, 97*(7), 212–214.

Maughan, T. S., Finlay, I. G., & Webster, D. J. (2001). Portfolio learning with cancer patients: an integrated module in undergraduate medical education. *Clinical Oncology (Royal College of Radiologists (Great Britain)), 13*(1), 44–49.

Mayor, V. (2006). Long-term conditions. 3: Being an expert patient. *British Journal of Community Nursing, 11*(2), 59–63.

McGrath, K. M., Bennett, D. M., Ben-Tovim, D. I., Boyages, S. C., Lyons, N. J., & O'Connell, T. J. (2008). Implementing and sustaining transformational change in health care: lessons learnt about clinical process redesign. *The Medical Journal of Australia, 188*(6Suppl), S32–S35.

McLeod, M. E. (2003). The caring physician: a journey in self-exploration and self-care. *The American Journal of Gastroenterology, 98*(10), 2135–2138. doi:10.1111/j.1572-0241.2003.07719.x

McNicholl, M. P., Dunne, K., Garvey, A., Sharkey, R., & Bradley, A. (2006). Using the Liverpool Care Pathway for a dying patient. *Nursing Standard, 20*(38), 46–50.

Meadows, L. M., Lackner, S., & Belic, M. (1997). Irritable bowel syndrome. An exploration of the patient perspective. *Clinical Nursing Research, 6*(2), 156–170. doi:10.1177/105477389700600205

Muir, F. (2007). Placing the patient at the core of teaching. *Medical Teacher, 29*(2-3), 258–260. doi:10.1080/01421590701291477

Peterson, H. E. (2006). From punched cards to computerized patient records: a personal journey. *Yearbook of Medical Informatics,* 180–186.

Pope, C., Ziebland, S., & Mays, N. 1999, E. B. B. (1999). Analysing Qualitative Data In Pope C & Mays N (Eds.), *Qualitative Research in Healthcare* (Second ed.). London: BMJ Books.

Powell-Tuck, J. (2009). Teams, strategies and networks: developments in nutritional support; a personal perspective. *The Proceedings of the Nutrition Society, 68*(3), 289–295. doi:10.1017/S0029665109001311

Richardson, S., Casey, M., & Hider, P. (2007). Following the patient journey: Older persons' experiences of emergency departments and discharge. *Accident and Emergency Nursing, 15*(3), 134–140. doi:10.1016/j.aaen.2007.05.004

Rigaux, N. (2005). [Journey to dementia]. *Psychologie & Neuropsychiatrie du Vieillissement, 3*(2), 107–114.

Rockwood, K., Wallack, M., & Tallis, R. (2003). The treatment of Alzheimer's disease: success short of cure. *The Lancet Neurology, 2*(10), 630–633. doi:10.1016/S1474-4422(03)00533-7

Sikes, P. (2007). *Auto/biographical and narrative approaches.* Retrieved from http://www.bera.ac.uk/autobiographical-and-narrative-approaches/

Storli, S. L., Lindseth, A., & Asplund, K. (2008). A journey in quest of meaning: a hermeneutic-phenomenological study on living with memories from intensive care. *Nursing in Critical Care, 13*(2), 86–96. doi:10.1111/j.1478-5153.2007.00235.x

Sturmberg, J. P., & Martin, C. M. (2006). Rethinking General Practice - Part 1: Far from Equilibrium. Disease-Centred and Econometric-Oriented Health Care and General Practice/Family Medicine. *Asia Pacific Family Medicine, 5*(2).

Sturmberg, J. P., Reid, A., & Khadra, M. H. (2001). Community Based Medical Education in a Rural Area: A New Direction in Undergraduate Training. *The Australian Journal of Rural Health, 9*(Suppl 1), 14–18. doi:10.1046/j.1440-1584.9.s1.6.x

Sturmberg, J. P., Reid, S., & Khadra, M. H. (2002). A Longitudinal, Patient-Centred, Integrated Curriculum: Facilitating Community-Based Education in a Rural Clinical School. *Education for Health, 15*(3), 294–304. doi:10.1080/1357628021000012787

Thorne, S., Armstrong, E. A., Harris, S. R., Hislop, T. G., Kim-Sing, C., & Oglov, V. (2009). Patient real-time and 12-month retrospective perceptions of difficult communications in the cancer diagnostic period. *Qualitative Health Research, 19*(10), 1383–1394. doi:10.1177/1049732309348382

Vegni, E., Mauri, E., & Moja, E. A. (2005). Stories from doctors of patients with pain. A qualitative research on the physicians' perspective. *Supportive Care in Cancer, 13*(1), 18–25. doi:10.1007/s00520-004-0714-2

Ventegodt, S., Andersen, N. J., & Merrick, J. (2003). The life mission theory II. The structure of the life purpose and the ego. *TheScientificWorldJournal, 3,* 1277–1285. doi:10.1100/tsw.2003.114

Venter, J. A., & Hannan, S. J. (2009). A complex case management system provides optimal care for all patients. *Journal of Refractive Surgery (Thorofare, N.J.)*, *25*(7Suppl), S655–S660.

Wales, A. (2005). Managing knowledge to support the patient journey in NHS Scotland: strategic vision and practical reality. *Health Information and Libraries Journal*, *22*(2), 83–95. doi:10.1111/j.1471-1842.2005.00572.x

Wales, A. (2008). A National Health Knowledge Network to support the patient journey. *Health Information and Libraries Journal*, *25*(Suppl 1), 99–102. doi:10.1111/j.1471-1842.2008.00818.x

Walker, R. D., & Hurt, C. D. (1990). *Scientific And Technical Literature: An Introduction To Forms Of Communication*. Amer Library Assn.

Wray, J., & Maynard, L. (2008). Specialist cardiac services: what do young people want? *Cardiology in the Young*, *18*(6), 569–574. doi:10.1017/S104795110800317X

Chapter 7
Patient Journey Record Systems (PaJR) for Preventing Ambulatory Care Sensitive Conditions:
A Developmental Framework

Carmel M. Martin
Trinity College Dublin, Ireland

Rakesh Biswas
People's College of Medical Sciences, India

Joachim Sturmberg
Monash University and The University of Newcastle, Australia

David Topps
Northern Ontario School of Medicine, Canada

Rachel Ellaway
Northern Ontario School of Medicine, Canada

Kevin Smith
National Digital Research Centre, Ireland

ABSTRACT

This chapter articulates key considerations for the translation of the concept of the Patient Journey Record Systems (PaJR) into real world systems. The key concept lies in the 'discovery' of the use of patient narratives to locate the phase of illness in a patient journey. We describe our developmental framework of in the context of Ambulatory Care Sensitive Conditions (ACSC) for older patients with multiple morbidity, who are at a high risk of hospitalizations and other adverse health outcomes. The framework addresses the feasibility and usability of an information technology based solution to avert adverse outcomes of hospitalization when this is potentially avoidable by activities in primary care.

DOI: 10.4018/978-1-60960-097-6.ch007

Key considerations in the PaJR knowledge systems are the design and implementation of robust expert knowledge and data support systems. The patient, caregiver, physician and care team perspectives drive clinical usability and functionality requirements. Experts from computer science domains in artificial intelligence, expert systems, and decision support systems ensure the requirements for the functionality of underlying systems architecture are met. We explore this transdisciplinary perspective and ways in which coherence might be achieved among the many practitioners and expert domains involved in a developmental framework for PaJR. We make a case for the implementation of PaJR systems as part of a universal move to electronic user driven health care.

INTRODUCTION

In this chapter we explore the translation of explicit and tacit knowledge (J. P. Sturmberg & Martin, 2008) about the patient journey into real world systems – the *Patient Journey Record System (PaJR)*. The exploration described in this chapter is from a clinical perspective. We propose a developmental framework to encompass knowledge translation from implicit information to explicit knowledge utilizing many existing developments in health services use of information technology, supporting self care and clinical care. Increasingly, ongoing developments in information technology can, if appropriately designed, provide a way forward for patient-centered user-driven care, particularly for patients with chronic conditions at high risk of decline, or where they or their families have sustained inputs and an ongoing active role in their care.

TRANSLATING NEEDS, IDEAS AND KNOWLEDGE FOR AN INFORMATION TECHNOLOGY-BASED SOLUTION

Understanding Knowledge Translation: A Brief Introduction

Knowledge translation (KT) is the process of transferring research-based knowledge to daily practice. Moving knowledge between users, researchers, inventors, innovators and consumers

should benefit society by improving the well being for its members, and enhancing the economic rewards for its goods and services (Graham & Tetroe, 2007). Knowledge comes in many forms and Lane and Flagg (2010) have identified three stages of development from the concept to operational design to implementation and marketing (Figure 1) (Lane & Flagg, 2010).

The development of a human information knowledge-based system (Kendal & Creen, 2007), involves: "Assessment of the problem; Development of a knowledge-based system shell/structure; Acquisition and structuring of the related information, knowledge and specific preferences for usability and functionality; Implementation of the structured knowledge into knowledge bases; Testing and validation of the inserted knowledge and Integration and maintenance of the system and Revision and evaluation of the system." ("http://en.wikipedia.org/wiki/Knowledge_engineering#cite_note-3," 2009).

Based on this theoretical framework and the PaJR conceptual framework, (Carmel M Martin, Biswas, Joshi, & Sturmberg, 2010) we are developing a prototype IT-solution to integrate patient, carer and clinician knowledge for ongoing close monitoring and more timely intervention for patients with chronic and/or unstable conditions.

A workable prototype implies the development of potential applications that form the basis for intellectual property and claims through patenting. Inventions are more tangible than discoveries,

Figure 1. Stages of knowledge translation from discovery, to invention to innovation.(Lane & Flagg, 2010) with the PaJR knowledge translation steps

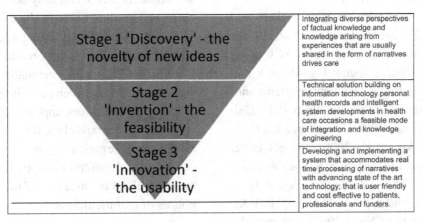

although inventions are still malleable and open to shaping in different ways (Lane & Flagg, 2010). A technology-based solution may be feasible and novel in a controlled setting, but utility is achieved only when the solution addresses the economic and operational constraints of the target user's problem in the context of the marketplace.

The Problem and Context for the PaJR Developmental Framework for Chronic Illness in Relation to Ambulatory Care Sensitive Conditions (ACSC)

"Chronicity" implies ongoing asynchronous and heterogeneous journeys of individuals through disease, illness and care encompassing health promotion, preventative care, diagnosis, self management and self-care support, disease management and control, treatment and palliation (C. Martin, 2007).

We argue that there is an immediate need for a frame of reference in order to design patient journey systems for individually tailored care that can address unmet needs in current and future health and e-health systems. Building on existing knowledge in areas such as chronic disease management (Dorr et al., 2007) and complex adaptive

chronic care models (Martin CM & Sturmberg JP, 2008) is necessary.

Ambulatory care sensitive conditions (ACSCs) are those conditions for which hospital admission could be prevented by interventions in primary care, the majority of which occur in complex phases of chronic care (U.S. Agency for Healthcare Research and Quality, March 12, 2007). Hospital admission may resolve acute destabilization of current health status, but does not necessarily resolve the underlying problem for which people are admitted, and many admissions result in harm due to unintended consequences of interventions including cognitive decline, mental distress, hospital acquired infections and inappropriate use of hospital resources. (Gillick, Serrell, & Gillick, 1982; Htwe, Mushtaq, Robinson, Rosher, & Khardori, 2007; M. Martin, P. Y. Hin, & D. O'Neill, 2004; Podrazik & Whelan, 2008; Shepperd et al., 2009). The problem of ACSCs is increasing in size, as the population ages, which underscores the importance of developing, adopting and implementing innovative programs (Falik, Needleman, Wells, & Korb, 2001). While an adequate supply of primary care services are required to provide interventions to prevent avoidable ACSC events, even in countries with well-developed universal and comprehensive primary care services such as the UK, Canada and Australia, there is, at the individual level, unpredictability in timing the need for an early intervention.

Internationally, health decision makers and service providers are seeking mechanisms for timely interventions to prevent ACSCs using predominately disease-focused guidelines and protocols, selected aged care team programs and/ or and fairly expensive telehealth models (Cai, Johnson, & Hripcsak, 2000; Celler, Lovell, & Basilakis, 2003; Darkins et al., 2008; Fursse, Clarke, Jones, Khemka, & Findlay, 2008; Kim & Oh, 2003; Krumholz et al., 2006) (Bronagh, Helen, & Jane, 2007; Laditka, Laditka, & Mastanduno, 2003; M. Martin, P. Hin, & D. O'Neill, 2004). Although the concept of early intervention may be promising, many inventive/innovative programs to prevent ACSCs are not cost-effective (Armstrong et al., 2008; Gravelle et al., 2007; Malcolm Battersby, 2007). For instance, the Australian Coordinated Care trials have involved a high level of human resources in order for a team to intensely follow a cohort of high risk individuals and have not proved to be cost effective.(Esterman & Ben-Tovim, 2002) Arguably, this is due to intense interventions being continuously deployed to the at-risk population over long periods of time which include a considerable amount of time when they are relatively well rather than distributing intense resources to people only when they are needed. Using linear models of health services research, there is an ongoing view that innovation is concerned with adding new services, rather than reconfiguring existing services. The result are larger teams are the answer making care more complicated and expensive, and more process orientated rather than focused on the individual journey based on affective as well as cognitive knowledge ((Carmel M. Martin, Biswas, Topps, Joshi, & Sturmberg, 2010)

While the use of narrative in electronic records is not in itself new (Kay & Purves, 1998), the *PaJR* approach is 'exploring and discovering' in its combination of multiple narratives around a patient's journey as a temporal framework into which more

or less structured data and services are connected and contextualized. Not only does this provide a more human dimension to the creation and use of health information, it integrates the patient as an active rather than passive participant and helps to reduce some of the inequalities intrinsic to data- and schema-driven models (Kay & Purves, 1998). Our framework supports chronic disease self-management and clinical interventions across all phases of the patient journey, and addresses the need to provide complex adaptive chronic care for those involved in unstable and multidimensional phases of chronic illness.

Development of a Knowledge-Based System Shell/Structure for the PaJR Developmental Framework

We propose that the input of patient and caregiver narratives and semi-structured data will be analyzed with intelligent knowledge systems that provide feedback to physicians and care teams. Identifying the state of "self rated health" or "health" from the patient and care giver narratives is a first step. (See Key Terms and Definitions) (Idler & Benyamini, 1997; J. Sturmberg, Martin, & Moes, 2010) The trajectory of self reported health and personal support arrangements provide the basic knowledge base that would be acquired by the analysis of self reports using various input modes, including text (both email and/or SMS), voice and mobile phones. These data would be coded and analyzed by intelligent agents and developed into a system to track the illness.

The Development of an Expert System

Expert systems are designed to carry the intelligence and information found in the intellect of experts and provide this knowledge to other members of the organization for problem-solving purposes. Problem solving is a mental process and has been defined as higher-order cognitive process that requires the modulation and control of more routine or fundamental skills. Problem solving occurs when an organism or an artificial intelligence system needs to move from a given state to a desired goal state.

In the PaJR project clinical experts, typically primary care physicians and nurses with many years of experience on "narratives and symptoms of decompensation" are asked to provide "rules of thumb" on how they evaluate the problems, both explicitly with the aid of experienced systems developers, and implicitly by evaluating evaluate case vignettes and using computer programs to examine the test data and (in a strictly limited manner) derive rules from their processes. Generally, expert systems are used for problems for which there is no single algorithm or "correct" solution which can be encoded in a conventional algorithm such as in a clinical pathway

Simple systems use simple true/false logic to evaluate data. More sophisticated systems are capable of performing at least some evaluation, taking into account real-world uncertainties, using such methods as fuzzy logic and complexity science. Such sophistication is difficult to develop and still highly imperfect. http://en.wikipedia.org/wiki/Expert_systemaccessed8/03/2010

Expert Systems Shells or Inference Engines

A shell is a complete development environment for building and maintaining knowledge-based applications. It provides a step-by-step methodology, and ideally a user-friendly interface such as a graphical interface, for a knowledge engineer that allows the domain experts themselves to be directly involved in structuring and encoding the knowledge base. http://en.wikipedia.org/wiki/Expert_systemaccessed8/03/2010

Issues to Consider In the Development of the PaJR System

Kevin Smith – IT –knowledge translation and systems design expert

User requirements and functionality are always the key drivers in the designing of intelligent systems for health care.

Firstly – it is important to develop partnerships among the clinicians and the intelligent systems experts. An intelligent system must be derived from multiple perspectives –initially - according to user requirements that then determine functional requirements that shape system design. This is always a non- linear iterative process. In order to derive the user requirements and functionality requires the clinician to engage with AI specialists and natural language processes. – AI or knowledge engineering specialists don't see patients, physicians don't design IT systems. Partnerships and joined up expertise, thus, builds innovation.

PaJR represents a journey, not only of the patient and the caregiver and care team, but also through multiple disciplines. The phases involved in the translational research framework are described below. These disciplines involved in these phases range from clinicians and psychologists to linguists and computational linguists to knowledge engineers and clinical evaluators and researchers.

Assess
  Identify physical, psychosocial and practical needs and problems
Provide
  Structural support - personal and practice continuity, access
  Information/advice on drugs, treatment, lifestyle
  Emotional reassurance and psychosocial counseling
  Appraisal and practical support

Mobilize

> Caregiver and or social agency to enhance physical, psychosocial and practical support
>
> Coordinated and integrated appropriate sources, facilitate structure of support

Training an Expert System for Patients with At Risk of an Ambulatory

The PaJR expert system will be 'trained' to monitor patient and care giver narratives by physicians and nurses who are experienced in the triage and management of people with multiple morbidity and at risk of an ACSC. The training set will be based on real cases and case vignettes of the patient journey as reported by the patient and/or care giver(s), the decisions made in clinical practice and the outcomes observed. Patients and care givers would be trained to record any concerns as soon as they occur and well before they might consider calling their physician or nurse. The expert system would be trained to monitor these narratives to detect changes predicting the need for early intervention.

The advantages of using an expert systems approach in PaJR includes the extension of outreach to multiple patients in an at risk cohort and the provision of early and/or continuous monitoring of individuals by the team on an as needed real time basis, 24 hours a day, 7 days a week. It will achieve this by provision of consistent processing and the maintaining of continual monitoring. However, expert systems are essentially cognitive and they lack 'common sense' and the everyday knowledge of care. They cannot draw on the vast patterns of experience from outside the narrowly focused expert system to address atypical profiles or unusual profiles. Experts need to express both explicit knowledge and implicit knowledge which may be difficult to articulate. Hence there is a need to see such systems as providing sophisticated extensions to facilitate timely access to clinical care and thus earlier decision making care rather than replacing the cognitive and affective skills of clinicians.

The PaJR framework describes a proposal for an innovative user driven, low cost, real time information adaptive solution for the prevention of ASCS (See Figure 2 for the PaJR 'discoveries'). The long-term patient-physician relationship and organizational structures of General Practice and Primary Care ideally provide the nexus for ongoing linking of multiple trajectories. In particular it has been shown that patients can benefit from information and communications technology (ICT) support of self-management (Green, Fortin, Maclure, Macgregor, & Robinson, 2006). Chapter 15 identified the importance of patient and care giver narratives, as they provide physicians and other health care professionals with knowledge

Figure 2. PaJR 'discoveries' are using the framework of Lane and Flagg. (Lane & Flagg, 2010)

'Discovery' State of Knowledge

Patient Journey Record systems (PaJR) as a technology-based solution to the specific problem of Ambulatory Care Sensitive Conditions (ACSC) requires the creation of new knowledge or 'discovery.'

PaJR 'Discoveries'

- **New formulation of existing knowledge and a transdisciplinary approach to ACSC**
- **New Conceptualizing the patient journey in primary care to ACSC**
- **New connections between self rated health perceptions and illness experience literature, new biomedicine models, complex systems knowledge**
- **New methodological approaches linking narrative analysis and intelligent information systems knowledge**

---

about the patient's journey in order to provide timely and appropriate user diver health care (Carmel M. Martin, et al., 2010). Self-rated health and patient perceptions of illness are better predictors of mortality and morbidity than disease-specific parameters (Bayliss, Ellis, & Steiner, 2009; Hubbard, Inoue, & Diehr, 2009; Idler, Russell, & Davis, 2000). (See Key Terms and Definitions)

The patient journey, using a complexity science perspective, can be understood as a journey towards the cusp of a 'catastrophe' of an ambulatory care sensitive condition.(Guastello, 2005)

The risk of an avoidable ACSC remains low while the individuals' health state and their overall sense-making are stable. However, if important factors in biopsychosocial domains change slowly, the individual and their social and care networks usually adapt. However, once these destabilizing factors reach a critical point, a sudden change to high risk, and hence the need for an ACSC alert, occurs. Subcritical risk levels are gradients to the high risk state. Because of the unpredictability of the timing of triggers and enablers of decline on the individual trajectory towards an ACSC adverse event, prior "learning of the system" from real-time data is required to "teach the system" to detect triggers and gradients of decline. A successful system will minimize false positives as well as negatives, and identify changes towards improvements or deterioration. The system will mainly function between the chronic and subacute complex phases in order preempt unstable phases of illness and acute care. It will not be involved if change is very rapid and in acute or very stable stages when narratives and patient data are not recorded.

Currently, prediction theories related to complex nonlinear systems are infrequently used in health research. In fact, complexity theory states that it is not possible to accurately predict outcomes in complex systems, although methods such as Bayesian probability theory, cusp catastrophe theory and the use of mathematical techniques including catastrophe and growth mixture analyses, vector auto regression (VAR), Bayesian VAR and Variance decomposition provide better estimates than simple linear models (Enders, 2003; Guastello, 2005).

Real-time self monitoring of symptoms and experiences is becoming common in specialized areas such as oncology that increasingly relies on sophisticated patient reported outcome measures (Basch et al., 2005; Jones, Snyder, & Wu, 2007). The PROM (patient-reported outcome measures) movement increasing seeks to obtain patient feedback through patient centred measures of experiences of care, in a whole range of areas from prostate surgery to psychological counseling. (Marshall, Haywood, & Fitzpatrick, 2006) Yet, in the US and other countries' primary care, delivery systems are not alerted by real-time patient reported deterioration patterns to intervene cost-effectively in primary care patients who contribute the bulk of ACSCs. Our conceptual framework provides the concepts to build such systems – in this case PaJR.

Expert support and advice, for example, on lifestyle changes such as diet and exercise, are central to health promotion, as is practical advice from individuals, family and peer supports (Ball, Costin, & Lehmann, 2008). Ongoing developments in ICT can provide a way forward for physician supported patient-centered user-driven care, particularly for patients with chronic conditions. Patients and caregivers who take a more active role in care can identify early deterioration patterns to assist timely interventions (Bodenheimer & Grumbach, 2003). Informatics, knowledge systems and complexity science (Darkins, et al., 2008; Mikhail Prokopenko, 2008) are developing fields which offer innovative ways to more effectively manage current health system problems.

Identifying Worsening Illness in Patient and Care Giver Narratives

Narratives of people at risk of ambulatory care sensitive conditions are to be obtained and qualitatively and semantically analyzed in order to develop algorithms to determine phases of illness using expert inputs. A clinical study will test patient and care giver, and clinical team usability. The development of a semantic engine will trawl patient narratives and extract warning signals that indicate that a patient may need early intervention.

In order to identify early warning signs of ill health leading to hospital admissions and develop mechanisms to facilitate early intervention requires

- setting up a patient/caregiver narrative and semi-structured database
- data structuring and semantic analysis of structured data from patients about the journey to emergency medical admissions
- feedback systems to the care team

Evidence is emerging about care at home through telehealth or other information technology modalities to support those who need ongoing health care as they journey through more unstable and complex phases of illness (Darkins, et al., 2008). In relation to health applications, there has been a broad adoption of Web 2.0 technologies and approaches in the form of professional and personal use of electronic health records - EHR and PHR (see Key Terms and Definitions for discussion of terms). The use of Web 2.0 technologies and/or semantic web and virtual reality approaches can enable social networking and health learning within and between these user groups and clinical care (Eysenbach, 2008). These developments are based on a wide range of research and knowledge management disciplines from knowledge engineering, semantic analysis, social constructionism to mathematical modeling of complex systems, and are usually beyond the scope of the majority of clinicians. Nevertheless, clinicians are beginning to engage, and need a developmental framework as an important starting point.

Developing a Real World System: Functionality

There is a requirement to integrate PaJR knowledge generating components into computer systems in order to solve complex problems normally requiring a high level of human expertise. How should user driven (patient and care giver) IT monitoring be designed that alerts primary care teams to the need for early interventions in order to prevent avoidable ACSCs? Can it be done without unnecessarily worrying people, alerting physicians and the team unnecessarily, and missing important changes in health?

The PaJR expert system prototype will be developed to demonstrate that the intelligent system will be established that would continue to learn, under the supervision of experts and with feedback from the outcomes of the patient journey, as more narratives and structured data are added to the PaJR system.

We make the case, building on emerging evidence, that we can, by taking complexity science approaches utilizing semantic analysis techniques, identify patterns of unstable states in the patient journey. We can then identify those phases of the patient journey that are linked to increasing risk for an ACSC in electronically provided self-recorded patient/caregiver information. Katerndahl recently described this approach in the management of patients with anxiety disorders (Katerndahl, 2009).

In order to develop a system that puts the patient and their caregiver at the centre of their care, we need to consider the feasibility of the use of electronic input modes like keyboard or voice by older patients and their care givers. Prototypes, such as the Heartphone where patients use their phone to relay their daily weights to a server that pattern processes their data to detect fluid retention for Congestive Heart Failure Patients, indicate the feasibility of the PaJR concept[1] from a user perspective. ("National Digital Research Centre - Heartphone," 2010). People who would be suitable for the PaJR submit their daily weightings through a mobile phone and both clinicians and patient/caregivers are comfortable with data entry and feedback mechanisms. Similar successful innovations are emerging everyday in a wide range of applications with accumulating evidence of success in major programs associated with cardiovascular, respiratory, diabetes and mental health programs (Darkins, et al., 2008; Department of Fusion Technologies and Nuclear Presidium, 2009; Eysenbach, 2008; Morris, 2005). These programs include disease focused and person-centred approaches. Yet it is often the subjective rather than the objective disease measures which are linked to mortality, morbidity and hospitalization.[2] Ongoing design and development is needed to streamline and operationalize these concepts. Social networking analysis and semantic and computational linguistic analysis (Eysenbach, 2008) are providing potent tools for the analysis of natural and disease related language (Morris, 2005; Zeng et al., 2006) and health concepts (Choi, Jenkins, Cimino, White, & Bakken, 2005). These tools have demonstrable potential for the electronic sharing of narratives in chronic illness (Jui-Chih, 2009), detecting instability in disease patterns such as cardiac disease with weight and symptom monitoring (Goldberger et al., 2002; Jordan, McKeown, Concepcion, Feiner, & Hatzivassiloglou, 2001; Salvador et al., 2005) (Molinari et al., 2004; Scherr et al., 2006) and in the care of elderly in the community (Bendixen, Levy, Olive, Kobb, & Mann, 2009; Bottazzi, Corradi, & Montanari, 2006; Chan, Campo, & Esteve, 2002; Tech, Radhakrishnan, & Subbaraj, 2009). Thus technological advances are converging to deliver more sophisticated and adaptive systems to support our patient journey systems - PaJR.

Developing a Real World System: Usability

Are the users ready? Early adopter physicians and health care professionals have enthusiastically embraced technological and knowledge services (Schoen et al., 2009), although the diffusion, uptake and enthusiasm among the mainstream is uneven and a slower process (Greenhalgh et al., 2004). Will older patients and their caregivers embrace technologies, which provide secondary and tertiary preventive and/or supportive care in chronic disease management (see Table 1)? There is emerging evidence about acceptance of a range of programs, particularly telehealth in heart failure programs (Ralston et al., 2007; Tang, Ash, Bates, Overhage, & Sands, 2006). When people develop unstable chronic disease and illness, their family usually become highly motivated to participate in their relatives or their own health care (C. M. Martin, Peterson, Robinson, & Sturmberg, 2009). On the other hand *"perceived health status"* is a second important influence for adoption, and refers to the patient's expressed physical and mental well being and motivation to improve (Goh, 2008; Venkatesh, Morris, Davis, & Davis, 2004), while a third health ability is defined as the individual *'resources, skills, or proficiencies'* (Venkatesh, et al., 2004), thus making it necessary that PaJR recording be coordinated by family members, if the patient does not have the necessary skills or motivation. Ideally all technological solutions need to take account of the patient and caregiver capacity and health ability.

Testing and Validation of the System

Having demonstrated the feasibility and usability of an expert system in the clinical sense, there is a need to test the reliability and validity of such a system in a real world context. The final stage in the developmental framework is to determine the robustness, functionality and usability, comparing our system assessment of risk with the presence or absence of admissions, visits to the emergency room and visits to primary care. This will involve comparing the real journeys of participants, caregivers and primary care providers with the predicted patient journeys. Did the PaJR system provide timely and usable feedback? Positive

Table 1. Framework for knowledge transfer from theory to practice

1. Assessment of the problem *Ambulatory care sensitive conditions occur partly due to problems of timely intervention for older people with multi-morbidity and un-predictable interactions among physical, psychological, social and environmental factors. While disease monitoring can identify changes in disease states, avoidable admissions and adverse outcomes are a result of nonlinear dynamic interactions among many factors. Research indicates that self rated health and health perceptions are better predictors of adverse outcomes than disease parameters.*
2. Development of a knowledge-based system shell/structure *We propose the input of patient and caregiver narratives and semi-structured data will be analyzed with intelligent knowledge systems that provide feedback to physicians and care teams. Self rated health in the context of patient and care giver narratives provides the basic knowledge base that would be acquired by self reports using mobile phone inputs. This would be coded and analyzed by intelligent agents and developed into a system to track the illness.*
3. Acquisition and structuring of the related information, knowledge & specific preferences for usability & feasibility *Narratives of people at risk of ambulatory care sensitive conditions are to be obtained and then qualitatively and semantically analyzed in order to develop algorithms to determine phases of illness using expert inputs. A clinical study would test patient and care giver, and clinical team usability. The development of a semantic engine to trawl patient narratives and extract*
4. Implementation of structured knowledge into knowledge bases The PaJR expert system prototype would be developed to demonstrate the: - Setting up a patient/caregiver narrative and semi-structured database - Data structuring and semantic analysis of structured data from patients about the journey to emergency medical admissions - Feedback systems to the care team An intelligent system will be established that will continue to learn, under the supervision of experts and with feedback from the outcomes of the patient journey, as more narratives and structured data are added to the PaJR system.
5. Testing and validation of the inserted knowledge and Integration and maintenance of the system The PaJR system would undergo functionality testing - Testing of all features and functions of a system [software, hardware, etc.] to ensure requirements and specifications are met. It focuses solely on the outputs generated in response to selected inputs and execution conditions. Usability testing is a combination of user interface testing and manual support testing to test ease of use, look and feel, ease of access.
6. Revision and evaluation of the system An iterative activity of testing in practice to refine the usability, functionality and reliability in the clinical setting. Because of the unpredictability of the timing of triggers and enablers of decline and the individual trajectory towards an ACSC adverse event, real time intervention around early detection of triggers and enablers of decline will be tested. Such an approach has to deal with early detection, false positives and rapid regression or early resolution.

findings would confirm that the system indeed is able to alert primary health care teams in a timely manner to facilitate and prioritize required care to older patients at risk of ACSCs. Negative findings would inform the field that primary care systems require more development or that the concepts underpinning health IT systems need to be refined, or indeed indicate that the direction of health related technology development must be changed. This is an iterative process and we will endeavor to refine the system until it is deemed functional, usable and robust.

Implementation and Commercialization

The widespread move to electronic health systems will ensure commercial viability of well developed PaJR systems. Major industry players such as Microsoft have embraced the patient journey idea in the design of electronic health information systems - http://www.mscui.net/PatientJourneyDemonstrator/ as have Intel - http://www.itnews.com.au/Event/166187,the-patient-journey-what-role-for-it.aspx amongst many others. Personal health records are proposed as a key mechanism for patient or user driven or at least person-centred health care http://en.wikipedia.org/wiki/Personal_health_record. Personal health records (Bourgeois, Taylor, Emans, Nigrin, &

Mandl, 2008; Detmer, Bloomrosen, Raymond, & Tang, 2008; Winkelman, Leonard, & Rossos, 2005) and mobile phone technology (Bielli et al., 2004; Farmer et al., 2005; Jayaraman, Kennedy, Dutu, & Lawrenson, 2008; Kaplan, 2006; Revere & Dunbar, 2001; Ryan, Cobern, Wheeler, Price, & Tarassenko, 2005; Scherr, et al., 2006) can link to electronic medical records and people can send information and ask questions directly through these technologies. After development and implementation, traditional health service feedback and evaluation and continuous improvement of the system will take place to strengthen the PaJR system.

DISCUSSION

The PaJR for people with complex chronic care must reconfigure new knowledge from narrative based medicine, chronic disease management, chronic illness care theory and complexity science. Clinical research is emerging to support this new approach using patient experience over disease based information to track the phase of illness and stage of care needs.

Currently health information systems are predominantly shaped by professional, organizational— and business-centered ideologies in which the role of the patient is that of a passive subject rather than an active participant (Detmer, et al., 2008). An individual's care pathway is unique, traversing dynamic experiences of health and illness, disease and treatment (Charon, Wyer, & for the NEBM Working Group, 2008). Empowering individual patients by enabling them to take control of their health, illness and disease, significantly improves their outcomes (Wallerstein, 2006). An ICT system that has direct input from and is constructed around the individual patient with chronic disease should enable them to take greater control of their journey. There are numerous care relationships, predictable and unpredictable, as well as positive and negative influences and

feedback loops, through which the patient must pass, hopefully making sense of them as they go.

The informational needs of the primary care team in partnership with other primary care and secondary and tertiary care providers should be supported by the *PaJR*. This meta-system will interdigitate with existing health information systems including the Personal Health Record and the Electronic Health Record, on the one hand supporting self-management and peer support programs and on the other, enabling patients' self-care and self-management of their chronic diseases even in the complicated, complex and chaotic stages of care.

The integration of the patient narrative into more formal informational processes also seeks to reverse the separation that clinical technologies have created between the clinician, caregivers and patient. Heeding subjective meanings and interpretations of their health journey and integrating them with more positivist and instrumentalist data and techniques (Sochalski et al., 2009) allows a degree of humanity and individuality to be reintroduced to an otherwise impersonal and often dehumanizing environment. Sense making is the pivotal concept that emerges in this developmental framework. Sense making at the level of the individual journey is a human activity conducted by the individual in their networks and context. Sense making takes place at different levels by different agents. At the level of care, sense making is essentially a human activity by clinicians that relies on knowledge and relationships with patients with decision making informed by evidence from medical and other knowledge sources. Sense making processes are tacit and explicit. Intelligent systems seek to build upon and replicate elements of the human processes of sense making to improve care. Intelligent systems can support human sense making, the core activity to detect shifts from stable to unstable phases in the patient's illness trajectory that includes their resources for adapting. PaJR must identify critical points in a timely fashion to prevent the deterioration into chaotic phases of the patient's illness journey, so that self management can be enhanced or appropriate and decisive clinical interventions can be taken.

Finally, the provision of and participation in patient care needs to be dynamic and adaptive to an individual's journey through stages of disease and illness. Human support enables patients to make sense of their experiences and optimizes their quality of life. Better planned and more human-focused care supported by electronic expert systems can prevent unnecessary costs which do not contribute to improved personal health experience and quality of life in the phases of end stage chronic disease.

The development of a PaJR-system requires a transdisciplinary approach to seamlessly integrate many layers of different types of knowledge, from clinical need, clinical and health related theory, to evidence systems, and must be able to make sense of natural language inputs to be a robust, usable, functional and marketable system. This outcome can only be achieved iteratively through continuous feedback and evaluation (see Figure 3).

CONCLUSION

Patient Journey Record Systems (PaJR) is an innovative project. The key concept is the use of patient narratives to make sense of the phase of illness of a patient in the context of ambulatory care for older patients, with multiple morbidity, who are at risk for the adverse consequence of hospitalisation. The framework addresses the feasibility and usability of an information technology based solution to avert Ambulatory Care Sensitive Conditions which are potentially avoidable by activities in primary care.

Key features include information feedback to support and enable self management and timely adjustments to care. PaJR architectures, thus, need to encompass self-recorded patient narratives, messages to and from the care team, potentially feeding into electronic health records of different types and configurations. In such a framework patients and clinical experts interact through social networking and sense making occurs through participation in group activities such as learning among hospital teams, primary care teams, patient and caregivers, peer groups and learners at all levels. As an additional layer of

Figure 3. The developmental phases of PaJR with different inputs

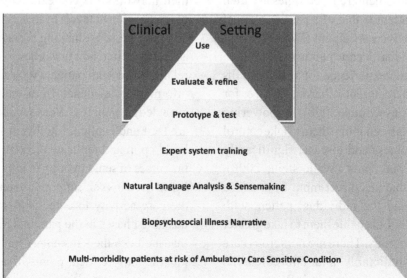

knowledge processing to the human networking, intelligent knowledge systems underpin this by *sense making* using intelligent agents employing advanced pattern processing and reasoning systems to continuously review and analyze the information generated by the narratives and other data in the PaJR.

Key considerations in the implementation and commercialization of PaJR knowledge systems are the design and implementation of robust intelligent knowledge and data support systems. While patient, caregiver and physician and care team perspectives drive usability and functionality requirements, experts from computer science domains such as artificial intelligence, expert systems, and decision support systems ensure the requirements for the underlying systems architecture are met. A transdisciplinary perspective and ways in which coherence might be achieved in the many practitioners and expert domains involved in a developmental framework for PaJR are highlighted. The commercialization of well developed PaJR systems as part of a universal move to electronic user-driven health care is assured if usability, feasibility and functionality are addressed.

REFERENCES

Armstrong, C. D., Hogg, W. E., Lemelin, J., Dahrouge, S., Martin, C., & Viner, G. S. (2008). Home-based intermediate care program vs hospitalization: Cost comparison study. *Canadian Family Physician Medecin de Famille Canadien, 54*(1), 66–73.

Ball, M. J., Costin, M. Y., & Lehmann, C. (2008). The personal health record: consumers banking on their health. *Studies in Health Technology and Informatics, 134*, 35–46.

Basch, E., Artz, D., Dulko, D., Scher, K., Sabbatini, P., & Hensley, M. (2005). Patient Online Self-Reporting of Toxicity Symptoms During Chemotherapy. *Journal of Clinical Oncology, 23*(15), 3552–3561. doi:10.1200/JCO.2005.04.275

Bayliss, E. A., Ellis, J. L., & Steiner, J. F. (2009). Seniors' self-reported multimorbidity captured biopsychosocial factors not incorporated into two other data-based morbidity measures. *J Clin Epidemiol, 62*(5), 550-557 e551.

Bendixen, R. M., Levy, C. E., Olive, E. S., Kobb, R. F., & Mann, W. C. (2009). Cost effectiveness of a telerehabilitation program to support chronically ill and disabled elders in their homes. *Telemedicine Journal and e-Health, 15*(1), 31–38. doi:10.1089/tmj.2008.0046

Bielli, E., Carminati, F., La Capra, S., Lina, M., Brunelli, C., & Tamburini, M. (2004). A Wireless Health Outcomes Monitoring System (WHOMS): development and field testing with cancer patients using mobile phones. *BMC Medical Informatics and Decision Making, 4*(1), 7. doi:10.1186/1472-6947-4-7

Bodenheimer, T., & Grumbach, K. (2003). Electronic technology: a spark to revitalize primary care? *Journal of the American Medical Association, 290*(2), 259–264. doi:10.1001/jama.290.2.259

Bottazzi, D., Corradi, A., & Montanari, R. (2006). Context-aware middleware solutions for anytime and anywhere emergency assistance to elderly people. *IEEE Communications Magazine, 44*(4), 82–90. doi:10.1109/MCOM.2006.1632653

Bourgeois, F. C., Taylor, P. L., Emans, S. J., Nigrin, D. J., & Mandl, K. D. (2008). Whose Personal Control? Creating Private, Personally Controlled Health Records for Pediatric and Adolescent Patients. *Journal of the American Medical Informatics Association, 15*(6), 737–743. doi:10.1197/jamia.M2865

Bronagh, W., Helen, R., & Jane, H. (2007). Emergency hospital admissions for ill-defined conditions amongst older people: a review of the literature. *International Journal of Older People Nursing, 2*(4), 270–277. doi:10.1111/j.1748-3743.2007.00093.x

Cai, J., Johnson, S., & Hripcsak, G. (2000). Generic data modeling for home telemonitoring of chronically ill patients. *Proc AMIA Symp*, 116–120.

Celler, B. G., Lovell, N. H., & Basilakis, J. (2003). Using information technology to improve the management of chronic disease. *The Medical Journal of Australia, 179*(5), 242–246.

Chan, M., Campo, E., & Esteve, D. (2002). Assessment of elderly mobility using a remote multisensor monitoring system. *Studies in Health Technology and Informatics, 90*, 72–77.

Charon, R., & Wyer, P.NEBM Working Group. (2008). Perspectives, Narrative evidence based medicine. *Lancet, 371*(9609), 296–297. doi:10.1016/S0140-6736(08)60156-7

Choi, J., Jenkins, M. L., Cimino, J. J., White, T. M., & Bakken, S. (2005). Toward Semantic Interoperability in Home Health Care: Formally Representing OASIS Items for Integration into a Concept-oriented Terminology. *Journal of the American Medical Informatics Association, 12*(4), 410–417. doi:10.1197/jamia.M1786

Darkins, A., Ryan, P., Kobb, R., Foster, L., Edmonson, E., & Wakefield, B. (2008). Care Coordination/Home Telehealth: the systematic implementation of health informatics, home telehealth, and disease management to support the care of veteran patients with chronic conditions. *Telemedicine Journal and e-Health, 14*(10), 1118–1126. doi:10.1089/tmj.2008.0021

Department of Fusion Technologies and Nuclear Presidium. (2009). *Meta-Knowledge Engineering & Management (MKEM)*. Research Server for High-Intelligent Socio-Cognitive Systems.

Detmer, D. E., Bloomrosen, M., Raymond, B., & Tang, P. (2008). Integrated personal health records: Transformative tools for consumer-centric care. *BMC Medical Informatics and Decision Making, 8*(1), 45. doi:10.1186/1472-6947-8-45

Diez Roux, A. V. (2007). Integrating social and biologic factors in health research: a systems view. *Annals of Epidemiology, 17*(7), 569–574. doi:10.1016/j.annepidem.2007.03.001

Dorr, D., Bonner, L. M., Cohen, A. N., Shoai, R. S., Perrin, R., & Chaney, E. (2007). Informatics Systems to Promote Improved Care for Chronic Illness: A Literature Review. *Journal of the American Medical Informatics Association, 14*(2), 156–163. doi:10.1197/jamia.M2255

Enders, W. (2003). *Applied Econometric Time Series* (2nd ed.). John Wiley & Sons.

Esterman, A. J., & Ben-Tovim, D. I. (2002). The Australian coordinated care trials: success or failure? The second round of trials may provide more answers. *The Medical Journal of Australia, 177*(9), 469–470.

Eysenbach, G. (2008). Medicine 2.0: Social Networking, Collaboration, Participation, Apomediation, and Openness. *Journal of Medical Internet Research, 10*(3), e22. http://www.jmir.org/2008/2003/e2022/. doi:10.2196/jmir.1030

Falik, M., Needleman, J., Wells, B. L., & Korb, J. (2001). Ambulatory care sensitive hospitalizations and emergency visits: experiences of Medicaid patients using federally qualified health centers. *Medical Care, 39*, 551–561. doi:10.1097/00005650-200106000-00004

Farmer, A., Gibson, O., Hayton, P., Bryden, K., Dudley, C., & Neil, A. (2005). A real-time, mobile phone-based telemedicine system to support young adults with type 1 diabetes. *Informatics in Primary Care, 13*(3), 171–177.

Frostholm, L., Ornbol, E., Hansen, H. S., Olesen, F., Weinman, J., & Fink, P. (2010). Which is more important for outcome: the physician's or the patient's understanding of a health problem? A 2-year follow-up study in primary care. *General Hospital Psychiatry, 32*(1), 1–8. doi:10.1016/j.genhosppsych.2009.08.004

Fursse, J., Clarke, M., Jones, R., Khemka, S., & Findlay, G. (2008). Early experience in using telemonitoring for the management of chronic disease in primary care. *Journal of Telemedicine and Telecare, 14*(3), 122–124. doi:10.1258/jtt.2008.003005

Gillick, M. R., Serrell, N. A., & Gillick, L. S. (1982). Adverse consequences of hospitalization in the elderly. [doi: DOI: 10.1016/0277-9536(82)90175-7]. *Social Science & Medicine, 16*(10), 1033-1038.

Goh, J. M. (2008). *Taking Charge of Your Health: The Drivers of Enrollment and Continued Participation? in Online Health Intervention Programs.* Paper presented at the Proceedings of the 41st Annual Hawaii International Conference on System Sciences (HICSS 2008), Hawaii.

Goldberger, A. L., Amaral, L. A. N., Hausdorff, J. M., Ivanov, P. C., Peng, C. K., & Stanley, H. E. (2002). Fractal dynamics in physiology: Alterations with disease and aging. *Proceedings of the National Academy of Sciences of the United States of America, 99*(Suppl 1), 2466–2472. doi:10.1073/pnas.012579499

Graham, I. D., & Tetroe, J. (2007). CIHR Research: How to Translate Health Research Knowledge into Effective Healthcare Action. *Healthcare Quarterly (Toronto, Ont.), 10*(3), 20–22.

Gravelle, H., Dusheiko, M., Sheaff, R., Sargent, P., Boaden, R., & Pickar, S. (2007). Impact of case management (Evercare) on frail elderly patients: controlled before and after analysis of quantitative outcome data. *BMJ (Clinical Research Ed.), 334*, 31–34. doi:10.1136/bmj.39020.413310.55

Green, C. J., Fortin, P., Maclure, M., Macgregor, A., & Robinson, S. (2006). Information system support as a critical success factor for chronic disease management: Necessary but not sufficient. *International Journal of Medical Informatics, 75*(12), 818–828. doi:10.1016/j.ijmedinf.2006.05.042

Greenhalgh, T., Robert, G., Macfarlane, F., Bate, P., Kyriakidou, O., & Peacock, R. (2004). Diffusion of innovations in service organizations: systematic review and recommendations. Storylines of research in diffusion of innovation: a meta-narrative approach to systematic review. *The Milbank Quarterly, 82*(4), 581–629. doi:10.1111/j.0887-378X.2004.00325.x

Guastello, S. J. (2005). Nonlinear methods for the social sciences. In Wheelan, S. (Ed.), *The handbook of group research and practice* (pp. 251–268). Thousand Oaks, CA: Sage.

Htwe, T. H., Mushtaq, A., Robinson, S. B., Rosher, R. B., & Khardori, N. (2007). Infection in the Elderly. [doi: DOI: 10.1016/j.idc.2007.07.006]. *Infectious Disease Clinics of North America, 21*(3), 711-743.

Hubbard, R. A., Inoue, L. Y., & Diehr, P. (2009). Joint modeling of self-rated health and changes in physical functioning. *Journal of the American Statistical Association, 104*(487), 912. doi:10.1198/jasa.2009.ap08423

Idler, E. L., & Benyamini, Y. (1997). Self-rated health and mortality: a review of twenty-seven community studies. *Journal of Health and Social Behavior, 38*(1), 21–37. doi:10.2307/2955359

Idler, E. L., Russell, L. B., & Davis, D. (2000). Survival, functional limitations, and self-rated health in the NHANES I Epidemiologic Follow-up Study, 1992. First National Health and Nutrition Examination Survey. *American Journal of Epidemiology, 152*(9), 874–883. doi:10.1093/aje/152.9.874

Jayaraman, C., Kennedy, P., Dutu, G., & Lawrenson, R. (2008). Use of mobile phone cameras for after-hours triage in primary care. *Journal of Telemedicine and Telecare, 14*(5), 271–274. doi:10.1258/jtt.2008.080303

Jones, J., Snyder, C., & Wu, A. (2007). Issues in the design of Internet-based systems for collecting patient-reported outcomes. *Quality of Life Research, 16*(8), 1407–1417. doi:10.1007/s11136-007-9235-z

Jordan, D. A., McKeown, K. R., Concepcion, K. J., Feiner, S. K., & Hatzivassiloglou, V. (2001). Generation and Evaluation of Intraoperative Inferences for Automated Health Care Briefings on Patient Status After Bypass Surgery. *Journal of the American Medical Informatics Association, 8*(3), 267–280.

Jui-Chih, C. (2009). *Multi-user Narrative Sharing System for Children with Chronic Illness.*

Kaplan, W. (2006). Can the ubiquitous power of mobile phones be used to improve health outcomes in developing countries? *Globalization and Health, 2*(1), 9. doi:10.1186/1744-8603-2-9

Katerndahl, D. A. (2009). Power laws in covariability of anxiety and depression among newly diagnosed patients with major depressive episode, panic disorder and controls. *Journal of Evaluation in Clinical Practice, 15*(3), 565–570. doi:10.1111/j.1365-2753.2009.01166.x

Kay, S., & Purves, I. (1998). The Electronic Medical Record and the "Story Stuff": a narrativistic model. In Greenhalgh, T., & Hurwitz, B. (Eds.), *Narrative Based Medicine: dialogue and discourse in medical practice* (pp. 185–201). London: BMJ Books.

Kendal, S. L., & Creen, M. (2007). *An introduction to knowledge engineering.* London: Springer.

Kim, H. S., & Oh, J. A. (2003). Adherence to diabetes control recommendations: impact of nurse telephone calls. *Journal of Advanced Nursing, 44*(3), 256–261. doi:10.1046/j.1365-2648.2003.02800.x

Krumholz, H. M., Currie, P. M., Riegel, B., Phillips, C. O., Peterson, E. D., & Smith, R. (2006). A Taxonomy for Disease Management: A Scientific Statement From the American Heart Association Disease Management Taxonomy Writing Group. *Circulation, 114*(13), 1432–1445. doi:10.1161/CIRCULATIONAHA.106.177322

Laditka, J. N., Laditka, S. B., & Mastanduno, M. P. (2003). Hospital utilization for ambulatory care sensitive conditions: Health outcome disparities associated with race and ethnicity. *Social Science & Medicine, 57*, 1429–1441. doi:10.1016/S0277-9536(02)00539-7

Lane, J., & Flagg, J. (2010). Translating three states of knowledge - discovery, invention & innovation. *Implementation Science; IS, 5*(1), 9. doi:10.1186/1748-5908-5-9

Lett, H. S., Blumenthal, J. A., Babyak, M. A., Strauman, T. J., Robins, C., & Sherwood, A. (2005). Social support and coronary heart disease: epidemiologic evidence and implications for treatment. *Psychosomatic Medicine, 67*(6), 869–878. doi:10.1097/01.psy.0000188393.73571.0a

Battersby, M., Harvey, P., Mills, P. D., Kalucy, E., Pols, R. G., Frith, P. A., et al. (2007). SA HealthPlus: A Controlled Trial of a Statewide Application of a Generic Model of Chronic Illness Care. *The Milbank Quarterly, 85*(1), 37–67. doi:10.1111/j.1468-0009.2007.00476.x.

Marshall, S., Haywood, K., & Fitzpatrick, R. (2006). Impact of patient-reported outcome measures on routine practice: a structured review. *Journal of Evaluation in Clinical Practice, 12*(5), 559–568. doi:10.1111/j.1365-2753.2006.00650.x

Martin, C. (2007). Chronic Disease and Illness Care: Additional Principles of Family Medicine are needed to address ongoing health system redesign. *Canadian Family Physician, Dec;53(12):2086-91.*

Martin, C. M. (1998). *The Care of Chronic Illness in General Practice. PhD Thesis.* Australian National University, Canberra.

Martin, C. M., Biswas, R., Joshi, A., & Sturmberg, J. (2010). Patient Journey Record Systems (PaJR): The development of a conceptual framework for a patient journey system. Part 1. In Biswas, R., & Martin, C. (Eds.), *User-Driven Healthcare and Narrative Medicine: Utilizing Collaborative Social Networks and Technologies (Vol. 1).* Hershey, PA, USA: IGI Global.

Martin, C. M., Biswas, R., Topps, D., Joshi, A., & Sturmberg, J. (2010). *Patient Journey Systems (PaJS): Narratives and evidence for a paradigm shift. Part 1* (Martin, R. B. C., Ed.).

Martin, C. M., Peterson, C., Robinson, R., & Sturmberg, J. P. (2009). Care for chronic illness in Australian general practice - focus groups of chronic disease self-help groups over 10 years: implications for chronic care systems reforms. *Asia Pacific Family Medicine, 8*(1), 1. doi:10.1186/1447-056X-8-1

Martin CM, & Sturmberg JP. (2008). Complex Adaptive Chronic Care: a framework for health, health care, health systems and policy. *Journal of Evaluation in Clinical Practice.*

Martin, M., Hin, P., & O'Neill, D. (2004). Acute medical take or subacute-on-chronic medical take? *Irish Medical Journal, 97*(7), 212–214.

Martin, M., Hin, P. Y., & O'Neill, D. (2004). Acute medical take or subacute-on-chronic medical take? *Irish Medical Journal, 97*(7), 212–214.

Mikhail Prokopenko, F. B. A. J. R. (2008). An information-theoretic primer on complexity, self-organization, and emergence. *Complexity, 9*(9), NA.

Molinari, G., Valbusa, A., Terrizzano, M., Bazzano, M., Torelli, L., & Girardi, N. (2004). Nine years' experience of telecardiology in primary care. *Journal of Telemedicine and Telecare, 10*(5), 249–253. doi:10.1258/1357633042026297

Morris, M. E. (2005). Social networks as health feedback displays. *IEEE Internet Computing, 9*(5), 29–37. doi:10.1109/MIC.2005.109

National Digital Research Centre. (2010). *Heartphone.* Retreived from http://www.ndrc.ie/projects/heartphone/

Podrazik, P. M., & Whelan, C. T. (2008). Acute Hospital Care for the Elderly Patient: Its Impact on Clinical and Hospital Systems of Care. [doi: DOI: 10.1016/j.mcna.2007.11.004]. *Medical Clinics of North America, 92*(2), 387-406.

Ralston, J. D., Carrell, D., Reid, R., Anderson, M., Moran, M., & Hereford, J. (2007). Patient Web Services Integrated with a Shared Medical Record: Patient Use and Satisfaction. *Journal of the American Medical Informatics Association, 14*(6), 798–806. doi:10.1197/jamia.M2302

Revere, D., & Dunbar, P. J. (2001). Review of Computer-generated Outpatient Health Behavior Interventions: Clinical Encounters "in Absentia". *Journal of the American Medical Informatics Association, 8*(1), 62–79.

Ryan, D., Cobern, W., Wheeler, J., Price, D., & Tarassenko, L. (2005). Mobile phone technology in the management of asthma. *Journal of Telemedicine and Telecare, 11*(Suppl 1), 43–46. doi:10.1258/1357633054461714

Salvador, C. H., Pascual Carrasco, M., Gonzalez de Mingo, M. A., Munoz Carrero, A., Marquez Montes, J., & Sosa Martin, L. (2005). Airmedcardio: a GSM and Internet services-based system for out-of-hospital follow-up of cardiac patients. *IEEE Transactions on Information Technology in Biomedicine*, *9*(1), 73–85. doi:10.1109/TITB.2004.840067

Scherr, D., Zweiker, R., Kollmann, A., Kastner, P., Schreier, G., & Fruhwald, F. M. (2006). Mobile phone-based surveillance of cardiac patients at home. *Journal of Telemedicine and Telecare*, *12*(5), 255–261. doi:10.1258/135763306777889046

Schoen, C., Osborn, R., Doty, M. M., Squires, D., Peugh, J., & Applebaum, S. (2009). A Survey Of Primary Care Physicians In Eleven Countries, 2009: Perspectives On Care, Costs, And Experiences. *Health Affairs*, *28*(6), w1171–w1183. doi:10.1377/hlthaff.28.6.w1171

Shepperd, S., Doll, H., Angus, R. M., Clarke, M. J., Iliffe, S., & Kalra, L. (2009). Avoiding hospital admission through provision of hospital care at home: a systematic review and meta-analysis of individual patient data. *Canadian Medical Association Journal*, *180*(2), 175–182. doi:10.1503/cmaj.081491

Sochalski, J., Jaarsma, T., Krumholz, H. M., Laramee, A., McMurray, J. J. V., & Naylor, M. D. (2009). What Works In Chronic Care Management: The Case Of Heart Failure. *Health Affairs*, *28*(1), 179–189. doi:10.1377/hlthaff.28.1.179

Sturmberg, J., Martin, C., & Moes, M. (2010). (in press). Health at the Centre of Health Systems Reform – How Philosophy Can Inform Policy. *Perspectives in Biology and Medicine*.

Sturmberg, J. P., & Martin, C. M. (2008). Knowing - in Medicine. *Journal of Evaluation in Clinical Practice*, *14*(5), 767–770. doi:10.1111/j.1365-2753.2008.01011.x

Tang, P. C., Ash, J. S., Bates, D. W., Overhage, J. M., & Sands, D. Z. (2006). Personal Health Records: Definitions, Benefits, and Strategies for Overcoming Barriers to Adoption. *Journal of the American Medical Informatics Association*, *13*(2), 121–126. doi:10.1197/jamia.M2025

Tech, M. M., Radhakrishnan, S., & Subbaraj, P. (2009). Elderly patient monitoring system using a wireless sensor network. *Telemedicine Journal and e-Health*, *15*, 73. doi:10.1089/tmj.2008.0056

U.S. Agency for Healthcare Research and Quality. (2007, March 12). AHRQ Quality Indicators— Guide to Prevention Quality Indicators: Hospital Admissions for Ambulatory Care Sensitive Conditions. Retrieved from http://www.qualityindicators.ahrq.gov/downloads/pqi/pqi_guide_v31.pdf

Venkatesh, V., Morris, M. G., Davis, G. B., & Davis, F. D. (2004). User acceptance of information technology: Toward a unified view. *Management Information Systems Quarterly*, *27*(3), 425–478.

Wallerstein, N. (2006). *What is the evidence on effectiveness of empowerment to improve health? Health Evidence Network report*. Copenhagen: WHO Regional Office for Europe.

Wikipedia (2009). *Knowledge Engineering*. Retrieved from http://en.wikipedia.org/wiki/Knowledge_engineering#cite_note-3

Winkelman, W. J., Leonard, K. J., & Rossos, P. G. (2005). Patient-Perceived Usefulness of Online Electronic Medical Records: Employing Grounded Theory in the Development of Information and Communication Technologies for Use by Patients Living with Chronic Illness. *Journal of the American Medical Informatics Association*, *12*(3), 306–314. doi:10.1197/jamia.M1712

Zeng, Q. T., Crowell, J., Plovnick, R. M., Kim, E., Ngo, L., & Dibble, E. (2006). Assisting Consumer Health Information Retrieval with Query Recommendations. *Journal of the American Medical Informatics Association, 13*(1), 80–90. doi:10.1197/jamia.M1820

KEY TERMS AND DEFINITIONS

Ambulatory Care Sensitive Conditions (ACSCs): ACSCs are those conditions for which hospital admission could be prevented by interventions in primary care, the majority of which occur in complex phases of chronic care (U.S. Agency for Healthcare Research and Quality, March 12, 2007).

Electronic Medical Record (EMR): A dataset of the patient's health information that is usually specifically generated, and sometimes owned, by one organization such as a medical clinic, hospital or HMO. This dataset is often more complete is certain areas but tends to be of a less standardized data format. While the patient may to some degree determine who has access to the record, this tends to be coarse grained, with the patient having little control over what is included or excluded from the record.

Health Record Systems: The nomenclature around health record systems varies from region to region. For our purposes, we have adopted the following names and abbreviations but recognize that this is not universal. We hope that clarifying this will help to explain how PaJR interacts with some of these systems. Electronic Health Record (EHR): a subset of the patient's entire information on health related issues. This subset consists of major items that are for general use across multiple systems and organizations, such as allergies, medications, major problems, blood type etc. Because of the broader scope of data

systems, this subset is necessarily simplified and adheres more closely to data standards.

Multimorbidity: (Bayliss, et al., 2009; Boyd et al., 2007; Fortin et al.) Can be defined as the simultaneous occurrence of several medical conditions in the same person. While definitions vary, prevalence varies from up to 27% in early adult hood to over 90% of GP attenders in the older age groups. In primary care settings multi-morbidity is the rule rather than the exception.(Carmel M Martin, 1998) Ambulatory Care sensitive conditions predominantly occur in older patients with multiple morbidity.(U.S. Agency for Healthcare Research and Quality, March 12, 2007)

Personal Health Record (PHR): Also known as 'Personal Health Application Platforms' and 'Personally Controlled Health Records', this is a new concept, not yet widely accepted, where the dataset may be generated by a wide range of providers or organizations but the key feature is that the patient has control over what is included or excluded, usually with the consent of the originating authority, and that the patient has complete control over who has access to this information, with ownership residing in the patient's hands. Data storage is often managed by a secure third-party, not related to the originating authorities. Personal Health Application Platforms and Personally Controlled Health Records' such as Google Health, Microsoft Health Vault, and Dossia. "Medicine 2.0" applications, services and tools, are defined as Web-based services for health care consumers (that is caregivers, patients,) health professionals, and researchers. (Eysenbach, 2008)

Self-Rated Health, Illness and Outcome Prediction: Self-rated health and illness perceptions are better predictors of morbidity and mortality than disease specific measures.(Hubbard, et al., 2009; Idler & Benyamini, 1997) Additionally, GPs' perceptions of their patients' understanding were accurate in 82% of the consultations, but when the patients had a both physical and psychological understanding of their health problem, the GPs were right in only 26% of the consultations.(Frostholm et al., 2010; Hubbard, et al., 2009)

Social Support: Social support can be simply defined as the availability of people on whom patients feel that they can depend.(Diez Roux, 2007; Lett et al., 2005) It comprises the following support domains – intimate, emotional, informational, structural, practical, appraisal and companionship and friendship.(Carmel M Martin, 1998)

ENDNOTES

[1]   Heartphone is developing a web-based system to support the management of chronic Ilnesses, using mobile technology in the home to measure and report on vital patient data including blood pressure, weight and medication levels. The project will allow medical professionals to get real-time information on patients, presenting the prospect of more timely intervention

[2]   Personal communication from heartphone is that the self assessed health status better predicted adverse outcomes than disease based measures in a population with cardiac failure.

Chapter 8
Multiple Paths in Health Care

Susan D. Ross
Consultant Internal Medicine, USA

ABSTRACT

The personal experience of Medicine by each physician is the product of a large number of dynamic and diverse factors: inborn talents and deficiencies, social and cultural environments, type of schooling, exposure to teachers and mentors, colleagues, family and friends, and of course, perhaps most important of all, encounters with patients. Many of these influences are beyond the direct control of the physician, and nearly all continue to change throughout a lifetime. Out of this seemingly random and chaotic mix of influences, each physician develops his or her own highly unique, and ever evolving understanding of what it means to practice Medicine today.

INTRODUCTION

If a thousand different physicians were to write their stories, you'd have a thousand different experiences of Medicine. If one physician were to write her story several times during her career, you'd likely have several different understandings yet again. Yet in all cases, perhaps some common lessons could be discerned. This chapter relays a few selected lessons learned by one physician over many years in practice.

DOI: 10.4018/978-1-60960-097-6.ch008

There Are Multiple Career Paths In Medicine

This advice was first given to me by my future father-in-law, a pediatric psychiatrist practicing for many years in Philadelphia. He told me this as I approached my graduation from university. I was trying to figure out what to do with my undergraduate bachelor's degree in experimental psychology. Although I had originally chosen it purely out of interest in the subject, when it came time to graduate and find a job, it appeared to be a useless degree. My only option seemed to be to continue on in academia to pursue graduate studies in psychology, but this option just didn't interest me.

While I knew what I *didn't* want to do, I had no idea what I *did* want to do, until my boyfriend's father suggested a career in Medicine. Yes, it is a good living in this country, but he also emphasized the intellectual and human rewards of studying and practicing Medicine. And he underlined the flexibility it affords women in particular, in terms of type of practice and hours of practice. He sold me on the idea.

Luckily I had already taken nearly all of the required subjects, except one, Organic Chemistry. So this course I took at a different university near my home town, while I lived in my parent's home and worked in a warehouse putting price tags on fancy women's clothing to be sold in high-end shops. (That was a unique educational experience too, but that is another story!). I did well in the chemistry course, and took my Medical College Admission Test (MCAT). My Verbal score was stellar, but my Science score was not. So I continued to study while working my warehouse job, followed by a dull office job, both of which convinced me more than ever that I just *had* to gain admission to medical school. Eventually, I succeeded in raising my MCAT Science score, and I was granted admission to the Faculty of Medicine in Toronto. And that open door changed everything, forever.

I have now been out in the world, practicing Internal Medicine, for twenty-six years. I have practiced in both Canada and the U.S., in both a hospital practice as well as an office practice, in a country with universal health care and in a country with free-market health care. I have worked as a clinical investigator writing protocols and treating patients on clinical trials. I have been part of senior management in a biotech company. I have been an entrepreneur in co-founding another company, MetaWorks, a consultancy specializing

in systematic reviews and meta-analyses. I have been the Medical Director of an AHRQ Evidence-based Practice Center (at MetaWorks), and more recently, an independent consultant in Evidence-based Medicine. And I have worked as a volunteer physician in a local clinic for uninsured people.

None of the paths I have taken over my many years in Medicine were planned at the beginning of my career. Not one. I never had a master plan for my life in Medicine. Perhaps some do, but I didn't. Instead, I have pursued paths that opened up to me along the way. And those paths have been many and diverse.

All this is to say that I am living proof that my father-in-law was right - there *are* multiple career paths in Medicine. To those contemplating a life in Medicine, my advice is simple – do it! In Medicine, there are countless opportunities throughout your career to go in whatever direction your talents, interests, and energy might lead you. Cliché? Perhaps. But nonetheless true. If you seek purely financial rewards, get an MBA and work in business. But if you seek a deeper understanding and experience of life, get a medical degree and choose your paths.

Beware of Dogma!

In the Spring of my final year of residency in Internal Medicine at a downtown teaching hospital in Toronto, I met with my residency program advisor. These meetings were required of all senior residents, and intended as a forum to advise residents regarding professional career paths after completion of training. Dr. C exuded confidence and great skill at the bedside, and I admired his clinical acumen. I looked forward to our discussion of my plans for life after residency. Not that I had anything definite in mind. I'd hoped that maybe I'd be invited to stay on in the teaching hospital, as a junior faculty member. But that hadn't materialized. Although I had excelled at the bedside, my Chief of Medicine had told me that she didn't believe I had shown due deference to my superiors, that my skeptical attitude was not appreciated. This surprised me, for in general I honored the academics who had been my only role models in Medicine to date. But I was not always readily accepting of what I perceived to be dogma. So, feeling somewhat rejected and worried about my upcoming transition to real-life clinical Medicine, I was job hunting.

Dr. C. read me like a book. He opened the conversation by saying that the academic life wasn't all it's cracked up to be. I was genuinely surprised to hear his comments about the petty politics, tedious administrative tasks, and ivory tower mindsets of academia. And he promised me that I would love real-life clinical practice in the community. He was right, at least regarding my eventual jump into a community hospital-based practice of Internal Medicine. From these new trenches out on the 'front line', the foibles of academics back at 'headquarters' seemed almost humorous at times. But I rarely thought about the academic world I'd left behind until many years later, after I'd relocated to Boston.

Soon after arriving in Boston, I joined an outpatient practice in an upscale suburban community, but I soon tired of dealing with the 'worried well'. And the financial transactions inherent in American-style practice both confused and repulsed me. So I jumped into a clinical research position at a local biotech company. I loved the basic science, and the challenge of developing a useful evidence base from a clinical trial program that we designed. And I was able to continue to see patients in a center-city hospital, only now as a clinical researcher.

Working with an advisory group of nationally recognized academic experts in the treatment of kidney cancer, my biotech colleagues and I designed a randomized controlled trial of the company's experimental immune treatment. This was a make-or-break study for our group, and would provide a pivotal piece of evidence in support of FDA approval. These academic advisors were quite dogmatic, and gave their very strong and nearly unanimous opinions about what the control treatment should be in our trial, and what the expected median survival time with that treatment should be. Suitably impressed with their collective gravitas, we believed them, and designed the trial accordingly.

I left the company shortly thereafter, to pursue independent consulting in clinical research–Boston was a hotbed of biotech start-ups at the time, so there was plenty for me to do. (And the hours–no call–were ideally suited to the requirements of mothering my young family). But three years later I heard that our kidney cancer trial had failed. And it failed for an unexpected reason, not because the experimental treatment failed, but because the control group outcome was better than predicted by the experts. The control group median survival time was a few months longer than estimated by the experts, which was great news for those patients, but which effectively voided the trial design. For now, with the between-group differences in survival time smaller than originally planned, the sample size was clearly insufficient for the observed difference between groups to reach statistical significance.

When I heard this news, I'd already joined forces with Dr. Thomas Chalmers from the Harvard School of Public Health to form a consultancy called MetaWorks. We performed systematic reviews and meta-analyses for our early clients–hospitals, drug companies, and non-profits, mostly– in order to provide the 'best available evidence' for healthcare decision-making. My old biotech employer asked us to retrospectively perform a literature review of relevant studies published up to the date of the planning stage of their failed trial. They were hoping to show that the trial's control group result was an unpredictable aberration. But no, that was not what we found. Instead, our literature review and analysis showed that the control group outcome could've been predicted much more accurately – at the time - using these tools of Evidence-based Medicine rather than relying upon the advice of those academic experts.

Why did the experts get it wrong? Perhaps because as physicians we are all trained to be willing to make decisions in the face of uncertainty. The experts were comfortable trusting their opinions, opinions informed by their own experience, and so was I. But perhaps their opinions could've been better informed ? In a seminal publication in JAMA (Antman, Lau, Kupelnick, Mosteller, & Chalmers, 1992), the authors provided several case examples of exactly this problem – expert opinion lagging behind the evidence. Unfortunately, the company ran out of funds to continue with more clinical trials, so the experimental program was closed down. There were many lessons from this failure, not the least of which is that not even academics are infallible. Dogma typically lags, and sometimes even rejects, what is knowable.

At MetaWorks we were often challenged by very intelligent people working not in academia, but in drug and biotech companies, to extend our thinking to solve new analysis problems. I learned first-hand that some of the most creative, outside-the-box thinkers are located not in academia, but outside of it. I won't speculate as to reasons why this is so, but I would like young medical students to realize that while there may be much that is attractive about academic Medicine, it is also true that academics do not have a monopoly on creativity or brilliance, nor do they necessarily have the steady stream of opportunities for creative problem solving that present to those in clinical practice or industrial research settings. I believe that the need to solve real-world problems forces creativity in finding solutions. Application advances theory. And I believe that the inter-disciplinary cross pollination that is fostered by our wired global community increases the likelihood that great leaps forward in the human scientific knowledge base, Medicine included, will happen

outside of those academic settings where, all to often, creativity doesn't get funded and conformist attitudes are required for advancement.

This experience only served to reinforce my life-long predilection to reject thinking that is overly authoritative. (I am a baby-boomer, after all!) And it fueled my excitement about the promise of Evidence-based Medicine (EBM), a promise I sought to develop and apply for over ten years at MetaWorks. At its core, EBM is a skeptic too. I admire its "show-me-the-facts" attitude. But when EBM proponents treat EBM itself as dogma, they ruin it. EBM experts currently threaten their own foundations when they close their minds to new and evolving, but non-traditional, sources of evidence in Medicine. With the advent of social networks and global telecommunications, the possibility of coupling the power of collective experience with the power of EBM is a potential 'force-multiplier' for healthcare.

Although Never Easy, it is Indeed Possible, and Enriching, to Juggle Family and Career in Medicine

During my third year as a medical student I started to experience strange bodily symptoms that were new to me, and worrisome. Since medical students sometimes do imagine that they've contracted whatever new disease they're reading about, this was not altogether unusual. I noted that I had all the symptoms of pregnancy, but of course, that was not possible, as I was using an IUD for contraception. My husband laughed at this newest condition to add to my growing list of imaginary conditions. Yet, the symptoms persisted. So off I went to my gynecologist, the one who had originally placed the IUD. He examined me, and did some tests, and told me that I was definitely not pregnant, just 'stressed out'. I was relieved, but puzzled, as I didn't really feel any more stressed out than usual. Another month went by, and still no period, so back I went to my doctor's office. And again, he assured me this was 'all in my head'. I just needed to try to relax a bit more. Instead, I stopped by a drug store on my way home, for I was not quite willing to believe him. I picked up a urine collection kit for a pregnancy test. I brought my little sample back to the store later that day (that was before self-testing kits were available), and called them the next afternoon for the results. "Honey, your test says you are pregnant." "What?" "You're pregnant! Understand?"

I hung up the phone, reeling with the news. I was shocked, but at the same time, not completely surprised, for I just knew *something* unusual had been happening to my body for the past few months, and it hadn't all been 'in my head'. My immediate fear was that this would put an end to my medical career, before it ever really had a chance to get started. I loved Medicine, and the thought of giving it up was crushing. But then, with my ever optimistic husband cheering me up, I gradually believed him. We *could* handle this. We *would* manage. And manage it we did.

I delivered a healthy baby – and that useless IUD! - on the night before my Urology final exam. I'd been studying so hard all day that I never even realized I was in labor until my water broke and flowed like Niagara Falls out our bedroom door, across the slanted hallway, and down the stairs, puddling in the parlor below. Post-delivery complications kept me in the hospital for ten more days. Being a patient was miserable, humbling, and truly eye-opening for a young doctor-in-training. Luckily, by the kindness of an assistant dean at my medical school, and other relevant faculty, my final exams were either delayed for a few months, or commuted permanently. Without really missing a beat, I eventually resumed my fourth year, one of rotating clinical clerkships at a downtown hospital, after an eight week 'elective' period that had been worked into the start of my year's schedule. To get credit for this elective, I'd spent it at home with my new daughter while writing a research paper - on breastfeeding, of course!

So I was thrilled to still be on track to graduate with my class, but each morning was excruciating for me, leaving my baby with her nanny, so I could go off and spend untold hours away from her, at the hospital. And while at the hospital, every time I heard an ambulance come screaming into our Emergency Room, I had a panic attack. I was convinced that something horrible had happened at home to my baby. I knew this was ridiculous, but I couldn't help myself. Sometimes I just had to stop what I was doing and call home to ask our nanny about her. Sometime I would just run down to the ER to be sure my worries were unfounded.

My private distress must have been noticeable. One day the attending physician on my current rotation, in-patient Psychiatry, invited me to lunch with him at a little Italian restaurant across the street from the hospital. As expected, he asked me for feedback on the rotation thus far, and wanted to know how well I liked, or disliked, Psychiatry. He then proceeded to tell me his rather unusual professional path. He had started out as a surgeon, but after several years, he had decided he was missing that sense of satisfaction he expected from his work. He wanted to talk to people, not cut them. So he switched into Psychiatry, and never looked back. He had found his true calling.

I was impressed by his willingness to open up like that with me, a lowly medical student. So I reciprocated, when he asked me how things were going with my clerkship overall. I told him how hard it was to spend so much time away from my baby daughter, even though I really loved what I was doing at the hospital. I guess he could see I was seriously conflicted, quietly suffering. He was thoughtful for a moment, and then gave me some wonderful advice, based upon his own experience as a single father raising two daughters. I'll paraphrase what he said, "Medicine is a huge time commitment. There's no getting around it. Since you can't be with your kids all the time, the best advice I can give you is this: be there for the most important moments of each day. And what are those? Mealtime, bathtime, and bedtime.

That's it. Focus on those times. Those are the most important times for any child, so be there as much as you can for those times, and don't feel too bad for missing the other times. Your kids will grow up just fine. They don't need Mommy there while they're sleeping, or during every waking moment. Just remember that. Your life will be easier, and mark my words, I am right on this." And he was.

I followed his advice as best I could. And it seemed to work. As the months went by, I could see that my daughter was happy and thriving, and I no longer felt so anxious and unhappy. I continued to follow his advice, as I went on to have another baby during my second year of residency, and two more later, when I was in practice as a hospital-based Internist in Toronto. As much as I love Medicine, I must say that raising these four children with my husband has been the absolute best endeavor of all.

So here is my particular advice for all you present and future medical women who may be reading this: Once you and your partner *know* that you would like to 'someday' have children, do not delay. 'Someday' is now. Forget your plans to wait until a better, more convenient time. There will *never* be a perfectly *convenient* time. I know what you are thinking, "This lady is advising professional suicide." But I speak from experience. I have learned through that unplanned first pregnancy early in my career that there is *never* an impossible time to have a baby, unless of course you wait until your biological clock ticks out. All times are workable, but sooner is definitely better. Don't listen to those who advise you to wait until your formal training is finished and you are established in practice. I highly doubt they speak from personal experience.

And my advice to everyone of both genders? When your colleagues are kind and generous to you, recognize it for the precious gift it is, and pay it back in kind, at every opportunity. That respect and love of your colleagues is at the very core of this profession's age-old practice of professional courtesy. Do not let that tradition die.

Respect Your Position as a Member of an Ancient and Honorable Profession: A Physician is, First and Foremost, a Healer

I recently returned to the land of clinical Medicine after a long time away as a co-founder and chief scientist at MetaWorks, a consultancy in Evidence-based Medicine. Like any traveler coming home after a long absence, seeing a familiar landscape with new eyes, I notice things now that I didn't see before. One of the more obvious changes is in physician attire. I see that doctors - at least in outpatient settings - rarely wear white coats anymore. Why is this?

I hesitated to ask my colleagues, in case the answer was so patently obvious that I'd be instantly judged a fool for even asking. So I went to the literature instead, and performed a completely unsystematic review. Nevertheless, what I found was enlightening.

First, I learned that my impressions are probably true. In 1991, more than 70% of hospital doctors and medical students wore a white coat more than 75% of the time (Farraj & Baron, 1991) whereas a study in 2004 showed that only 13% of physicians chose to wear a white coat (Douse, Derrett-Smith, Dheda, & Dilworth, 2004). I also found several studies of various designs that showed the majority of patients prefer their physicians to wear white coats (Brase, 2006; Cha, 2004; Dunn, 1987; Gooden, 2001; Nair, 2002) and this includes children (Matsui, 1998; Barrett, 1994) and their parents (Gonzalez Del Rey & Paul, 1995). And it's not just hospitalized or ER patients. Some of the strongest evidence comes from out-patient settings (Rehman, Nietert, Cope, & Kilpatrick, 2005). These studies have also shown that these patient preferences apply to both male and female physicians. And it appears that patient preference for the white coat is not necessarily a factor of a particular healthcare system, as this effect has been reported in the U.S., England, Canada, and Australia.

So if patients clearly prefer their physicians to wear white coats, why don't doctors wear them anymore? It has been said that fears of transmitting infection are the main reason, but I don't buy this. A neck tie or wristwatch might also transmit infection, yet I don't see these items dropping by the wayside as white coats have. Despite no good evidence supporting infection risk (Bazaz & Brown, 2007), the National Health Service in the U.K., in its effort to control hospital-acquired infections, recently outlawed the white coat (along with wristwatches!) in its "bare below the elbows" policy (BMA Central Consultants & Specialists Committee, 2007).

Are there other reasons why white coats are unpopular among physicians? Perhaps it's attributable to one of several different "white coat effects", such as negative effects upon the therapeutic milieu in psychiatry, or blood pressure measurement in the office. But I doubt these are the reasons most docs have abandoned their white coats. I expect they are just trying to level the playing field with their patients, trying to remove any perceived barriers that the white coat, as a symbol of authority (and power), might induce. But isn't authority what patients seek from their caregivers? Sure, they also seek warmth and friendliness, a caring attitude, but authority and compassion are not mutually exclusive. If leveling the relationship removes the trust in expertise that is at the heart of the therapeutic relationship, how could that be a good thing? Delivering patient care is a service, to be sure, but it is not the same as other types of service delivery models in our consumer society. When people who are sick or worried come to the doctor for help, their expectations are not the same as when they go to Macy's to buy a sweater, or to a fast food joint to buy hamburgers. Or are they? In our market driven culture, perhaps some would argue that these service delivery models should be the same. And perhaps for those trapped in assembly-line clinical practices, it feels like they already are!

Of course, the more obvious advantages of white coats to those old school physicians like me who actually like wearing them is a) the big pockets hold manuals, a source of portable knowledge (although with PDAs and point-of-care computers, this may not be as important as it used to be); b) they protect your own clothing; c) they help patients readily identify you as 'the doctor'. But even if we discount all these reasons for wearing a white coat, we cannot discount the fact that – rightly or wrongly - the white coat conveys authority and expertise to patients. Some might scoff at the idea that something so seemingly trivial might have a healing effect. But I suspect those who scoff are doing so from a position of health and confidence. Who are we to assume that the white coat has no meaning to the sick, the worried, the debilitated? Studies like those referenced above suggest otherwise. Isn't this what white coat ceremonies at medical schools are all about?

At my medical school, I don't remember having a white coat ceremony. But I remember well the bedside teaching I received from a senior internist who seemed to be the embodiment of wisdom. He said we must always do four very simple things in our encounters with patients: 1) *sit*, no matter how busy you are, even if only for a couple of minutes; 2) *touch*, however briefly– a handshake, or a handhold, makes a human connection; 3) *listen* – your patients will *always* tell you their diagnoses, if you let them; 4) *look* like a doctor – meaning grooming, speech, and attire – for your very presence is powerful and therapeutic. These simple lessons I have tried to apply in patient encounters ever since, whether in the office or in the hospital. I have no data to prove it, but I believe those small gestures go a very long way in establishing a connection that is necessary to patient trust, which in turn is critical to establishing a therapeutic relationship.

We worry a lot nowadays about losing our professionalism in Medicine, and blame external forces for our declining morale. But as far as I can tell, no one is forcing us to abandon the powerful symbols of our profession (except in the U.K.!). Doctors are doing this of their own volition. I would counter with this: If physicians really want to help patients – 'putting patients first' – shouldn't we strive to establish strong therapeutic relationships? The white coat may be 'only' a symbol, but knowing the power of this particular symbol to strengthen the therapeutic relationship, shouldn't we put our white coats back on?

If you are convinced of your goals, push as hard as you can. But your plans? Those are what make God laugh. Relax and let the currents take you - they probably will anyway. To paraphrase John Lennon: Life is what happens when you're making other plans.

In 1986 I was in my third post-residency year of practice. I had a part-time office practice, primarily for endocrine patients, but most of my time and energy was spent in a hospital-based Internal Medicine practice in a Toronto suburban hospital. I took all emergency medical admissions every fifth day/night, which usually totaled between five and ten new patients with diabetes out-of-control, myocardial infarctions or unstable angina or heart failure, COPD exacerbations, drug overdoses, and so on. That practice kept me incredibly busy, and seven days a week I was at the hospital.

Although it was a very demanding practice, I loved everything about it, except the lack of any real time to be completely 'offline' with my family. On weekends my two oldest children even accompanied me to the hospital, just to have some 'Mommy time'. They'd wait happily at the nursing station, eating candy supplied by kind nurses, or drawing pictures, while I quickly rounded on my ward patients. But this was a band-aid solution to the need for more family time. The need to be constantly available, even if only by phone or pager, started to wear me down.

I was in that weary state when the Ontario doctors went on strike to demand higher pay.

This event shook my world to the core. I think most physicians anywhere cannot imagine turning people away from the hospital, standing on the sidewalk outside the ER sending ambulances away. But that is exactly what happened. And all elective procedures were cancelled as a strict 'work to rule' practice was implemented. I was asked to join in, but I could not bring myself to do it. I was asked to join the doctors marching, carrying signs and chanting slogans, up University Avenue to Queen's Park, home of Ontario's Parliament. I could not do it. I was so disheartened by the strike. It went against everything I had so recently internalized about the nobility of the practice of Medicine. Luckily, the strike did not last long, but my joy and pride in the profession were seriously damaged.

Why did the doctors go on strike? In Ontario, there was universal healthcare, run by the government. On the one hand, I really liked never having to worry about monetary transactions with patients. The doctor-patient relationship was pure. But, on the other hand, there were indeed serious problems with Ontario's system. Pay rates for doctors were low and not rising with inflation. And the availability of services for patient care was quite poor for a Western nation, and getting worse as the years went by. Politicians of the ruling party determined healthcare budgets year to year, and it seemed there was a constant ratcheting back of everything. At my suburban hospital, there was always insufficient staffing, leading to bed closures, leading to inability to move admitted patients out of the ER, leading to the all-too-frequent need to divert ambulances trying to bring sick patients to our hospital. I always had some of my admitted patients staying on stretchers in hallways in the ER for two, sometimes three, days at a time. It was like a MASH unit on the front lines of battle. And it was particularly frustrating because there were beds aplenty upstairs on the medical wards, just not enough nurses to staff them. Some of my patients received all of their needed care in the

ER over several days, and were discharged home before they ever made it upstairs to a ward bed.

But my tipping point was reached shortly after the doctors' strike. One night when I was on call, a 36 year old man with multiple acute and chronic renal, metabolic, cardiovascular, and neuropathic complications of long-standing Type 1 diabetes was delivered by ambulance to our ER. That is where he died, after spending a day and a half on a stretcher in the hallway waiting in vain for an ICU bed. Our ICU beds were all occupied by equally sick patients, so, after temporarily stabilizing him, the nurses and I got on the phone and tried desperately to find another hospital anywhere in the city that had an open ICU bed he could be transferred to. But not one could take him. They were all completely maxed out. So, when this young man died, right there in the chaotic hallway, I gave up on Canada.

I decided I'd had enough of trying to practice good Medicine in that environment, and I moved back south of the border from whence I came. I moved to Boston, and started practicing office-based Internal Medicine in a suburban HMO practice. And I was amazed at the differences in service availability. For instance, every little town in the suburbs around Boston had its own MRI. Waiting times for scans were mere hours! When I left Toronto, there were but two MRIs in the entire city, and waiting times for non-emergent scans were over six months! I had jumped from famine to feast.

Yet so many patients were not admitted to this feast. I soon learned that in the U.S., healthcare is no less rationed than in Canada. In the U.S., access is limited by lack of health insurance. In Canada, access is limited by lack of services. The result is the same. In both systems, healthcare is effectively rationed. I don't know the solution, but suspect that as long as resources are finite, and demand is essentially infinite, there is no solution that will satisfy everyone. Some type of rationing may thus be necessary, but neither Canada nor the U.S. have got it right yet.

So while, the serious inequities in Americans' access to healthcare came as another rude awakening for me, what made me most restless and unsatisfied with clinical practice was the pervasive emphasis on healthcare as a financial transaction. I didn't understand the byzantine complexities of billing and payments in the U.S. - I still don't. I looked around for alternative paths, and found there were many.

I decided to try something completely new and different, yet still in Medicine, so I jumped into a salaried clinical research position at a venture-funded immunotherapy clinic at a Boston hospital. This nascent enterprise quickly morphed into a full-fledged biotech company, riding the explosion of knowledge about the immune system. I rode this biotech wave for four exciting years. It was my 'residency', so to speak, in immunology, in clinical research methods, and in entrepreneurship. And I was still seeing patients, albeit now as a researcher. Monetary transactions with patients did not enter my day-to-day world, and I was happier for it.

But as a researcher, I quickly realized the constant difficulty of getting my hands on the best information, and getting it when I needed it. I spent a lot of time in the library, and talking to experts, but never was confident in the information I culled from these sources. I needed the best available information to design the best clinical research protocols. And I realized that I'd experienced very similar frustrations when I was in clinical practice in Toronto. There too I had fought a losing battle trying to stay current with the latest information as it rapidly evolves in Medicine. Having personally experienced this unpleasant sense of never having the right information at the right time, I was primed to appreciate the new music of Evidence-based Medicine when I first heard it in 1992.

At that time, I happened to read two amazing articles (Antman et al 1992; Lau et al 1992) from Dr. Thomas Chalmers and colleagues at Harvard's School of Public Health that opened my eyes to the possibilities of using information better in Medicine. That message was so strongly appealing that I soon departed my clinical research work entirely and started MetaWorks – an EBM consultancy - with Dr. Chalmers. We aspired to develop the infant science of systematic reviews and meta-analysis to better inform decision-making in Medicine, in both practice and in research. And what a ride that was (Ross, 2009)!

Now EBM is well-accepted, but then, it was new, and we were missionaries. Now, we are faced with new challenges of getting evidence into practice. Evidence from systematic reviews and meta-analyses has narrowed the gap between evidence and practice, but not closed the gap. It will *never* close the gap, for such evidence by its nature addresses populations of patients, and provides average results for groups, not for individuals. Patients approach the evidence gap from their own unique positions, and may well wonder how those group averages from clinical trials relate to them as individuals. Physicians bridge this gap all the time, by making inferential leaps from evidence to patient, and the narrower the gap, surely the more accurate the leap. But it is still a leap. Once we have moved the clinical studies evidence as close as we can towards the patient (by using systematic review and meta-analysis methods), the next challenge is to narrow the gap further by moving patients closer to the evidence. We have to somehow factor in their unique preferences, values, and circumstances, the unique features of disease as it impacts them. This is my imperfect understanding of User-Driven Healthcare, as a way to employ the collective intelligence of individuals in real-life circumstances to narrow that evidence gap, to make our provider inferences for the care of individual patients more accurate than ever.

Recently, after being inspired by some old friends at a 25th reunion of my medical school class, I resolved to get back into clinical practice again. But what really inspired me to acting on this resolution was seeing the enthusiasm my son

radiated as he has moved through his courses in medical school. His excitement and his stories brought back many happy memories, and re-energized me to really get back into practice, but a practice on my own terms. I decided I still didn't want to practice clinical Medicine as a business transaction, and I was admittedly a bit 'rusty' on the latest developments in Internal Medicine. So I studied hard to catch up, and then volunteered my services at a Free Care Clinic for the uninsured. The very kind Medical Director at that Clinic helped ease me back into the saddle. I found that my clinical skills were still good – like riding a bicycle, you don't ever forget – and my patient encounters were immensely satisfying, so after two years, I decided to get back in a bit deeper. I took a position at a government-run clinic for military veterans. I've been at this now for nearly two more years, and have found it has satisfied my need to interact as a physician with real patients with very real, and often neglected, healthcare needs. And keeping my hand in clinical practice keeps me grounded in my EBM consulting work. It also shows me glimpses of a new path in Medicine, that of User-driven Healthcare. Where this path might lead, I cannot see, but I am tempted to wander down a little way to see what might lie just over the horizon.

Remain Humble, Willing to Fail, and Open to New Ideas (Even Many Years out of Training): Keep Moving forward on Whichever Path You are On

I believe sticking with one path for an entire professional career puts practitioners at the risk of stagnation. True, dogged persistence to one path sometimes leads to truly admirable expertise and remarkable careers, but more often I've seen too many one-path colleagues grow stale, bored, and dissatisfied with their work, and their lives. I would advise young physicians and medical students (my two sons included) to stay open to new ideas, to stay aware of how healthcare and Medicine are evolving around you, to be willing to change paths and to be unafraid to fail. Fear keeps people in ruts. When you enter Medicine, you enter an amazing enchanted forest, and you can hardly go wrong in choosing any of the many paths that will open up before you as you travel through it. As long as you stay true to your best instincts, you will honor your patients, this profession, and yourself.

I am now 26 years in practice, and can honestly say that Medicine has never grown stale for me. For the last fifteen years I've been immersed in EBM (Ross, 2009). At MetaWorks, my consultancy specializing in systematic reviews and meta-analyses, we struggled with ways to bring the best available evidence from the literature to the front lines of clinical research and clinical practice. One of our ideas was to build a database of treatment results in different patient subgroups. For instance, if in a systematic review of the efficacy of drugs A, B, and C in congestive heart failure, we could glean results not just for study groups, but also for relevant subgroups, such as people over age 75, or African-Americans, or those with ejection fractions <30%, this might make the evidence more relevant to a particular patient or patient's doctor trying to choose among treatments A, B, and C. We had already developed Internet accessible and easily navigable, queryable databases of extracted data from systematic reviews, but it was organized by treatment group, not at the more granular level of subgroups. And it was, by and large, data from the artificial world of clinical trials. And although we prided ourselves on its 'user-friendliness', it was really intended for use by savvy researchers, not primary care providers or patients.

It seemed to me if we could build such a database that included all subgroup results too, that would be a powerful way to narrow further the inferential gap that now exists between average results in the clinical trials literature and individual patients. And if we could include results from real-world observational research, and if we could make the database interface even more user-friendly, such as permitting natural language queries, it could be even more useful to patients cruising the Internet in their living rooms, or to doctors at the bedside. Unfortunately, MetaWorks could never raise the necessary capital to make this idea a reality. In my opinion, it is still much needed as a way to narrow that inferential gap that exists today in Evidence-based Medicine. It has been gratifying to see a recent renewed interest in subgroup results in the context of discussions about Comparative Effectiveness Research (CER) as a component of healthcare reform in the U.S. Perhaps it is an idea whose time has finally come.

In the meantime, the Internet has enabled several disruptive applications to emerge. Social networking communities such as Facebook and Twitter were first, and have taken off globally. Next came cyber-communities for healthcare professionals, like SERMO, with over 110,000 physician members in the U.S. at the time of this writing. SERMO offers traditional 'curbside consults' in a secure cyberspace environment. The clinical content of SERMO is invariably anecdotal, at the case-by-case level. And it is no more or less so than the content available in online patient communities, such as Patients-Like-Me, that have arisen at the same time. The focus on individual experiences of illness that these patient and provider communities offer may one day help to narrow the gap that now exists between individuals and the group averages that are typical of summarized trials from the literature. The challenge now is to find ways to harness the power of their collective intelligence about disease, diagnosis, prevention, and treatment, and to build bridges between them and the best available evidence from the literature. I cannot imagine how this post-EBM world will evolve, or what it might look like – the path leads ever onward through this beautiful forest. But there are definitely footprints on that path already.

REFERENCES

Antman, E. M., Lau, J., Kupelnick, B., Mosteller, F., & Chalmers, T. C. (1992). A comparison of results of meta-analyses of randomized control trials and recommendations of clinical experts. Treatments for myocardial infarction. *Journal of the American Medical Association, 268,* 240–248. doi:10.1001/jama.268.2.240

Barrett, T. G., & Booth, I. W. (1994). Sartorial eloquence: does it exist in the paediatrician-patient relationship? *BMJ (Clinical Research Ed.), 309,* 1710–1712.

Bazaz, R., & Brown, C. (2007). War on white coats. *Lancet, 370,* 2097. doi:10.1016/S0140-6736(07)61891-1

BMA Central Consultants and Specialists Committee. *Uniform and dress code for doctors: guidance from the central consultants and specialists committee, 2007.* Retrieved from http://www.bma.org.uk/ap.nsf/Content/CCSCdresscode051207?OpenDocument&Highlight=2,ccsc,bare,below,elbows

Brase, G. L., & Richmond, J. (2006). The White–Coat effect: physician attire and perceived authority, friendliness, and attractiveness. *Journal of Applied Social Psychology, 34,* 2469–2481. doi:10.1111/j.1559-1816.2004.tb01987.x

Cha, A., Hecht, B., Nelson, K., & Hopkins, M. (2004). Resident physician attire: does it make a difference to our patients? *American Journal of Obstetrics and Gynecology, 190,* 1484–1488. doi:10.1016/j.ajog.2004.02.022

Douse, J., Derrett-Smith, E., Dheda, K., & Dilworth, J. P. (2004). Should doctors wear white coats? *Postgraduate Medical Journal, 80,* 284–286. doi:10.1136/pgmj.2003.017483

Dunn, J. J., Lee, T. H., & Percelay, J. M. (1987). Patient and house officer attitudes on physician attire and etiquette. *Journal of the American Medical Association, 257,* 65–68. doi:10.1001/jama.257.1.65

Farraj, R., & Baron, J. H. (1991). Why do hospital doctors wear white coats? *Journal of the Royal Society of Medicine, 84,* 43.

Gonzalez Del Rey, J. A., Paul, R. I. (1995). Preferences of parents for pediatric emergency physicians' attire. *Pediatr Emerg Care, 11,* 361-364.

Gooden, B. R., Smith, M. J., Tattersall, S. J., & Stockler, M. R. (2001). Hospitalised patients' views on doctors and white coats. *The Medical Journal of Australia, 175,* 219–222.

Lau, J., Antman, E. M., Jimenez-Silva, J., Kupelnick, B., Mosteller, F., & Chalmers, T. C. (1992). Cumulative meta-analysis of therapeutic trials for myocardial infarction. *The New England Journal of Medicine, 327,* 248–254. doi:10.1056/NEJM199207233270406

Matsui, D., Cho, M., & Rieder, M. J. (1998). Physicians' attire as perceived by young children and their parents: the myth of the white coat syndrome. *Pediatric Emergency Care, 14,* 198–201. doi:10.1097/00006565-199806000-00006

Nair, B. R., Attia, J. R., Mears, S. R., & Hitchcock, K. I. (2002). Evidence-based physicians' dressing: a crossover trial. *The Medical Journal of Australia, 16,* 681–682.

Rehman, S. U., Nietert, P. J., Cope, D. W., & Kilpatrick, A. (2005). What to wear today? Effect of doctor's attire on the trust and confidence of patients. *The American Journal of Medicine, 118,* 1279–1286. doi:10.1016/j.amjmed.2005.04.026

Ross, S. (2009). *Travels with Shubh: A Memoir of the MetaWorks Journey.* Bloomington, IN: iUniverse.

Chapter 9
Medical Student Perspectives:
Journey through Different Worlds

Binod Dhakal
Medical College of Wisconsin, USA

Susan D. Ross
Consultant Internal Medicine, USA

ABSTRACT

This chapter traces the learning experiences of a medical student through his career journey in medical training from two different world settings of Nepal and US. The chapter sketches the author's interactive learning with his patients through his case notes right from his medical student days in Nepal to residency in the US. The juxtaposed commentary from a senior physician provides a longer view lens through which these learning points may be considered. These case notes and narrative insights from the health professional's perspective thus aim to demonstrate and stimulate experiential learning in medicine, a valuable means of obtaining expertise.

INTRODUCTION

Illness is deeply embedded in the social world, and consequently it is inseparable from the structures and processes that constitute that world. For the practitioner, as for the anthropologist, an enquiry into the meanings of illness is a journey into relationships (Kleinman 1988).

My aim during this process of learning has been to document the journey where I came across a few issues of human life beyond the scope of modern

medicine as it is often taught. These were not only stories of human suffering from disease per se but stories of social, economical and psychological pressures. These narratives have been published earlier in a different platform. (Biswas, Dhakal 2003)

Learning Journey from Pokhara, Nepal to Evanston, a City North Of Chicago, USA...Binod Dhakal

In my early medical student life in Pokhara, I found child labor, alcoholism and cultural practices to be an important determinant in the genesis and

DOI: 10.4018/978-1-60960-097-6.ch009

evolution of certain so called disease problems that I came across. The narrative below is about a common and important social problem in that part of the world where I began my journey.

"You must have seen a lot of deliveries by now, you are in third year, aren't you?" my mother asked me with extreme sense of pride in front of my relatives." Yeah mom but we will see all of them in final year of medical school." Whenever I was on vacation my mother always used to show an interest in my subject and I tried to change the subject.

My mother always had the greatest dream to see me become a doctor. Maybe it is a matter of pride for her in front of her peers. When she found me being interested in medicine more than physics, she was happy to realize that her dreams would be fulfilled.

It seemed to me as if I was what Einstein would label a lone ostrich trying to bury its head in the sand of physics (the subject of my interest) to protect myself from the evil quanta of medicine! In fact I never wanted to become a doctor but as bad luck would have it there was no way to escape...

Initially I didn't want to go to medicine because I hated biology. I thought it is just memorizing the facts that others have developed, with no use of concepts and imagination like mathematics. The beauty of equations and mathematical concepts were for me the main attraction of physics.

Commentary: Susan Ross

It is interesting to see the roads we travel to arrive at this field of medicine. I also took a somewhat circuitous route before arriving here. In high school, advanced mathematics came easily to me, but I hated it. In undergraduate university, my first love was literature, but Shakespeare and poetry seemed an impractical major. So instead, I majored in Experimental Psychology because I loved the idea of bringing more objective science to the study of behavior and the mind. It seemed 'cool'. And somehow it seemed more practical too

(i.e., conducive to getting a job after graduation). However, I soon learned that it was not conducive to anything other than more post-graduate study of the same thing. So I eventually came to consider medicine. The science was fascinating, and with a medical degree I knew I could choose from many different career paths. I was the first in my family ever to attend medical school, and my mother was thrilled, although worried about how a woman would be able to manage in this arduous calling. In any event, although Binod and I hail from very different backgrounds, I see these similarities in our roundabout journeys to medicine.

Binod Dhakal's Narrative Continued

Time passed on. Eventually I managed to reach the final year of medical school and the much awaited day (of course not mine) arrived, that is the day of labor room posting. My spirits had already sunk. Nonetheless I had to attend the thing at least to tell my mother about the process of giving birth and the role of much glamorized human interventions. We were made into groups of two and posted in one of the regional hospitals of the country.

My other friend was a brilliant chap with tremendous interest in the subject; I was feeling ashamed of myself to protect the unnecessary ego that has crept into me over the years.

On the way I was engrossed in Steven Weinberg's "The First Three Minutes" that tried to lessen my frustrations to some extent. We reached the hospital at 8:00 clock and the whole night we had to stay there seeing and conducting deliveries if lucky enough. We entered the first stage room which welcomed us with unfashionable furnishings and a peculiar odor. I was feeling happy to see the empty beds but the sleepy intern instructed us to wait as somebody may show up soon. We came back to the examination room and waited.

On the wall I found something written in nice handwriting:

From the unreal Lord lead me to the real From the darkness Lord lead me to the light From death O Lord lead me to immortality.

Oops! The futile reassurances!! How could one deny death, which is inevitable? Exasperated, I again opened Weinberg's book and tried to enjoy the dance of muons and kaons.

After one hour a fat lady came accompanied by her husband. We took her to the examination room. The intern asked me to examine the lady while he was busy writing the sheet. I tried to behave as if I was a good doctor (not a student) and started to do the general examination followed by abdominal. I put my hands on the abdomen but could elicit nothing when I suddenly realized that the lady's sweetheart was giving me a hostile look from outside. Seeing this, my buddy told him to go out for a while and latched the door from inside. Finally the intern finished the examination and she was to be taken to the first stage room and to be started on an intravenous line. Two sisters came, one carrying an IV set with her. They asked me, "Will you try?" I hesitatingly said," Okay" I gave a prick but blood didn't come, again pressed hard but the lady made a painful cry "Aaa...". I was searching for another point but the sister who now knew my abilities said sarcastically, "The lady is delivering soon". I found myself sweating. Within a few minutes she was taken to labour room where I could hear the sisters shouting in chorus," Push" "Push" "Not in the neck, push down".

Finally the lady delivered a male child following which she shed a few tears of happiness.

Mundane work load! Disgusting cries, dirty birth passage and the bloody field, I suffered... I saw the devilish facade of humanity behind the glamour of childbirth that made me feel suffocated.

Next day I went again but with much lesser zeal than what I had had the previous day. The beds were full with different crying faces. The intern asked me to assist a delivery, I agreed (again driven by ego) and put on gloves.

After sometime in one lady the baby crowned and she was taken to the labor room flanked by the sisters. We followed them.

The lady was short, in her twenties and seemed to be economically deprived gauging from her physique and attire. She did not put much effort to push as others and much to my surprise she gave a big blow to the intern's hand when he wanted to put his finger inside." If so why did you come here?" the intern shouted. The lady delivered a female child assisted by me.

Her face became expressionless; no signs of satisfaction which I had seen in each and every mother after delivery since yesterday. She sniffed instead and dabbed the corner of the eyes turning her head to one side. The moment became unfathomable.

I came back to the examination room and tried to concentrate on Weinberg's book but every moment my thought went with the lady and every moment I was haunted by a question, "Why she did not want to deliver?"

I saw the lady being taken on a trolley outside, she was later accompanied by an old man and a small lady. From the room I could hear some murmuring reassurances, when somebody in the crowd shouted, "Unmarried!"

A moment of silence... I threw the book and rushed towards the crowd to understand the situation and they told me that the lady whose delivery I conducted was in fact unmarried.

Her boyfriend after having spent time with her married somebody else.

I met her father (a short man with shabby attire) who appeared ecstatic at having a grandchild. He promised to leave no stone unturned in bringing up the child! "There is no fear in love but perfect love casteth out fear"...I learnt a new lesson.

Life would never become same for the lady and her father who had to undergone all embarrassment and humiliation to bring up the illegitimate child in the midst of so called civilized people. And so would be mine. I felt ashamed of myself of being quite oblivious to the world in which I function everyday!

Thoughts changed from funny quarks to human sentiments, from Heisenberg to Hutchison and Osler and from equations to care and service to humanity!

Susan Ross Commentary

Perhaps it is clichéd, but it's nonetheless true to say that patients and their families are the best teachers in the world of medicine. This is true whether you are a medical student or 25 years in practice! And what is it about these patients who really teach us, the ones we remember, that makes them so different from all the others we soon forget? I suppose all patients have something to teach us, but only when we are both present and actively receptive do we learn. As doctors, it is all too tempting to just be prescriptive, and not receptive. But to be truly receptive, we must be willing to acknowledge that a particular expression of disease, in the context of a particular life, might somehow add to our storehouse of useful information. For instance, I'll never forget a middle-aged Vietnamese man I cared for in Toronto, when I was a medical resident. With recurring fevers, and vague abdominal complaints, he presented a particular diagnostic puzzle. Only by taking a very careful history – and learning about his unusual weekend practice of butchering and roasting goats for communal meals with other Vietnamese émigrés - did I eventually diagnose Q fever after several physicians before me had been stymied. This patient taught me an awful lot about the value of taking a good history yourself, and not relying upon the histories that other doctors have recorded. He also taught me a whole lot about granulomatous hepatitis!

But beyond clinical methods and medical facts, if we are lucky, our patients might also teach us how to be a little bit wiser or kinder or braver or stronger. I will never forget a young woman I cared for early in my career, when I had a hospital-based practice in Internal Medicine. My patient was a young single mother from Jamaica who'd come to Toronto for a better life. She was admitted to hospital for a work-up of fever, hematuria, and flank pain. She had a beautiful three year old daughter who would stay with her mama in the hospital room as long as possible each day. The diagnosis wasn't that difficult – she had renal cell carcinoma – but it was already widely metastatic at the time of diagnosis. Her prognosis was abysmal, six months survival, at most. It was excruciating to have to tell her all this. It would have been a difficult conversation for any doctor, but at the time, I was also a young mother, with my own three year old daughter, I identified with this patient very strongly, for despite our differences, we shared the joys and hopes of motherhood. But she showed me how to be brave when faced with such cruel news. I have never forgotten that young woman's strength, and her example helped me to maintain perspective when immersed in my daily struggles to juggle work and motherhood.

That is the real gift of patients, and we as physicians are truly blessed to have such privileged access to this realm of human experience.

The scientific method of abstraction is very efficient and powerful but we have to pay a price for it. As we define our system of concepts more precisely, as we streamline it and make the connections more and more rigorous, it becomes increasingly detached from the real world. Ordinary language is a map, which due to its intrinsic inaccuracy, has certain flexibility so that it can follow the curved shape of the territory to some degree. As we make it more rigorous, the flexibility gradually disappears, and with the language of mathematics we have reached a point where the links with reality are so tenuous that the relation of the symbols to our sensory experience is no longer evident. This is why we have to supplement our mathematical models and theories with verbal interpretations, again using concepts, which can be understood intuitively but which may be slightly ambiguous. (Capra 1976)

There are many ways you can take care of patients in medicine, from lab technicians to superspecialists, but for me internal medicine has its own charm. Since medical school, I was very impressed by the way internal medicine physicians used to treat the patients, from history taking to coming to diagnosis. Using your pure thought process and at the same time listening to patient's stories, while taking care of the patients, were two main things that attracted me to this subject.

Commentary: These are the same reasons I chose Internal Medicine: the human interaction and the diagnostic puzzle solving.

The following case description has been earlier published in a concept paper by my erstwhile teacher in Nepal (Biswas 2002). Our teacher had one day asked us to take an unconventional route to history taking by not just focusing on usual clinical problem solving, anatomical disease localization but also taking into account the other dimensions of illness that possibly may have been unearthed in an exploration of life events surrounding any given patient's past and present.

Binod Dhakal Narrative

Case Description Written 8 Years Back When I Was a Third Year Medical Student

A 40 year old man was admitted to our hospital with a history of burning sensation in his stomach, shortness of breath, and swelling of the entire body for 17 months. His symptoms started 17 months back when he was working as a security guard in India. Breathlessness was of a progressive nature, initially only on exertion but later on even at rest which kept him awake throughout the night. Swelling then followed, initially his limbs and later his entire body swelled up to such an extent that he was completely bed ridden.

For these complaints he was taken to a hospital in Agra, India, where he stayed for two months.

His symptoms subsided except for mild residual breathlessness. He also contracted malaria during his stay at hospital for which he was given chloroquine. He remained OK for almost one month after which his old symptoms again recurred.

He made many futile attempts to get relief, even tried alternative medicine but the symptoms remained all the same. Eventually he came to our hospital thinking that if he had to breathe his last it should be closer home, in his own country.

On examination he was propped up in bed and his whole body appeared edematous. His pulse rate was 70 beats per minute, regular and of a peculiarly collapsing nature.

His blood pressure was 118/90 left arm supine and Hill's sign (difference in the upper and lower limb BP more than 60) was positive. The jugular venous pressure was raised 5 cm from the sternal angle. There were widespread pulsations both in his precordium and epigastrium. An ill sustained apex away from the mid clavicular line on the 6th inter costal space along with a parasternal heave was felt on palpation. On auscultation an early diastolic murmur; high pitched, blowing, decrescendo was heard best in the third intercostal space near the left sternal border. An ejection systolic murmur was also found in the aortic area. Other signs included a pistol shot sound over his femoral artery, dancing brachii and prominent carotid pulsations. Palpation of the abdomen revealed tender hepatomegaly.

Out of some of the investigations the Chest X Ray showed a large heart and echocardiography showed an incompetent aortic valve.

He was given the diagnosis: severe Aortic Regurgitation with Congestive Cardiac Failure.

There are many instances in my medical school life that changed my attitude toward medicine. Of all these one of the most important was the mystery behind human body and mind and the opportunity to explore truth of its existence. Consider the life events of this patient:

He was born in a small village of Myagdi (a place near Pokhara, Nepal) in what could be labeled as a very poor family in terms of economic status. Being economically deprived from the beginning, his family had to eke out a living that could be described as a bare minimum existence and this he felt created an intense desire in his mind to make money.

He studied up to fifth standard but could not pursue his studies as he had to support his parents to alleviate the burden of his family. He spent almost all his adolescence in inner turmoil of ignorance, needs and expectations. To wake up in the morning, toil almost the entire day in the fields and eat whatever was available at home was his life.

He was married at 21, had three children and that he felt made it more difficult for him to bear the brunt of economic family pressures.

He was perfectly healthy during his youth other than infrequent body ache which he felt may have been due to over exertion.

There was no history suggestive of rheumatic fever that could explain his present condition. Or it may be that the symptoms (probably minor) might have failed to attract his and his parent's attraction in front of his greater responsibilities.

With high hopes to sustain his family he decided to go abroad as most of our countrymen do. He went to India and started working as a security guard. The salary was minimum about 40 US dollars per month and he couldn't save any money. So he left the job after 2 years and started living with sadhus where he had no problem of food but again couldn't make any money.

During this period he started noticing a mild burning in his stomach. He left his sadhu companions and started working as a night guard.

One day he developed acute shortness of breath and was taken to a hospital in Agra, India.

What was the cause of his present condition? Was it Rheumatic fever? Or was it a result of his bare minimum existence, overcrowded surroundings and poor access to Health?

Medicine might take great pride in taking a giant step toward cloning designer babies but it must take into account that there is still a large population who because of poor access to health are forced to an untimely death.

Now there were two options for the patient: either to wait for a time when he would develop an acute heart failure or severe arrhythmia that could finish him or get the incompetent valve replaced that at this point of time was clearly beyond his economic reach (and even then the chance of the complications would not lessen although it may reduce his breathlessness and provide symptomatic relief).

My future plan is to practice medicine in a broader manner focusing not just on internal medicine but on external medicine as well.

Susan Ross's Commentary

Even in the prosperous country in which I presently live, the U.S., it is not at all uncommon for people to suffer the ill effects of deprivation and neglect of basic healthcare. In a Free Clinic south of Boston – which is, ironically, the medical mecca of the U.S. – I recently volunteered for two years seeing patients who were often migrants or illegal immigrants with no health insurance. They could stop into the clinic for free care, but diagnostic testing and treatment were a real challenge, given their circumstances, and there was little continuity of care. At present, I work in a different clinic in Boston that cares for marginalized patients, many of whom have been homeless and spent their life 'on the streets'. They suffer multiple morbidities as a result, and just as at the Free Clinic, testing and treating these people is a real challenge because of their lack of social support and meager financial resources. In addition, their health is also often compromised by serious mental health issues and substance abuse. Physicians cannot ignore the 'back story' of their patients, for it will inescapably impact the diagnosis, treatment, and outcome. Healthcare is inextricably tied to socioeconomic status, no matter what country you practice in.

Binod Dhakal Narrative

This case report was interestingly well received and commented on in the same issue of the journal (Leavitt 2002) providing the much needed encouragement for a medical student.

As this medical student author made his journey from one of the economically deprived countries of the world to one of the most powerful economies, he realized a big difference in the way medicine is practiced. The availability of modern technological resources had made the practice of medicine in this part of world almost seem a different branch of science. Also from my personal experiences in residency and in my personal opinion, litigation and fear associated with it here had made medical practice more like a stereotyped science with very less freedom to think!

Patient profiles changed from Pokhara to Evanston and yet there was something that remained unchanged in the following narratives.

A 64 year old Hispanic male was admitted to our hospital in Evanston with sudden onset of painful swelling of right calf of one day duration. The patient was otherwise in good health except for diabetes mellitus of 10 years duration which was poorly controlled. The patient was not taking any medications and also not on diabetic diet.

The patient was working when he had a sudden pain and swelling in his right calf along with dizziness. Pain in his right calf and was 8-9/10 in intensity with no radiation. He did not have any fever, chills, and shortness of breath or loss of consciousness.

On examination the patient was average built and in distress due to pain.

The temperature was 98.8F, pulse was 82 and the respirations were 20. The blood pressure was 108/67 and the pulses were palpable all over the major arteries. The right calf was swollen and tender to touch. Mild erythematous changes developed over few days. The vibratory and proprioception were normal and the babinski was negative.

His complete blood counts and hemoglobin along with electrolytes and creatinine were normal. His blood sugar was 287mg/dl along with an HbA1C of 11.2 and creatine kinase of 2458 which were grossly raised. The sedimentation rate, CRP and ANA were negative. Bilateral venous Doppler of legs ruled out a deep vein thrombus. The patient was negative for HIV. CT scan of right calf shows diffuse low attenuation within mid to lower portion of medial head of gastrocnemius. No abscess or fluid collection was noted.

The patient was started on aspirin; vicodin and prophylactic lovenox. Antibiotics which were started initially were stopped. On the fifth day biopsy of right gastrocnemius muscle was performed which showed myonecrosis, hemorrhage and atherosclerotic changes of small vasculature suggesting ischemic necrosis of the muscle.

The patient symptoms improved over days with medications. He was discharged after 8th day of admission.

Life Events of the Patient

He was born in a small place in Mexico in a large family. When he reached his adolescence he saw his friends immigrating to USA for money and he followed suit. He started working in small places, sometimes construction worker, sometimes in farms picking apples and eventually as dish washer in a restaurant. He forgot that he is more of human being with flesh than money making machine during this course when one day he started having nausea, vomiting and dizziness for which he was brought to the emergency room by his friends. He was given the diagnosis of diabetes at the age 50 and was given some medicines. He never followed with any doctor afterwards and never filled any prescription as he had no insurance. He continued to neglect his health till he landed up in our hospital with an infarct in his leg.

The real world is not linear. Human life is chaotic where present outcomes are extremely sensitive and non linearly responsive to initial conditions and so unpredictable.

We made a diagnosis in the patient that may not have been possible if he had been in his small village but could we provide him the ultimate care he needed?

After I came into medicine, and after interacting with patients as human beings, I found all the facts mentioned in medical text books full of life. Actually it is the patients and their stories that inspired me.

Binod Dhakal Narrative

Another Patient Story
A 72 year old male with past medical history of HTN, Psoriasis, Carcinoma Prostate and Grave's disease was admitted in our hospital due to increasing shortness of breath that started over the past 3 weeks. The patient was asymptomatic before 3 weeks when he started getting short ness of breath which made him visit one of his doctors who found his oxygen saturation to be low for which he was prescribed home oxygen and antibiotics.

He denied any fever, cough, chest pain and swelling of legs. The symptoms did not get better despite these, rather progressed, forcing him to see his Primary care physician who got an imaging done of his chest (CXR and CT) and referred him to our hospital after the results.

He was on Hydrochlorthiazide/Lisinopril, crestor, levothyroxine and Efalizumab (raptiva) for his psoriasis. A previous smoker he claims to be pretty independent before these episodes.

On examination the patient was in respiratory distress using his accessory muscles but was oriented and alert. Admission vitals were T 96.8, BP 144/75, P 92, RR 32 and he was saturating 88% on Nasal Canula which improved to 95% on venti mask. The systemic examination showed dull percussion note on both chest with coarse crackles all over the chest. There was no clubbing and lymphadenopathy.

The initial blood count showed a WBC count of 12.6 with normal differential and normal electrolytes with LDH of 245. The initial blood gas showed respiratory alkalosis with hypoxemia (Sao2 83%). There were bilateral interstitial and alveolar opacities in chest X-ray which was similar to the one done with the Primary care physician. The pulmonary consultation was made at this time and the patient went for bronchoscopy and got transferred to the unit. Efalizumab (Raptiva) was stopped considering one of the side effects of the medicine having been reported earlier as interstitial pneumonia. The patient condition remained the same with oxygen, nebulizations and multiple antibiotics started by the Emergency Physician. The bronchial biopsy showed bronchial mucosa and lung parenchyma with chronic inflammation. The cultures for virus, bacteria, fungus and Pneumo cystis carinii PCP all were negative. The patient then went for open lung biopsy and in the mean time Intra venous steroids were started. The biopsy showed interstitial inflammatory fibrotic process suggestive of Ususal Interstitial PneumoniaUIP which was confirmed by second opinion.

The patient started showing significant improvement in his status shown by his decreasing oxygen requirements. The IV steroids was continued for few days and then changed to oral. He was discharged home on oral steroids for 4-6 weeks. The final impression of his clinical condition was a possible Raptiva induced Interstitial pneumonia that recovered on discontinuation of the drug.

On follow up the patient was found to be doing much better with very little oxygen requirement and significant improvement in the chest x-ray. The patient was asked to continue steroids for 4-6 weeks.

Life Events of the Patient
He was born and brought up in the States. He was up-to-date with all his health screening from the beginning and used to have good knowledge of health made possible by the internet. He enjoyed playing golf and running in his treadmill, which was restricted recently due to his condition. He developed psoriasis in late 60s with plaques around his limbs that were cosmetically unappealing!

He had been a happy man with Efalizumab (raptiva) as the disease went into remission.

I saw him months after his Efalizumab (raptiva induced illness and he appeared significantly improved although still needing oxygen for his daily activities. He was asking me when he could play golf.

Initially there was some problem with communication with my patients when I came to the US. But surprisingly I found all my patients very pleasant and never complaining despite the poor communication. Slowly as I started to learn more about them and their culture, it never remained a problem.

Doctors are viewed by Nepali society as different creatures. The trend is changing in the cities but in the rural areas they still think a doctor is god. I remember one incident when as undergrads we were attending a community based camp that was performing cataract surgery. There was one lady with mature cataract who had not been able to see for years. After the surgery when she could see, the first thing she told to our ophthalmologist was that he is god. In US also doctors are highly valued, but I feel money is the main attraction behind it. The patients here also give respect to doctors, but not like god as in Nepal.

Susan Ross Commentary

No matter what country you live in, the motivation to enter Medicine is complex and variable, I am sure. Perhaps it is strictly monetary for some, but I think this must be the exception and not the rule, and is not limited to a single country or culture. Judging from the medical students I have met, I suspect their main motivations are love of the science and love of people. But I agree with the observation that physicians are not treated as gods in the U.S. That is a good thing. I suspect

wherever the general populace is well educated, Medicine is understood as the science that it is, rather than as some unfathomable mystery practiced by magicians. So while not gods, doctors are still treated with great respect in this country. But I do fear their status could fall as Medicine becomes transformed from a noble profession serving humankind into just another service business catering to consumers.

In conclusion, as Hippocrates said, "life is short, opportunities fleeting"...Medicine has grown so vast that it's almost impossible to master everything. But if you can listen carefully to your patients and take good care of them, regardless of which culture you are working in, I think that is the most rewarding thing you will ever achieve as a physician.

REFERENCES

Biswas, R. (2002). Developing Holistic health care in the third world: A working study proposal. *Eubios Jl Asian Intl Bioethics (Tokyo)*, *12*(4), 143–147.

Biswas, R., & Dhakal, B. (2003). Medical student narratives for understanding Disease and social order in the third world. *Eubios Jl Asian Intl Bioethics(Tokyo)*, *13*(4), 139–142.

Capra, F. (1976). *Tao of Physics*. UK: Fontana.

Kleinman, A. (1988). *The illness narratives*. New York: Basic Books.

Leavitt, F. J. (2002). What is Bioethics? Commentary on Harris & Sass on The Eubios Declaration, Biswas on Holistic Health Care, Yu Kam Por on Futile Medical Treatment. *Eubios Journal of Asian and International Bioethics; EJAIB*, *12*, 162–164.

Chapter 10
Stories of Illness and Healthcare from a Physician Perspective

J. Huw C. Morgan
Consultant in International Medical Education, UK

ABSTRACT

Doctors have unique and privileged opportunities to observe and participate in the illness narratives (stories) that patients present with. Hearing, understanding and respecting the patient narrative is as important as correctly practising the technical aspects of medical diagnosis and treatment, and yet traditionally has received much less emphasis during medical education. The stories below (which have all been altered to preserve patient confidentiality) illustrate how attention to the patient's narrative enables a richer and deeper interaction with them that enhances the therapeutic aspects of the consultation.

INTRODUCTION

We shall not cease from exploration And the end of our exploring Will be to arrive at where we started And know the place for the first time. (Eliot 1967)

A doctor spends the majority of his working life in face to face contact with people. Every year he has thousands of consultations with the members of his practice population. He shares their pains, their sorrows, their fears, hopes and (sometimes) their joys. Whilst many of these consultations

may not involve issues of any great consequence or significance, there are a number that do. They may not occur every day or even every week, but over the course of a month there will certainly be a few occasions when both patient and doctor feel that together they have touched on something profound; that the nature of their communication has resulted in a degree of real human contact that transcends the mundane. The way the patient uses (or fails to use) the resources of themselves, their religious faith, their family, community and friends will become apparent and will have a great influence on how the doctor and others are able to provide of health care.

DOI: 10.4018/978-1-60960-097-6.ch010

All doctors will know this, although they may not put it into concrete thought or word. It is probably what most of us find the most enjoyable and rewarding aspect of practice, as well as being the hardest to define. It is what I refer to in a number of places in what follows as the 'spirituality' of the consultation, in an exploration of a number of accounts of 'embodied minds and failing bodies'.

Pregnancy and Childbirth

And he who gives a child a home Builds palaces in Kingdom come. (Masefield 1988)

Few issues in human life have the same emotive power as the conception and birth of children. Problems in this area are quite common, and can cause deep-seated turmoil, particularly, but by no means exclusively, for women. I will describe two patients of mine who found their own solutions to difficulties here.

Santosh was a young Asian lad who had recently married by arrangement, as is common in his community. He was happy with his new wife, but came to see me six months or so after the wedding to say that he was concerned that his wife was not yet pregnant. I was about to explain to him that this was not necessarily a cause for concern and within normal limits still, when a bell rang distantly in my mind. Several years before when he was in his mid teens, Santosh had developed a Lymphoma presenting with enlarged inguinal lymph-nodes. It was high grade, and he was apparently cured following radio and chemotherapy. However, I thought I remembered a letter in the notes from the radiotherapist warning that although every effort had been made to shield his genitalia, his future fertility might have been compromised by the radiotherapy. I didn't say anything about this to him there and then, but suggested that it would be advisable to check his sperm count, and sent him off with the appropriate instructions. I then checked back though the correspondence in his notes, and found the letter which did indeed give the above warning.

The semen analysis was returned reporting the complete absence of spermatozoa, and I prepared myself for a session of breaking bad news to Santosh. As one might expect, he was devastated by the news, the more so as in his community it brought shame on all his family if he could not father children. After several long explanations, he sat weeping quietly, saying: "It's a hard thing to accept".

"A very hard thing," I agreed.

"Is there nothing at all that can be done?" he asked despairingly.

I talked gently about A. I. D., but said there was no way of reversing the damage done to his testicles so that they would again make spermatozoa. At his request, I agreed to refer him to a Urologist for a second opinion.

"Alright, Thank you doctor," he finally said, and left abruptly.

A few days later his wife and his brother came to see me together. His wife spoke only limited English, so the brother explained that he was present to interpret. He said that Santosh had come back very distressed after his consultation with me. Was it true that he would never be able to father a child? I agreed that unfortunately it was true; deciding that on this occasion there was no point in withholding information which was clearly of significance to Santosh's wife. (The brother had already told me that Santosh knew they were coming to see me to talk about his problem, and was happy about it.)

There was a brief exchange in their own language between the brother and wife. Was it true that I had referred Santosh to a specialist, they wanted to know? I said that it was, but that there was no treatment for the condition. The wife could conceive by means of A.I.D. if they both agreed to that. There was a further native language exchange between them, and then they thanked me for seeing them and left.

A few weeks later I was routinely checking through the day's returned laboratory results when I came across a positive pregnancy test with Santosh's wife's name on it. I thought it must be a mistake in the labelling of the form, which is always a possibility with Asian names handled by non-Asian practice staff. I checked the address and date of birth, and they both corresponded with Santosh's wife, and further research revealed that her notes had an entry by one of my partners indicating that she had attended for confirmation of pregnancy a couple of days previously. I mentioned it to my partner at the next opportunity, and she remembered seeing Santosh's wife but knew nothing of his problems.

A few days later Santosh and his wife came to see me, both grinning from ear to ear.

"You're pregnant then!" I said to his wife.

"Yes doctor," she said, and gave me a meaningful look before lowering her eyes and blushing becomingly.

"Great news isn't it Doctor!" said Santosh enthusiastically. I agreed that it was, and proceeded to discuss arrangements for ante natal care and delivery. As they left, Santosh's wife gave me another meaningful look.

I don't know definitely, but I assume that she and the brother must have agreed to conceive the child together to spare Santosh the indignity and shame of infertility, and the uncertainty of A.I.D. with an unknown donor. Whether Santosh was consciously aware of what happened I don't know.

Nine months later a little girl was born, to Santosh's delight.

This story is an interesting example of how people find meaningful solutions to their problems when given some basic information by the doctor. I may have unwittingly planted the idea in Santosh's mind (assuming he was an informed participant in the drama between his wife and his brother) when I initially talked to him about A.I.D. He had commented that it wouldn't really be his child, and I *think* (I can't actually remember) that I had said that perhaps it was possible for his

brother to donate sperm so that it would be kept in the family. Whatever the case, a suitable solution was found without further medical intervention.

The second case I will describe does not have such a happy ending, and concerns a young woman called Tania. Tania became pregnant by her stable partner for the first time when she was aged twenty five. All went well for the first few months, and then she developed high blood pressure. I managed to control this satisfactorily for a couple of weeks, but at thirty two weeks she went into premature labour and gave birth to a dead child. Post mortem chromosome analysis showed that the child had an extremely rare chromosomal abnormality that was incompatible with life. Tania was naturally extremely upset, and her relationship with her partner broke down a few months after the still birth.

She eventually worked through her grief and returned to normal life, getting a great deal of support from her mother. A few years later she was in another relationship and became pregnant again. Her obstetrician monitored this pregnancy closely in view of the previous history, and once again for several months everything appeared to be fine. At thirty five weeks disaster struck again, with another still birth following an intra-uterine death. Once again the child had the chromosomal abnormality. History repeated itself further in that Tania's boyfriend left her shortly after the still birth. She was extremely depressed and required antidepressants for many months, as well as much supportive counselling.

During this time she saw a consultant geneticist for investigation of her own chromosomes, which revealed that she carried a faulty chromosome responsible for the problems of the two babies she had conceived, but that would not necessarily be passed to each child that she conceived. The geneticist considered it highly unfortunate that two consecutive pregnancies should have inherited the defect, and whilst it may occur again it was statistically far more likely that she would have a normal child next time.

Tania was by now beginning to recover from her depression, and her solution to the problem was clear: she wanted to be sterilised. She told her obstetrician this at a follow up appointment, and he point blank refused, saying it was out of the question as she didn't even have a partner at the present time, a remark to which she took great exception.

She presented her case for sterilisation to me, saying that she understood all that the geneticist had said (she had had several sessions with his counsellor afterwards), but the trauma of two still births was so great that she could not contemplate conceiving a child again, knowing there was any risk at all of it happening on a further occasion.

I indicated that I understood her feelings, but that I was not keen to re- refer her until she was totally recovered from her depression and clear that she still felt the same way. She accepted this and some three months later when she was in much brighter spirits we returned to the issue. I presented all the possible arguments against sterilisation and she answered them all with unflinching determination. Accordingly I wrote back to her obstetrician supporting her decision, and he sterilised her in due course. Since then she remained in good mental health, held on to her demanding job, and had no regrets about her decision.

Tania's case is interesting in that it was again she herself who proposed sterilisation as the solution to her problem. The production of dead babies had become a very negative part of herself image that she could only get rid of by ensuring that she was made incapable of producing babies at all. Once this was achieved, she was free to get on with her life, as its meaning was no longer centred on her being a bearer of dead children.

Both these cases illustrate how people sometimes find their own solutions to difficult problems, given some basic support from the doctor. It is always interesting, and a privilege, to observe such triumphs of the human spirit over adversity.

Past Trauma, Present Reality

Time present and time past Are both perhaps contained in time future, And time future contained in time past. If all time is eternally present All time is unredeemable. What might have been is an abstraction Remaining a perpetual possibility Only in a world of speculation. What might have been and what has been Point to one end, which is always present. (Eliot 1967)

Sometimes people experience events of such magnitude and significance at one particular point in their lives that the whole of the rest of their life is lived in the shadow of them. This seems particularly to apply to those who lived through traumatic experiences in war. I was born in the lean post world-war two years and my early childhood memories involve air raid shelters, siren testing and old army equipment of my father's, so I have always been interested in the experiences of those who were involved at first hand in that long conflict. The narratives below illustrate how conflict related events can shape the whole of a person's subsequent life and reactions to ill-health.

Stanley was a small, rather hairy man with somewhat pointed ears, in his early sixties when I first met him. He suffered from clinically proven Ischaemic Heart disease giving him Angina, *and* Oesophagitis, so it was always difficult to sort out what his chest pain was due to. He also had Chronic Bronchitis, having smoked twenty a day for forty odd years, and was a frequent attender. He always had a faintly apologetic air about him, and although I found him rather irritating because he refused to stop smoking but expected instant treatment for his many smoking related diseases, it was hard not to like him too.

One day he seemed less chirpy and talkative than usual, and said he didn't really know if I could help with this problem, but he was feeling a bit depressed. Gentle enquiry led to the statement that he thought the depression was due to "bad dreams". I asked what the dreams were about, and he was a bit evasive at first, referring vaguely to unpleasant experiences in the past. I continued to press him gently for details, and finally it all came out.

The previous week he had taken part in a memorial parade and service for members of a local regiment that he had been in during the War. They had been in some disarray on the retreat to Dunkirk in 1940, and he was part of a group of about eighty men who were caught by the advancing German army. They were herded into a large barn in a field near their point of capture, sprayed with sub-machine gun fire, and then a number of hand grenades were tossed in and the doors closed. (As he spoke, I remembered seeing an item about this event on the regional TV news a few days previously). He had been one of only twelve young men who escaped from the barn alive, and in his case actually uninjured physically. Having been involved in the preparation and carrying out of the memorial event, the awful memories had been re-evoked. As he spoke, I realised that he had suffered from what is now termed Post Traumatic Stress Disorder for the last fifty years, and suddenly saw him and his whole demeanour in a new light. He suffered from the classical survivor's guilt, and in some ways the whole of his life from that point onwards had been an apology for being alive. He actually went on to talk about this even as I thought it.

"I should have died with my mates back there really," he said, shaking his head sadly. He had received no counselling or follow up help after the event, (presumably 'Counselling' didn't exist in the armed forces in 1940!), although he was in touch with some of the other survivors and they still met up once a year, but it seemed they usually had a hard drinking session and didn't talk about the event that dominated their lives ever since that awful day.

It was a long consultation, and at the end he thanked me, saying it was funny but he'd never told anyone else about it before. He did not consult again about his mood or his dreams, and in fact

consulted less frequently about his other illnesses after that. After seeing him, I reflected on how fortunate I was never to have been involved in war. How could anyone ever really get over an experience such as Stanley had suffered? Never a day passed without him thinking about it, he had said. It was an event whose meaning over shadowed the whole of his life, and profoundly affected his need for medical attention.

Arthur was a man of similar age to Stanley, whom I first met when he developed Atrial flutter. He came under control with Digoxin, later changed to Amiodorone, but as the years passed he developed Left Ventricular Failure requiring Diuretics and Ace Inhibitors. All this required regular consultations for review, and I would see him every few months in the surgery except on those rare occasions when he was too ill to attend. Despite the relative severity of his illness he was always cheerful, always uncomplaining, and unfailingly courteous. He used to bring books with him to read in the waiting room (unusual behaviour in my practice population), and I discovered we had similar tastes in popular fiction. Over the years we discussed the relative merits of Frederick Forsyth, Jack Higgins, Ted Albuerry, Leslie Thomas and many others, for a few minutes at the end of the consultation.

One day he had Len Deighton's book "Bomber" under his arm (a sort of drama documentary about a night bombing raid on a German town). I had read it years before and still remembered how gripping it was. "Bit of a busman's holiday for me actually," he said when I commented on it.

"Oh yes?" I enquired.

"Used to fly Lancasters myself in the war. Shot down over Berlin in '45 in fact".

By now I was hooked, and urged him to go on and tell me the whole story.

They had just completed a bombing run when they were hit by anti-aircraft fire, he explained. (He was a good story teller and his description was vivid.) They couldn't work out the full extent of the damage in the darkness but he realised the plane was loosing height fast, so he struggled to hold it steady once they were away from the probing search lights, and told the crew to bail out. By the time they'd all got out he was down to a few hundred feet and too low to get out himself, so he had to go for a crash landing. Knowing his life depended on his skill in the next few minutes he tried to keep the plane to as gentle a descent as possible. Suddenly he saw that he was above one of the forests north of Berlin, so he cut the engines and put the plane down gently on the tree tops (apparently a standard emergency procedure). It had not quite lost momentum when it reached the edge of the trees, so it tipped forward and hit the ground nose first, but he was saved by his harness and was unhurt. He scrambled out, set fire to the plane, and got away as quickly as he could. He went on to describe how he'd relied on his survival gear and training to keep out of the way of the retreating German army, living off the land, and eventually got picked up by advanced units of the Allies making the final push for Berlin.

"And here you are forty years later telling me about it!" I said when he'd finished.

"Doesn't seem that long," he said. "Always thought I'm lucky to be alive since then."

Suddenly I could understand his cheerful acceptance of his heart disease. He regarded every day of life since surviving the crash as a bonus to be accepted with gratitude. Rather unprofessionally I had let the consultation over run by twenty minutes while he told me his story (which was not essential from a medical point of view), but I considered it time well spent to gain a greater insight into how Arthur understood his illnesses and indeed the whole of his life. He would never forget that he had almost miraculously survived as a result of his own skill and bravery, and looked on it as a privilege to be alive still to tell the tale.

Both Arthur and Stanley illustrate how a major life event can form the focus of meaning for people many years after it occurred. It is helpful for the doctor to learn about his patients' past, for much of the present can then be understood in new light.

Heartsinks Revisited

I was much too far out all my life And not waving but drowning. (Smith 1988)

All doctors are familiar with patients who consult repeatedly for ill-defined problems that defy accurate medical classification, or make a big deal out of every minor ill, or who require inordinate amounts of emotional support. The sinking of the doctor's heart when they walk into the room or when their name is seen on the appointments list has been used as a descriptive tool that gives permission for the doctor's reaction to these people. It does not, however, help much in getting to the root of their troubles, which in a *few* cases (I would by no means claim all) is actually possible. This does not necessarily alter the patient's behaviour much, but it does change the doctor's attitude to them and render the consultations more rewarding, as he or she understands the factors that have shaped the patient's need for recurrent seemingly inappropriate medical attention. I will describe one such case in some detail.

Fran was about thirty when I first met her. She and her new husband had met when they were both in-patients in a psychiatric hospital, and they had been re-housed in a block of flats next to my surgery. The diagnosis attached to her was "Depression with underlying Sociopathic Personality Disorder." She was an overweight, rather unkempt lady who seemed to have a simmering underlying anger and resentment against the world in general. She consulted frequently with upper abdominal pain in the early days, and to my surprise a barium meal showed some Oesophagitis. No sooner had this diagnostic triumph been celebrated (she and her husband were pleased that a doctor had "found something actually wrong" with her), then she started to have what looked like Grand Mal fits. I was a little suspicious of the exact nature of these, as they occurred only when others were in attendance and were not associated with incontinence or tongue biting, nor any post-ictal drowsiness. However on one occasion she was admitted to hospital after a 999 call by her husband, and kept in for a couple of weeks for thorough investigation. An EEG recording during a fit showed no abnormality, and it was decided that the fits were due to a "Dissociative state", or, to use an older term, were Hysterical. This finding was to cause endless problems for Fran through the years, not least because of junior hospital staff failing to appreciate the difference between dissociation and malingering.

The next thing that happened was that Fran became pregnant, and sadly had an intra-uterine death at twenty four weeks. It was around this event that I first started to develop some real empathy for Fran. She wanted to have a proper funeral service for her dead baby, but this posed problems for the hospital as the child officially was not yet "capable of being born alive" and so would normally be destroyed like the products of an early miscarriage. After consultation with the pathologist and the hospital chaplain, a sympathetic undertaker was found and the baby buried in an unmarked but special plot in a local cemetery. What impressed me during my efforts on her behalf to sort this out was her insight into the need to grieve properly for her child, and how this would be helped by the carrying out of the normal rituals surrounding death. She clearly appreciated my attempts to help her with this, and some kind of breakthrough in our relationship occurred.

She still had fits periodically (anticonvulsants having been tried and found useless) and continued to consult frequently. She became pregnant again, and this time carried to term to produce a little girl. Shortly after this, the family moved to a council house and left my list, although they were still within my practice boundary. I had interesting mixed feelings, of relief that a difficult patient had left, together with disappointment that someone I felt I had an improving relationship with had moved away.

For two or three years I had no more contact with them, but then by chance I met Fran's husband

(himself a rather vulnerable and immature man) at a railway station where he was working as a porter. He was effusively warm in his greetings and insisted on bringing me up to date with the family news. A few weeks after this I was visiting a patient who lived near Fran, and found on emerging from the house that Fran was waiting to greet me like a long lost friend. She gave me a photograph of her daughter (now a lively toddler) and said that she and her husband had been talking about me and would like to rejoin my list, as I was the best doctor they'd ever had (and so on!); I could hardly refuse.

Fran now was fatter than ever, and had added mild diabetes to her other problems, as well as nocturnal incontinence of urine. Her fits now were more like narcoleptic attacks, sometimes leaving her deeply asleep for fourteen to sixteen hours. All of this was being investigated in hospital out-patients, but with little progress. There were periodic admissions when Fran was 'unconscious' for longer than her husband could cope with. They both remained unable to really grasp the concept of dissociation (fits and sleepiness arising from the sub-conscious mind, I tried to tell them), and this was not helped by Fran being admitted to a hospital in another area of the country whilst on holiday with a diagnosis of "Status Epilepticus".

By now they had a real grievance against the hospital where Fran was normally admitted, that she was regarded as a 'psychiatric case', and once her old notes were obtained the attitude of the staff changed from one of concern to one of dismissal. Fran was also annoyed that her physicians at the hospital always wanted reports from the psychiatrist whose care she was still under from time to time with recurrent severe depression requiring admission. In the midst of all this, I started to learn a little bit about Fran's early life, which was to give me a new and deeper understanding and respect for her many problems.

The first opening up about her childhood came when she heard that her father, from whom she was estranged, was terminally ill. He had been a hospital administrator, and had apparently used his power and influence to keep Fran confined in hospitals for much of her adolescence, because she was "difficult". Later, I learnt that he had also physically and sexually abused her in early childhood. Whilst he was dying, Fran struggled with the mixed feelings of grief, anger and revenge against him, and used to phone me regularly to talk about it. It was only after he died that she discovered the full extent of his abuse of power in hospitalising her, and her mother's complicity with the events. Her recurrent dissociative states now seemed easy to understand, and fitted the pattern not infrequently seen in people who've suffered from severe childhood abuse.

She could not remember a lot of what happened in her early childhood, and found it extremely difficult to talk about her parents, but when she had recovered to some extent from her father's death, she and her husband decided to pursue legal claim against the hospital where she had been kept as a teenager, as a way of dealing with some of her anger and resentment. She was also by now wanting to sue her psychiatrist and some of her other medical advisors for negligence. I remained in favour with her, and had to tread a very delicate line between acknowledging her legitimate anger at some of the treatment she'd received in the past, and cautioning that some of her complaints were projections of her continuing inner turmoil onto her doctors.

I continued to see Fran fairly regularly, to help sort out some new symptom or be given an update on her solicitor's progress with medical reports from independent doctors about her past treatment. Sometimes weeks or even months would pass with no contact from her, and then there would be a flurry of phone calls and consultations. What happened that I no longer perceived her as a "heartsink" patient? It is surely just that as I learnt more about the traumas of her past, I felt more able to be understanding of the deep seated psychological turmoil that she endures, and that manifests itself in diverse physical symptoms. She is not "waving"

(indulging in attention seeking behaviour for self gratification), but "drowning" (desperately struggling with profound inner distress), because, in the words of the poem, she's been much too far out all her life. I also felt that I was one of the very few doctors she has had contact with that she actually trusted, and that is a very important role for a person who has suffered the abuse that she has.

Perhaps very few "heartsinks" provoke any degree of real empathy from their doctors (perhaps very few deserve it!). Fran's case illustrates that there are some where knowledge and understanding can actually change the doctor's perception of the patient, enable him to cope in a more satisfying way with their demands, and help the patient to have more appropriate attitudes to the medical system.

Tragedy

What I had not foreseen Was the gradual day Weakening the will Leaking the brightness away, The lack of good to touch The fading of body and soul like smoke before wind Corrupt, unsubstantial. (Spender 1988)

No doctor is a stranger to tragic events in the lives of his patient. These may strike like a bolt from the blue, or creep gradually and stealthily but with equal devastation into the everyday reality of any one of us. If he is to be of any help, the doctor has to hold that difficult middle ground of genuinely empathising with his patient, whilst not being so overwhelmed with sorrow and grief that he cannot continue to function as a clinician whose support the patient depends on. This is not easy, and makes considerable demands on the doctor's emotional resources. He would be less than human if he was unscathed by some of these events in his patients' lives, and yet they can be occasions when that indefinable heart to heart spiritual contact between patient and doctor is at its deepest, bringing their own reward.

I met Terry and Kay during my first week in the practice. A couple in their late twenties (about my age at the time), they had found happiness together after difficult previous marriages for both of them. Terry was one of those people who virtually never attended the doctor, but his notes showed that about a year previously he had seen my predecessor complaining of a strange heavy feeling in his central chest and occasional difficulty in swallowing. She had arranged a barium swallow, but he never attended the appointment. Now he was back with the same symptoms worsening, and Kay had come to make sure that he went for the tests this time.

The X-rays showed a widened mediastinum with enlarged hilar lymph nodes and the radiologist advised urgent referral to a chest physician. I duly arranged this, telling Terry and Kay "straight" at their request that it looked as though Terry had got a tumour. The physician did a biopsy which showed a highly malignant mediastinal sarcoma, and passed Terry on to a thoracic surgeon. The surgeon rang me immediately after the exploratory thoracotomy to say that unfortunately the sarcoma was totally inoperable, and whilst they would try some radiotherapy the outlook for Terry was bleak.

I can still remember the consultation with Terry and Kay when he'd come out of hospital (where they had been told little). They were too high on the tide of their new happiness together to really believe that Terry was going to die, and clung desperately to the straw of hope offered by radiotherapy. This did in fact improve Terry's symptoms for a time, and for a couple of months things were alright. Then Terry developed a pain in his lower thigh, and examination showed bony swelling and tenderness. An X-ray confirmed a metastasis in the lower femur. Terry was now on Morphine and NSAID's for the pain, and more radiotherapy was tried. The pain settled but he was unable to walk properly, so at Kay's request I obtained a wheelchair urgently for him.

It became clear that something was now happening to Terry's mind. He couldn't concentrate well and could no longer fix mechanical things around the house. I suspected cerebral metastases but said nothing to Terry. We were however now talking about death, and he expressed a fear of not being able to cope with his deteriorating physical condition, and of leaving Kay. Nursing help was soon needed for Kay, who was determined that Terry would die at home. Nurses and support workers from the local hospice were involved too, to give emotional support to them both.

Terry's last few weeks were difficult, "the gradual day weakening the will". He gradually slipped into more or less permanent unconsciousness, requiring Morphine suppositories for pain relief (no syringe drivers then). Then he started to have fits. I felt at the limits of my skills as a very new principal in General Practice, but managed to get him stable with Diazepam suppositories which Kay had to administer, as the nurses could not call frequently enough to give both drugs at the necessary intervals.

I gave Kay my home phone number, knowing that she would not abuse free access to me, and remained on permanent call for Terry for the last couple of weeks of his life. When the end came, their flat was filled with relatives who had gathered to help Kay, who by now was extremely stressed and nearing collapse from exhaustion. After confirming that Terry had died, it seemed natural to hug Kay, who cried inconsolably on my shoulder for several minutes, until led away by her sister. I felt the need afterwards to seek out my district nurse who had been closely involved with Terry's terminal care, and talk to her for a few minutes as we both tried to discharge our own grief at the death of a man of twenty nine, who had just begun a new and happy chapter in his life.

I saw Kay a few times afterwards, and the nurses and myself received a moving written tribute from her both personally and (suitably edited) in the local paper. Kay was numb with grief, and ceased consulting me not long after Terry's death. She returned on the first anniversary with a hoarse voice, which with great insight she attributed to re-surfacing emotions. We talked about Terry, and how happy they had been together. "It just seems so bloody unfair!" she said, shaking her head in sadness.

She did not consult me for several years after that, and I learnt that she had told one of my partners that she felt I had become almost like a member of the family whilst looking after Terry, and that she did not feel right about seeing me as a doctor. I felt, and still feel, that this was a heartwarming recompense for a case that had taken me to the limits of my clinical and emotional resources.

I met Pamela for the first time at the ante-natal clinic, a bright, attractive young woman, smiling in anticipation of planned motherhood. She was a fairly unusual patient for my practice area, being a nurse who was obviously from a wealthy background. The pregnancy proceeded uneventfully, and at about thirty four weeks she moved to another area of the country where her husband (a hospital administrator) was going to be based for several months. I never did learn the full details, but there were problems around the birth (by emergency caesarean section), and when they returned to my area to live it was clear that the little boy (Peter) was far from right. There was evidence of gross developmental delay, and he was seen regularly by a local paediatrician. It was soon clear that he had severe Cerebral Palsy, and was having regular problems feeding and breathing.

Pamela's life became centred on caring for Peter, who would scream incessantly whenever there was anything distressing him. The local paediatric unit was very supportive and operated an open door policy for Peter. Often Pamela would take him straight there when he was clearly ill. She would consult me for less dramatic problems, but given the level of his handicap I saw little of him in the first two or three years of his life.

Pamela became pregnant again when Peter was three, and fortunately this time all was well, and she had a baby girl who grew into a lively and obviously intelligent child. Peter was a continuing drain on Pamela's resources, as with every passing year he got bigger but did not develop at all in any other way. He had to be fed through a naso-gastric tube, and be kept strapped into a chair or lying on the floor. The stress of all this had put a severe strain on Pamela's marriage, and her husband would leave and then return in an episodic manner.

When Peter was about six, for the first time Pamela started consulting me about herself and her feelings about all that had happened as a result of Peter being the way he was. It was clear that her dedication to Peter's care had taken an enormous toll, but she was so driven by both her concern for him and her sense of duty that she made minimal use of respite admissions to hospital, and her support family who could have Peter at weekends. I would try and persuade her to give herself more time, but she was always reluctant. Slowly it emerged as she talked to me over several weeks, that she greatly feared that Peter would die, and that this concern obsessed her. She felt guilty whenever she was not with him, as she felt that only she really understood his needs. Her life was totally centred around him, and she felt guilty about that too, as she knew it wasn't fair on her daughter and her husband, and yet she could not bear to do less than her total best for Peter all the time. This emotional strain, plus the twenty four hour physical demands of Peter, had turned the young woman I met seven years before into a prematurely aged lady who was close to breaking point.

There was no solution to or resolution of this situation. I continued to offer what emotional support I could to Pamela, painfully aware that she really needed much more practical and psychological help than she would allow herself to have. In the eighth year of Peter's life, the family moved back to the area where he had been born, and I never saw them again. I did hear later that Peter had died, and could not help wondering how Pamela coped with this, her greatest fear.

Few people know the strain of caring for a severely handicapped child. Those who do may talk of the hidden resources within oneself that it brings out, and the capacity for love that even the most damaged human being may show to those who care for him. Pamela knew these things too, and helped me to learn about them. I can only hope that they have been enough to comfort her through the grief of loosing Peter, whose short life shattered so much of hers.

It is when tragedy strikes in the lives of his patients that the General Practitioner's role of 'being there' is perhaps at its most important. In one sense he is standing helplessly by while events of enormous import unfold in front of him, producing profound reactions in those they affect. But in another sense he is there as someone outside the engulfing tragedy for the patient, who understands its significance for them, and is able to offer support. This is always a humbling experience for the doctor, as together he and the patient confront some of the ultimate mysteries of the human condition, and can do little but be present with respect and awe.

Crisis

It - may jolt the Hand That adjusts the Hair That secures Eternity From presenting - Here. (Dickinson 1988)

The doctor is often consulted by people who perceive themselves to be beset by a crisis that is affecting their physical or mental health in some way. Although the crisis is real enough to them, it is not always confirmed by the objective judgement that the doctor brings to the situation to be as real as they thought. Whatever the case, a particular intensity is added to the consultation if it's meaning is framed in crisis terms by the patient.

The Chinese word for crisis apparently means a mixture of danger and opportunity, and often these occasions prove to be like that for those experiencing them. Sometimes there is positive and life enhancing change after a crisis; sometimes there is the beginning of a breakdown of some kind. Once again, the doctor's most important role seems to be to *be there* for the person in the midst of the crisis.

Linda was a woman in her mid thirties, the wife of a publican, with a teen-age daughter at school. I was called urgently to see her at home in the middle of the day by her husband, who said she was suffering from chest pain and breathlessness. When I arrived, I found Linda sitting at the foot of the stairs hyperventilating and crying: "Help me, help me, I'm dying!"

Her husband told me that she had called him from a 'phone box in town to say that she had developed pains in her chest whilst driving in busy city traffic, and that he had to come and collect her as she couldn't drive home. He had picked her up and she had become steadily more distressed, so he had called me.

Examination confirmed that she was hyperventilating but there was nothing to suggest any physical disease. As I stepped back after examining her she flung her arms around me and said, "Don't go away, I'm sure I'm going to die." (I was glad that her husband was there!) Re-breathing in a paper bag calmed her down a bit, and I gave her a short acting Benzodiazepine tablet to take. I explained to them both that she had had a panic attack and that although these were very frightening, she was in no actual physical danger, her heart and lungs were fine. I asked her to see me in the surgery the next day.

She was initially apologetic and embarrassed when she came the following day, but then went on to talk about the fact that she and her husband faced eviction from the pub they managed and lived in, as the brewery that owned it were not satisfied with the money they were making. This had been playing on her mind and getting her into a state, and she had finally "flipped" whilst driving into the city the previous day. She was still on edge and worried about her physical health, requiring further reassurance that panic attacks could not be fatal. We talked about action she could take to prevent recurrences, and that tranquillisers were not a good idea when there was a specific cause for her anxiety.

These two consultations proved enough to be the turning point for her. She started to take positive action to find alternative accommodation for the family in the event of the worst happening, and with her husband went through their finances to work out what they could actually live on, making enquiries about other employment for them both. Several months later they did actually have to leave the pub, but re-settled happily, and she had no further disabling anxiety. In the crisis, she had changed the danger into an opportunity.

Reg was a man in his mid fifties who had not consulted a doctor for over ten years. He came in a rather apologetic manner, saying he didn't know if there was anything really the matter or not. He commuted to work in a town some twenty miles away, and recently he was having increasing trouble getting up in the morning, feeling that he couldn't face the day. That morning he'd rung in to say he just couldn't make it, and his supervisor had told him to: "get down the doctor's and get yourself sorted out!" It was soon clear that Reg had significant clinical depression which he had been fighting for months. This related to management changes at work that reduced his job satisfaction and left him feeling unappreciated, whilst having to put in more hours.

I recommended that he had at least two weeks off sick, and started him on antidepressants. I soon wondered whether I'd made a mistake, as he took to the sick role with enthusiasm, and consulted frequently with a symptom and mood diary. Eventually I confronted him about this, and he admitted that he was terrified that I would say he was fit for work again, so he was doing his best to remain unwell. That led to a longer discussion about his work, and the possibility of early retirement on medical grounds. He reflected on this for a while, and then decided to go for it.

A protracted period of correspondence with his personnel department followed, and eventually he was offered a reasonable early retirement package. He was still having sickness certificates, and had become fairly doctor dependant. After nine months of antidepressants I suggested we tail them off and stop, although he was still quite anergic and low in the mornings. I was wondering whether I had made the wrong move in supporting him in the sick role, as he now complained of purposeless-ness and boredom at home.

A few more months drifted past before I persuaded him that he was not really sick any more, and should not have further certificates. He could live fairly comfortably on his retirement pension and was not inclined to "sign on" as he did not want to work again despite his claim of boredom. He stopped seeing me eventually (some eighteen months after the initial crisis), and I did not see him again for several years. When he consulted me then about a straightforward physical problem, I asked how things were going, and he said nothing much had really changed since he last saw me, but he had got used to "a quiet life".

In Reg's case, the crisis had been an occasion that precipitated a withdrawal from life rather than an opportunity for constructive change and growth, but that is perhaps not unusual in men in their mid to late fifties who have simply had enough of the struggle to hold down an increasingly demanding job, and are content to settle for a more contemplative existence whilst still in sound enough physical health to enjoy it.

A crisis loosens the fabric of our everyday lives and confronts us with hidden possibilities that we generally prefer not to think about, disrupting the routines and patterns that we have woven around us to prevent "eternity from presenting - here -". It is the doctor's privilege to be present at times of crisis for many of his patients, a familiar figure for them to relate to as the storms of uncertainty and fear rage around them.

Rare Disease

Common diseases commonly occur.

The above is a catch phrase often retold in medical school. Once or twice in a lifetime the doctor may stumble across a rare illness. The effect of this is likely to be beneficial to his relationship with the patient, as he will be more than usually interested in the condition and may have to spend a fair bit of time explaining the nature of the disease to the patient, who is unlikely ever to have heard of it. He is likely also not to forget the patient, who probably has the only case of whatever it is that he is going to see in his professional life. This may result in a special kind of bond between the patient and the doctor, partly because the meaning of the patient's life will for a while be bound up with the fact that they have a rare disease.

Doreen was a large, cheerful, hardworking lady in her late thirties who had married for the second time in her late twenties, having had no children in her first marriage. I knew her only through consultations with her children when they were small. She acted as secretary and accounts manager for her husband's building business, and worked from home, looking after the children at the same time. She consulted me for the first time about herself some seven years after I had first met her. The children were all at school now and life was easier, but she had noticed that she seemed to be lacking in energy and feeling weak. She would feel her legs were tired after walking up the stairs, and her hands didn't seem to have the strength that they used to. Also, her husband was complaining that she sounded a bit drunk after she'd been talking for more than a few minutes; her speech would get slightly slurred. I sensed immediately from my past knowledge of her that this was not going to be a psychological illness, and proceeded to examine her carefully. She was just slightly dysarthric as she told me her story, but I found no objective weakness on examining her muscle groups (she was a big, strong lady,

and said her grip used to be a lot firmer). There was no muscle wasting and her nervous system seemed to be normal. Feeling the challenge of the diagnostic chase, I took blood for a full count and differential, viscosity, thyroid function, electrolytes, tissue antibodies and CPK, and tested her urine (negative for sugar, protein and blood). I asked her to come back in a week, and consulted the textbooks and my partners. The most likely possibility seemed to be Myasthenia Gravis.

Surely not, I thought. Probably it will turn out to be some non-specific viral myositis. However, as the lab results came back I found all was normal apart from raised antibodies to acetyl choline receptors. According to the book, this fitted the picture of Myasthenia. When I saw her the following week, I explained what the tests showed, and that the next logical thing to do was to try an injection of a special drug to see if it got rid of her symptoms. The chemist would have to order this especially as it was such an unusual condition. She went off with a prescription for Edrophonium, and arranged to see me again in a few days time. I very rarely think about work when I'm not actually working, but as I got up on the morning she was due to come back I must admit to feeling a sense of anticipation; was my diagnosis going to be correct?

It was a tense moment as she lay down on my examination couch and I prepared the injection. As it the drug slipped into her circulation, she experienced slight dizziness, but then sat up and said, "I feel normal again!"

"Squeeze my hands," I said. She almost crushed me with her large hands, now restored to their full power. She stood up, still holding my hands, and said: "That's incredible!" We didn't actually dance around the room like the anonymous patient and her fiancé who originally discovered the effect of neostigmine, but it was a moment of celebration. I explained again that the effect of the Edrophonium would wear off in few minutes, but that now we knew what we were dealing with, we could start treatment with the appropriate drug to control her symptoms. I started her on Pyridostigmine and wrote a referral letter to a neurologist. She rang me on her way home to say that the effects of the injection had worn off completely.

She improved a bit on the Pyridostigmine, and in due course got to see the neurologist. It was amusing hearing her tale later of how the hospital doctors were practically falling over in amazement that a general practitioner had managed to diagnose Myasthenia. After a time she was started on steroids, and eventually had a thymectomy, but despite the necessary input from specialists she saw me periodically for explanations of what was happening with her treatment. She was eventually stable on Pyridostigmine and although never quite returned to her previous levels of strength and energy, she could function satisfactorily. She and her husband moved away from the city a few years later, but she thanked me effusively the last time she came to see me for my help with her care. "I'll never forget when you gave me that injection," she said. I reflected that I'll never forget it, either. I don't expect a similar diagnostic triumph again in my career.

Cilla and Bert were a couple in their late forties whom I hardly knew when Cilla consulted me in a very distressed state. She had been married to Bert for over twenty five years, they'd had three children, and she'd just discovered that Bert's father had died in a mental hospital of a hereditary disease, and that Bert had an older brother that she'd never known about who was now in a mental hospital with the same disease. She was sure that Bert had the disease too, because he was starting to make funny movements that he couldn't control, and her sister in law (that she'd only just met) told her that was how it started. "It's called Hunting something or other, "she said.

"Huntington's Chorea," I said.

"That's it. You've heard of it then doctor?" I said that I had, but I knew very little about it. I got a textbook of medicine out and looked it up, reading out a suitably paraphrased account to her.

"I'm sure Bert's got it," she said tearfully. We discussed what to do next. Bert totally refused to come to see me, but she thought that she might persuade him to go to see a specialist. Then there were the children to think of; they had to know about it, none of them were married yet but they were growing up fast. I referred Bert to a neurologist, giving a full family history and explaining the situation. He saw Bert, confirmed that he did indeed have the disease, and arranged genetic counselling for the children (all daughters).

Over the next several years I started seeing Bert once a year, as his choreo-athetoid movements meant he could no longer work as a filling station attendant. His decline was very gradual, but he slowly became more ataxic so that he couldn't go out, and life was getting more stressful for Cilla, who worked full time. She could also no longer tolerate sexual intercourse with Bert, which of course he found frustrating. I arranged for a Community Psychiatric Nurse to see him regularly so he could talk about his feelings (not something he found easy), and for a while he attended a day centre for disabled people. Slowly the home situation started building towards a crisis. Bert was falling frequently and was really getting unsafe to be left alone. I feared that long term admission was soon going to be required and got him seen by a psychiatrist. Then Cilla got the address of a nursing home in another county which specialised in caring for people with Huntingdon's and similar diseases, and took Bert there to see it. It seemed to be just the answer; he could stay there in the week and come home at weekends whilst he was still well enough. Money wasn't a problem as Cilla was earning well and her daughters would also help. However, Bert started to get difficult, and refused to go. This precipitated a few more crisis consultations with Cilla, who had to get to the point of seeing that she had to be firm with Bert for her own sanity's sake. In a sense she needed permission from me to do this, and finally she got Bert admitted there, some thirteen years after the diagnosis had initially been suggested by herself.

That resolved the problem. Bert was happy once he was there, and Cilla was far less stressed. Over the years I had got to know them both quite well, and again a particular kind of bond was formed because of the rarity of Bert's disease.

Rare diseases rarely occur, but occur they do, and they offer unusual opportunities for the doctor to be involved in the long term care of people who are particularly needful of the information and emotional support that the he is in a unique position to give. This can lead to a very rewarding relationship with the patient and their principal carer, as once again the family doctor is the available and approachable figure who can help them cope with the medical system on which they must rely.

Romantic Love

All the rocket ships are climbing through the sky, The holy books are open wide, The doctors working day and night, But they'll never ever find that cure for love. There ain't no drink, there ain't no drug, There's nothing pure enough to be a cure for love. (Cohen 1988)

Probably nothing in human life has the power to inflict as much pleasure or as much pain as the overwhelming and essentially mystical experience of what is called romantic love. It remains popular as a subject for songs, books and films even in societies that are fast abandoning lifelong marriage as the appropriate vehicle for its consummation and nurturing. Indeed, it is often used as the justification for the breakdown of marriage, when one of the partners has 'fallen in love' with someone else. Like birth and death, the expression of sexuality in love is one of those core human experiences that are profoundly spiritual, involving the greatest depths of our being, enabling us to transcend ourselves in union with another.

In his daily work, the doctor will come across many people who are wounded in love, and sometimes too some of the fortunate few whose lives are transformed by finding reciprocated true love with a compatible partner. The stories below are about occasions when the presenting problem itself was the pain of love.

I had known Jean for many years, a woman then in her late thirties who rarely consulted. I was surprised to see her name added as an urgent extra to my appointment list one afternoon. She was (fortunately) the last patient. She came in and said: "I don't know why I'm here, really". I waited in silence, and she slowly started to cry. When she had controlled her initial spasm of weeping she managed to say: "I've just found out my husband's been carrying on with someone else." A long story finally emerged of how she'd suspected this for some time, but whenever she challenged him he had plausible excuses, and obviously she wanted to believe him. What particularly hurt her was that a few years before she'd been very attracted to a man at work, but had told her husband about it and had resisted the temptation of an affair because she wanted their marriage to be strong, even though at the time they'd "been going through a rough patch."

She was deeply hurt by feelings of anger, loss and resentment, which with minimal prompting she poured out. Eventually I asked gently what she planned to do, but she was unable to see any way forward. I asked her to see me again in a couple of days, as I felt she needed emotional support and from my previous knowledge of her knew that she would soon be on her feet again.

She was already much calmer when I saw her again, saying that she had confronted her husband with choosing between the other woman and her, and that if he wanted the other one he had to leave immediately. This had shaken him a lot and he'd promised to end the affair, having been (she thought) truly surprised at her level of distress which made him realise how much she cared about him. She thanked me for listening to her and said she felt she could cope with things satisfactorily now.

I didn't see her again with reference to this episode, and as far as I am aware her marriage has continued. She continued to consult rarely, although she lived near the surgery and I often saw her in the streets around. The sharing of her emotional pain had produced a deeper bond between us, an example again of the spirituality of the consultation emerging because of an event highly charged with meaning for the patient.

Tina I had known since she was in her early teens, now an unmarried mother in her twenties.

She came to see me one day with bruises on her arms and face. "How did you get these?" I asked, already having a pretty good idea.

"It was my boy friend," she said, "he hits me sometimes when he gets drunk." The boy friend, I knew, was the father of her child, but they did not live together all the time because of his drinking and violence. I actually knew this from Tina's mother who was also my patient, but Tina had never told me herself until this occasion, so I had to listen as though receiving new information. Despite her distress at the treatment he dished out from time to time, Tina still had some feelings for the man that she was not able to put aside, and did not want to end the relationship. "There's still something there, you know?" she said to me sadly. I couldn't help reflecting that a few years earlier, when I had less experience of the remarkably powerful effects of romantic love in people's lives; I would have failed to understand how she tolerated a man who hit her. As it was, I could only offer her support whilst suggesting that for her own good she should see he police about charging him with assault. She wanted me to document the bruising in case she did decide to press charges, but (as I thought) she did not do so, and I think continues to tolerate periodic beatings from a man with whom she has known the pleasure as well as the pain of love. Tina usually consulted one of my partners after that, as though embarrassed that she had revealed an intimate secret to me that somehow betrayed her boy friend.

Although it is more common for women wounded in love to come to the doctor, it does also happen with men. Darren was an apparently rather rough young man who was often in trouble with the police for drug offences (he took Amphetamines) and seemed to live on the edge of various criminal fraternities in the area, altogether not the sort of man one would have thought likely to get in a state over a girl. However, appearances can be deceptive, and it was with surprise that I found him telling me one day that his romantic pre-occupation with a girl who'd ditched him for some underworld gang boss was "doing his head in." He'd had a relationship with the lady in question that had lasted a couple of years, and then he'd suddenly found out she was also dating the gang boss as well. He couldn't do anything about it as the man had more power in the scene they both frequented and could arrange "an accident" if he made any trouble. To cap it all, it was rumoured that the girl was pregnant and he didn't know if the baby was his or not. It was a strange experience seeing this tough, tattooed, unshaven hard man breaking down in tears because he'd been betrayed in love. In matters of the heart, it seems no one is immune to the power of love. Darren was actually wanting me to give him 'a tablet' to stop him feeling as he did, and I had to virtually quote the lines of a song to persuade him that no such product exists.

Eventually time did its healing work and Darren "got it together again", but I saw him many times over this episode and learnt a lot about not being prejudiced by people's appearances. Underneath the hard man image lay a sensitive and bleeding heart.

When people show their wounded hearts to the doctor, the consultation always moves into that area where its spirituality is apparent, for the doctor and patient together are encountering one of the profoundest realities of the human condition. It is an insensitive doctor, who is denying aspects of his own humanity, who does not treat such occasions with great respect.

CONCLUSION

The previous stories illustrate some of the ways in which people afflicted with real or perceived illness react and use a variety of resources to cope with their problems, and how their requests for medical care are affected as a result. The doctor needs to listen to his patient's stories, understand the pattern of the narratives and respond accordingly, acting in accordance with his patients wishes as far as possible. In this way, by 'being there' for and with the patient through each episode of illness and perhaps for many years in the case of a chronic disease, the doctor can offer support, comfort and appropriate counsel in ways that go beyond purely clinical management. To do this is a great privilege and is central to the vocation of medicine. This important truth must be just as much a part of medical teaching as the key elements of the clinical syllabus if the profession is to live up to its reputation and status with the public. Every consultation with a patient is like a journey of exploration, and after many years in practice it starts to become possible to say that, although we are just where we started, we are perhaps beginning to 'know the place for the first time'(Eliot 1967) as we gradually learn more about the nature of being human.

REFERENCES

Cohen, L. (1988). *Ain't no cure for love*, I'm Your Man, CBS Records 1988

Eliot, T. S. (1967). *Little Gidding*. Four Quartets, New York: Faber and Faber.

Masefield, J. (1988). *Pompey the Great*. Oxford, UK: Oxford Library of English Poetry.

Chapter 11
Lived Experiences in Cardiothoracic Surgery:
A Personal View

Anjan Kumar Das
Stempeutics Research Malaysia, Malaysia

ABSTRACT

This chapter narrates the story of patients with cardiac illnesses requiring surgery and reveals how the physician-surgeon tries to reconcile a low resource setting patient care narrative with resource demanding modern scientific medicine and the areas of disconnect that this generate. This chapter is written in three parts. The first part is a narrative of training that the author received and the development of his philosophy of medicine. The second part describes his experiences in the government health services in the State of West Bengal in India and the third describes how we worked in a remote location in Nepal, the author was able to set up a cardiothoracic unit. The chapter narrates the problems, solutions and outcomes of surgery in these circumstances and how it was possible to overcome difficulties to offer a service to the patients which, while having many flaws, did offer treatments that would have never been possible for them to access otherwise.

INTRODUCTION

Early Life

I was born in a very typical middle class family in Calcutta, then still the first city of India. I belong to the Midnight + 10 generation, meaning that I was born a decade after the coming of independence changed the lives of everybody in the

subcontinent and particularly those of the people of Bengal where I was born. This was because the British succeeded in dividing the country before they went, a tried and tested formula that they had used in Ireland with success a few decades earlier. All other considerations apart, what this meant was that there was an exchange of population that surpassed anything that had ever taken place in human history earlier and a large proportion of the Hindu population of what became East Pakistan fled to a truncated state of West Bengal.

DOI: 10.4018/978-1-60960-097-6.ch011

Calcutta was cut off from its economic and cultural hinterland and our childhood was the time that the Western half of Bengal, which remained a part of India, tried to come to terms with this. My mother's family was part of the exodus: her family left their East Bengal home to come to Calcutta where my parents were married in 1955.

I however was privileged in that we were in the upper reaches of the middle class and I went to one of Calcutta's leading English Medium schools, run by the Salesians, an order of Catholic monks who originated in Turin in the nineteenth century. This meant that the teaching was in English and we learnt our own language as a second language. I passed out from school in 1974 and was able to successfully compete in the stiff admission tests to the Medical College, Calcutta.

The Medical College had a proud inheritance. It was the first institution to be set up in Asia to teach Western Medicine, and it was here that the first human dissections took place in the subcontinent, a practice which was strictly taboo in the India of the early nineteenth century. By the time I joined in the middle of 70's, decay had set in, as it had in all institutions in Bengal. This was partly because of the shift in economic priorities; the democratic government of India was now more concerned about the vote bank states of the Hindi heartland and the major Southern states. Bengal, now truncated, with its major part lost in the vivisection that followed Independence now counted for little in the new dispensation. This slow decay was aggravated by the Naxalite movement which blew through West Bengal like a cyclone in the mid sixties. Hailed by Communist China as the "Spring thunder over India" this movement, which supported a Maoist type communist uprising, closed institutions, caused a flight of capital and began the brain drain from West Bengal that continues to this day. The violence came to an end when the movement was eradicated by an equally brutal state intervention, but it left the state ripe for a communist takeover, albeit of the constitutional kind. Ever since 1977

West Bengal has been ruled by communists and while this led to some land reforms in the rural areas, and ensured a better life for the rural poor, it also meant a cynical degradation of all institutions of higher learning which were derided as elitist. The 30 + years of Communist rule have left West Bengal's institutions in a state of paralysis. There has been little progress and the State has progressively fallen behind all the leaders in India today. This is a humiliating comedown for a state that prided itself in "thinking today what India thinks tomorrow".

However when I joined the Medical College it was still a name to conjure with. It was even then one of the leading medical colleges in India. The college buildings were built on a grand scale, the Corinthian columns of the principal Medical College Hospital building still awed in its magnificence. The Anatomy Museum and the Pathology museum were still the best in India and teaching was excellent. The biggest advantage was the rush of patients. The number of patients and the variety that we could see in the wards and the OPD enabled us to perfect our clinical skills. Though we did not realize it at the time, medicine was becoming more and more technology dependent and we were still learning the medicine of the past. This had two effects one good and one bad. The bad part was, of course that we fell more and more behind when technology driven medicine became the face of modern medicine. But the obverse was that we were capable of handling patients with little equipment and back up that stood us in good stead when we went out to the real world that was the Indian health care system.

I was influenced by the system. I remember my first "Boss ", under whose tutelage I did my initial house job in surgery, was very skeptical of what he called unnecessary and new fangled interventions. He laid immense emphasis on the clinical eye and tailoring the surgery to the patient. This meant that he would never recommend gall bladder surgery for a 65 + patient (In the seventies, this was considered old). Neither did he allow us to prescribe antibiotics that were not available at the Hospital drug store at no cost to our patients. He preferred to counsel patients in any cases of what we call "bad" Cancers, e.g. gall bladder cancers rather than jumping in to operate. He would always prefer a good palliation rather than a major, hopefully curative, resection procedure that had a high mortality. I was very much influenced by him. I practiced a generation after him, but I found that in the public health care system his principles were valid and have remained valid to this day. This is a sad reflection perhaps of the lack of progress in modern medical facilities in our country. Moreover he taught me the importance of cutting your coat according to your cloth and that surgery is for the patient and not for the greater glory of the surgeon, an important truth that is often forgotten in today's technology driven virtuosity that leaves the patient with a large bill and little improvement in results than a simpler, less costly, intervention would have given.

I started my working life after my post graduation in a private hospital but soon shifted to the Government Health system. My ambition was to become a teacher, and to do that one had to join the public health care system. I was posted initially in a health centre in the North Bengal district of Malda. Here I worked in a Primary Health Centre in a remote part of the district, bordering Bangladesh. The largely Muslim populations of this area were agriculturists and Bidi workers. The making of bidis (a form of cigarette) was a cottage industry in those parts and this organized industry was a valuable addition to the income of this poor population.

It was an adventure for a city bred person like me. I had to travel on a bus from the district headquarters and then by a horse drawn tonga for the last five kilometers to the Health centre. Here I had one senior colleague, a public health nurse and four other nurses and sundry other health workers to cater to the needs of a population of more than half a million. There was a post office at about 2 kilometers distance, but no other educated person

except the school masters who lived far away. The panchayat system had just been promulgated by the State government and for the first time local politicians had a say in the developmental expenditure of their areas. This led to an initial burst of enthusiasm and much microlevel development took place, including roads, tube wells, school building construction and the like. Later, unfortunately the Indian disease of corruption became all pervasive and today Panchayats are a byword for corruption, though localized in form. But of the time I write, (1989) the panchayats were still a force for change in the rural areas and the energy of the local representatives was infectious.

I enjoyed my time there. Living separated from my family was a novel and not always enjoyable experience, I saw rural India from close quarters and this has coloured my perceptions ever since. I am not one of those who blindly subscribe to Cowper's "God made the country and man made the town "thesis. I experienced the pettiness and factionalism of village life and its stifling parochialism. The villagers were greedy for free official handouts, willing to turn into an ugly mob at the blink of an eyelid and often stubbornly unwilling to understand why their children needed immunization. But having said that, I also saw, for the first time, the extent of privations that they suffered. The poverty was not as spectacular, if I may use the term, as those of the slums of Calcutta, they were all pervading, grinding them into dust in its inexorability and often accepted with a sense of fatalism that never failed to infuriate me. I began to perceive why this population did not cooperate with the authorities to stop over the border smuggling and why they were so resistant to the idea of sending their children to school.

I was a trained surgeon, but I did not know anything about anaesthesia! So I was forced to teach myself ether anaesthesia: we held down patients as one of us administered ether drop by drop on a pad held over the patient's face. I soon realized that this was a fairly safe method of anaesthesia and this enabled me to operate on a wide variety of conditions including intra abdominal conditions like cholelithiasis and appendicitis and we even did a cesarean section on a patient with obstructed labour who refused to be transferred to the District headquarters. We, thankfully never lost a patient and I still remember the effusive gratefulness of a father whose daughter had a cleft lip when we managed to give her a (fairly) normal looking lip postoperatively. It was here that I first began to innovate in ways that came in handy even when I was later working in a tertiary care setting. I realized that though I was a specialist (by training) I could turn my hand to everything if I wanted, with at least a moderate level of competence and this was vital if I wanted to work in a government setting and truly this was the need of the day in rural India. This stood me in good stead when in Calcutta I was needed to do the work of a perfusionist or even as a scrub nurse if necessary.

I was transferred out from the district to the Medical College (my alma mater) after about a year. I was lucky. There were many colleagues who had worked for years, even decades in the districts before they managed to get a coveted transfer. I was luckier because I intended to work in cardiac surgery, a specialty that was ignored by most other aspiring surgeons in those days, at least in West Bengal. This was probably the reason for my good fortune.

Experiential Learning in Cardio Thoracic Surgery

It is now common knowledge that India provides some of the best and most sophisticated health care facilities in the world. It has always been a destination for medical tourists from the Middle East as well as from the neighboring South Asian countries, but now it is also the port of call for many Western patients who prefer Indian Hospitals for their low costs and better services. And there is really every reason for this influx. Indian hospitals have today facilities and services that

in many cases rival their Western counterparts in their outcomes. It has been estimated that In Indian hospitals earned Rs 4500 crores (Approx $ 900 million) during this year. These earnings are projected to rise to $ 4 billion in 2012.

I had the privilege of working on a fellowship in one such hospital. The Escorts Heart Hospital was then perhaps India's leading cardiac hospital, led by one of the most dynamic heart surgeons in India, Dr Naresh Trehan. Trained in New York, Dr Trehan was among the first in India to see the possibilities of an American Hospital transplanted onto Indian soil and his hospital was then the busiest in India, doing almost as many surgeries every day as the Cleveland Clinic which was supposed to be the busiest in the world. The infrastructure was, in a word, world class. The consultants were publishing regularly in major world journals and the results were outstanding by any outcome measures.

After the stint there was over I returned to my hospital, the Calcutta Medical College Hospital where I had been working for about 9 years. We had an academic department, housed atop the David Hare Block, named after the famous 19th century teacher and social reformer who started life as a watch maker in Edinburgh. Our facility was arguably the best in the Government sector in West Bengal. We operated five days a week, doing a total of just about 100 open heart surgeries a year, a number that the Escorts Heart Hospital did in a week. This was only one of three centres in West Bengal in the Public sector that had a fully fledged cardiac surgery unit and no other hospital had these facilities in a population base of about 70 million. Even here the difficulties were legendary: poor facilities, lack of drugs and even on occasion, oxygen; and poorly trained nurses and technicians made our life that much more difficult forcing us to do work that could easily be done by less trained personnel, wasting our time and energy. The OPD which functioned thrice a week saw at least 100 patients in each session, most of them in dire need for surgery. We were, after all, the only one of three referral centres catering to not just West Bengal, but to a substantial portion of Bangladesh, Orissa, the then Bihar and Nepal as well as most of the north eastern states. There was a disconnect here that was disconcerting; I seemed to have traversed from the first world to the third in a matter of a few hours of travel.

This disconnect did not confine itself to just the facilities, but even the patients we saw were completely different. Our patients were in the main congenital heart diseases which had not been treated in the early part of their illness. Most of them were adult congenital, to use the prevailing lingo. As a consequence most of them had pulmonary hypertension and a significant number were inoperable and most had become high risk subjects. Another large segment was the "valves". We had a large population of rheumatic heart disease patients who had tried the gamut of therapy from modern medical practitioners, local quacks, and homeopathy before they came to us for help. There was an entity that we described jokingly, though we never published, a Water Pot heart which meant a huge dilatation of both the left atrium and the right ventricle following mitral valvular disease complicated with tricuspid valve disease. Again most of these patients were at the border line of inoperability and results of surgery were understandably poor.

The point I am trying to make is that in India there are two worlds in healthcare. There is the world of major private hospitals where the patients suffer from diseases peculiar to the well fed classes, coronary artery disease being the most common. Valve diseases were uncommon and most of the mitral valve disease that we saw there were mainly a result of ischemic heart disease and not the stigmata of rheumatic disease as in the public hospitals. There we had the best nurses, all well trained, as well as technicians who did many of the chores that are necessary during cardiac surgery. Here we had to start by setting up the transducers and laying out the necessary

instruments as well. It was a form of Snow's two cultures, only here it cost lives.

Narratives of Valvular Heart Disease

Narrative 1

Mira Sarkar was born into a family of share croppers in the Malda district of West Bengal. Their condition had improved considerably following land reforms which followed the election of a communist led government in the State. However while they were spared the hunger that had been a common accompaniment to their existence earlier, they still were desperately poor; improvement in their condition was only relative. One of five children, Mira developed rheumatic fever at the age of 11. The fever and joint pains resolved in a couple of weeks, she was treated only by "some tablets from the *dactar babu* (Doctor, in this case, the local quack)". These were presumably analgesic tablets which reduced the pain and inflammation. Nobody auscultated her heart and she barely rested after the illness as she had to resume her work in the fields and at home to enhance family income. She was married at the age of 16, and became pregnant after about 3 months. During the course of this pregnancy she first noticed that she was breathless and often dizzy. This she blamed on her pregnancy and she was delivered of a boy at the local Health centre. Here she was never seen by the doctor, but was given a Tetanus Toxoid by the nurses in charge and prescribed some iron tablets.

Life resumed, but now it was obvious to her that she could not do the hard work of bringing water from the local tube well and she was often dyspnoec while doing the washing. She managed to conceal this from her husband's family successfully for about two years but on one occasion she woke up in the middle of the night gasping for breath and according to her "about to die". However this resolved when she sat up in bed, but her husband took her to the Health centre where she was seen by the doctor in the OPD and diagnosed provisionally to have a valve disease. She was referred to a physician in the District Town of Malda where she was told that one of her valves had gone "bad" and she needed surgery. She was advised to go one of the Calcutta teaching hospitals. She could only come after her husband had sold her only piece of jewellery, a necklace that had been a present from her parents during her marriage. She came to the Medical College on a Monday which was not an OPD day and spent the night on the footpath on College Street. The next morning she was seen in the OPD and advised to be tested. The tests, she was told would only take place in batches. A series of blood tests on the same day, an ECG also the same day, but she would have to come back after three weeks for an echocardiogram. After much pleading, a sympathetic house surgeon changed her date to three days later and she had the Echo done on that day. She spent the weekend on the footpath once again and then was seen in the OPD once more and this time the consultant spoke to her and her husband and told them that she had a valve disease which needed early surgery and this would entail the replacement of the mitral valve which would cost about Rs 60,000 ($ 1200) and she would be expected to recruit at least 5 blood donors. When she asked for alternatives, she was told that she could continue having drugs and a three weekly injection of penicillin s rheumatic fever prophylaxis, but this was not really an alternative, she had to have surgery to think of a long term survival. Mira went back to her village, stopped her diuretics and long term penicillin after three months. She had repeated bouts of heart failure and died suddenly one evening. She was 19.

Narrative 2

Sankar Ghosh was a born in a tea garden worker's family in the North Bengal District of Jalpaiguri. His father was a member of the powerful communist led union. When he began to complain of breathlessness after play in school, he was referred to a physician who immediately diagnosed a mitral valve disease from an unnoticed rheumatic fever in his childhood. He too was referred to Calcutta, where fortunately he had a relative who could give them shelter. He too attended the OPD in Medical College and was duly advised Mitral Valve replacement. He was more fortunate in that his father's connections ensured the sanction of the cost of the valve from the Chief Minister's Relief Fund and his father raised the rest from his fellow workers who donated generously. His father was also able to borrow from his Provident Fund account. The surgery was successful and he was discharged on the tenth day after surgery and was advised to continue some drugs including anticoagulants which, he was told, were vital. He did very well postoperatively, becoming completely asymptomatic and resuming his school work. He failed his school leaving exams and was offered a job in a local factory that made a local brand of confectionary. He began to work here but was laid off when business was bad. By now he had been taking his anticoagulant drugs for 3 years though he had stopped his penicillin injections. When he was laid off, he stopped the anticoagulants also. One morning, two years later he suddenly suffered a stroke that left him paralysed on the right side. He was admitted to the District Hospital in Jalpaiguri where he developed pneumonia and died after three weeks.

What is the Problem?

Both these patients would have had a good long term result if they had no constraints in their treatment. In the first case (Mira), she was unable to afford the treatment required and died basically without treatment, despite the availability of a nominally free health care system in the State of West Bengal. The second was luckier, in that he had the family and other resources to utilize the system in order to have the surgery that he required despite the high costs involved. However the social system in which he lived and lack of local heath care resources prevented the proper follow up which is an integral part of the treatment in these conditions and resulted in an adverse outcome.

If we look at the results of mitral valve surgery that are reported by centres in the West (and these results are now routinely duplicated by most major Indian hospitals), it is evident that the public hospitals which are the principal teaching hospitals have a much poorer outcome. This however is not due to any lack of expertise or sometimes not even the lack of modern equipment as most such hospitals have modern equipment, but social factors which appear to be well nigh impossible to remedy.

I speak from experience. I spent the first two decades after graduation in public hospitals, and most of this time was spent in three major teaching hospitals of Calcutta. These were the Institute of Post Graduate Education and Research, The Calcutta Medical College and The NRS Medical College. All these hospitals were major hospitals, their bed strengths ranged from 1500-2000. They had large departments of Thoracic and Cardiovascular Surgery, each with a 50 bed inpatient unit, ICUs and dedicated Operation Theatres, Radiology Facilities and Pathology laboratories. They participated in Undergraduate training, Postgraduate and superspeciality training as well. The IPGMER ran Daily OPDs, while the other two hospitals had OPDs thrice a week. Two operating rooms functioned for five days a week for planned surgery and as and when needed for emergencies.

The staffing pattern was based on the West Bengal Heath Service guidelines. There were three consultants who admitting privileges and several other trained surgeons assisted by medical officers and house officers. Nurses and technicians were allotted from the hospital pool but usually were part of the department for long periods. The nurses were poorly trained. They were graduates from the nursing schools of the Government which were scattered among the Teaching Hospitals and District Hospitals of West Bengal. At that

time none had any specialized training in cardiac nursing or Operation room (OR) nursing, though many had been trained on the job and were extremely competent. The technicians also had a similar background. They too had not been trained especially in the function of the Cardiac Unit, but as members of the team for a long time, had obtained a competence that made them integral and important team members.

The patient pool was drawn from the lower middle and the poor classes. This meant that the vast majority of patients were totally dependent on government funding for their treatment. Cardiac surgery is notoriously expensive and thought the government paid for most of the disposables and drugs used for surgery, there was a proportion that had to be paid for by the patient. Unfortunately valves were one of the items not provided. Consequently the patient had to spend about Rs 10000 ($500) and the cost of the valve if it was needed (Rs 25000-60000) ($500-1200). It was an impossible proposition for many of the patients especially if they had no contacts among the local politicians who wield immense power in their areas. This fate befell Mira, who simply could not have surgery and died untreated. Others were luckier, especially if they could manipulate the system. There are several government schemes to provide financial help for such patients. The Relief Funds associated with the Prime Minister's, Chief Minister's and the Governor's offices could help with fairly large amounts. However the paperwork needed and the follow up that was needed was not possible without connections in the local political bureaucracy, some education and persistence. Even then there was no provision for proper follow up in the vast hinterland from where the patients came, and this led to avoidable tragedies of the type that befell the patient in our second narrative.

Thus, working in these conditions led to changes in practice from the best practice guidelines of text books and the large professional bodies. In the real world, a surgeon soon learnt that it is necessary to relearn many things, cut corners and accept some unpleasant consequences as inevitable, though avoidable. As a point of fact, there were two principal themes that we had reconciled ourselves with.

Cost Cutting

There was an inexorable need to cut costs. It became one of the principal mantras in our hospitals. Unfortunately this often meant cutting corners as well!

Narrative 3

Swapan Ganguly 23 year old male came to the Medical College Hospitals with an atrial septal defect. His mother had been warned that he had a heart defect during his childhood, but as he was almost symptom free, she did not pay much attention. Now he had recurrent bouts of fever and chest infection and had been referred for surgery. He was told that he would need to spend about Rs 10000($ 200) for drugs and disposables not supplied by the hospital, but was unable to procure the amount for about 4 months. Finally he came to the concerned consultant and said that he had collected Rs 6000($ 120) from various sources and he could by no means procure any more money. The consultant then admitted him and corners were cut by reusing the cannulae used for surgery after sterilization and by using a suture for his sternum rather than stainless steel wires. The patient had a good result and was well for at least two years after follow up. He is presumably doing well.

The reuse of disposable cannulae is strictly prohibited in all guidelines. It is associated with infections and possible haemolysis and is something that most surgeons working in private hospitals would never consider doing. However it was a routine practice in my Department as a cost cutting measure. This saved the patient almost Rs 5000 ($100) and made it possible for many patients who would otherwise be unable to afford surgery, have their operations. This worked fairly well in

congenital heart conditions, particularly those patients who needed only one surgical procedure. Swapan was one such patient. However this could lead to infective complications in patients who had valve replacements or had patches left behind in the heart. The results of surgery were inevitably worse than the published results elsewhere, and through no fault of the surgical or ICU team.

Similar cost cutting was a normal part of the anaesthetic and ICU management as well. For instance when propofol first became available, we were unable to use it because of the cost. Changing IV lines daily, a routine practice in ICUs could never be done as it would have added to patient costs, similar cutting of corners were commonplace and if research is to be believed must have led to less than optimal results.

Lack of Support Systems

The patient often lacked the most basic support systems at home that are taken for granted in more prosperous societies. For instance the patients were often unable to take enough time off from work, or in the case of women had to resume housework very soon after their surgery. The nutritional requirements were often not met. Ay best of times the patients lived at the edge of sustenance and a major surgical operation could tip them onto a form of malnutrition which had implications regarding their survival and morbidity after surgery. Even transport to the hospital in the immediate postoperative period for complications like minor wound infections and the like could be impossible to organize because of a lack of funds or logistics and what was a minor complication might in time flare up to a major one.

Narrative 4

Rinku Sonar was operated for a ventricular septal defect. She came from a family of reasonably prosperous farmers and could afford to have the surgery done, though her family sold a plot of land to enable them to pay all the expenses. She had a minor swelling in the region of one of the sternal wires which she ignored because this was the harvest season and nobody in the family could be spared to make the journey to Calcutta. Ignored, the infection spread to several other sutures and she had a full blown sternal wound infection that led to another hospitalization and major surgery to resuture the sternum and a greater omental graft. This cost the family another piece of land, though she did well after this and was well on her last follow up.

This story ended on a comparatively happy note though it could have had fatal consequences. Here the problem was not money; the family could afford to pay, though they had to sacrifice land. But a simple matter of lack of support led to a neglect of her minor wound infection that could have led to mediastinitis and death in the long run. Several other narratives ended with a much worse outcome and again these unfortunate outcomes would never have occurred in the presence of a good peripheral health system or a system of logistical support to patients as is considered routine in developed societies.

Strategies Developed to Meet These Deficiencies

The surgical teams working in this field soon learnt techniques to deal with these deficiencies.

These can be considered in several heads:

a. *Changes in surgical techniques*

There included using valve repair techniques in patients who would ideally need a valve replacement in order to save on the cost of the valve. Mitral valve repair techniques are an integral part of cardiac surgery. Several investigators have designed and validated techniques for repair in order to avoid the complications and costs of valve repair. However most Western observers have used these techniques in non rheumatic

hearts and the results in rheumatic valve disease is much worse than in ischemic or degenerative disease. We were forced on occasion to accept a less than ideal repair to obviate the necessity for a valve replacement. This in turn led to a less than ideal result, but the reasoning was that we were buying time for 5-10 years and tailoring the surgery to the patient's pocket. While this would seem to be ethically dubious, it is also a fact that the alternative was often death as epitomized by our first narrative.

All colleagues in the team had to change techniques to suit the conditions. The anaesthesia team also had to modify their techniques to the situation on the ground. This often meant using drugs that were not ideal, or more properly being unable to use drugs that were available and shown to ensure better results; depending on clinical expertise rather than, say, blood gas reports to monitor the patient and so on. While these were not necessarily associated with worse outcomes, it did entail committing more human resources to a patient and necessarily reduced the output of the clinician.

b. *Reusing " disposables"*

It was a routine practice in our department to reuse disposable canulae, as well as monitoring lines and transducers after sterilization. It has been shown that this practice is likely to lead to greater infection levels and the transmission of various diseases like Hepatitis B, Hepatitis C etc, it was considered impractical to adhere to these guidelines. The cost of disposable lines and cannulae amounted to about 35% of the cost of surgery and reducing this amount made surgery affordable to a large proportion of patients. In fact adhering to the standard guidelines would probably have meant that about 40-50% patients would have been unable to afford surgery. It was felt that this was the lesser of two evils and to tell the truth we managed to get good results with, to my knowledge, no reported adverse events.

However as our follow up was very incomplete, this statement must be treated with caution.

c. *Counseling*

We found it useful to counsel patients regarding discharge medication in a manner that would probably raise the hackles of any patient rights groups in the west. The second narrative records an event that was extremely common. Patients who had a valve replacement went home and after the convalescence period felt so much better that they considered themselves cured. Unfortunately, though surgeons and cardiologists like to propagate the myth that patients are cured by cardiologic or cardiac surgical interventions this is rarely the case. All patients need careful follow up and regular medication and often reintervention after a period of time. To our patients, the intervention that had been done was a onetime affair. They could not dream of having another such intervention, both because of the costs involved and the massive expenditure of social and family resources and good will. Thus, a patient with anticoagulant therapy was told that he needed to have the anticoagulant every day. If he stopped for a single day, he would die. Thus was obviously not true but such counseling often conveyed to them the sense of urgency which we felt was essential. We often did not prescribe regular P time tests. We were aware that this would never be done. Nobody from a village would travel to the District town, perhaps 70 km away and get the test done. So we took a calculated risk. If the P time was raised, a warning bleed would be more likely to bring the patient for follow up and then it would be possible to correct the problem, the converse would not be noticed and the patient would present with a stroke or die suddenly from a non functioning valve. This was a reality that had to be faced and techniques developed accordingly to deal with it.

Follow up was also scheduled accordingly. They were scheduled at long intervals, solely because the patients would never have followed the schedule otherwise. Even with these modifications, follow up was never complete and patients came to the OPD for follow up only if there was a specific symptom, or more tragically, they reported to the Emergency Room (ER) with a life threatening complication.

What are the Ethical Issues?

To the present author there are no ethical issues involved. I do not think that I am any less endowed with moral values than most. However I think I speak for many, if not all my colleagues as well when I say that we felt no moral dilemma at all when we changed the rules of the game to suit our patients and us.

There are well laid out guidelines, set up by professional bodies, almost all of which we violated in our practice. This is the stuff of ethical nightmares. But in practice, "it is a war out there" and we felt that our practices could easily be justified, at least to ourselves, because the benefits far outweighed the drawbacks. Our patients were totally dependent on us. Their personal resources were few, their education levels low and their expectations so high that it was not possible to disappoint them, at least unless we were prepared to refuse surgery to the large majority of the patients. This was often tantamount to a death sentence, and we felt justified in taking calculated risks in order to offer the patients a chance and we felt that this was justified by the results.

Concluding Remarks

Tertiary care in a government setting is the stuff of nightmares. The reason is not a lack of facilities; it is simply a lack of funds. With the a total absence of any form of social security system, patients are totally dependent on the government run health care system for their needs. While there are many concerns about the Government run systems and many valid criticisms are made it is necessary to recall that a major cardiac surgery costs about Rs

100,000-Rs 225,000($ 2000-$ 4500) in the best run cardiac centres. This is not inclusive of the cost of infrastructure. Thus the government spends a very large sum on setting up the infrastructure, an equally large amount for the salaries and allowances of the personnel working there and then understandably the system fell short when paying for the costs of disposables for the patient. In any government run facility in West Bengal (of which I have personal knowledge), this amounts to about Rs 30,000-50000 ($ 600-$1000) for each patient. Operating on 100 patients a year means a cost of Rs 5 million ($100,000) a year only for patients undergoing open heart surgery. It is well to be reminded that each of these departments also catered to the needs of patients undergoing thoracic and vascular surgery and emergencies. These made up the majority of their work, thus costs were further increased and the patient did not pay for any of these procedures as well. To my mind, though I never worked out the sums, this was obviously not sustainable. And indeed the Government grants often did fall short, forcing cancellation of surgery for such reason as a lack of reagents to run the blood gas machine. There has also been occasion for surgeons to organize oxygen cylinders form another department so that a planned surgery was not cancelled.

The solution to this problem is well known. The only solution is a good quality health insurance paid for by taxes or by individual subscriptions. It seems incredible that while we can afford to spend enough money to have state of the art space research, atomic research and the largest rural employment scheme in the world, we are unable to set up a proper health system that can be paid for by subscriptions or by the government if need be. The only consolation is that neither has the United States! Until this is done, heath care providers will be forced to innovate and scrimp to save patients. The techniques that we have used will be used in order to save patient lives, though in some cases they may lead to a loss of life as well.

Note

The prices are true for the decade of the nineties of the last century when I worked in Government hospitals and at this time the per capita income In India was approximately $ 390 rising to approx $ 490 by the end of the decade. Subsequently the income growth has been more impressive, rising to $ 749 by 2008. However these statistics conceal the unevenness of the growth, as poverty (defined as an Income < $ 1 / per day per person was as high as 42% according to World Bank estimates. It is also to be noted that the eastern States of India, which includes West Bengal lags behind the national average in both GDP growth as well as reduction of poverty levels.

PART 3

I have always been in love with the mountains. I fell in love in 1978 when I visited Darjeeling for the first time and have been enamoured ever since. The Himalayas are my first love and I have walked the hilly trails of this mighty chain from Kashmir to Arunachal Pradesh, a swathe of India and Nepal that is almost 3000 kilometers long. It was a seasonal love affair. Twice a year without fail, I bad my family goodbye, gathered together my rucksack and my climbing boots and set off on a trek. I have also been on several climbing expeditions. I had a completely different set of friends who were my companions in these expeditions. We have walked the mountainsides for more than 20 years now together. In the autumn of 1998 we walked the round Annapurna trail. This trail entails crossing the Thorang La, a pass 5416 meters(approx 18,000 feet) high set in the Annapurna range of mountains connecting it with the gorge cut out in the hills by the Kaligandaki River. Over the pass is the famous Hindu pilgrimage site of Muktinath which has been a destination for holy men and householders for aeons. Further down is the town of Jomsom which has an airstrip which is connected to Pokhara. It was here that I met Dr Amitabha Basu, who was working at the Manipal College of Medical Sciences in Pokhara. I had not even heard of the college but as soon as I reached there I fell in love with the place. About 8 months later I joined the faculty there.

Pokhara is one of the most beautiful places in the world. This is not only because of the views, which is unique in that as you look north the entire horizon is filled with snow clad mountains, at the centre of which is the Macchapuchare. This mountain stands like a sentinel over what for me was the enchanted valley of Pokhara and its people. There are several lakes in vicinity, including the famous Fewa Tal in Pokhara itself. The entire valley is full of green fields and hills and trails and mountains and is home to some of the most hospitable people in the world. Somehow I felt that I had come home. To me it remains the hometown of my dreams.

The Manipal College of Medical Sciences had been started here by India's Manipal group, which had a long experience of running medical schools in various Indian locations. The students were half local and half foreigners including a large proportion of Indians, but Srilankans, Bangladeshis, Americans, Kenyans and South Africans and the odd Iranian student lent colour to the campus

And it was here that I, being the only cardiothoracic surgeon within 200 kilometers, really began to appreciate the odds of working in this sort of environment. MCOMS had a tertiary care hospital, but was this was just starting. We were in at the birth of the hospital with all its attendant disadvantages and advantages. The advantage was that we could mould our departments to our liking, but the disadvantages were also of a daunting nature. There was little trained help, while we had very sincere and active colleagues in the medicine and other departments; they too were hampered by a lack of many facilities that we took for granted in big cities.

I summarized the difficulties of working in such an environment in a presentation that I had made at an invited presentation at the Bhopal Hospital in 2003. There were three principal disadvantages. First was the lack of trained nurses and technicians. I had to train the girls to manage a chest drain as they were not familiar with even a simple water seal drain. We set up a surgical care unit where we managed to train the nurses in ICU management, but with a dearth of equipment there was always a tug of war in order to be able to utilize simple equipment like the Pulse oxymeter and a cardiac monitor which had to be shared with the physicians. The use of inotropes and drugs like nitroprusside and nitroglycerine was being just introduced to the hospital by our physician colleagues.

A second difficulty was the lack of suitable equipment. I was lucky enough to have a trained cardiac anaesthetist; this was because I had married one and she had joined the Institution with me! But she did not manage to get a double lumen endotracheal tube until 2003, three years after we first started working here. We had no invasive monitors, at least in the initial phase and had to depend lot on clinical skills to manage patients intra and post operatively. It was now that our special skills, honed in the government hospitals of Calcutta, really came in useful. We were not fazed by the lack of modern equipment as many of our other colleagues trained in major institutes were. We could make do with much less equipment and were used to relying on clinical skills.

I had no colleagues with whom I could discuss clinical problems or rely upon to help me during surgery. My other surgical colleagues had never even seen an open chest in their careers. When I did my first case (a lobectomy) it was the first time that both my assistants had ever seen a live human lung! The first surgery for mitral stenosis got me a standing ovation from the students when it was reported at the weekly clinical meeting, but while this was good for my ego, it only underlined how undeveloped the surgical services were in Pokhara.

Another difficulty was that the first patients that were referred for surgery were precisely the sort of cases that a fledgling department would like to avoid. For instance, I got a referral of a patient who was exsanguinated from haemoptysis and almost in extremis. The patient survived an emergency lobectomy but died in the post operative period, an incident that left me depressed and my physician colleagues with queries about my surgical prowess! I have reported elsewhere about my experiences with constrictive pericarditis in this hospital. The mean right ventricular pressure was so high that most would have been considered inoperable in most departments. But here we were forced to operate on such patients. This was a catch 22 situation: if the patient died, referrals would stop, but if in order to improve results we refused patients, referrals would stop anyway!!

Narrative 5

Sunita Gurung a 22 year old young woman was diagnosed to have mitral stenosis at the Western Regional Hospital when she was 19. This happened when she was pregnant with their first child. She was told to go to Kathmandu, the capital of Nepal for surgery, but this was impossible for her considering the poverty in which her family was mired. She was referred to me for surgery in 2000. I decided to do a closed mitral valvotomy for her. This operation which I have heard described as the most important cardiac procedure ever invented, was done in an hour long surgery in November 2000. I was able to get a good split and despite severe pulmonary hypertension she made a good recovery and became symptom free in six weeks time. She followed up regularly until 2004 when I left Pokhara and she was completely well and was taking her anti rheumatic fever prophylaxis regularly. Her life style changed completely and she felt better than she had ever done in her adult life.

Closed mitral commisurotomy was first done by Souttar in 1925. The operation became more used in the forties when Bailey in the United States and Brock in the UK made it a standard surgery. It came to India in the fifties and by the eighties; surgeons had series of as many as 3000 odd cases. I have personally operated on at least 800 patients. It fell from grace in the seventies with the advent of open heart surgery and in Western textbooks it was no longer described when we were students. However it remained and remains one of the most effective surgical operations for the commonest valvular disease in developing nations. Mitral stenosis is ubiquitous in the Indian subcontinent. Up to about 50% of patients who have rheumatic fever may go on to develop mitral stenosis. In the initial phases of the development of cardiac surgery, closed mitral commisurotomy using the Tubb's dilator was a very effective means of intervention in this condition and resulted in excellent palliation in such patients. However with the advent of open heart surgery, Western writers told us that this operation was outdated as even mitral stenosis patients should have an open mitral commissurotomy. This, despite several reports from India and South Africa testifying to the excellent results obtained by this procedure. When we were students, even in India, centers which were more developed than us began to lecture Indian audiences on the need for OMC.

I have always been skeptical about this thesis. Closed mitral commisurotomy needed only one competent surgeon, a reasonably well trained anesthetist and standard surgical equipment augmented with some clamps and the Tubb's dilator to treat effectively a condition that was the cause of the biggest chunk of valvular heart disease in India. Why then should we abandon this procedure for OMC which needed the use of the heart lung machine, major infrastructure development and advanced equipment which was not available (and still is not) in most parts of India or the rest of the subcontinent? In fact I felt that it was possible to do closed operations in patients who were, to use strict criteria, inoperable by the closed technique, and we presented our work at the International

College of Surgeons meeting in Kathmandu in 2003 to acclaim. Unfortunately, I did not publish my work because reasons beyond my control. I did a total of about 30 closed mitral commissurotomies while I was I Pokhara. This was with no mortality and one patient who developed mitral regurgitation. I felt that these results would rival any series from a big centre using open techniques. It is unnecessary to follow Western guidelines in all situations and my work in Pokhara confirmed this. Similar results were obtained in constrictive pericarditis, operating on patients that no western surgeon would have touched with a barge pole.

CONCLUSION

I have now at least temporarily ended my career in Cardiovascular Surgery. I now work with stem cells in a shiny laboratory filled with the most advanced equipment, in a field that is the latest in medical science. I am at home here, publishing in high impact journals and setting up clinical trials that will, if completed successfully be landmark studies. This sudden change came when I was offered a post by an old colleague of mine who had worked with me in one of my hospitals. I was initially reluctant to leave clinical practice, as in common with all true surgeons, cutting was the mainstay of my existence. But now that I am here, I am enjoying it. There is a fascination in going where few men (or women) have been before. I wish I had such a laboratory at my disposal when I was doing clinical surgery. It might have taught me to reflect, to try out ideas and perhaps prove many things that I now believe only by instinct. But I am a firm believer of not crying over spilt milk and I hope that I will still be able to contribute, perhaps not to a patient directly as I was doing earlier, but by increasing knowledge that will contribute to reduction of human suffering, after all that is what we are here to do: our entire education and training was for this end and I strive to do it with as much dedication as I am capable of. The results are for others to judge!

Chapter 12
Smaller Heroes I Didn't See

Brendan O'Shea
Trinity College Dublin, Ireland

ABSTRACT

The theme of this chapter explores aspects of professional blindness in the family practice setting. The exploration uses the vehicle of an exercise in practice audit, which resulted in a more meaningful level of interaction between the GP and a particular group of individuals in his practice. What set out as a quantitative exercise in audit inadvertently threw up valuable qualitative insights and reflections on how this family doctor had previously viewed this group of individuals in the past, and more importantly, would do so in the future. In particular, the exercise challenges us to look for and see the ambitions and hopes of those individuals who attend us for medical care, in order to properly respect these important aspects of their humanity, and to assist us in more easily rising beyond the confines unwittingly imposed and accepted by a passive acceptance of disease defined horizons and the medical model. The audit outcomes include improved levels of achievement in the relevant markers of good care, easily and unremarkably measurable in the standard manner. A key outcome, rather more difficult to measure, included an increased respect and recognition of the difficulties, efforts, challenges, fears, hopes and varied realities experienced by this most particular group of eclectically selected individuals.

INTRODUCTION

I believe in professional blindness. It can happen to very dedicated health care professionals. It can happen to health care professionals who are chronically too busy. It can even more easily happen to not so dedicated health care professionals, and burnt out health care professionals. Like the flu, sometimes 'there can be a lot of it about,' as we often say to our patients.

It happens when we simply fail to see the outstanding humanity of a case or a cohort. We might lose sight of the poor while caring for the rich. We might become deaf to the quieter sounds of

DOI: 10.4018/978-1-60960-097-6.ch012

suffering due to the clamour of the more articulate worried well. We might just get too tired.

I came across some smaller heroes a few years ago.....

I am a General Practitioner in Ireland. My interest lies in ongoing personal care to individuals and their families over time. I am in a small family practice, now almost 20 years in the same town, just outside Dublin, on the east coast.

In 2004, I engaged myself with a broad quality assurance process then owned and delivered through The Royal College of General Practitioners, the FBA (Fellowship by Assessment) process. It has since been discontinued, having been run for 12-14 years. I was among the last of the 300 odd souls to complete it, and in 2004, completion of the process required submitted evidence of satisfaction of 64 specific criteria, exclusively relating to the care provided to patients attending my practice. Embedded in this included the requirement to complete full audit cycles on care provided to patients in 8 conditions, 'concerned with the care of diseases which are selected according to national and local priorities.' One could nominally select the 8 conditions, bearing in mind that at least 5 had to closely reflect major killer diseases (eg Diabetes and Hypertension for example), but that left the other 3 you could truly select yourself. This caused me to wonder.

I was still wondering several months later.

'...and do you know I have to cook in the dark now as well?'

She said this to me as she backed out the door after a very busy and almost chaotic consultation. Despite arriving in consultation without much time at all in the waiting room, she and he arrived breathless and stressed. He was, as usual, inarticulate with excitement and some pain. He was significantly overweight, stocky, perpetually restless and loud. Despite his 5 years and his most peculiar habits of socialising and interacting, he was on familiar territory. On bursting into the consulting room, he sharked over to the Mayo table where minor surgical instruments and kit

were awaiting the next gash, lump, ingrowing toenail or IUCD. He knew this would immediately make me jump up with all the residual athleticism I had remaining. I did, and he beamed back at me (there are many ways to say hello!). Then he opened and closed all the presses, before retiring to rock on the examination couch.

We quickly established he had a further middle ear infection, and addressed this. Our 3-4 minutes were almost up, that being the current timeframe he could endure being in the room. I had a moment to enquire, in a professional, formulaic manner, '....and how is everything?' as we all began to decamp.

'Oh its fine, ' she replied, in a loud and floridly melodramatic manner, rolling her eyes upwards and shaking her head. 'It's just fine....' she continued as he shot out the door ahead of her. '..... and do you know I have to cook in the dark now as well?'

She and he left.

Of course I didn't know she had to cook in the dark. I didn't know what it was to cook in the dark in a small council house, provided and maintained in an overwhelmingly indifferent manner by the local authority. Both she and her son were loud and forceful individuals, and the sentence kept ringing in my head, banging around my brain in the weeks afterwards, until it met up with that other thought banging around in there, the need to identify the subject for the eighth audit cycle of the FBA process.

Our young man was living his life from the quixotic perspective of operating on the more challenging end of the autistic spectrum. That is to say he had fairly severe autism, diagnosed some 3 years previously. He was boisterous, loud, energetic, and feisty. It was at this point, a cause of deep and grave concern to his parents, his older sister and I, that he was thus negotiating his way through life from this most inconvenient perspective, but of course it was of no concern to him at all whatsoever.

He was already overweight, and would not allow his hair to be cut. He was vigorous, quick and strong, so he presented as a formidable force, with a shock of long thick jet black hair. Despite his steadfast refusal to engage with polite society on anything approaching our own terms, there was no way whatsoever he could be set aside or conveniently ignored. He imposed his own eclectic and wayward will upon everything he encountered, with an admirable and steadfast focus that bordered on the ferocious. You know the type.....?

At this point, in his wild journey of development, he was engaged with light switches and ritualistic toast making. He was gaining weight fast on the basis of toasted sliced pan, and given his penchant for turning off all light switches, we were all in the dark about this, in many ways. Hence his mother's delightful throwaway statement as she tore out of the consulting room, in pursuit of him, as he raced out, and into the car park ahead of her. Of course she would be chasing him until the day she died.

I thought about this boy and his mother. They caused me to think about some other cases that made me feel a profound admiration whenever I stopped to think of their situation. They were cases that had no easy endpoint. They were never going to be 'cured.' They were probably not going to die anytime soon either, as in a palliative care case. They were going to go on. They came to see me as younger patients with their main carers, usually their parents. They were labouring under some large medical imposition that profoundly affected their ability to live what would ever be considered 'normal' lives. Following any of their consultations, it was truly easy to be filled with an admiration for them, for their families, and to feel a heightened sense of luck, gratitude and forbearance at my own very good fortune. They crashed through the surgery appointment system, picked up a fix, and blazed out again, often lurching from one crisis to the next. I felt that I knew them. They and their carers were very loyal patients of the practice. But did I really know them, and was I doing the best I could for them holistically? Could I continue in my 'best practice' and intermittently evidence based medical odyssey, and recruit them into the eight audit cycle?

Surely I could. It would be an audit cycle, on the care afforded to Smaller Heroes.

The amateur scientist within whispered to me. 'But how can you satisfactorily define inclusion criteria for these cases...' A colleague described them as NECNOS (*pronounced 'neck knows'*)- in the terminology of ICD, "not elsewhere classified and not otherwise specified." I grappled with this for a few weeks, even as many other cohorts in other audit cycles fell conveniently and most obligingly into place. The hypertensive patients did so with systolics and diastolics, cholesterols and creatinines. The diabetic patients were simply dripping with figures, lab values, BMIs and a plethora of measured characteristics. Perhaps that is what happens when we, as family doctors, surrender these patients into a style of medicine really conceived and owned by specialists and epidemiologists. When we get them back, they have been so wrapped up in numbers their personal selves become opaque to us and are, forever branded, packaged and delivered as a neat bundle of figures, which is what their 'care' becomes, and by which figures we tend to judge them irrevocably, all traces of humanity in our care lost and made unnecessary.

'This study....'

Irrespective of these considerations, in the final analysis, there was a need to get on with it and for the purposes of the exercise, ie completing the FBA Programme, there was a need on my own part to make this particular audit cycle work. I considered my disease register for my practice, which I had been compiling for 4-5 years. It included the usual categories, the neat hypertensives, the demarcated diabetics, the malignancies, the psychiatric categories etc. Scattered among them were the heroes, the key defining feature crystallising in my mind was that of the prospect of most of a life ahead of them afflicted with a significant medical issue which would markedly impair their ability to lead a 'normal' life in the usual and nominally independent manner we all take for granted.

These patients were difficult to tightly define, and were medically a very heterogenous group within the practice. They were certainly not going to comply with my selfish, transient but increasingly urgent need for a couple of rows of nice neat figures. A further unhelpful feeling I had was that the areas I might wish to improve in their care were unlikely to be easily measurable, and therefore not amenable to an audit cycle, even if they could be satisfactorily defined as a group. A further negative thought flitting through my mind as the project quickened was that it was relatively easier for my specialist colleagues to do nice neat case series, given that they were usually seeing a lot of a relatively few conditions, whereas the this patient group in my own practice represented a spread of wildly differing pathological diagnoses. Perhaps they and their carers and siblings could be presented as a case series of absolute heroes? (no classification for 'hero' in ICD 9). Perhaps heroism might be the defining characteristic, as opposed to a fasting serum cholesterol of greater than 5.0 mmol?

After some consideration, I decided to opt for an audit cycle on the care received by this group, whoever they were. I believed that it would afford me the opportunity to explore and improve my own role as their Care Coordinator. More importantly, I allowed myself to believe that the exercise would surely improve the care provided, and would therefore benefit the individuals themselves. My forming suspicion was that while the kind perception my patients had of me as their GP might well be good, I also strongly suspected that in reality, my care largely consisted of fire brigading, and that their care was fragmented among many other agencies, without any firm hand on the tiller.

Add a bit of science, but not too much.........

Target Population

The target population was defined as children, adolescents or adults (together with their parents / carers) who had special needs. They were taken to include all individuals within the practice, who by virtue of a significant diagnosis, had an ongoing and permanent deficit in the areas of physical activity, social interaction and / or intellectual functioning. The method of case identification included reference to the practice disease register, where their section in the Register had now been maintained for 2 years preceding.

The key inclusion criteria here was that the individuals concerned would never be capable of leading an independent life in the community, without ongoing and intensive social support from their carers. These individuals would be affected by their conditions indefinitely going forwards, ie unlike the case of a terminal malignancy for example, where there would be a likely end point in the short term.

These were long term heroes:

1. 32 yr F Tuberous sclerosis
2. 9 yo M Downs' syndrome
3. 3 yo M Non specific developmental delay
4. 13 yo M Dyslexic / several additional schooling difficulties
5. 9 yo M Aspergers' syndrome
6. 5 yo M Optic nerve hypoplasia / speech delay / moderately low IQ
7. 10 yo M Complex congenital heart disease
8. 5 yo M Autism
9. 8 yo F Downs' syndrome
10. 1 yo F Severe generalised developmental delay / hypotonia
11. 30 yo F Generalised / non specific low IQ
12. 11 yo F Autistic (mild spectrum)
13. 8 yo F Moderately severe developmental delay / absent corpus callosum
14. 9 yo M Attention span deficit hyperactivity disorder / dyslexic

15. 39 yo F Low IQ / epilepsy / calcified basal ganglia
16. 38 yo M Moderately low IQ
17. 30 yo F Moderate low IQ / epilepsy
18. 11 yo F Mild low IQ / dyslexic
19. 10 yo M Cystic fibrosis / asthma
20. 14 yo M Attention span deficit hyperactivity disorder / mildly low IQ

Audit Process

The defined audit process included a retrospective evaluation of care received at time of first diagnosis, following which the more typical first and second surveys of care were carried out, with reference to a 'gold standard.'

Where ever would I find a 'gold standard ' for this lot? Unlike the British Thoracic Society infallibly guiding for Chesty Patients or indeed the Irish Diabetic Federation doing likewise for Diabetics, there was no obvious convenient equivalent for smaller heroes and NECNOS. Likewise, I looked to the Irish and Royal Colleges of General Practitioners, and could find no mention of any such individuals, or any reference to such personal attributes among any patient groups defined in the pages of their guidelines. I did come across a useful reference provided by a colleague in paediatrics, which was entitled 'Basic Medical Surveillance Essentials for people with Down's Syndrome (Guidelines of the Down's Syndrome Medical Interest Group DSMIG (UK & Ireland) Irish Edition (2001)' (www.dsmig.org.uk)(2), and this provided a useful set of standards, several of which were applicable and relevant in partly evaluating care provided to my own group of patients.

The Audit

The first survey included a chart review, which confirmed a fairly average set of files. It confirmed that the care provided was reactive, largely related to crisis management and the management of minor medical issues. It was also evident from the notes that the reality of the level of disability was never meaningfully recorded for any of these individuals at all. Secondary care was merely hinted at in the notes, as opposed to being properly recorded in depth. Most of all, there was no sense of personality evident in the records. I did believe that I carried this within my own self, but on reflection, this was not really adequate, and certainly of no assistance to my practice colleagues, or any unfortunate locum covering the practice in my absence.

Following a reflection on this, I then set out, in the time honoured way, to define a gold standard prospectively, and set targets for the second survey. This would be based on a year of clinical care delivered, and augmented by a prospective scheduled consultation with the patient and their principal carers, in order to reach those places which were clearly not being explored in regular care provided, and to take up any tasks that were being currently neglected because they belonged in the 'important but not urgent category' of life's jobs (Doctors are particularly bad at these!).

Criteria

Clear diagnosis documented appropriately in medical record
Date of diagnosis clearly noted
Detailed diagnosis documented
Main care details comprehensively noted (ie all services / specialists referred to)
Disability defined with reference to gross/fine motor, co-ordination, socialising, intellectualising, hearing and vision
Clear listing of all associated medical problems
Height and weight recorded with reference to expected centiles
Detail evident regarding current educational situation / work situation
Documentation regarding the carers' ambitions / concerns
Documentation regarding the patients' ambitions

In addition, I also took the opportunity to survey carers in these key areas.

What services / facilities have you found really useful?

What services / facilities have you found to be disappointing?

Are there any changes we could make to your GP service?

In the course of the second survey, any appropriate interventions identified were acted upon.

The Main Outcomes

The files were tidied up. They certainly passed muster as a decent set of Problem Orientated Medical Records. This was pleasing, and ticked the requirement of the exercise in Audit.

Some other harder and indeed 'impossible to define' things also occurred. In the course of the year of the second cycle, and especially as a result of the prospective longer consultations, the three of us, including then patient, their carer and myself, developed a much better understanding of each other. I feel (what a suspect thing for a Doctor to ever admit to!) that we moved our relationships onto a better plane. The Carers were amazed, delighted and frankly astounded at being invited and respectfully requested to spend an hour of their time to reflect on the care and the experiences of their loved one.

One had the distinct impression that despite the high complexity of their cases, they had never had the undivided attention of a Doctor for a full hour. Ever. There was a modest amount of 'getting things off their chest.' I learnt much detail about the local support services such as Dietetics, Speech Therapy, and Occupational Therapy. I thought I knew about these things in my locality, but it was all a bit abstract. I learnt in a different, more meaningful way which of these services actually delivered to my patients and which ones did not. I developed a feel for the local schools, and which Principals and Teachers had an empathic feel for these patients, and which ones did not. I

learnt a great deal about 'working the system,' not ordinarily contained in text books, and ordinarily well beneath the radar of impossibly busy health care professionals, especially Doctors. I learnt in detail about several additional layers of benefits and grants, as opposed to having a vague (and therefore useless) knowledge of such things. An 'in house' in formation pack was easily drafted, garnering the experience gained from these longer consultations.

In the course of the second survey, I diligently set about disseminating and sharing these various pearls of wisdom throughout the group, and improved the Practice Referral Directory based on information gleaned from the experiences of the group of patients and their carers. The second survey resulted in many specific actions carried out on a case by case basis. In seven instances, Patients and Carers were put in contact or 'twinned,' where typically a family coping well with Autism for example were socially introduced to one that was struggling with it.

These things, good as they were, were actually not the real benefit of the process. From my own selfish perspective, the real benefit came from my own formal expression of interest in these people, who I was seeing in a different and more holistic manner. In particular, the last two items in the survey grid caused me to reflect. These were the questions regarding the hopes and ambitions of the patients and their carers.

In future....

Ambition is a curious thing. I would care to believe that it is a distinctly human characteristic, particularly when we think our way beyond today's dinner, tomorrow, to next week and beyond. As health care professionals, we tend to be quite organised, and think well into the future, planning for promotions, projects, further degrees, doctoral theses and climbing the rungs of our various career ladders. Likewise, in our personal lives we tend to be ambitious, given that we have the organisational characteristics of individuals who have achieved ourselves into third and fourth level education, have significant status in our own social communities, and in most instances a very decent living.

Perhaps it is that all of this regard and respect causes us to become blind in a basic human sense to the experiences of individuals who are arguably at the very other end of this spectrum of autonomy and privilege. Perhaps it is also that the stigma of the afflicted adds to our blindness; fear of asking because of fear of the answers.

In setting up the second survey, I understood for the first time that whereas in routine consulting, I often asked people, including younger and older ones, what were they planning as part of routine consultation chatter (and often noted it down), I never asked this group, and I had no real idea what anyone of them aspired to. Perhaps it was an oversight, or due to the often chaotic nature of many of their consultations, but I suspect it had more to do with an unspoken dread of what their answers might be, or the fear of opening a vast pandora's box of frustrated ambition. Perhaps it was a personal arrogance, based on the assumption that these individuals could have no ambitions worth considering.

The omission to ask and enquire was probably a most unpleasant mix of all of these things; but whatever it came from, it was unacceptable. It was at the heart of my own professional blindness in this instance.

When our original character had exhausted the possibilities of the light switches and the toaster, what would he like to do then? What did his mother fear, hope and think? Did he fear, hope and think? I had no idea.

So, I asked. The world did not stop. Now I know.

This is what I found out, and have never forgotten in all my subsequent contacts with these individuals.

Personal Ambitions

That I will get really good at swimming. That I will always get my own way. That I will get to read all the Barney, Mr Bear and Gruffaloe stories. That I will join the army and be a soldier (less reading and writing there). That I will get to do science, and make everyone the same as myself, and have total control over mammy. That *I* will have Mammy all to myself, all of the time. That I won't be afraid of dying and there will be no more surgery ever. That I will grow up and be a comedian. That I will be a hairdresser, get married, and later on be a beautician, because I want to make people more beautiful. That I will be hugged and play with the other boys. That I don't know. That I get to drive Tractors and be *in the middle* of the family. That I won't be dribbling. That I keep on running. That I get to keep working (stacking shelves 10 hours a week in a sheltered work scheme). That I will get to work at building like Daddy, be a Vet, a Beautician and a Lifeguard. Be an Accountant. Be a Carpenter, like Daddy.

Certain attributes make us more human. We laugh. We have ambitions. If my system of care for my patients ignores their ambitions, it is inhuman.

All known patient ambitions in this group are now known to me, and recorded (100%).

And by the way....

Other more concrete and less ethereal interventions along the way included the following.

Referrals

7 Referrals to specialist colleagues (Paediatrics(growth clinic, gastroenterology, orthopaedics))
4 Referrals to Educational Psychology
9 Referrals to Occupational Therapy
4 Referrals to Speech Therapy
2 Referrals to Literacy Classes
3 Referrals to Early Intervention Childcare Service
1 Referral to Radiology
2 Referrals for Audiometry

Additional miscellaneous correspondence included queries to psychiatry (1) regarding medication management, to ophthalmology regarding monocular vision, to cardiology regarding fitness to participate, to maxillofacial surgery regarding intervention for persistent dribbling (the dribbling is stopped!), and one to the Chief Medical Officer at the Military Hospital regarding dyslexia and fitness to work as a soldier, who kindly said 'maybe.'

Assistance with work placements (3), a referral to the National Rehabilitation Board (1) and networking directly between patients (7) were also carried out. The latter is the practice of putting one patient / carer in contact with another patient / carer for a specific reason, which process is set up in a formal and supervised manner. Every case was reported systematically and registered on the National Disability Database. Much correspondence was generated towards schools, in relation to obtaining Special Needs Assistants in classes, and to the local Council in relation to improving accommodation. Several individuals were coached in relation to better management of school issues. One hero and their carer were advised to change GP, because they had moved 14 miles away.

This would be a nice place to end this story. It would be the wrong place. We need to consider what things worked well for these people, and more importantly what did not work well.

In asking about parts of the health service which worked well for them, many responded in the expected manner, and generously praised a variety of agencies. Two of the twenty answered 'Nothing,' and 'Nothing – its all been a struggle.'

When asked what things they found to be disappointing, there was a longer list of responses.

Three had moved schools because of bullying. One family had moved house / town because of bullying. Four reported they were unsupported by the headmaster / school because of bullying. 'No one seems in control,' was observed by one couple, and 'slow diagnosis' was related by several also.

A further disconcerting observation was made in relation to the service we were providing at the surgery. When asked were there any changes they would like us to make to the service at the surgery, 19/20 said no, and one said yes, specifying shorter waits in the waiting room. At this point, having completed the first cycle of the audit, I truly understood that the service had been deficient.

This too is a contributing factor in our own professional blindness, that our patients have a fatal acceptance of the mediocre, and we can't reliably rely on them to point out to us when we miss things. If we are nice, they will tolerate average and bad care. They will be grateful for what they get, much more often than not, and largely irrespective of whether it is good enough or otherwise.

I believe in professional blindness. It can happen to very dedicated health care professionals....

REFERENCES

Basic Medical Surveillance Essentials for people with Down's Syndrome (2001). *Basic Medical Surveillance Essentials for people with Down's Syndrome*, Guidelines of the Down's Syndrome Medical Interest Group DSMIG (UK & Ireland) Irish Edition Retrieved from www.dsmig.org.uk

Chapter 13
Practical Pointers in Medicine Over Seven Decades:
Reflections of an Individual Physician

Richard James
Davidson, USA

ABSTRACT

This chapter illustrates a life in medical practice and emphasizes the importance of lifelong learning in medicine through sharing of lived experiences. The life narratives display the authors own observations of what he has learned and unlearned over the years. Also added are observations about his retirement project - editing and publishing abstracts of the current primary care medicine literature - that exemplifies the need for health care professionals to continue sharing life-long.

INTRODUCTION

Early Life

Dr. Wertman was our family doctor. His office was in his home on Main Street in our small Eastern Pennsylvania town. We seldom went to his office. He came to our home when my parents called him to attend to our usual childhood illnesses. I remember the large black bag he carried. It contained, in addition to his stethoscope and other instruments, rows of bright pills in little bottles lining both sides of the bag. This amazed us. After the usual history and examination, he would

open one or two pill bottles and dispense what we needed. I did not know what the pills were, but we recovered with their help, or in spite of them.

After the formality of the visit, he would relax and chat with us. He seemed to be part of the family. He talked with a heavy Pennsylvania Dutch accent. On one occasion he described a camping trip he and his family enjoyed. Insects were the only down-side of the week. With his accent, he did not call them insects or bugs; he called them "buks". I innocently asked him "What's 'buks'"? My family howled with laughter at my innocence and Dr. Wertman's chagrin.

When he got ready to leave, my brother and I would ask him to give us another pill. He would solemnly take two little pills out of one of the

DOI: 10.4018/978-1-60960-097-6.ch013

bottles and present one to each of us. We did not know what the pills were. Later we suspected they were a mild laxative.

As we grew, he began to call my brother "the preacher" and call me "the doctor". He became my role model. At the age of 12, I decided to become a doctor. This smoothed and straightened my life-path. I did not waiver. I worked and studied hard, and was admitted to a prestigious medical school at an early age.

I am still grateful for this early opportunity to decide my life-path.

Medical School and Internship: 1940-44

Medical school was intense. Some days I would arrive home exhausted. My habit then was to go to bed for a few hours. My mother would prepare a late supper. I would then study into the wee hours of the morning, go back to bed for a few hours more and then on to school. This system worked well for me.

We were awed by our professors. We placed them on a high pedestal. We believed they were all-knowing. They were kind, but strict in demands for our learning. Only occasionally would we detect a touch of hubris. They spoke with authority. Now, of course, I realize that what they taught, although the best of the day, was based on personal opinion and experience. No one had heard of evidence-based medicine.

Ward rounds were hierarchical. Professors led the line, instructors followed, then residents, and students. Emphasis was on the disease, not the patient with the disease; on getting the diagnosis and treatment right. The patient was treated respectfully, but objectively. It was impersonal. I do not recall any mention of the patient's feelings or personal life.

I was a second year medical student at the time of Pearl Harbor. I remember sitting in pathology lab listening on a small portable radio to President Roosevelt give his "day of infamy speech" and announce the declaration of war with Japan. The war adversely affected my medical education. Half of the school's medical and surgical faculty formed a hospital unit and was posted to India. Our instruction schedules were accelerated. We graduated early. For good or ill, during a curtailed internship, we performed interventions for which we were inadequately trained. I gave spinal anesthesia, and performed minor surgery. I remember delivering four babies in one night when on call. I was the only representative of the university hospital Ob-Gyn staff present at the time. All residents and chiefs had left. Fortunately, excellent nurse anesthetists came to my rescue. All eight patients survived. But I did not develop any personal connection with the mothers. I scarcely knew their names. On the days after delivery, I did not visit to check on them to ask about how they felt and how their babies were doing. I believed my work was done. I presume I felt I was too busy. I still regret this oversight.

On another occasion, I was removing an ingrown toenail under local anesthesia. The patient, rightfully concerned about my youth, said, "Don't you cut off my toe." I responded, "Never fear Madam, I don't know how."

When it came my turn to scrub with an internationally known surgeon, I was excited. The patient was a slim teen-age girl with presumed appendicitis. (It turned out not to be appendicitis. He was hacked.) The patient was under spinal anesthesia. She remained alert and interested in all that was going on. During his examination of the pelvis Dr. R asked the patient if she would like to see her ovary. She said yes. He lifted the ovary out of the incision and showed it to her. She was one of the few women in the world to see her own ovary.

Looking back on those early days, I realize medicine, as compared with medicine today, was rudimentary. (Believe it or not, when I first studied biology as an undergraduate, I was taught that the human cell contained 48 chromosomes.) Of the medical school subjects, only anatomy resembled that of today. Physiology was in a formative stage. The normal systolic blood pressure was 100 plus your age. Biochemistry did not deserve to be called "chemistry". It focused mainly on carbohydrates, fat, and protein. Pharmacology presented few really effective drugs. Insulin was the only drug available for treatment of diabetes. Diabetes was diagnosed when symptoms of thirst and polyuria appeared. No one knew the function of lymphocytes.

Penicillin

I had a front seat at the penicillin revolution. When I began medical school, few people had heard of penicillin. Sulfadiazine was the major antibacterial agent. Sulfa drugs were a major advance, but were toxic.

Robert Bud, Head of Information Research at the Science Museum of London, in his recent book about the history of penicillin (2007) recounts admirably and in detail the oft-told, still fascinating, story of the discovery and development of penicillin. According to Bud, penicillin's discovery in 1928 by Alexander Fleming was quite serendipitous. Fleming noted an unusual pattern of growth inhibition of bacteria in an agar plate contaminated with a naturally ubiquitous mold. There was little scientific interest in this discovery, and it took several more years before the substance was purified. It wasn't until World War II that the antibacterial substance – now called penicillin after the *Penicillium notatum* mold strain – was used to treat a human patient. Albert Alexander, a policeman, had severe septicemia. The amount available was minuscule by present standards. At first he improved, but the supply ran out, and he relapsed and died.

Shortly thereafter, as more patients received it and had good results, news spread about the new miracle drug, which was being developed in England. The drug's effectiveness was self-evident. Randomized trials for efficacy (had they been known at that time) were not neces-

sary. But funds for research were limited in the UK because of the Depression and the war. Production of large quantities was not possible. Other scientific problems were considered more important. The British sought help from the U.S. In early 1941, a representative of the Rockefeller Institute visited London and was so impressed by penicillin's potential, that he paved the difficult way for a remarkably coordinated country-wide effort of U.S. pharmaceutical and fermenting industries, and even the mushroom industry, to increase production dramatically. Pfizer, a small drug company specializing in production of citric acid for the soft-drink industry, began to produce penicillin. Pfizer is now one of the world's largest pharmaceutical companies.

By 1943, small quantities became available. It was reserved for the military. Actually, at first, some in the armed services were not enthusiastic about its use. Then, in 1943, came the remarkable observation that penicillin cured gonorrhea and syphilis. The traditional treatment with arsenic was suddenly displaced. (Early in my career, I gave intravenous injections of an arsenic compound – arsphenamine - to several patients.)

By the time of the Normandy invasion (June 1944) there was a plentiful supply, but not for civilians.

By this time, word had spread across the world. It was electrifying. There were many heart-rending pleas from civilians to obtain a small supply. By 1945, penicillin became freely available. What was originally priceless eventually cost pennies. Penicillin became available at the onset of my medical career, and I remember well the excitement at the time as news spread.

Warfarin

Also at the start of my medical career, I had the privilege of witnessing another major advance in therapeutics. As the developmental history is recounted in Wikipedia ("Warfarin," 2010), in the early 1920s, veterinarians in Canada noted that cattle were bleeding excessively, sometimes fatally. They determined the cause was feed containing spoiled sweet clover. In 1929, it was noted that these cattle had a low prothrombin time.

In the early 1940s, Karl Link and students at the University of Wisconsin finally crystallized the anticoagulant. It took five years. It was a coumarin. They named the chemical "warfarin" (Wisconsin Alumni Research Foundation + arin. The foundation had supported the research.) It was first used as a rodent poison, but by the early 1950's, use as a therapeutic anticoagulant in humans had begun. President Eisenhower received it to treat his myocardial infarction in 1955. It was not until 1978 that inhibition of vitamin K was understood to be its mechanism of action. Warfarin has continued to this day as a major therapeutic drug. It may soon be supplanted by direct thrombin inhibitors.

Army Service

Immediately after conclusion of an abbreviated internship, along with my colleagues, I entered the Army Medical Corps as a first lieutenant. I became a Flight Surgeon, posted to the 19th Troop Carrier Squadron, stationed at Hickham field in Hawaii. This was after the war ended. Although my tour of duty was uneventful overall, I recall several unforgettable happenings. The mission of the squadron was to maintain communications with the entire South Pacific, as far as Australia. Some of the crew members, shortly after returning, appeared at my dispensary with a urethral discharge. My job was to diagnose and treat. (By that time penicillin was freely available.) I would take the smear to the field hospital and ask the lab technician to stain it. She was a mighty pretty and smart young lady. I maintain that I am the only man in the world who met his wife-to-be over a gonorrhea smear.

On another occasion, I asked my colonel to let me join a flight to the far reaches of the South Pacific - to Aitutaki atoll in the Cook islands

about 1500 miles east of New Zealand. We were evacuating the few remaining troops. I did not have to go on the flight. I asked to join because it seemed to me to be an adventure. We island-hopped, flying in an ancient, but presumably safe, high-wing four-engine Liberator bomber. Navigation was primitive. Our navigator was not much older than a teen-ager. But, he was good! After over 1000 miles of dead reckoning, he guided the plane over the center of the small atoll. After completing the mission in several days, we took off to return. There was no gasoline on the atoll. About 100 miles out, the pilot noted some indication of trouble in one of the engines. He turned the plane around and landed back on the atoll. The crew chief opened the engine to discover the trouble. He found nothing but a small piece of metal at the bottom of the cowl. Not knowing where it came from or what it was for, he threw it away. We took off again, heading for Christmas Atoll (now Kiritiami). Our radio operator was not able to raise the radio on the atoll. (Later we learned the crew there was partying.) We knew gas was running low. Fortunately we finally picked up their beacon, which they had left turning. We landed with a few gallons of gas left.

My purpose in telling this story is not simply to recount an adventure, but to point out something much more important. Our actions may have grave consequences on others. If I had not survived the flight, my parents would have been destroyed. They had already been devastated by the loss of my brother, a very young Ensign in charge of a gun crew on a freighter carrying supplies for the invasion of North Africa. His ship was lost off the coast of Casablanca in December of 1942. His body was never recovered.

At the time, I never thought of this possible consequence of my actions. It never crossed my mind. As I finally matured, I began to consider. I have thought about it ever since.

So - advice to the young - consider the consequences of your actions. They may have a profound and destructive effect on others.

GI Bill

One of the wisest decisions of our Federal Government was to create the "GI Bill" after the war was over. This enabled millions of service personnel to gain additional education and to retrain at the school of their choice as they returned to civilian status. Tuition, books and a small stipend were supplied. I took full advantage of the bill, receiving over three years of postgraduate training, including two years of residency at a major medical school and hospital. I witnessed, at a distance, one of the earliest and most significant randomized trials—streptomycin treatment of tuberculosis. This training prepared me for a career as an internist—a primary care physician for adults.

Panama Canal

By the end of my post-graduate training, I had married. We were broke. To gain funds to start a practice, I accepted a salaried post in the department of medicine at Gorgas Hospital in the Panama Canal Zone. The canal was still under the jurisdiction of the United States. We treated many patients with amebiasis. I saw my first, and only, case of Chagas disease. There was no malaria in the Canal Zone thanks to the early work of Gorgas. Jeeps periodically roamed the streets at night spraying DDT.

This service, although short, was pleasant and rewarding. I had the opportunity and pleasure to work beside many high-ranking medical officers who were still in the U.S. Army. The Grace Steamship Line graciously offered canal employees a free passage on one of their many ships transiting the canal. I marveled at the engineering marvel. It is still impressive after 100 years.

Early Private Practice: 1954-55

At that time, few internists were sub-specialists. We covered almost all the sub-specialties ourselves. There were no emergency room physicians; no hospitalists. We made house calls regularly. The standard fee for an office call was $3; for a house call $5.

Up to that time, medicine was, by present-day standards, backward. "Normal" systolic blood pressure was 100 plus your age. Treatment was primitive—relatively few effective drugs. Malignant hypertension was treated by sympathectomy or a "rice diet", extremely low in sodium. Diabetes was diagnosed when symptoms occurred. Diabetic coma was common. We successfully treated many coma patients and believed we had cured them.

On a brighter note, prevention of rheumatic fever with penicillin treatment of streptococcal infections became possible. We conducted rheumatic fever clinics to prevent recurrence with monthly injections of long-acting penicillin. At that time, rheumatic fever and rheumatic heart disease were major public health problems. The local health department set up rheumatic fever clinics. Patients with a history of the disease came in monthly to receive an injection of long-acting penicillin. Along with the use of penicillin to treat strep throat, and prevention of recurrence, rheumatic fever became an extreme rarity in the U.S. Most younger clinicians have never seen a case. It persists in developing countries.

It was becoming clear that cigarette smoking was deadly, due to the pioneering epidemiological studies of Richard Doll and Bradford Hill. The first study appeared in the British Medical Journal in 1950 (Bradford & Hill, 1950). "The risk of developing the disease (lung cancer) increases in proportion to the amount smoked. It may be 50 times as great among those who smoked 25 or more cigarettes a day as among non-smokers." (Bradford & Hill, 1950)

During the war, smoking was tacitly promoted. Many young men became addicted. Four years later, Doll published the British study of over 40, 000 doctors. This confirmed that cigarettes did indeed cause lung cancer. The science of epidemiology was established.

Unfortunately, the public paid scant attention to the danger of cigarettes. And still pays scant attention. I have wondered, however, if there is anything good about cigarettes. Did smoking give some relief from the extreme stress experienced during combat? Did cigarettes help us win the war?

My aim, after saving some money for a start, was to enter private practice. We chose Charlotte, North Carolina as our home because it seemed to be a pleasant, small city with a potential for growth. Young internists usually started solo. There were no large clinics to offer immediate employment at a substantial salary. Office space was tight. I was on my own. Fortunately, George Black, a kindly, elderly general practitioner, rented me a few rooms in his small office building. He even offered the help of one of his nurses to help me if I ever had a female patient. Things were tough. One afternoon, I remained in the office waiting for the phone to ring. It did not ring. As I left for the evening, I noted it was off the hook.

The county medical society maintained a phone number for sick people who did not have a physician. Many of the calls were at night, which were regularly referred to the lowest doctor in the pecking order. I was it. The older doctors in town preferred not to be disturbed at night. I visited the most deprived areas of the city. I was never accosted. On one occasion a call at 2AM awakened me. The caller's wife had severe abdominal pain. I noted the address and sleepily drove to the house. When I approached the house, I noted there were no lights on. This was unusual. I rang the doorbell, awakened the occupant, and learned that I had come to the wrong address. What to do? I went back home and tried unsuccessfully to go back to sleep. About 5 AM the phone rang. The husband asked where I was. I told him the story. He then replied, "That's all right, Doc, she is better and we don't need you to come".

Gradually, more local practitioners offered me the opportunity to take call for them on weekends or when they were on vacation. After about six months, Dr. Bill Matthews, who was well known and had a large practice, asked me to join him as a partner. My life became easier, but a lot busier.

I did not realize at the time that we were on the verge of the most prolonged and fruitful era of scientific medicine.

Practice Years

Over the past half century, I witnessed the most amazing and productive advances in medical history. Penicillin, warfarin, control of rheumatic fever and polio, and beginning control of TB (due to the expanding efforts of our Public Health system) were just the start. The list is so long it is impossible for me to mention them all:

- Ability to control hypertension, including self-measurement of blood pressure at home
- Earlier diagnosis and better control of diabetes
- Cure of peptic ulcer disease. (Who would have believed that peptic ulcer disease could be cured by antibiotics? Kudos to our colleagues in Perth, Australia.)
- Advances in endoscopy, permitting visualization of the GI tract
- Introduction of statin drugs, a giant step in ability to reduce atherosclerotic disease
- Use of radio-active isotopes in diagnosis and treatment
- Thrombolytic therapy
- Cognitive-behavioral therapy
- More (modestly) effective psycho-active drugs
- Expanding sophistication of laboratory testing
- Hospice, a giant step forward in compassionate end-of-life care. Palliative care for better control of pain and suffering
- Growing attention to ethical issues in medicine
- The growing presence of women in primary care practice

- Statistics: All original investigations published in major journals now contain a statistical analysis. This is new to us oldsters. I am not well versed in statistics. I have learned a few basic principles: sensitivity, specificity, predictive values, likelihood ratios, confidence intervals, and pre- and post-test probability. And a bit about Bayesian statistical analysis. This is all I needed to know. Clinicians do not have to be expert statisticians to understand and apply new research.
- Generic drugs: The recent availability of generic drugs at several large pharmacies at a low price ($4 for a supply of one month and $10 for three months). This increases the benefit / harm-cost ratio of drugs. (If the patient cannot afford the drug, then the best application of evidence-based medicine is useless.)
- Evidence-based medicine: stressed the importance of absolute risk reductions in trials comparing treatment vs. control. And the number of subjects needed to be treated to benefit one (NNT), instead of relative risk reductions (e.g., a 20% reduction). The latter is clinically meaningless and misleading. The randomized, controlled trial is the strongest scientific tool we have to determine the value of various therapeutic interventions. But it is far from perfect. One great deficiency is the lack of generalizability. There may be many reasons why an intervention is not applicable to an individual patient. This is where the "art" of medicine is applied. Primary care practice is especially concerned with this problem. We must know the life-style and the social circumstances of the individual patient, his individual concerns and willingness to accept and comply with treatment recommendations. We must share and negotiate a treatment plan.

In early years, we covered emergency room calls, had full responsibility for hospitalized patients, and took turns taking week-end and night calls as well as full patient coverage in the office. We became too busy--at times to the point of near-burnout. If I had to do it over again, I would try to cut down and do a better job of pacing myself. I would restrict the number of patients in my practice, and have the privilege of spending a little more time with each patient and gaining a better understanding of their personal fears, hopes and concerns, taking time to listen to their narrative, and empathizing. I think I would have more fully enjoyed practice and been a better doctor.

Internal medicine became increasingly specialized. More cardiologists, rheumatologists, infectious disease specialists, allergists, gastroenterologists entered practice. Then came the emergency care physicians and later, hospitalists. Those of us who called ourselves internists gradually became primary care, point-of-entry physicians for adults. We also had the privilege of continuing to care for some patients and their families over two generations. We felt we were underpaid compared with our specialist colleagues. We commented that we did not have any "procedures" for which we would be reimbursed handsomely. Merely talking with the patients and establishing an empathetic relationship was underappreciated and underpaid. Primary care internists responded by increasing their patient load.

Gradually, the approach to the patient began to change. In later years, physicians began to abandon the authoritative-paternalistic approach, which had governed the doctor-patient relationship for centuries. We realized that patients must participate in their own care, and do their own part in maintaining their health. They must act in many ways as their own physician. As more effective therapies became available, patients began to have more choices in treatment, and had to be actively involved in those choices. We heard more about "patient-centered medicine", "patient preference", "shared decision-making", "evidence-based" medicine, and the primary care "medical home".

Now, we stand on the brink of a new kind of scientific medicine, which will revolutionize medicine - the genome and all its applications. Advances in epidemiology, imaging, and surgery were equally startling. Epidemiology has expanded its boundaries and gained a predominant place in medical science. It has presented bed-rock guidance to primary care medicine as studies repeatedly established that maintenance of health depends on a healthy lifestyle. Dyslipidemia, obesity, lack of exercise, smoking, high salt intake, hypertension and poor diet were proved to be major risk factors, emphasizing the need for individuals to take charge of their own health. I believe the greatest health-related failure of medicine and our society is our inability to lead the general population to assume responsibility for their own health. Unfortunately, some physicians fail as role-models.

Imaging advances I have witnessed include CT scans and MRI; interventional radiology with balloon angiography and stenting; radioisotopes in therapy and diagnosis; ultrasound as a standard diagnostic tool; mammography; and angiography. (We were amazed when we first viewed opacification of the coronary arteries by injected dye.)

With regards to advances in Surgery in my lifetime, there were also many. Early on, post-surgery patients were kept in bed for days. Hernia repair was followed by at least a week in bed. Patients were admonished to avoid lifting and strenuous physical activity for several months. In 1970, Lichtenstein introduced careful repair under local anesthesia, with immediate ambulation. His suggestion was met with derision by the surgical community. Some called it "laughable". Other advances in surgery have been astounding: joint replacement, organ transplantation (the world was electrified when hearing news of the first heart transplant), heart surgery, urological surgery, and laparoscopic surgery are outstanding examples. Our surgical colleagues (bless them)

are highly skilled. Few persons in the U.S. reach my age without some surgical intervention, which lengthens life and reduces disability.

Lastly, the computer age deserves mention. To us elders, the advent of the computer and the World Wide Web is the most startling innovation. I believe this ability of individuals to freely communicate will greatly improve understanding between diverse persons and cultures around the world. It will do much to promote universal peace.

Years ago, we could not have believed that instant communication between individuals around the world would be possible. Transfer of documents, commentaries, scientific studies became routine and easy. Add to this the remarkable search engines, which facilitate instantaneous access to a vast variety of information. Consulting textbooks (often out-of-date) for needed information became passé. The laborious need to go to the library and search for the pertinent journal article was no longer necessary. It became much easier and quicker to obtain dictionary definitions of words than using the dictionary itself. I trust our young students and colleagues fully appreciate this tremendous advantage. They should learn more, and learn more quickly than we oldsters could.

Post Active Practice

After retiring from active office practice, I did not really consider myself "retired". I went on to other challenges. The two most important were participating in "free clinics" and editing and publishing abstracts of journal articles of importance to primary care clinicians.

Physicians in most communities in the US collaborated in forming and running free clinics to serve disadvantaged, homeless, and uninsured individuals. No questions asked—no limitations to enrollment, never any charge. Admittedly, service was suboptimal, but I believe helpful to many. Generic drugs were supplied free of charge. (Our patients seemed to do very well on generics.) Continuing care was made available with weekly visits. Some specialists in the community offered free consultations. Hospitals offered limited free laboratory and X-ray service. We were able to obtain some specialty drugs from pharmaceutical companies. When I finally resigned from this service, three years ago, I had completed 62 years as a licensed physician. I was proud of that.

During my years of active practice as a primary care internist, I had little time for keeping up with the current literature. I subscribed to several journals. They would pile up, most unread, many unopened, until I discarded them to make room for another pile. I am convinced that most busy clinicians, trying to balance a demanding practice with a semblance of family life, cannot adequately keep up.

Shortly after leaving active office practice, I began to review journals, abstracting articles I believed would be of interest to my former group of internists. I would meet with them every month and make an oral presentation accompanied by a written summary. They enjoyed it and encouraged me to continue. I then began to review each issue of JAMA, BMJ, NEJM, Lancet, Annals of Internal Medicine, and Archives of Internal Medicine and abstract articles of interest to primary care internists in the community, and publish them monthly.

I select articles on the basis of my own "clinical appraisal". Does the article present anything of practical importance? Can it be applied immediately to practice? Would it lead to a change in practice? I abstracted systemic reviews, editorials, and commentaries in addition to original investigations. I also included reports on new concepts (including ethical issues) that a well informed primary care internist should know as a basis of care and caring. Each month I included a "highlights" section containing a short summary of what the abstract contained to which I added editorial comments based on my experience. I was encouraged by a statement written by Robert H. Moser, M.D.:

"I am convinced the volume of pertinent new information that finally becomes available each year—the meaty stuff that a physician needs to know in order to provide optimal care to his patients—is not overwhelming. It is finite; it is tractable. But it is difficult to pin down. The problem lies in separating the wheat from the incredible amount of chaff." (Moser, 1978, pg. 350).

With the advent of e-mail, I was able to send monthly issues to a growing number of "subscribers". As the World Wide Web became available, I was able to publish the abstracts on the Internet, which could be downloaded by anyone interested. Because circulation was growing and the expense of publishing grew, I formed a corporation under the laws of the State of North Carolina to permit a tax deduction as a free, public-service, non-profit organization. There is never any charge for the publication. It contains no advertising. It is completely without bias. Monthly publication continues to this day. The web site (http://www.practicalpointers.org) receives about 10,000 "hits" a month from individuals around the world.

Beyond trying to absorb current information from the literature, one must be able to remember (or perhaps more importantly, to quickly retrieve and recall) information in order to apply it, should the occasion arise. Because of the need for easy retrieval, I compile a semi-annual index of all abstracts based on medical subject headings (e.g., diabetes; hypertension). Each MeSH is linked to the highlights section and editorial comments, and then on to the full abstract and the citation. The entire contents can be read in one or two evenings to refresh memory of what is new and clinically important for primary care.

For example, in the 2009 January-June Index, I included eighteen "practical clinical points" which primary care clinicians may wish to advise patients about, consider, and be aware of. To illustrate, I've excerpted five of these points, with their citations, below:

- Use aspirin for secondary prevention of vascular disease. Use in primary care is debatable.

    Antithrombotic Trialists' Collaboration Aspirin in the primary and secondary prevention of vascular disease a collaborative meta-analysis of individual participant data from randomised trials. Lancet May 30, 2009; 373.

- Avoid inhaled long-acting beta-agonists alone for asthma. Use combined with inhaled corticosteroids.

    Kuehn, B.M. FDA panel advises banning 2 popular asthma drugs. JAMA January 28, 2009; 301: 365-66.

- Reduce risk of hypertension by increasing potassium intake and decreasing sodium intake.

    Cook, N. R. Joint effects of sodium and potassium intake on subsequent cardiovascular disease Archives Internal Medicine. January 12, 2009; 169: 32-40.

- Life-style factors to reduce onset of type-2 diabetes, even in older patients.

    Mozaffarian, D. Lifestyle risk factors and new-onset diabetes mellitus in older adults. Archives Internal Medicine. April 27, 2009; 798-807.

- Patients to self-monitor BP.

    McManus, R.J Blood pressure self-monitoring "Clinical review" BMJ January 3, 2009; 338: 38- 42.

CONCLUSION

In describing my personal journey related to primary care medicine, I omitted the most important part, my relation to my patients. Early on, and throughout my practice career, emphasis was on the disease, not missing a diagnosis, and getting the treatment right. The approach was paternalistic and authoritarian. There were wise commentators who wrote about "caring for the patient", but, in my experience, this was not emphasized. The physician's reputation rested on skill at diagnosis.

I did indeed develop close empathetic relationships with some patients, but they were in the minority.

I was very conscientious in taking a careful medical history. Completing a careful and inclusive physical examination was a primary application of good medical practice. The physical examination was a cornerstone of good practice. There were few imaging and laboratory tests to confirm a diagnosis. Now, diagnosis is much easier and quicker; treatment is more specific. This could allow more time to develop a personal connection with each patient.

If I could start over, what would I do differently? I would try to:

- Conduct a more relaxed practice style to avoid any risk of burnout
- Extend office appointment times to at least 30 minutes
- Continuously sharpen my listening skills
- Spend some office-visit time socializing with my patient as means of understanding their "stories", concerns, and the factors in their lives that may impede adoption of healthy lifestyles
    - Understand what the patient hides has a profound effect on her health
    - Have no hesitancy in relating some of my own "story" if it were related to the patient's story.
    - Take full advantage of palliative care and Hospice services, not waiting too long to request their help.
- Gratefully accept the help of hospitalists and emergency room doctors
- Continue to visit my hospitalized patients and check on their progress
- Attend funerals. Make calls on the family after a death
- Make house calls

- Be concerned about costs of drugs. The best drug suggested by the best of evidence-based medicine is useless if the patient cannot afford it.
- Order generic drugs whenever possible. Teach patients to use a pill cutter to extend the life of a prescription
- Emphasize justice—the neglected 4th leg of medical ethics
- Remember that communication with the patient must be prompt and continuing. A patient waiting for a test report is an anxious patient
  - Accept as gracefully as possible the patient's refusal or inability to change adverse lifestyles (e.g.smoking, poor diet) and keep trying as gently to help the patient change
  - Recognize that many patients are health illiterate. Treat them with respect and patience
  - Continue to do the best I can to accept that I am imperfect, make mistakes, and will experience tragedies as well as triumphs
- Avoid regret that I will not be around to witness the next 68 years in the ongoing history of medicine.

REFERENCES

Bud, R. (2007). *Penicillin – Triumph and Tragedy*. Oxford, UK: Oxford University Press.

Doll, R., & Hill, A. B. (1950). Smoking and carcinoma of the lung. *British Medical Journal, 221*(2), 739–748. doi:10.1136/bmj.2.4682.739

Moser, R. H. (1973). Mission Possible. *Journal of the American Medical Association, 226*, 350. doi:10.1001/jama.226.3.350b

Wikipedia (2010, January 28). *Warfarin*. Retrieved February 11, 2010, from http://en/wikipedia.org/wiki/Warfarin

Chapter 14

Learning Medicine:
A Personal View

B. M. Hegde
Manipal University, India

ABSTRACT

This is a personal view on experiences in learning medicine from a physician academic and erstwhile vice chancellor of an Indian university. It summarizes his lessons learnt in a medical career that has made him explore medical traditions primarily to refute false dogmas that in his view continue to permeate the sciences to this day.

It is some time ago that Mr. Ron Paul, Congressman from Texas, predicted that the US economy would soon collapse, in his historic speech in the Congress. He was laughed at and ridiculed for those statements. Today he is being remembered by ordinary Americans who are on the verge of losing everything. Similarly, I have been writing to warn our fraternity that our system is doomed to fail and collapse sooner than later, thanks to its obsession with making money at any cost for which we have joined hands with the pharmaceuticals and technology manufacturers (and recently with craze for "health" insurance, another of those American flops) almost from the late 1960s when I wrote a paper on *How to avoid*

DOI: 10.4018/978-1-60960-097-6.ch014

modern medicine? "Never make money in the sick room" was the warning given by Hippocrates himself. People ridiculed me and laughed behind my back. There was even an attempt to get me out of my department! Recent IOM audit in the US has shown that the US medicine as the worst among the 14 industrialised countries and the medical establishment there as one of the leading causes of death and disability! Story would repeat elsewhere, if audited.

My colleagues think that I am coming in the way of their making money. That is very far from the truth. I would be the happiest person if they make any amount of money by the right royal way. I was only trying to tell the medical profession that the drug companies and the instrument manufacturers are taking us for a ride using our goodwill with patients to bleed the latter of their hard earned money. In the name of regular screening the ignorant people are made to believe that if they went for a regular check up they will live happily ever after. This is another ruse to net more people to take drugs. Recently it was recognized that in the US healthy young people, by the time they reach the age of thirty, are already on at least one tablet daily for some fault or the other in their check up reports. Mind you, this is in addition to multivitamins, baby aspirins and what have you!

The anti-propaganda against the innocent cholesterol, a life saving chemical in our system, mostly manufactured by our own body for its survival, has reached its pinnacle in that most Americans look at least a decade older than their chronological age and are looking famished with their skin coming off its moorings. Cholesterol lowering drugs are a big business hit. Most Americans today hardly eat anything and look sickly! Poor cholesterol, it is having a tough time trying to keep man alive with billions of new cells being formed daily to replace the dead ones. Every cell wall is made up of hydrophobic cholesterol. Lowering cholesterol unnecessarily could result in faulty cell wall which is an invitation for cancer growth!

My daughter always asks me why I write what I write. She is very critical of my quoting US statistics to prove my point in my articles. She is an internist in practice in the US. US is one country where there is total freedom of speech and expression. That should never be misconstrued as freedom to write anything one wants to write and criticize anyone or any country. As long as one knows that one is upholding the truth as is known at that point in time, one need not be worried about anything else. I have a very simple principle in life. Any human activity should be for the common good of people and society. There are so many myths in the field of modern medicine that need to be demolished for the common good. This could never be done with authenticity from anyone outside the field of modern medicine

although there have been attempts by great writers to look inside the medical field from outside and point out the mistakes. Unfortunately, most, if not all of them, blame the malady on doctors and not the system.

George Bernard Shaw is a noted name here. His play, *Doctors Dilemma,* was the one that changed the practice of medicine in England forever. Up until that play was enacted in London many of the *illustrated* doctors there, like many of our *illustrated* doctors today, have been doing whatever they thought was good for the patients irrespective of the consequences of their action. Unfortunately, no one from inside the system tried to undo the damage. Bernard Shaw took upon himself to correct the system having observed the stupidity of many medical interventions of his time. One example will suffice. Sir Arbuthnot Lane was a great surgeon in London at that time. No one could dare to talk to him about what he does. He had a hypothesis that all people with vague symptoms, which today is being labeled as *chronic fatigue syndrome,* had bad toxins emanating from their large gut as the cause of the disease!

His remedy was simple, total colectomy for such patients. Though this was resented by many patients they subjected themselves to the procedure as they had implicit faith in Sir Arbuthnot. Result was that almost half of the rich and famous Londoners was walking with an open drain on their abdomen making the city really stink. The play by Shaw put an end to the procedure and Sir Arbuthnot's practice as well. My efforts are to see that similar fate does not befall us today. Let us try and put our heads together to see how we could get back our position of authority and respect in society as in the distant past, where doctors were looked up to as next only to God. After all, patients could certainly live without doctors, as they had done for ages in the past but, doctors cannot hope to live without patients. Unlike in the 19th century London, information gets round pretty fast these days, thanks to the internet. Before patients leave us and go elsewhere, let us put our house in order.

Ivan Illich also did make an attempt to set things right in the medical field in the US in the 1930s, without much success.

While there could be a few greedy doctors in every society at any time, as there are greedy people in every other walk of life, majority of doctors in the US, India and elsewhere work with a mission of doing good to others. Despite all that US statistics do show that the medical profession has become a bane to society in the present milieu. This is a very serious matter to be brushed under the carpet. We should never have an ostrich like approach to difficult problems thinking that the problem does not exist or would go away. We should face the challenge head on to start a debate to get into the core of the matter to set things right, if we could. If we inside do not do that it will soon fall into the hands of outsiders like Sir George Bernard Shaw, Illich and others who did not know of the trials and tribulations that the majority of doctors have to, per force, go through to survive in this hostile atmosphere.

I think I am qualified to look into the system from within as I have been in this business of understanding the human body and its perils for more than half a century, if I were to start from the day I entered the Stanley Medical College in the then Madras city in India where East India Company had started one of the first three medical colleges in India. Interestingly, all those three cities have since changed their names but the content and the curriculum brought by the British MBBS degree has changed very little in medical education even to this day. Ever since that time I have been a curious student of the working of this enigma, the human body, both in times of illness and wellness. I must admit that I am as curious today as I was fifty years ago.

I became a doctor serendipitously although I had dreamed of becoming a teacher and doctor right from my childhood as I had our family doctor who was a God incarnate. My teachers were so good that one could easily make them one's role models. Unfortunately, I came from

a remote village in India far away from the big city of then Madras where the medical college was situated. When I passed my inter science from MGM College in Udupi with very good marks, I was asked to apply for medicine by my loving teachers led by Late Professor UL Achar, a great physicist. Unfortunately, I had not asked for the application forms in time and the last date for submission was fast approaching. Only four days were left for submission when I received the forms from Madras, thanks to the vagaries of our postal system although it was the only department without any corruption!

After filling the form I went over to Mangalore, a distance of 90 kilometers from where I lived (Hiriadka) to see if I could get someone going to Madras to personally take the forms. Providentially, there was a gentleman at the Railways Station (Late Kula Srinivas Shetty) who offered to do just that. That was Sunday and the next day the form had to be registered at Madras Medical College. The gentleman went from the Railway Station in Madras, the following morning at 9am, directly to the Madras Medical College, opposite the Central Station to register the same on time. Thank him and thank God, I eventually got selected and became a doctor only to be thrown out of Madras when I graduated with Gold Medal, special prize in surgery and distinctions because, by then, our district was taken away from Madras State to form the new Mysore state which eventually became Karnataka.

The British had taught our "great" leaders the fine art and the great benefits of divide and rule philosophy. They divided India on language as if the existing divisions on caste, colour, race, and religion were not enough to destroy peace on earth. I had to sit an all India test to get selected for DGHS scholarship for my postgraduation, a decent sum at that time. I went over to King George's Medical College in Lucknow where I had the luck now to be under a great researcher and teacher, Late Professor SS Mishra, who instilled research hunger in me when I was still young and impressionable. He also taught me, by example, to be one hundred per cent honest about research data. May his soul rest in peace. I have been following him faithfully ever since. He was the one that wanted me to go abroad and study in the UK to get my Royal College of Physicians membership by passing the tough MRCP (UK) examination. He was so pleased when I came back with my training in cardiology at the National Heart Hospital, Middlesex Hospital Medical School and Harefield Cardiothoracic centres in England and the MRCP (UK) degree. He regularly used to write handwritten letters enquiring about my progress up until his last breath.

London was a great eye opener for me. My Chief, Late Walter Somerville, was a great cardiologist, a CBE, editor of the British Heart Journal for thirty years, and a great thinker and writer par excellence. He honed my writing skills, if I have any, when I assisted him with the journal. My Indian English was refined by him. He never used to find fault but, would suggest a better way to convey the same message. My other teacher, Late Richard Emanuel, also took me under his care for research as also to look after his private patients at the London Clinic. This exposed me to the rich and the famous of the world in addition-Kings, Presidents, Prime Ministers and the lot. It was a great education to see the so called great men also had feet of clay when it came to their own mortality.

Walter wanted me to have some exposure to American cardiology and he arranged for my training under Nobel Laureate Bernard Lown at the Harvard Medical School, another eye opener to bench research in addition to clinical bed side enquiry. All these men were great teachers from whom I have imbibed many tricks of the trade. While at the Harvard another great teacher took a liking for me. Lewis Dexter was the father of investigative cardiology and he used to take me along to follow his footsteps in whatever he did, even to occasional dinners in restaurants where we used to discuss life in addition to cardiology.

The other teachers that influenced my thinking and clinical acumen were TA Watkin Edwards, Malcolm Towers, Marvin Sturridge, Jack Belcher, Jane Somerville, CJ Stewarts, Michael Barry, Miss Mary Sheppard and a few others.

My teaching career started very early in life at the Kasturba Medical College Manipal/Mangalore. Although I had been teaching almost all over the world at different times, my base was Mangalore where I have been teaching for nearly 40 years from the day I started as a tutor in 1962 till I retired as the Vice Chancellor of Manipal University in 2003. Since then I have been examining for the Royal Colleges of both UK and Ireland which incidentally started way back in 1988. Teaching is my first love. Teaching is in my blood. I enjoy talking even to school children. While I was PG student at Lucknow one of my junior teachers, SN Pandeya, picked me up for teaching his BDS students which I did, I was told, very well. I enjoy teaching even now when I get an opportunity.

My experiences have taught me a few lessons. Mistakes all of us make and there is no one who has not committed mistakes. Human beings are fallible. The first lesson I learnt was never to make the same mistake twice. I had a fair share of my troubles dealing with my colleagues, students, patients and seniors. The second lesson I learnt was that anyone could fool you. If they fool you once it is shame on them, but if you let them fool you for the second time it is shame on you. The third lesson I learnt was that only when you go out of your way to help others they will turn out to be your worst enemies for obvious reasons! But then, the pleasure and happiness of helping others far outweighs this risk. I had gone out of my way, even risking my own future, to be of help but that was never appreciated. The lesson is never to expect anything in return, when you do good except to get the pleasure of helping others. The all time best lesson I learnt was this world and the people there are not what they appear to be or proclaim to be. Each of them has his/her own agenda although they mask it most of the time.

My life taught me one other lesson which I would like to let the younger generation know. Although money is absolutely necessary to live, medical profession should not be used solely to make money. Your due share will come. There will be times when people will cheat you but, that is how it should be. If all people are good world would be a monotonous place to live. Variety is life's best spice. I had bad times and good times, the latter always followed the former. The great lesson I learnt was that nothing abides; all things flow. I learnt from my teachers, my patients, my colleagues, but more than them all, I learnt and keep learning from my students.

I became a Head of the Department, then Dean of the medical school and, finally a Vice Chancellor of the university and all these experiences have shaped my thinking to a great extent. I have burnt my fingers several times trusting all people all the time. At the end of all that I would like to treat everyone as good until proven otherwise. People could fault me for my lapses but no one could honestly cross their heart and say that I deliberately harmed any of them using my power and clout. I am absolutely clear about that. My fault was that I used more heart than head in dealing with sub-ordinates forgetting what Jesus said: "Be ye, therefore, wise like a serpent but harmless like a dove." My sorrow is that despite my giving my best and being nice to my superiors, many of them have not been able to see my true worth. History will judge men and matters better than one's peers. I followed the dictum that it is only small minds that talk and worry about individuals; greater minds think of events while, the greatest minds think of issues concerning mankind as a whole.

My second love was research which I define as "organized curiosity coupled with logical skepticism." It was Ralph Waldo Emerson who once wrote that to be a doctor gives one a great training to be a writer as it is only the doctor,

practising on the bed side, who gets to see human emotions totally naked! I started writing for the first time in the early 1960s mainly because I had an urge to let the common man know what is good for him to live well and let others live as well. Although my hate-mail file is much thicker than the fan mail, I have no doubt that I had started a new tradition in health education of the common man taking him away from the usual *health care system* to the true health care system. I believed in what Churchill once said: "he has a right to criticize who has a heart to help."

Medical research for me is bed side thinking-having a question in my mind on the bed side, at times stimulated by my thinking (vanishing breed) students, to go as far away from the bed as I could to get the right answers. In doing so I soon fell into a large trap where I found that the whole medical world was being converted into a trap from which the hapless patient could never escape unscathed! My first paper in lay press entitled *"how to avoid medicine"* got me into real trouble with the medical world as also my immediate colleagues in the medical school and the pharmaceutical lobby! I quickly realized that the scientific basis of modern medicine, leaning heavily on statistics is anything but true science. While the human physiology is holistic, non-linear and dynamic our mathematical base of medical science is linear, static, and reductionistic. I have been proving that for decades but, lately people in very high positions in western countries have opened their eyes to this truth. A recent editorial in the Archives of Internal Medicine of October 26th, 2009 would take your breath away when it condemns our bench mark RCTs (randomized controlled trials) as unacceptable as science in no uncertain terms.

"Knowledge advances NOT by repeating known facts, but by refuting false dogmas," wrote Karl Popper years ago. I have been pursuing that line of thinking in all my research and have been able to demolish many myths in medicine. To list all of them would be futile exercise here for want of space; suffice it to say that most of them have been published in peer reviewed conventional journals. (Hegde 1975-2003)

When I started the campaign to bring out the truth about cardiac revascularization procedures way back in 1995 in the Journal of the Royal College of Physicians of Edinburgh people started hating me. The truth is now dawning on every one who cares to know the truth. My article *Unconventional wisdom in medicine,* published in 1992 in the Glasgow Royal College Bulletin was another shocker. Many others followed suit. Rest is history. However it is a single handed campaign against the iron wall of medical care industry which has a greater agenda to keep the gullible public under the myth of secrecy has not been very effective but I think I have been able to start a debate. Recent audits in the US and 14 other industrialized countries in the west have corroborated my writings of the last four decades.

Since my retirement from the routine 9-5 job in 2003, I joined a group of scientists led by the all time great Professor Rustum Roy of Penn. State University in the USA to start our own research organization, *World Academy of Authentic Healing Sciences,* with the parent body, *Friends of Health,* headed by Professor Roy who has been spearheading a movement for *Whole Person Healing* (WPH), a word now accepted by the Academy of Sciences in the USA. We have also started a new International Science Journal, *Journal of the Science of Healing Outcomes* (www.thejsho.com) of which I have been made the editor-in-chief with Professor Roy to guide me. We have an editorial board of very eminent scientists from all over the world, including some Nobel Laureates. This is a purely charitable venture.

One of my prime duties is to go round the world with a begging bowl to collect money to keep our research and the journal afloat. Good hearted infracaninophiles do help, but more help is needed. Hope to continue this as long as God gives me the stamina. I need your prayers as well. In this effort God has blessed me with an elder brother, (not

biological) a senior at medical school, Professor CV Krishnaswami of Chennai, an internationally acclaimed diabetologist and a true scientist. He has been a great source of inspiration and we work together in this great task. As he has lots of big contacts in Chennai, he gets me money and we are starting a centre for research soon there with money from his friends and patients. I remain ever grateful to him.

Another humane friend is my class mate in school, the son of our then headmaster in school, Mr. Pundalik Kini, a nuclear scientist turned engineer consultant, who has a flourishing business in San Francisco. He helps me to collect money for this worthy cause. Kini's life motto is to help others. I can't thank him enough for all that he is doing for me. When in need I always draw upon the munificence of Professor Rustum Roy, another God's gift to me.

I am happy that our new effort to authenticate healing outcomes in many complementary systems is proceeding well. Our research efforts have started yielding fruits. We have many of them published in our own journal which has a new super peer review (only specialists in the area of research like physicists, chemists etc. review papers) system in place. In closing, I have a true confession to make. I never ever planned any one of the multifarious activities that I reported above although I am aware of the dictum that "if you fail to plan, you will plan too fail." I did not know that dictum till very recently!

REFERENCES

Emanuel, R., & Hegde, B. M. (1975). Association of Secundum Atrial Septal Defect with Abnormalities of AV Conduction of Left Axis Deviation. *British Heart Journal, 30,* 1085–1092. doi:10.1136/hrt.37.10.1085

Hegde, B. M. (1985). How to detect early splenic enlargement? *The Practitioner, London, 229,* 857.

Hegde, B. M. (1988). *Blood Pressure and Meals.* The practitioner, London, 232, 224-225.

Hegde, B. M. (1992). Materia Paramedica. *Journal of the Royal College of Physicians & Surgeons of Glasgow*, 18.

Hegde, B. M. (1993). Need for change in Medical Paradigm. In *Proc Roy Coll Phy Edin., 23,* 9-12.

Hegde, B. M. (1993). The state of Internal Medicine. In *Proc Roy Coll Phy Edi., 23,* 511-18.

Hegde, B. M. (1994). *24, 228.* Miscellanea Medical. In Proc Roy Coll Phys Edin.

Hegde, B. M. (1994). Auscultation for MVP. *Lancet, 344,* 1446–1447. doi:10.1016/S0140-6736(94)90619-X

Hegde, B. M. (1995). Auscultation for MVP. *Lancet, 345,* 29.

Hegde, B. M. (1995). *Unconventional Wisdom in Medicine* (p. 292). Glasgow: Bull.Roy.Coll. Phys.Surg.

Hegde, B. M. (1995). Coronary Artery Disease, Time for Reappraisal. In *Proc. R.C.P. Edin., 26,* 421-24.

Hegde, B. M. (1995). Mitralklappen - Prolaps? *Medical Tribune(German), 17,* 36.

Hegde, B. M. (1996). Hypertension Â– Past, Present and Future. *Kuwait Med. J.,* (suppl.), 194–198.

Hegde, B. M. (1997). Medical Humanism. *Proceedings of the Royal College of Physicians of Edinburgh, 27,* 65–67.

Hegde, B. M. (1997). Reductio Ad Absurdum. *Briti. Roy. Coll.Physi. Surg. Glasgow, 26,* 10–12.

Hegde, B. M. (1997). Heart of the Matter. *Bull. Roy. Coll. Physi. Surg. Glasgow., 26,* 14–15.

Hegde, B. M. (1998). Cardiological Examinations [letter]. *Jr.Roy.Coll.Physi. Lon., 32,* 83–84.

Hegde, B. M. (1999). Exercise Â– Sense Versus Non-Sense - Bull. *Roy. Coll. Physi. Surg. Glasgow, 28,* 13–14.

Hegde, B. M. (1999). Hypertension Â– the other side of the coin. *Jap.Soc. of Hyper. Int, 13-14,* 99–100.

Hegde, B. M. (2002, March). Health Care Delivery in India Today. *JAPI, 50,* 425–427.

Hegde, B. M. (2002). To do or Not to Do-Doctors Dilemma, Plea for Proper Audit. *JIACM, 3*(3), 236–239.

Hegde, B. M. (2002). Septmeber). Needless Interventions in Medicine. *JIMA, 5*(3), 153–15.

Hegde, B. M. (2002). Where is the Reality? *Kuwait Medical Journal, 34*(4), 263–265.

Hegde, B. M., & Chakrapani, M. (1991). Early Renal Involvement in Mild moderate hypertension. *Chinese Medical Sciences Journal, 6*(3), 46.

Hegde, B. M., & Rao, R. A. C. (1987). Long term Thiazide Therapy and Fat Profile. *Cardiovascular Drugs and Therapy, 1,* 310.

Rajendra, A., Hegde, B. M., Subbabba, B. P., Ashok, R., & Niranjan, C. U. (2002, September). Wavelet Analysis of Heart Rate Variability: New Method of Studying the Heart's Functions. *Kuwait Medical Journal, 34*(3), 195–200.

Wolf, G., & Hegde, B. M. (1976). Syphilitic Aortic Regurgitation. An appraisal of surgical treatment. *The British Journal of Venereal Diseases, 52,* 366–369.

Chapter 15
Descriptive Statistics with a Purpose

Ronan Conroy
Royal College of Surgeons, Ireland

ABSTRACT

A statistic is a data summary which provides useful information. I use the example of sex work research in Africa to ask the question "useful to whom?". In over 800 papers on sex work in Africa published over more than two decades, the focus has been on sex workers as spreaders of HIV, enriching the research community while further stigmatising the sex workers who participate in the research. In this study, partly run by sex workers themselves, the focus is on targeting micro-economic aid, and documenting the violent and abusive culture in which sex work is practised. The chapter illustrates the data analysis using Stata. However, it tries to place the descriptive statistics into their wider context in the research agenda, including a discussion of the ethics of research into vulnerable groups.

WHAT IS A STATISTIC?

Sir John Sinclair introduced the word 'statistic' into the English language. His explanation of why he did so is still useful to read:

"Many people were at first surprised at my using the words "statistical" and "statistics", as it was supposed that some in our own language might have expressed the same meaning. [...] the idea I annex to the term is *an inquiry into the state of a country, for the purpose of ascertaining the quantum of happiness enjoyed by its inhabitants, and the means of its future improvement.*"

Sinclair's idea of useful facts was not necessarily numbers; any information useful to describing the state of a country and planning for its improvement. Statistics are defined in terms of their usefulness.

A statistic, I propose, is a useful numeric summary of data.

DOI: 10.4018/978-1-60960-097-6.ch015

Now contrast this with the statistics lecturer who breezes into his first class of statistics 101 and says, with an air of enthusiasm that is palpably feigned:

"Suppose we measured the heights of twenty people – how could we summarise what we have found out?"

Now I cannot imagine any reason at all for measuring the heights of twenty people. I cannot imagine a hypothesis that might have driven me to do it, nor a burning question that can be answered with the data. For this reason, there are no statistics you can calculate – there is nothing in the data that answers a question, nothing that can be used to bring about the improvement of people, as Sinclair would have put it. The only question that comes to mind is the mental state of anyone who pops out one fine morning to measure the heights of twenty people.

Not every dataset I analyse is full of excitement, but in each case I cannot start work without understanding what it is that we need to know – what was the purpose of gathering the data. Indeed, I once wrote a paper about the process of finding exactly the way of analysing a very simple dataset that would provide useful information to patient and doctor, showing how only one of the many ways of looking at the data actually gave this information (Conroy, 2002).

I've been doing research out in Kenya for almost two decades now. In the course of this, I've made a lot of friends, met a lot of people, heard a lot of stories. These somehow shape my idea of what is important, what we need to know, what, in short, of a statistic is.

This chapter takes you through the rationale behind, the conduct and analysis of and my own reflections on the research. The results are published (Elmore-Meegan, Conroy, & Agala, 2004). This is more like the behind-the-scenes documentary.

This is a story about sex workers, some of whom are friends of mine. It is to them I would like to dedicate the chapter.

WHO NEEDS STATISTICS ABOUT SEX WORKERS AND WHY?

Before I introduce some descriptive statistics, I have to explain why we might need them. And to do that, I need to tell you something about sex work and sex work research in sub-Saharan Africa.

The Plague Bringers

Our story starts, as far as I can see, in 1986, with the publication of a paper in the New England Journal of Medicine (Kreiss, et al., 1986)

The acquired immunodeficiency syndrome (AIDS) is epidemic in Central Africa. To determine the prevalence of AIDS virus infection in East Africa, we studied 90 female prostitutes, 40 men treated at a clinic for sexually transmitted diseases, and 42 medical personnel in Nairobi, Kenya. Antibody to human T-cell lymphotropic virus Type III (HTLV-III) was detected in the serum of 66 percent of prostitutes of low socioeconomic status, 31 percent of prostitutes of higher socioeconomic status, 8 percent of the clinic patients, and 2 percent of the medical personnel. The presence of the antibody was associated with both immunologic and clinical abnormalities. The mean T-cell helper/suppressor ratio was 0.92 in seropositive prostitutes and 1.82 in seronegative prostitutes (P less than 0.0001). Generalized lymphadenopathy was present in 54 percent of seropositive prostitutes and 10 percent of seronegative prostitutes (P less than 0.0001). No constitutional symptoms, opportunistic infections, or cases of Kaposi's sarcoma were present. Our results indicate that the epidemic of AIDS virus infection has, unfortunately, spread extensively among urban prostitutes in Nairobi, Kenya. Sexual exposure to men from Central Africa was significantly associated with HTLV-III antibody among prostitutes, suggesting transcontinental spread of the epidemic.

You can see a number of key words in the title: *prostitutes, spread, AIDS, epidemic*. I have written them with commas between them, but this message was to be reinforced again and again in the intervening 20 years. Research into sex work (prostitution) in Africa has become an industry, with 815 published papers, innumerable conferences, reports, meetings and, of course, funded programmes.

Sex workers are seen as the motor of the AIDS epidemic in sub-Saharan Africa, the cess pool from which the disease spreads. This view was given a powerful impetus by the publication of a World Bank policy document, "Confronting AIDS" (Anonymous, 1997). The authors of the report did calculations of the effect of sex workers on the spread of AIDS. They published their findings using Figure 1.

They argued, on the basis of their calculations, that targeting low-income men was an inefficient way of preventing AIDS. Their rate of infection might be as high as 10%, but with only 4 partners

a year (one wonders if sex workers counted as partners) 500 low income men would generate only about 88 new cases of HIV infection a year. By comparison, the same number of sex workers, who had a high rate of HIV infection, would generate 10,000 new cases of HIV a year, assuming that each had four partners a day.

The frightening image of a core of 500 sex workers infecting 10,000 men a year provoked an intense focus on trying to change the behaviour of sex workers by getting them to use condoms, and trying to get their clients to accept condom use. The health promotion message was clear: the whores are spreading the plague.

Perhaps this message would have been more forgivable if it was true. But where had the underlying assumption of four clients a day come from? It had come from some published research on Nairobi sex workers and from 'author's calculations'. We don't even know whether it represents

Figure 1.

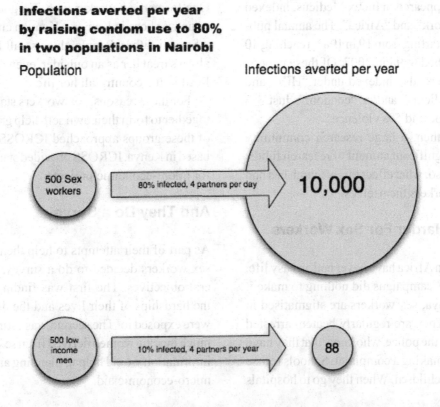

Infections averted per year by raising condom use to 80% in two populations in Nairobi

four clients a day, 365 days a year, or allows for days off now and then for holidays, visiting family, recovering from beatings or being detained without trial by the police. And we don't know, critically, whether these are four new, never-before-seen partners a day, or four partners. The only figure that seemed to dominate the debate was the one in the big circle: 10,000 new infections.

It's notable that the World Bank performed no sensitivity analysis to ask what would happen if they were wrong, and client numbers were lower than their estimate. For a large and powerful organisation to base a recommendation on a single estimate is a very big gamble with the lives and resources of others.

The World Bank report ushered in a spate of health promotion campaigns aimed at sex workers, based on the idea that they were the motor of the AIDS epidemic, and that preventing the rise of AIDS depended on changing what sex workers did.

The first effect of this intense interest in sex workers was to drive and fund a vast research agenda. In the two decades since the 1986, 1,276 papers have appeared in Index Medicus, indexed under "Sex work" and "Africa". The annual publication rate, starting from 19 in 1986, reaching 40 in 1989, climbed to 98 in 2007. Of these papers, 795 (62%) were also indexed under "HIV" and 535 under "Clients" and/or "condom". Just 3% mentioned rape and 5% violence.

There is, then, a large research community attracting a significant amount of research funds. We must ask, so, what effect this research has had on the sex workers themselves.

Life Gets Harder For Sex Workers

Sex workers in Africa have never had an easy life. And the AIDS campaigns did nothing to make it better. In Kenya, sex workers are stigmatised in many ways. They are regularly beaten, arrested and robbed by the police, who know that they have no chance of making a complaint. Schools refuse to admit their children. When they go to hospitals

clinics, staff will refuse to see them, or leave them waiting until everyone else is seen. They are also usually excluded from self-help groups.

Self help groups are everywhere in Kenya. Often run by women, they use seed money, often from donor organisations, to start projects which are then self-financing. For example, the group may provide land and labour and, with financial help, build chicken coops and buy chickens and feed. Once the chickens start laying, they can sell the eggs to finance feed, and when they can start selling hens the group is usually self-sustaining.

Kenyan self help groups are often hostile to sex workers. There are several reasons for this. The first is that Kenya has a large number of religious groups who might be called fundamentalist, and who disapprove of sex workers. Though even as I write this, I realise that you don't have to be in any way religious to discriminate against sex workers; it just seems to help. The second reason is that sex workers are often from outside the area in which they work, and may not be from the same ethnic group as their good neighbours. One former sex worker who is a good friend of mine was born in Kenya, a Kenyan citizen, but of a Somali father. People always call her Somali, always treat her as an outsider, even though she's lived in the country all her life.

For these reasons, sex workers started getting together to form their own self-help groups. Some of these groups approached ICROSS, and NGO based in Kenya. ICROSS provided start-up money for micro-economic projects.

And They Do a Survey

As part of their attempts to help themselves, the sex workers decided to do a survey. It had several objectives. The first was finding out about the hardships of their lives and the dangers they were exposed to. The second was estimating how much income women derived from sex work. This information would help in planning and targeting micro-economic aid.

The survey was done by interview. All the interviewers were sex workers, and they interviewed their co-workers in their native language. There were 9 different translations of the questionnaire, all back-translated to ensure their accuracy. By using peer networks, the interviewers were able to identify eligible sex workers, and because the women were interviewed by their peers, the degree of trust and openness was good.

LOOKING AT THE DATA

It has taken a while to get to look at the data, but the choice of descriptive statistics will depend on the purpose of the study. I wasn't sure how to present the data analysis. I use Stata, and it occurred to me that I should probably present the analysis exactly as I do it. You can think of yourself looking over my shoulder. The commands I write may not mean much to some readers (and I should point out that Stata is fully menu-driven - it's just that it's easier to document your data analysis if you use the keyboard, as I do). So what follows is a more or less actual Stata data analysis session, warts and all (some of the output looks a lot less nice than I would like, for example).

Numbers of Clients: The First Key Question

How many clients did the women see in the previous week?

(I habitually abbreviate Stata's summarize command to summ. You can abbreviate it to su, but that makes it harder for a casual reader to work out what it's short for. I will make occa-sional comments about working in Stata - if you don't use Stata you can bleep over them.)

The average number of clients per week is 5.5. This is a bit disconcerting. These 474 sex workers are supposed to see four clients a day, according to the World Bank. And yet the average, 5.5 clients a week, is less than one a day. How many of them did see four clients a day? Adding the detail option to the summarize command gives me extra descriptive statistics, including information about percentiles and extreme values. (see Table 2)

Look at the extreme values at the high end of the range: 75% saw 8 clients or fewer per week, while 90% saw 9 clients or fewer per week and 99% saw 15 clients or fewer per week. Indeed, the four highest values are 15, 16, 19 and 19.

In other words, not one single sex worker in the 474 surveyed saw four clients a day, whether you define this as 20 clients a week (allowing two days off) or 28 (making her work around the clock).

Confidence Intervals

Of course, the figure of 5.5 is the average for the sample of 474. The real average for Kenyan sex

Table 1. Summ clients

Variable	Obs	Mean	Std. Dev.	Min	Max
clients_in~k	474	5.508439	3.148363	1	19

Table 2. Summ clients, det

clients in last week				
Percentiles		Smallest		
1%	1	1		
5%	1	1		
10%	2	1	Obs	474
25%	3	1	Sum of Wgt.	474
50%	5		Mean	5.508439
		Largest	Std. Dev.	3.148363
75%	8	15		
90%	9	16	Variance	9.912191
95%	11	19	Skewness	.8967739
99%	15	19	Kurtosis	3.940713

Table 3. ci clients

Variable		Obs	Mean	Std. Err.	[95% Conf.	Interval]
clients_in~k		474	5.508439	.1446091	5.224283	5.792595

workers might be higher or lower than that. We can get the confidence interval using the ci command.

The confidence interval tells us that the average number of clients that Kenyan sex workers see each week might be as high as 5.8 or might be as low as 5.2, but is unlikely to be outside that range. And unlikely is defined as "less than 5% likely". So although our sample may have under-estimated or over-estimated the average number of clients, the error is unlikely to be grave. There is a margin of uncertainty of just ±0.3 around the mean. A sample of 474 women gives a precise estimate of the mean.

There is a slight problem, of course: clients come in multiples of one, and the number of clients per week is quite small. For this reason, the distribution has two properties that will make it unlike the smooth, bell-shaped curve in the textbook. We could re-run the calculation telling Stata that clients are a rare event (this is kind of ironic, given the frenetic frequency with which the World Bank thinks of sex workers' client turnover). (see Table 4)

The confidence interval is slightly, but not importantly different.

Stata can also estimate confidence intervals for quantiles, using qreg (quantile regression).

Running a regression with no predictor variables causes the regression to estimate just one value: the constant. In this case, I am estimating the 95th percentile, so the estimate is 11, just as

before, and the confidence interval is 9.1 to 12.9. In other words, it is unlikely that the 95th centile for clients per week is any higher than 13 (in round figures).

EVIDENCE BASED-POLICY?

Where does this leave the World Bank's calculations? Utterly unsupported. And this survey was not alone. We reviewed previous publications which reported on client numbers of sex workers in sub-Saharan Africa. The figures in this survey are in line with the other published reports we could trace on PubMed and in the 'grey literature' at the time, including data presented at conferences and not subsequently published (Gathiqi, et al.; Hawken, et al., 2002; Pickering, Okongo, Nnalusiba, Bwanika, & Whitworth; Pickering, Quigley, Hayes, Todd, & Wilkins). Indeed, the highest client levels we were able to find were those reported by Wilson, who reported an average of just over 10 clients per week in Harare bar-based sex workers (Wilson, Chiroro, Lavelle, & Mutero, 1989), and even this is far short of the World Bank estimate. And more recent data are no different: using a sophisticated client diary methodology, Ferguson reported that Kenyan sex workers had an average of 54.2 sex acts a month (that's less than two a day) and, more important, that the average number of different clients was

Table 4. ci clients, pois

Variable		Exposure	Mean	Std. Err.	Poisson [95% Conf.	Exact Interval]
clients_in~k		474	5.508439	.1078016	5.299157	5.723867

Table 5. qreg clients, q(95)

Iteration 1: WLS sum of weighted deviations = 905.40183							
Iteration 1: sum of abs. weighted deviations = 1029.3							
Iteration 2: sum of abs. weighted deviations = 364.3							
.95 Quantile regression			Number of obs = 474				
Raw sum of deviations	364.3 (about 11)						
Min sum of deviations	364.3		Pseudo R2 = 0.0000				
clients_in~k		Coef.	Std. Err.	t	P>|t|	[95% Conf.	Interval]
_cons		11	.9472633	11.61	0.000	9.138635	12.86136

only 13.6 (Ferguson & Morris, 2007). Clearly, the other factor that the World Bank's calculations did not take into account was that the four partners a day were probably not four new partners.

FINDING SUBGROUPS

Are there subgroups of sex workers with different numbers of clients? If we can identify subgroups with relatively small client numbers, these may be easier to target with micro-economic aid, because the amounts of money they earn from sex work

will be less, and so sex work will be easier to replace with other sources of income.

Here is where looking at numbers becomes tedious. We could look at quantiles for each of the areas in which the study was run, but there is an easier way: the boxplot.

Boxplots show key quantiles of the data. (see Figure 2)

The boxplots display descriptive statistics. You can think of a boxplot as a ladder. The rungs of the latter are descriptive statistics. (see Figure 3)

You will notice that some boxplots show dots above and below. These dots represent outliers:

Figure 2. Graph box clients, over (area)

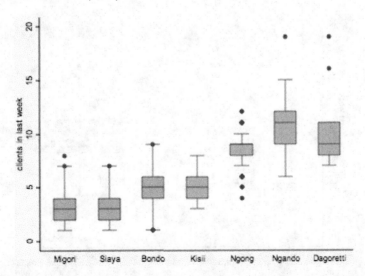

Figure 3.

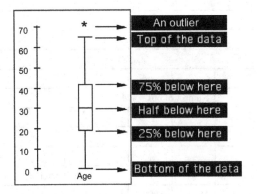

values so high or so low that they don't seem to belong with the rest of the data. There are a couple of very active sex workers in Ngong, and there are so few in Dagoretti that the boxplot is missing some of its bits.

Two Groups

You can see that there are two groups of locations: ones with lower client rates (Bondo, Kisii, Migori and Siayia) while the other three locations – Ngando, Ngong and Dagoretti – have higher client rates. This makes sense in terms of the demography of these locations. The first four

are rural towns, while the last three are townships on the outskirts of Nairobi. So rather than having seven locations, there appear to be two groups of sex workers: those in rural towns, and those in townships. When we plot numbers of clients in the two groups we can see there is quite a difference. (see Figure 4)

You can see that the sex workers in rural towns had low client rates. Three quarters saw five clients a week or fewer, and not one of them saw ten clients. On the other hand, the township women had a median of 10 clients a week, though three quarters saw twelve or fewer.

Seeing Descriptive Statistics and Data At Once

The trouble with boxplots is that they show descriptive statistics, but they do not show data, except for outliers. However, the stripplot command, written by Nick Cox, allows you to display the data and superimpose boxplots. (see Figure 5)

I have told stipplot to do separate dotplots for each area, to superimpose a boxplot (which I have lowered slightly to keep it from being overprinted by the dots using the boffset option) and the jitter the data. Jittering adds a small amount of

Figure 4. Graph box clients, over (township)

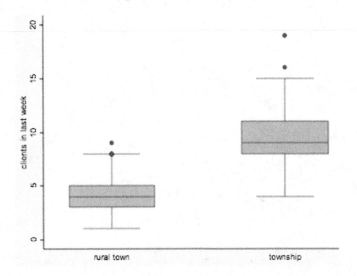

Figure 5. Stripplot clients, over (area) box jitter(3) boffset(-.2)

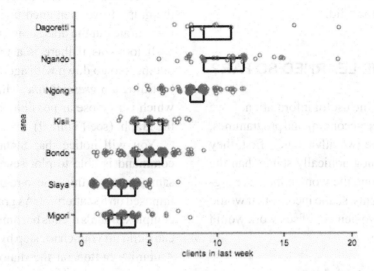

random noise to the data so that points which would have overprinted are now visible separately.

This is a reasonable compromise between the need to see actual data and the need to have descriptive statistics. It very clearly shows the two groups of areas: townships and rural towns. You will notice that the boxplots here show the 25th, 50th and 75th percentiles – they lack 'whiskers'. The lack of whiskers isn't really a problem when we can see the actual data.

We can also use stripplot to display means and their confidence intervals. (see Figure 6)

The dots show the means and the whiskers show the confidence intervals. We can see that the small sample size in Dagoretti has resulted in a very wide confidence interval, while the confidence intervals for the rural towns are small, reflecting the large samples. And, of course, in all of this it remains abundantly clear that not one of the almost 500 sex workers has see anything like

Figure 6. Stripplot clients, over (area) box jitter(3) boffset(-.2)

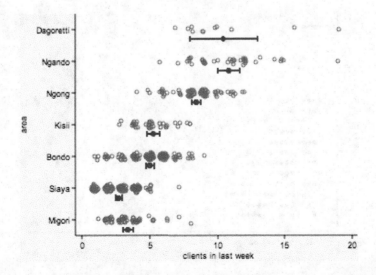

the number of clients that the World Bank's calculations assumed they did.

WHAT HAVE WE LEARNED SO FAR?

Already we have some useful information. It we are going to start micro-economic aid programmes, the rural towns have two advantages: first, they are much more demographically stable than the townships, and second the women there see significantly fewer clients, so the income that would be needed to keep women out of sex work would be substantially less.

Client Numbers and Age

We can look at how client numbers vary with the woman's age using a scatterplot. Our first attempt looks less than useful, though. (see Figure 7)

There are only three sex workers aged over 40, and they have half the graph to themselves. Furthermore, since clients and ages come as whole numbers, there are probably lots of dots on that graph printed one on top of the other.

A second look, this time using if to restrict the graph to women aged under forty and jitter to separate out the dots somewhat. (see Figure 8)

It looks as if there is a tendency for client numbers to go down with age. We can check this by fitting a *regression line*. This is a straight line which is as close as possible to all the points on the graph. (see Figure 9)

You will notice that Stata's twoway graph command is able to plot several graphs on the same chart – in this case, a regression line superimposed on a scatterplot. As graphs become more complex, Stata's menus become more useful. You can build up your chart, step by step, pressing the <submit> button on the dialogue to check the effect.

The regression line shows a sharp decline in client numbers. However, it does suggest something unusual: that by the age of 36, women see no clients at all. The problem is that a regression line is straight. Often, a straight line is a reasonable way of showing a relationship, but here the relationship isn't so simple. The next graph shows a smoother. A smoother is like a regression line – it tries to keep as close to all the data points as possible – but it has a certain amount of flexibility to bend to match the shape of the data.

Figure 7. Twoway scatter clients age

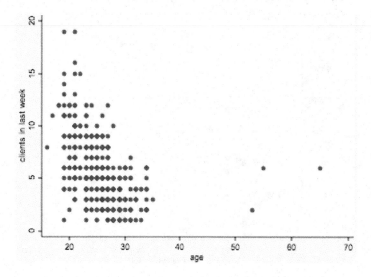

Figure 8. Twoway scatter clients age if age < 40, jitter(5)

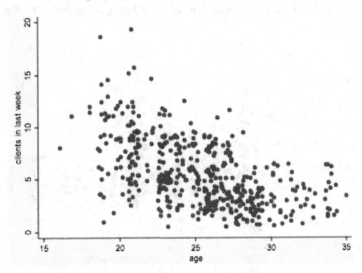

Figure 9. Twoway (scatter clients age if age < 40, jitter(5)) (lfit clients_in_last_week age if age < 40)

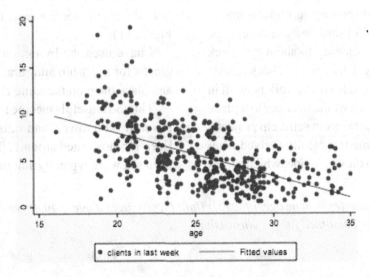

At this point, although I am continuing to show the Stata commands, you can take it that the graph was produced using the menu dialogue! (see Figure 10)

As you can see, the smoother (it's a fractional polynomial smoother) suggests that client numbers fall until late twenties, after which they level off at about three clients a week. Smoothers are lines which can inflect to fit complex shapes within the data. Some use the tactic of dividing the data up into segments and fitting a line to each segment,

with some clever manoeuvring to make sure that the lines join up. Fractional polynomials follow a different tactic, using a regression-based approach that makes use of all the data simultaneously, modelling the relationship using powers of the predictor variable. They were originally proposed by Royston and Altman, and introduced into Stata by Royston and Altman in the following year (Royston & Altman, 1995). They have now become part of 'official' Stata.

Figure 10. Twoway (scatter clients age, jitter(5)) (lfit clients_in_last_week age) (fpfit clients_in_last_week age) if age < 40, legend(order(1 "Clients in last week" 2 "Regression line" 3 "Smoothed fit"))

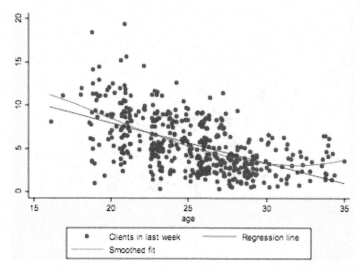

These results are encouraging. Older women– those between 25 and 35 – are seeing fewer clients, with typical numbers falling to about 5 a week at age 25 and 3 a week by age 30. This suggests that the income derived from sex work is small in older women, and that it would be easier to replace this income with income from self-help projects.

How much income is typically derived from sex work is shown in the next graph, which shows only the results for the rural town women. (see Figure 11)

I have used the by option to make separate graphs for township and rural town sex workers and place them on the same chart.

This too is useful - income from clients is much lower in rural towns, and falls slowly with age. Even for those aged around 20, weekly earnings form sex work typically amount to about 8 Euro,

Figure 11. Twoway (scatter income age, jitter(5)) (fpfit income age) if age < 40, legend(order(1 "Income (Euro) last week" 2 "Smoothed fit")) by(township)

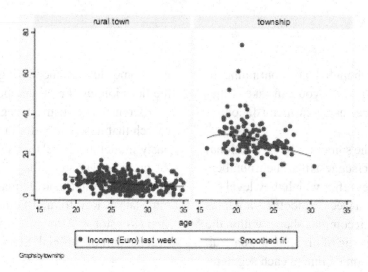

falling to about five euro at age 30. It's not a lot of money in European terms. Compared with the resources that have been spent on AIDS prevention by targeting sex workers, the amount of money that would have been needed to remove the necessity for sex work is small indeed.

On the other hand, income is considerably higher in the townships, where prices paid for sex are typically higher, though here, too, the income falls off with age. And it's more variable too. Note that I have, once again, used a fractional polynomial smoother. The very high variability in income among the younger township sex workers might have deflected a regression line quite significantly.

Social Stability

Another two key features which may influence our planning relate to the social stability of the sex workers - whether they have a regular partner, and whether they have children.

Among the 335 sex workers in rural towns, 60% live with a regular partner, 51% have some other job in addition to sex work (though many of these would have jobs in bars and hotels where sex work is implicitly part of the job) and 60%

have children. The profile of the township sex workers is slightly less settled-looking, with 48% living with a regular partner and 40% with another job, though 56% are supporting children.

By now a picture is emerging which suggests that tackling sex work with micro-economic aid in rural towns will be easier for a number of reasons: the women have fewer clients and, given that the cost of sex is also less, the total amount of money they will have to earn each week to allow them to move out of sex work is a lot less. They are also older, and more likely to be in a stable relationship and to have another source of income.

The Hazards of Sex Work

To be a sex worker is to find yourself without the protection of the law. My friend Julie, who earns a precarious living giving massages, is a former sex worker. Julie is a woman in her middle age. I suppose she won't mind me referring to her as a traditionally built African woman - we joke about it a lot. Julie lives in one of Nairobi's townships, and often has to travel long distances to clients' homes. Returning from a client whom she massages regularly - an elderly woman who seems to enjoy gossiping about politics at least as much

Table 6. By township, sort: ci lives_with_partner has_other_job any_children, bin

-> township = rural town					
				Binomial Exact	
Variable |	Obs	Mean	Std. Err.	[95% Conf.	Interval]
lives_with~r |	335	.6029851	.0267322	.5483768	.6557556
has_other_~b |	335	.5074627	.0273149	.4525732	.5622191
any_children |	335	.6089552	.0266614	.5544312	.6615348
-> township = township					
				Binomial Exact	
Variable |	Obs	Mean	Std. Err.	[95% Conf.	Interval]
lives_with~r |	139	.4820144	.042382	.3965342	.5682772
has_other_~b |	139	.3956835	.0414762	.3138276	.4820836
any_children |	139	.5611511	.0420911	.4745086	.6451316

as she enjoys Julie's massages - she was set upon by thieves who had evidently been waiting for her. They took everything: not just her money, little as it was, and her phone, and her shoes; they even broker her finger to force from it a ring of no great value that had been given to her many years before by her father. Then they beat and raped her, leaving her with broken bones and a cracked pelvis.

There was no point in calling the police. Sex worker or former sex worker, they don't care. One story I heard from another former sex worker still makes me shudder. She had a friend who had quit sex work and was living with her partner, expecting their first child, and working at a badly-paid but legitimate job. She was picked up by the police who recognised her from her sex worker days. There was no point in her protesting that she now had a 'proper' job. They beat her, kicking her pregnant belly repeatedly and taunting her that it would be better for the baby to die now than to be born to someone like her. 'Once a whore, always a whore!' they yelled when she tried to tell them she had a proper job. (The word they used was a lot more vulgar in Kiswahili.)

The police have a regular habit of picking up sex workers. The sex worker is held without charge at the police station where by day they are slave labour, cleaning and cooking for the police. At night one of the police may decide to take her home and rape her. After some weeks the woman is released without charge. Usually what happens

is that her friends or family find out where she is and pay the bribe. It costs something over €100 to have a sex worker released - a very significant sum of money in Kenya, as you can see from the typical weekly earnings of a sex worker. And yes, I've bribed the police to release a sex worker who was one of the data collectors for this study. Although I hate the idea of bribery, I know what happens to sex workers in police custody.

The survey contains data on some of the common hazards that the women face. We can use Stata's ci command to get rates and confidence intervals. (see Table 7)

The bin option tells Stata that the variables are binomial – they take on just two values: yes or no, 1 and 0. Stata has truncated the variable names, but we can see that 15% were arrested in the previous month, 14% had to bribe the police, 17% were beaten by a client, 35% raped by a client, 8% forced to have sex with a client who was clearly suffering from a sexually transmitted infection and that almost 70% had been treated for a sexually transmitted disease in the past six months.

One glance at Stata's documentation will show that there are a number of options for calculating confidence intervals for proportions. Extensive simulation work by Brown and Das-Gupta has resulted in the recommendation that you use Agresti-Coull confidence intervals for large sample sizes and either Jeffreys or Wilson methods for samples of 40 or less (Brown, Cai,

Table 7. ci arrested_in_last_month beaten_in_last_month raped_past_month infected_client treated_for_std, bin agresti

Variable		Obs	Mean	Std. Err.	Agresti-Coull	
					[95% Conf.	Interval]
arrested_i~h		474	.1455696	.0161989	.116543	.180295
beaten_in_~h		474	.1687764	.0172038	.1376464	.2052319
raped_past~h		474	.350211	.021911	.3086096	.3942207
infected_c~t		474	.0843882	.0127675	.062364	.1130947
treated_fo~d		474	.685654	.0213239	.6424824	.7258406

& DasGupta, 2001). But the choice of method is going to alter only the finer detail. The headline figure are what are shocking. What matter if the real monthly incidence of being beaten is 11% or 20%? Even our lowest estimate of the incidence is unacceptable.

While ci gives confidence intervals which are useful for constructing a table in a paper, the ciplot command, written by Nick Cox, is more useful for displaying them. As always, if you haven't installed ciplot, you can download it from the ssc archive. (see Figure 12)

Sex workers in Kenya have lives that are characterised by danger and exploitation, for less money each week than the cost of a Pizza in Ireland.

The Ethics of Research

Research into sex work in Africa has been largely driven by the agenda set out at the start of this chapter: sex workers spread AIDS. Sex workers are endlessly asked if they have been tested for HIV, if they use condoms, if they would continue working if they were HIV positive. On and on. The

first effect of this intense interest in sex workers was to drive and fund a vast research agenda. The thousand-plus papers that have appeared since since 1986 are the tip of an iceberg. How many researchers have drawn their salaries from this industry? How many have ridden the escalator of promotion up to professorships on the backs of the women they researched?

I was approached some years ago by a researcher who wanted me to help analyse some data. The paper was going to be called "Women selling sex in Kenya: would knowing their HIV status change their behavioural intentions?". The questionnaire is shown Table 8.

My heart sank. It ticks all the boxes for state-of-the-art sex work research. Clients per month? Check. HIV status? Check. Sex if HIV positive? Check. Reducing women to the status of reservoirs of infection, like public toilets or open wounds. Notice that the researcher doesn't seem to care why women might have started in sex work, or might have to continue even if they were sick. The participants were never asked about money, hardship, beatings, having children to support, being excluded from other jobs, being an immi-

Figure 12. ciplot arrested_in_last_month bribed_police beaten_in_last_month raped_past_month infected_client treated_for_std, binwil horizontal title("Exposure to occupational hazard") xtitle(Proportion (Confidence Interval))

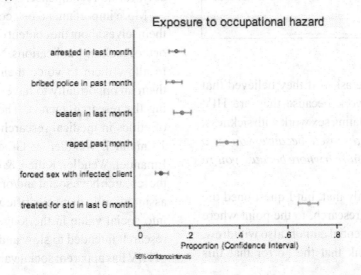

Table 8.

1) Age __
2) Place of work _____
a) How many clients do you see per month? ___
3) Do you know your HIV status? []
a) If yes, are you HIV positive? []
b) If no, are you interested in finding out? []
4) If you were found to be HIV+, would you continue to see clients? []
a) If yes, would it be more clients? []
b) Less clients []
c) Would you use condoms all the time? []
5) If you were very sick, would you continue to see clients?5 []
a) If yes, would it be more clients? []
b) Less clients? []
c) Would you use condoms all the time? []
6) Do you believe that women enter sex work for any of the following reasons?
a) They are widowed? []
b) They are HIV+? []
c) They are sick? []
7) Do you take breaks from sex work? []
a) If yes, how many per year? ___
b) For how long each break? ___
c) For what reason? _____

grant. But they were asked if they believed that women enter sex work because they are HIV positive, or sick. Equating sex work with sickness, explicitly. *"You're diseased because you're a whore"* becomes *"You're a whore because you're diseased"*.

I refused. Not only that, but I questioned the ethical value of the research, to the point where most of the other potential authors also withdrew. I would like to think that the horror that this

questionnaire evoked had a lasting effect on the researcher. Certainly, no paper was ever published.

It's not that this chapter was unusual either. It is part of a massive publishing enterprise – an industry that has sprung up around sex work intervention programmes has kept hundreds of academics employed, attracted large sums of money in funding and boosted the careers of many people, who are, almost without exception, white, men living in rich countries. But this research agenda has had the opposite effect on the sex workers themselves, driving them deeper into stigmatisation and social exclusion, making their lives more dangerous, making them invisible as people who are daily raped, beaten and ostracised.

The research itself has been published in publications that are inaccessible to the sex workers, written in a language that is stilted and formalised, available in journals that require the reader to pay to read the content; one of the articles cited in this chapter is available online at the staggering cost of US$37.50 plus tax – and ironically, it's an ethics paper (Shivas, 2004); Relate this to the weekly income of a sex worker, shown in the graph earlier. At current rates of about US$2.50 per sex act (Ferguson & Morris, 2007), a sex worker would have to have 15 men ejaculate in her to earn the right access to one journal article, to which they have contributed their data, probably, for no recompense.

More important, no one consulted the women themselves about the content of either the research or the resulting publications. No-one saw the need to allow them to voice their concerns, to give them an opportunity to have an input into defining the research agenda. The primary principle of ethics in medical research is that of value (E J Emanuel, Wendler, & Grady, 2000; Ezekiel J Emanuel, Wendler, Killen, & Grady, 2004) – that the research have social and/or scientific value (the assumption is that scientific value will translate into social value in the longer term). Certainly, research intended to slow and reverse the spread of HIV has apparent social value. However, when this research is justified by predictions made on the basis of the findings a single study – findings at odds with other research in the area – the research is in breach of the second principle: that of scientific validity.

Justice and Exploitation

The main criticism of the research, though, rests with the unequal distribution of risks and benefits. Exploitation occurs when one person in a relationship receives an unequally small share of the benefits or an unequally large burden of the risk (Ezekiel J Emanuel, et al., 2004). Guidelines for research in developing countries stress the need to minimise the risk of exploitation (Anonymous (Participants in the 2001 Conference on Ethical Aspects of Research in Developing Countries), 2002). For this reason, Emanuel and his colleagues place the requirement for collaborative partnership above all other ethical principles when planning multinational clinical research (Ezekiel J Emanuel, et al., 2004). By this they mean that the researcher has a moral responsibility to develop partnerships with the community, and to share with them the responsibility for identifying the important health problems and assessing the value of the proposed research. Researchers should ensure that recruited participants and communities benefit from the conduct and results of the research, and share the financial rewards equally.

This is one of the core principles of research ethics – justice: a fair distribution of the risks and benefits of the research. And it is this principle which is flagrantly violated by sex work research in Africa. The benefits go to those whose careers are founded on the study of sex workers, while the sex workers themselves who participate in the studies have their needs ignored. It's not so far from the casual enslavement of sex workers practised by the police. Indeed, one long term study of sex workers offers free health care to the sex workers and their children so long as they remain in the study. Since many are HIV positive, they are essentially entrapped into prostitution, unable to quit sex work and lose their free health care. This, as Andanda points out, invalidates informed consent and can amount to coercion to participate (Andanda, 2009).

Vulnerability

One of the important ethical principles here is that of respect for vulnerable individuals. To be vulnerable means to face a significant probability of incurring an identifiable harm while substantially lacking ability and/or means to protect oneself (Schroeder & Gefenas, 2009). Importantly, "vulnerability cannot be defined independent of [...] the relationships, power dynamics, and social and political circumstances of the particular protocol" (Shivas, 2004). That is, it is the relationships involved in the research and the social and political implications of the research which determine vulnerability. I am not suggesting that vulnerable groups should not be researched – quite the opposite. Vulnerable groups can potentially suffer by failure to research them, making their problems and the potential solutions to these problems invisible (Denny & Grady, 2007). I would argue that we have an especial duty of care to vulnerable groups, who are powerless to bring about the social change which would benefit them. This duty is to hear them, to be their voices. But to do that, we need to know what needs to be said. Good research starts with listening, as Emanuel and his colleagues point out (Ezekiel J Emanuel, et al., 2004).

There is a Buddhist story, told by Thich Nhat Hanh, which I always quote. A monk heard a fisherman praying before an ornate statue of a god decorated with jewels. "Please, dear God," the fisherman prayed, "hear the prayer which I make again today as I have made it every day for twenty years: let me be able to buy a boat, so that my sons may have a livelihood provided for them when I die." At this, the monk reached out and removed a jewel from the statue. "Your prayer is answered," he said, giving it to the fisherman.

The priests of the temple were angry. "Why did you take the jewel from the statue?" they asked. The monk replied "The God had heard the fisherman's prayer long ago. But he had no hands to grant his wish, so he used my hands."

A HAPPY END?

This story does not have a happy end, as yet. ICROSS helps start group projects. Some are simple, like the chickens. Others simpler still – one woman just needed money to buy a small charcoal stove, a couple of bags of fuel and some maize. She now sells roasted maize at a street corner. And one group wanders the beaches at a tourist resort. They will take top quality family photos with digital cameras, and email them to you so that they will arrive before you get home that evening. They have re-invested in better cameras and computers, and are one of the most cheering success stories.

But in the meantime, the research empire that branded these women as the spreaders of disease earns and spends large sums of money. And who has the research benefited? Clue: they are mostly white, almost all men. And no; they would never sleep with a prostitute.

A Note on Language

The language of science is nice clean stuff. You say *males* and *females*, not *men* and *women*, and you say *participants* (or, worse, *subjects*) not *people*. And you never say whore unless you're an anthropologist. The language of Stata is even cleaner still. It seems to be all about data manipulation, statistical inference and other activities that are value-free. But all of these languages are ways of talking about the same thing – the women (and men) whose lives we are supposed to be making better. And, as I hope to have shown, there is an essential link between the research agenda and

all of these languages. The items that appear on surveys, the statistical procedures we chose, the way we write up our results are all a function of a social agenda. And, in the case of sex work, it is a social agenda of which I am deeply ashamed.

I wanted to present the language of Stata, of Science, of Stigma all together, as all part of the same enterprise. I wanted to show that data analysis does not occur on a different planet to police rape. And a data analyst can't keep his or her hands clean.

REFERENCES

Andanda, P. (2009). Vulnerability: sex workers in Nairobi's Majengo slum. *Cambridge quarterly of healthcare ethics: CQ: the international journal of healthcare ethics committees, 18*(2), 138-146.

Anonymous,. (1997). *Confronting AIDS: Public priorities in a global epidemic: World Bank.* Oxford: University Press.

Anonymous. (Participants in the 2001 Conference on Ethical Aspects of Research in Developing Countries). (2002). Ethics. Fair benefits for research in developing countries. *Science, 298*(5601), 2133-2134.

Brown, L., Cai, T., & DasGupta, A. (2001). Interval estimation for a binomial proportion. *Statistical Science, 16*(2), 101–117. doi:10.1214/ss/1009213286

Conroy, R. M. (2002). Choosing an appropriate real-life measure of effect-size: the case of a continuous predictor and a binary outcome. *The Stata Journal, 2*(3), 290–295.

Denny, C. C., & Grady, C. (2007). Clinical research with economically disadvantaged populations. *Journal of Medical Ethics, 33*(7), 382–385. doi:10.1136/jme.2006.017681

Elmore-Meegan, M., Conroy, R. M., & Agala, C. B. (2004). Sex workers in Kenya, numbers of clients and associated risks: an exploratory survey. *Reproductive Health Matters, 12*(23), 50–57. doi:10.1016/S0968-8080(04)23125-1

Emanuel, E. J., Wendler, D., & Grady, C. (2000). What makes clinical research ethical? *Journal of the American Medical Association, 283*(20), 2701–2711. doi:10.1001/jama.283.20.2701

Emanuel, E. J., Wendler, D., Killen, J., & Grady, C. (2004). What makes clinical research in developing countries ethical? The benchmarks of ethical research. *The Journal of Infectious Diseases, 189*(5), 930–937. doi:10.1086/381709

Ferguson, A. G., & Morris, C. N. (2007). Mapping transactional sex on the Northern Corridor highway in Kenya. *Health & Place, 13*(2), 504–519. doi:10.1016/j.healthplace.2006.05.009

Gathiqi, H. W., Bwayo, J., Karuga, P. M., Kihara, A. N., Omari, M. A., & Plummer, F. A. *The socioeconomic status of prostitutes at a truck drivers' stop and their interaction with male clients.* Paper presented at the Int Conf AIDS. 1993 Jun 6-11;9(2):830 (abstract no. PO-D09-3672).

Hawken, M. P., Melis, R. D., Ngombo, D. T., Mandaliya, K., Ng'ang'a, L. W., & Price, J. (2002). Part time female sex workers in a suburban community in Kenya: a vulnerable hidden population. *Sexually Transmitted Infections, 78*(4), 271–273. doi:10.1136/sti.78.4.271

Kreiss, J. K., Koech, D., Plummer, F. A., Holmes, K. K., Lightfoote, M., & Piot, P. (1986). AIDS virus infection in Nairobi prostitutes. Spread of the epidemic to East Africa. *The New England Journal of Medicine, 314*(7), 414–418. doi:10.1056/NEJM198602133140704

Pickering, H., Okongo, M., Nnalusiba, B., Bwanika, K., & Whitworth, J. Sexual networks in Uganda: casual and commercial sex in a trading town. *AIDS Care, 9*(2), 199–207. doi:10.1080/09540129750125217

Pickering, H., Quigley, M., Hayes, R. J., Todd, J., & Wilkins, A. Determinants of condom use in 24,000 prostitute/client contacts in The Gambia. *AIDS (London, England), 7*(8), 1093–1098. doi:10.1097/00002030-199308000-00011

Royston, P., & Altman, D. (1995). Using fractional polynomials to model curved regression relationships. *Stata Technical Bulletin, 4*(21).

Schroeder, D., & Gefenas, E. (2009). Vulnerability: too vague and too broad? *Cambridge quarterly of healthcare ethics: CQ: the international journal of healthcare ethics committees, 18*(2), 113-121.

Shivas, T. (2004). Contextualizing the vulnerability standard. *Am. J. Bioeth, 4*(3), 84-86; discussion W32.

Wilson, D., Chiroro, P., Lavelle, S., & Mutero, C. (1989). Sex worker, client sex behaviour and condom use in Harare, Zimbabwe. *AIDS Care, 1*(3), 269–280. doi:10.1080/09540128908253032

Chapter 16
Medical Humanities

P. Ravi Shankar
KIST Medical College, Nepal

ABSTRACT

Medical Humanities (MH) provide a contrasting perspective of the arts to the 'science' of medicine. A definition of MH agreed upon by all workers is lacking. There are a number of advantages of teaching MH to medical students. MH programs are common in medical schools in developed nations. In developing nations these are not common and in the chapter the author describes programs in Brazil, Turkey, Argentina and Nepal. The relationship between medical ethics and MH is the subject of debate. Medical ethics teaching appears to be commoner compared to MH in medical schools. MH programs are not common in Asia and there are many challenges to MH teaching. Patient and illness narratives are become commoner in medical education. The author has conducted MH programs in two Nepalese medical schools and shares his experiences.

INTRODUCTION

Science is at the heart of modern medicine. The technique of scientific experimentation and subjecting treatments to modern scientific enquiry has resulted in significant advances in modern medicine. The shortcomings of a medical culture dominated by scientific, technical and managerial approaches however, were recognized in the 1960s and 1970s (Greaves & Evans, 2000). This lead to an increased focus on the 'human' side of medicine and on subjects traditionally considered as the humanities. In the United States (US) and the United Kingdom (UK) medical sociology, social history of medicine and medical ethics emerged as academically respectable disciplines.

At the end of this chapter the reader will:

a. gain a broad idea of what are the Medical Humanities (MH)
b. understand the advantages of teaching MH to medical students

DOI: 10.4018/978-1-60960-097-6.ch016

c.   be introduced to a selection of MH programs in developed countries

d.   know about MH programs in developing nations

e.   explore connections between medical ethics and MH

f.   gain an overview of MH in the Asian context

g.   know about the author's experiences with MH modules and

h.   be familiar with possible challenges and future directions for MH in developing nations.

WHAT ARE THE MEDICAL HUMANITIES?

Workers do not agree about what constitutes the Medical Humanities (MH). Dr. Kirklin from London, England, an international expert in MH defines it as 'an interdisciplinary, and increasingly international endeavor that draws on the creative and intellectual strengths of diverse disciplines, including literature, art, creative writing, drama, film, music, philosophy, ethical decision making, anthropology and history in pursuit of medical educational goals' (Kirklin, 2003). MH has the objective of helping learners to be good physicians. Another definition states MH as the application of the techniques of reporting, interpreting and theorizing developed by traditional humanities fields to phenomena within the traditional medical field (Evans, 2002). The humanities include subjects like history, literature, philosophy, ethics, anthropology, sociology, theology, psychology and others which explore the world as it appears from the point of view of frail, flesh-bound, human experience (Evans, 2002). MH are just those same subjects/studies concerned with the specific experiences of health, disease, illness, medicine and health care, the practitioner–patient relationship and, above all, the clinical consultation as an arena for human experiences (Arnott et al., 2001).

MH involves the human experiences of medicine seen through the humanities and reflected philosophically (Evans, 2002). An author states that the debate should be less about which disciplines to include and be more about the human experience of medicine (Coulehan, Belling, Williams, McCrary & Vetrano, 2003). Recently experts in the field of MH have tried to arrive at a pedagogical definition (Shapiro, Coulehan, Wear & Montello, 2009). According to these authors, MH teaching activities share several characteristics. They use methods from various humanities disciplines to investigate various aspects of medicine and healthcare practice. Health profession students are taught to better understand and critically reflect on their professions. It is intended that they become more self-aware and humane practitioners. The activities are interdisciplinary. An editorial states that MH does not fit into the traditional boundaries of disciplines and subjects but is a perspective whose concern is what it means to be 'fully human' (Greaves & Evans, 2000). MH supports the exploration of the human side of medicine and encompasses the intersection of the arts and medicine (Hooker, 2008).

WHY TEACH MEDICAL HUMANITIES TO MEDICAL STUDENTS?

MH can have both instrumental and non-instrumental functions in a medical school (Hooker, 2008). Instrumental functions are those which have a direct bearing on the daily work of doctors while non-instrumental functions lead to general education, personal development and new methods of thinking (Macnaughton, 2000), (Skelton, 2000). Nearly two decades ago, Professor Downie had suggested four types of connection between literature and medicine (Downie, 1991). One type benefits literature, the second provides entertainment and relaxation, the third provides insight into the standing of professions in the public perception and the fourth provides glimpses of 'whole person understanding' and is directly beneficial to the practice of medicine. 'Whole person understanding' requires a knowledge of the patient's (person's) personal biography beyond what is usually obtained during traditional history taking and some imaginative sympathy/empathy with that biography.

The arts, especially literature may provide insights into common shared human experiences, individual differences and the uniqueness of each human being and can enrich language and thought (Scott, 2000). Literature may serve to introduce students to problematic, unfamiliar life situations (Macnaughton, 2000). Drama can teach students to communicate well orally while philosophy can teach them the skills of analysis and argument. Literature can serve as a source of case histories for students. Painting can bring out the different non-verbal ways in which feelings or attitudes can be expressed. History of medicine emphasizes the transient nature of most medical knowledge and underlines the importance of staying up to date (Macnaughton, 2000). Sir William Osler, a pivotal figure in modern medicine is largely responsible for medical education within a university environment, strong roots in basic science, application of scientific methods to clinical medicine, emphasis on bedside learning, involvement of students in hospital routines, and the residency system after medical graduation (O' Rourke MF, 1999). The author states that personal encounters with patients, relatives, students and colleagues are precious. To enrich these encounters, we need the wisdom which comes not from knowledge alone, but from a breadth of educated experience, and from humility. "Evidence-based medicine" is being thrust upon us, with emphasis on large clinical trials, often cleverly designed, and supported by commercial interests. Results of individual trials are often considered more important than reason and logic as applied to individual patients. This may not be a welcome development. Sir Robert Hutchison, another important figure in modern medicine also stressed the importance of wisdom.

Knowing the limits of one's knowledge and where he/she or the patient can obtain more information is important in modern medical practice (Shankar, 2010).

Plays, poems and novels demand an emotional response from readers who obtain an opportunity to understand and challenge their biases and prejudices. The humanities may allow medical students to meet and interact with students and teachers from other disciplines and help build a 'better' relationship with the outside world. Stories have been used traditionally to bring home and reinforce among readers a 'moral' (Evans, 2001). The novelist or poet can stimulate the imagination of readers by suggesting new possibilities or understandings beyond those met with in daily life. Literature can expand on the limited scenarios encountered in day to day life. It is very difficult for doctors and healthcare professionals to understand what the patient is going through. A study of literature and art may help in the process of this identification and understanding.

MH teachers can employ literature to stimulate the practice of reflection among students (Evans, 2001). Character ethics and virtues can be analyzed and taught according to the authors of a recent paper (Bryan & Babelay, 2009). They propose a four step method of reflective practice including the details of a situation, the relevant virtues and values, ethical frameworks and the range of acceptable course of action. MH can help and support ethics teaching in medical schools, by promoting reflective thinking. An artistic or intellectual passion can provide doctors with a new focus for appreciating and recharging their daily work (Peterkin, 2008). Creativity encouraged by the humanities allows new ways to solve clinical problems and deal with uncertainty in clinical practice. Illness changes the way patients relate to their daily life and they struggle to find meaning. Patients expect help from their doctors and healers in their adjustment effort. Images, music and poems may help in finding the way (Peterkin, 2008). Medical biography offers physicians clues about how others have responded to tough intellectual or circumstantial challenges (Hooker, 2008). Medical biography details the human side of practitioners and can play an important role in humanizing medical practice. This is only a brief outline of the many ways in which MH can help in the education of doctors.

Medical Humanities Programs in Developed Nations

MH programs are common in United States (US), United Kingdom (UK), Canada, various European countries and Australia and New Zealand. Table 1 shows selected MH programs in developed nations. MH has been taught at the University of Rochester School of Medicine and Dentistry

in the US since 1987 (Spike, 2003). A ten week course titled 'The patient, the physician, and society' was conducted for students at that time. In 1991, the course was divided into two eight week courses titled 'Ethics and law in medicine' and 'The medical humanities seminars'. In 1998, the University adopted the 'double helix' curriculum which intertwines basic sciences and clinical medicine over all four years of medical school. A concentration in clinical ethics and humanities was approved.

At the Northeastern Ohio Universities College of Medicine in the US 'The human values in medicine' program was started in the 1970s (Wear, 2003). The required curriculum is 120 hours. Examples of topics discussed are 'Culture and medicine', 'On professionalism', 'History of

Table 1. Selected Medical Humanities programs in medical schools in developed nations

Medical school	Country	Brief description
University of Oslo Faculty of Medicine (Frich & Fugelli, 2003)	Norway	Literature, visual arts, architecture and music are used to explore MH
University of Rochester School of Medicine and Dentistry	United States	Two 8 week courses: 'Ethics and law in medicine', 'The medical humanities seminars'. MH concentration created
Dalhousie University Faculty of Medicine (Murray, 2003)	Canada	Broad concept of MH. Multiple approaches to humanities. Retreats, writing contests
Northeastern Ohio Universities College of Medicine	United States	'The human values in medicine' program. Various topics like culture and medicine, literature and medicine explored.
Stony Brook University School of Medicine (Coulehan et al., 2003)	United States	Medicine in contemporary society. Publishes 'Contexts' a quarterly newsletter.
Royal Free and University College Medical School	United Kingdom	Centre for medical humanities. Professional development spine, a course for medical students
University of California, Irvine College of Medicine	United States	Started with a literature and medicine elective. Poetry, prose, visual and performing arts, independent research projects.
University of Sydney (Gordon & Finkelstein, 2003)	Australia	Elective studies. Masters program in MH
Hamburg University Faculty of Medicine (Sammet, 2003)	Germany	Lectures on history of medicine since 1919. Institute for the history and ethics of medicine established. Syllabus constructed in 2003 for a MH course
Faculty of Medicine of the Technion-Israel Institute of Technology (Ber & Bar-et, 2003)	Israel	Elective on psychosocial aspects of medicine in 1970s. In 1994 elective in literature and medicine.
Weill Cornell Medical College (del Pozo & Fins, 2005)	Qatar	Readings in literature and philosophy. Focuses on nature and biology, the patient, the physician, the family, the hospital among others
Lund University (Wachtler, Lundin & Troein, 2006)	Sweden	Elective courses to medical and humanities students. Independent study projects

medicine', 'The physician as writer' and 'Literature and medicine' among others. Seminars are offered over lunch or during evenings. At the Stony Brook University School of Medicine the Institute for Medicine in Contemporary Society was started around 1990 to nurture interdisciplinary projects exploring relationships between medicine and other dimensions of contemporary culture (Coulehan et al., 2003). The institute publishes 'Contexts' a quarterly news letter which serves as a forum for MH. In the UK, the Centre for Medical Humanities is based within the Royal Free and University College Medical School (Kirklin, 2003). The centre aims to increase awareness of MH, develop teaching resources, and build an educational program supported by sound educational principles and innovative research. At the University College London the first MH course was offered in 1998. An optional two week full time undergraduate course called 'Living with and dying from cancer' was offered to third year medical students. Since then many optional MH courses have been offered to students at this medical school.

At the University of California, Irvine College of Medicine in the US the program in MH started informally in 1997 (Shapiro & Rucker, 2003). The program uses poetry and prose, narrative ethics, visual and performing arts and independent research projects to explore MH. Small group, interdisciplinary teaching and faculty development is emphasized. Evaluation of the program indicated a positive response among learners and an increase in empathy. A center for Medical humanities and Ethics was started at the University of Texas Health Science Center at San Antonio in the US in 2002 (Jones & Verghese, 2003). The center has the ultimate goal of developing and implementing a longitudinal and integrated MH curriculum in the medical school. The center has created a curricular blueprint for each of the four years of medical school.

A recent survey looked at MH programs in Canadian medical schools (Kidd & Connor, 2008). They listed 14 medical schools with MH programs. The University of British Columbia has a mandatory course taught over the first two years of the curriculum. The Universities of Alberta and Saskatchewan both have required courses in MH. The University of Manitoba is the only Canadian School with a formal, non-elective MH program. Other Canadian medical schools are also running MH programs. In the US, various MH programs were briefly described in a special theme issue of the journal 'Academic Medicine' (Various, 2003). MH programs at the University of Arkansas, Stanford University, University of California, San Francisco, University of South Florida, Southern Illinois University, University of Illinois at Chicago, University of Michigan, University of Montana, University of Nebraska, Davidson College, the Brody School of Medicine, Drexel University College of Medicine and University of Virginia were described.

The Auckland School of Medicine in New Zealand has emphasized the psychosocial aspects of the doctor-patient relationship since its founding in the late 1960s. In 1995 an interfaculty committee was formed to oversee the design and implementation of teaching MH (Grant, 2003). The course was started as an elective and in 2000 was made compulsory for all students. Students are taught in small groups using active learning approaches. The teaching is spread through all years of the course.

A recent qualitative study notes problems with the program and states that the humanities are constructed, defined and used within a medical frame of reference. Humanities students do not have a place in the program according to the authors. The Florence Medical School in Italy promotes the disciplines of history of medicine, bioethics, psychology and hygienics in the training of physicians and these subjects are together called the medical humanities (Gensini, Conti, Lippi & Conti, 2005). A web-based MH curriculum has been developed at the Georgetown University Medical School in the US (Wellbery & Gooch,

2005). The curriculum comprises of eight units. Each unit is explored through interpretation of art, literature, dance and music along with reflective interviews and scholarly commentaries. An arts library and a teacher's guide are parts of the website. The author has only described a selection of MH programs in developed nations. Table 1 describes selected MH programs.

MH programs have been conducted in Taiwan which can be regarded as a developed Asian country. In 1997, MH was interwoven into different phases of the medical course at the National Taiwan University College of Medicine (Wang & Lue, 2003). Lectures on medical history, ethics in medical research and small group discussions on social medicine topics have been introduced. Two six-week courses on family, society and medicine and life and death have been introduced during the clerkship years of training. At the Taipei Medical University in Taiwan, a community oriented curriculum design for MH has been conducted (Tsai, 2008). The concept of 'doctor as a mediator in the changing relationship with patients' has been introduced in the medical curriculum. Willing students and teachers from different schools interact with communities in programs that advance their health autonomy. The curriculum has two stages with the first stage of study being conducted in the classroom and the second stage consisting of field practice.

Medical Humanities Programs in Developing Nations

The Brazilian Society of Family Medicine conducts courses to enable students to develop a patient centered approach and become more humane doctors. Opera has been used to teach MH in Sao Paulo, Brazil (Blasco, Moreto & Levites, 2005). Students attend opera performances and reflect on their experiences. The opera performances act as a catalyst to encourage students to explore the human dimensions of being a doctor. Table 2 summarizes selected MH programs in developing countries. At the Marmara Medical School in Turkey the 'Human in medicine' courses are part of the preclinical curriculum. The program was evaluated as moderate or above moderate by 60-80% of students (Gulpinar, Akman & User, 2009). The program provided a contrasting perspective of the arts and humanities to the biological perspective of medical education.

A voluntary MH module has been conducted for interested pre-clinical and clinical students and faculty members at the Manipal College of Medical Sciences (MCOMS), Pokhara, Nepal (Shankar, 2008; Shankar, 2009). The module is described in detail in the section on my experiences with the Medical Humanities.

At the KIST Medical College (KISTMC), a new medical school in Lalitpur, Nepal a MH

Table 2. Selected Medical Humanities programs in developing countries

Medical school	Country	Brief description
Sao Paulo	Brazil	Opera used to explore MH
Hacettepe University (Elcin et al., 2006)	Turkey	Good medical practice course. Student projects on MH.
Marmara Medical School	Turkey	Human in medicine. Part of the preclinical curriculum
La Plata University (Acuna, 2003)	Argentina	MH program started in 1970s. Medicine and literature, anthropology, history of medicine and medical kalology
Manipal College of Medical Sciences	Nepal	Humanities 101. Medicine and the arts, ethics and medicine and contemporary issues in medicine.
KIST Medical College	Nepal	Sparshanam. Case scenarios, brainstorming sessions, role plays, debates and student activities. Paintings widely used

module named 'Sparshanam' (touch in Sanskrit, an ancient language) is conducted for first year medical students for around 90 minutes every Wednesday morning. The module is described in detail in the section on my experiences with the Medical Humanities. Table 2 describes selected MH programs in developing countries.

Medical Ethics and Medical Humanities

Medical ethics deals with the ethical principles of medical practice. Medical ethics programs are common in medical schools in western nations and as we will later examine appear to be more common as compared to MH programs even in developing nations. Kopelman in an article had examined various similarities between medical ethics (bioethics) and MH and concluded the two could be regarded as one field of study (Kopelman, 1998). Six related framework features unite these two fields. Both work in a systematic manner on certain important problems of the human condition and use interdisciplinary approaches to unravel and learn about them. Both employ cases and practical reasoning to understand and solve problems. They employ problem solving methods and find morally justifiable solutions to problems. Both seek interdisciplinary and collaborative scholarship, service and/or teaching (Kopelman, 1998). Another author however, has stated that bioethics as taught in medical schools should not be considered as part of or substituted for MH within the curriculum (Friedman, 2002). The author states that MH has become a hand maiden to bioethics. Bioethics falls within the broader domain of MH but has gained more acceptance and respectability and has evolved into a discipline dominated by rules and scientific method of reasoning while MH uses a more humanistic approach. MH supports individual questioning and collective probing which motivates students to examine fundamental questions about medicine and their own place in the field. The range of benefits and experience gained by studying MH cannot be obtained by studying bioethics. Bioethics at present seems to be more accepted and respected as a scientific discipline. Some authorities had suggested that we should concentrate on bioethics instead of developing and implementing a program on MH in our medical school.

Ethics concerns itself with rules of behavior and standards for various situations. In our MH modules we have concentrated on many ethical dilemmas and problems also. We discussed the importance of maintaining the confidentiality of patient information, the ethical implications of the changing nature of the doctor-patient relationship, the issue of declaring a patient dead, euthanasia and with holding treatment from patients who are brain dead among others. The ethical debate on abortion was also considered. At the Michigan State University in the US, ethics teaching is organized within a series of modules which help students understand the ethical and professional challenges facing the medical profession (Andre, Brody, Fleck, Thomason & Tomlinson, 2003). Students understand these challenges and place them in perspective during their future career. Students cannot be good doctors without understanding the social forces shaping medicine. There is a close link between ethics and MH throughout the course. I personally think that a broader approach to ethics can be offered immersing ethical dilemmas, problems and standards of behavior within a MH course.

Bioethics Teaching In Medical Schools

Now let us briefly review bioethics teaching in medical schools. Traditional medical ethics has developed since the 1950s into bioethics (Al-Umran, Al-Shaikh, Al-Awary, Al-Rubaish & Al-Muhanna, 2006). The authors of a recent article state that bioethics teaching is lacking in most medical schools in developing countries. The study at King Faisal University College of

Medicine, Saudi Arabia confirmed inadequate formal instruction in medical ethics and recommended that bioethics should be taught in clinical settings and the medical curricula should include the Islamic code of medical ethics. Assessment of the impact of the module on knowledge, attitude and practice of medical students and long term impact on their professional life are required. A paper published in 1999 had examined medical ethics curricula in Asia (Miyasaka, Akabayashi, Kai & Ohi, 1999). The authors mailed the questionnaire to a total of 206 medical schools and 100 schools responded. Eighty-nine schools reported offering some teaching in medical ethics. The authors concluded that medical ethics courses were widespread in the study area but the programmes offered were diverse.

In Sri Lanka, a developing country in South Asia all medical schools offer a certain amount of teaching in bioethics but there is a shortage of trained teachers (Sumathipala, 2006). In 2004 in the US a survey found that 71 of the 123 schools surveyed had medical ethics covered in the curricula (Lehmann, Kasoff, Koch & Federman, 2004). At the Queensland University of Technology in Australia health ethics was taught as relational engagement to paramedical students (Milligan & Woodley, 2009). The students were invited to produce their own creative composition in response to a short vignette describing the plight of a fictional patient. Students enjoyed the task and the authors found this to be a powerful tool which challenged and sensitized students to the deeper human dimensions of their practice. In India, the Indian Council for Medical Research is the central body for coordinating, formulating and promoting biomedical research. The council offers training programs and is formulating a core curriculum for teaching bioethics in different medical schools in the country (Kumar, 2006). In Iran a medical ethics research center was established in 1993. Seminars and courses on medical ethics for different healthcare personnel have been conducted in different regions of the country (Larijani, Zahedi & Malek-Afzali, 2005). In Turkey, 18 of the 39 nursing schools incorporated an ethics course into undergraduate nursing education programs (Gorgulu & Dinc, 2007). Class discussions, lectures, case studies, dramatization and demonstration were the different learning methodologies used.

Medical Humanities in Asia

Asia is a huge continent with the largest number of medical schools and the maximum percentage of the world's population. Medical schools have been opened in the private sector in many Asian countries recently. MH has been taught using small group, interactive learning techniques in programs in developed nations (Shankar, 2008c). A safe, non-threatening environment and a more egalitarian student teacher relationship are required for the success of MH teaching. According to an author, Asian cultures have a stiff and formal student-teacher relationship with the teacher being perceived as a distant authority figure (Eng, 2000). With increasing adoption of problem-based learning methodologies the relationship is slowly becoming more informal even in Asia.

Literature and art used to explore various aspects of MH are mainly from a western perspective. These may be difficult to use in an Asian context. Also English and other colonial languages dominate as the language of instruction in Asian medical schools. Most students have been educated in English medium schools in many parts of the Asian continent. Asia is a huge continent however, and there may be regional differences. Most students use a different language at home and in conversing with their patients (Shankar & Piryani, 2009a). Most of the literature used in MH courses worldwide has been in English. Asian students due to linguistic and other factors may find it difficult to identify with literature excerpts written in English. The literature, art and medicine database (http://litmed.med.nyu.edu) is a good source of annotated literature and art excerpts. We have used the database as a resource for teaching material for our MH courses. There is a need to create a similar database of resources for various Asian countries.

Asia being a huge continent has a multiplicity of languages and diversity of cultures. So MH courses and resource materials have to be developed and individualized to particular settings. In the west the Universities have a number of faculties and disciplines under one roof or in close proximity. In many parts of Asia linkages between medical schools and liberal arts colleges are not common. There is a physical distance between these facilities and an even greater mental distance. Medical schools are reluctant to accept the involvement of liberal arts faculty in teaching their students and liberal arts faculties may not be comfortable with such a role. Also many Asian medical schools have not developed the concept of a core curriculum and elective areas of study. New material is periodically added to the course but old and obsolete material is rarely deleted. This makes the curriculum and course material large and unwieldy. The huge amount of information to be mastered makes it difficult for students to find time and energy for learning MH. MH has been stated to be an interdisciplinary study and interdisciplinarity is essential for its contribution to knowledge and to teaching (Evans & Macnaughton, 2004). Collaboration across disciplines is not very common in a South Asian and maybe, an Asian context. This may have an adverse impact on development of MH. The author of the article (Evans & Macnaughton, 2004) warns about the risk of interdisciplinarity to the academic careers of those already recruited or those planning to join the field. This indicates that interdisciplinarity may not be a comfortable concept even in the west

In the west, strong administrative support for MH was and is present (Shankar, 2008c). A variety of subjects and methods were used to teach MH and learning is fun and interesting. The challenge for Asia is to develop the same degree

of administrative support and financial resources for developing MH.

Patient and Illness Narratives

The use of narratives including physicians' and patients' stories, literature and film is increasingly popular in medical education (Kumagai, 2008). The author of a recent article states that these efforts are often described as 'soft' and are placed at the margins or periphery of medical school curricula. An approach to patient-centered medical education and narrative medicine was initiated at the University of Michigan Medical School in the US in 2003. The approach involved home visits and conversations between medical students and patient volunteers and their families. The program aimed at fostering humanism in medicine. At the Harvard Medical School in the US an innovative longitudinal integrated clerkship was offered to medical students (Ogur & Hirsh, 2009). Students reported that the clerkship helped in creating a dynamic learning environment, helped them learn about the effects of illness on their patients' lives and connect more deeply with their patients. In Canada, an entire first year clinical skills program has been framed as an exercise in narrative construction and has been termed as 'narrative structuring' (Pullman, Bethune & Duke, 2005). Short essays on various materials presented in the course, written reports on ethical aspects of clinical case studies used and student journals were used for course evaluation.

A recent article describes narrative medicine as a patient-centered approach to the practice of medicine that rescues the patients' stories and integrates what is important into patient care and healthcare decisions (Pearson, McTigue & Tarpley, 2008). In an American medical school a narrative-based project was piloted among third year surgical clerkship students. Students produced a detailed narrative write up about a patient they had an opportunity to 'know'. Students opined that the experience was valuable and wanted narrative reflection to be used in medical education. The authors are planning a similar program for surgical residents. Patients are identified by their bodies while physicians' bodies are secondary to their minds according to two American workers (DasGupta & Charon, 2004). Doctors get little opportunity to deal with personal illness experiences or with illnesses in their loved ones. At the Columbia University in US, the 'personal illness narrative' offers students' opportunities to reflect on their own illness experiences and witness their colleagues' stories. The authors (DasGupta & Charon, 2004) state that narratives can lead to more empathic and self-aware practice of medicine.

At the Johns Hopkins University School of Medicine in the US Internal Medicine residents participated in a year long qualitative study about personal growth (Levine, Kern & Wright, 2008). They wrote narratives every 8 weeks and a final narrative at the end of the program. Writing promoted reflection and self-awareness. MH educators are frequently using narratives to teach and equip students for a meaningful and fulfilling relationship with their patients (DasGupta, 2007). Pediatric illness narratives have unique insights for physicians. These voices can help physicians adopt a medical practice which stresses not only diagnosis and treatment but also recognition and healing.

Biswas and colleagues had used medical student narratives for gaining a broader perspective of disease at the Manipal College of Medical Sciences, Pokhara, Nepal (Biswas, Dhakal, 2003). He had also used narratives at the Melaka-Manipal Medical College in Malaysia (Biswas et al., 2008)

MY EXPERIENCES WITH THE MEDICAL HUMANITIES

I first got interested in establishing a MH program at MCOMS, a Nepalese medical school as a curriculum innovation project while pursuing a fellowship in medical education offered by the

Foundation for the Advancement of International Medical Education and Research (FAIMER) (Shankar 2009a). The module concentrated on three core areas: medicine and the arts, ethics and medicine and contemporary issues in medicine. Critical analysis of literature and art, case scenarios and role plays were used to explore various aspects of MH. The sessions were held after regular class hours. The faculty participants acted as cofacilitators and added their experience and knowledge to the group deliberations and presentations (Shankar, 2008a). Detailed participant feedback was obtained about the module. Students and faculty enjoyed participating in the sessions (Shankar, 2009). They felt role plays were an enjoyable and effective learning modality. More literature and art from a South Asian context should be used according to participants. Sexual and reproductive issues were covered during the voluntary module. Sexual promiscuity, unprotected intercourse, teenage pregnancy, abortion, aphrodisiacs and enhancement of sexual performance and homosexuality were among the various topics covered (Shankar, 2008b). The article describes two scenarios dealing with sexual and reproductive issues covered during the module. The participants were of the opinion that sexual and reproductive issues are a grey area in the curriculum. The module was successful in sensitizing participants about certain of these issues and they felt the skills and knowledge acquired would be helpful in their future practice.

The module I facilitated at MCOMS was voluntary and the major challenge was to make learning interesting and fun and attracting and retaining participants (Shankar, 2008d). The sessions were held beyond the usual working hours; after dinner for students in the clinical years and during the lunch break for basic science students (Shankar, 2007). I had to be flexible to address participant requirements and at the same time fulfill the session and the module objectives. The sessions were conducted in small groups and were activity-based. In the evening sessions each group had both student and faculty participants.

The major challenges for me were to create case scenarios which were interesting and adequately explored the area under consideration. No formal assessments were held; assessments were formative and informal. The emphasis was on helping participants improve. A major challenge was finding literature and art excerpts for the module. The literature, art and medicine database maintained by New York University was especially useful. Certain literature excerpts were felt to be difficult. The excerpts were in English and described a western scenario and in certain cases participants found it difficult to identify with and relate to the excerpts. Among the literature and art excerpts used during the module were 'Tube feeding' by Richard Selzer, 'Uncle Curly's heart song' by Ron Moran, Cancer ward by Alexander Solzhenitsyn and photographs of the violent conflict in Nepal (Shankar, 2009). Four of the case scenarios used was also described in the article (Shankar, 2009). The stigma of homosexuality, the social stigma attributed to leprosy regarded as a course of God, the stigma of mental illness and neglect of mentally ill patients and compulsory rural service for all scholarship students were explored through role plays.

At KISTMC, a new medical school in Lalitpur district of the Kathmandu valley a module was conducted for faculty members and medical and dental officers. The sessions were conducted during Sunday afternoons and Dr. Piryani, an internal medicine specialist joined me as a co-facilitator (Shankar, 2009b). The basic approach followed was similar to that used in MCOMS. The faculty participants were uncomfortable with open discussion about issues of human sexuality and felt role-plays were childish (Shankar, 2009c). Based on the participant feedback changes were made to the module. Role-plays were reduced and group work and discussions were used to explore MH. Many literature excerpts were felt to be difficult by the participants.

The author and Dr. Piryani made a case for conducting MH programs for first year medical students. The management and especially the Principal, Prof. Dr. TP Thapa was supportive and the module was started in February 2009. The module is held every Wednesday morning from 8 am to 9.30 am. Case scenarios, brainstorming sessions, role plays, debates and student activities are widely used (Shankar & Piryani, 2009). Paintings were used throughout the module. Participants were asked to explore what they saw in the painting and what they felt, create and recite a song or poem about the painting, explore the issues depicted using role plays and create a short story of around 100 words about the painting. Informal feedback from the participants was positive. Literature excerpts were not used considering the experiences of the previous two modules. Considering the large student body other faculty members were involved as cofacilitators. Music and songs were a part of the session and an open space (Khula Manch) is provided where participants can share experiences, sing songs or recite stories and poems. In a recent article Shankar and Piryani have described three paintings and their associated activities in detail. The paintings were *Portrait of Dr Gachet* by Vincent van Gogh, *He can no longer at the age of 98* by Francisco Goya and *The glass of absinthe* by Edgar Degas (Shankar & Piryani, 2009). Students did not feel that the "western" paintings were out of place and not relevant in a Nepalese context.

CHALLENGES FOR MEDICAL HUMANITIES IN DEVELOPING COUNTRIES

In many developing countries MH is not a part of the medical curriculum. A strong case must be made for including MH in the curriculum. MH programs I feel can be started as an elective and after obtaining feedback and opinion from both students and faculty can be considered as a part of the curriculum later. A challenge will be developing linkages with liberal arts institutions and creating literature and art excerpts for MH from a regional context.

Most developing countries have a rich tradition of music and oral story telling which can be exploited for MH teaching and learning. The language of MH teaching may also require careful consideration. In most countries the medium of medical instruction is English. Many developing nations have a multiplicity of languages. A mixture of languages can be used for MH learning. In South Asia students for the undergraduate medical (MBBS) course have to study the subjects of Physics, Chemistry and Biology during the last two years of school (Shankar, 2008e). In Japan, entry to medical school is open to all high school graduates (Tokuda, Hinohara & Fukui, 2008). The entrance examination for admission is however, traditionally based on the contents of Mathematics and the Sciences. Because of this only few humanities students gain admission to medical school. Students study liberal arts during the first two years of the six year undergraduate medical course. This may give Japanese students a wider perspective. Restricted exposure to the arts may make it difficult for medical students to identify with the finer aspects of literature and other humanities subjects. This may be an especial problem while teaching the philosophy of medicine. I had tried to introduce students to a certain amount of philosophy during the MH module at MCOMS. The participants were interested in certain of the sessions but found it difficult to appreciate other aspects. Also I am not well trained in philosophy to be able to explain complex topics and ideas to a young audience.

Another challenge would be finding time in the medical curriculum for one more 'subject' or area of study. The examinations are mainly based on factual recall and reproduction of textual information. To meet the requirements of the assessment system students mainly resort to rote learning and cramming. The heavy curriculum and the familiarity of students with a rote learning style makes it a challenge to introduce MH which

as already stated is best learned in a small group activity based learning style.

The core competencies which a medical graduate should possess and how these should be developed should also be spelled out in greater detail. Even in the west there have been only few studies which have categorically studied the effect of a MH course on empathy and other characteristics of students. An eight week literature and medicine elective significantly improved empathy and attitude towards MH among participants at the University of California Irvine College of Medicine in the US (Shapiro, Morrison & Boker, 2004). Lancaster analyzed a four week literature and medicines course and showed that students had gained empathy (Lancaster, Hart & Gardner, 2002). DasGupta and Charon conducted a six week seminar which required reflective writing by students about personal experience of illness. They found that on conclusion of the seminar students self-reported greater empathy for patients (DasGupta & Charon, 2004). These studies had looked at these characteristics a short time after the completion of the seminar or module. Studies on the persistence and further development of these characteristics are required. It is more difficult to measure characteristics like empathy and self-awareness compared to a specific skill or ability to perform a particular task. Convincing curriculum planners and administrators about the need and importance of MH in the curriculum may require objective and easily quantifiable measures of effectiveness. Table 3 looks at challenges for MH teaching in developing nations and suggests possible solutions.

SUMMARY

Modern medicine has been dominated by scientific, technical and managerial approaches. The shortcomings of this approach have been recognized and the strengths of disciplines like literature, art, creative writing, and philosophy

Table 3. Challenges for Medical humanities teaching in developing nations and possible solutions

Challenge	Possible solution/s
MH not recognized as an essential part of the medical curriculum	Create a case for inclusion. Elective modules in beginning to demonstrate advantages of MH.
Lack of linkage with liberal art institutions	Greater exchanges between various types of institutions. Creating a forum for MH involving people from various backgrounds
Lack of art and literature excerpts	Efforts directed towards creating these resources. Multidisciplinary collaboration. Creating of a database like the literature, art and medicine database.
Language of MH teaching.	English or other colonial languages common media of instruction. Not likely to be commonly used with patients. English has the advantage of greater amount of resources. Debate needed
Entry to medical school restricted to students from science background	In the west students from liberal arts background allowed to take up medicine. Entry to medical school can be opened to all high school graduates. Humanities subjects can also be considered in the entrance examination.
Finding time for one more 'subject' in the curriculum	Delineation of core curriculum and electives. Reduction of questions requiring factual recall of information. Removing obsolete and less important material from the curriculum.
Lack of objective evidence of effectiveness of MH courses	Few studies have looked at impact of MH on empathy and other characteristics. More difficult to study impact compared to other areas. More MH programs should be started as pilot projects and both short term and long term effectiveness studied.

among others in offering an alternative perspective have been accepted. A number of definitions have been used for MH by authors in different countries. MH can have both instrumental and non-instrumental functions in the education of medical students.

MH programs are common in developed nations. Most medical schools in the US offer a certain amount of teaching in the humanities. There are strong MH programs in the United Kingdom, Europe, Australia and New Zealand. The author has briefly described selected MH programs in this article. Among developing nations MH programs have been conducted in Brazil, Turkey, Argentina, Malaysia and MCOMS and KISTMC in Nepal.

Medical ethics (also termed as bioethics) seems to have gained more acceptance and respectability compared to MH. An author states that both MH and bioethics share a number of common characteristics while another commented that bioethics has gained dominance over MH. The author of the present manuscript had explored ethical issues during the various MH modules he had conducted.

Bioethics teaching is more common in medical schools compared to MH. The authors of a recent article however, state bioethics teaching is lacking in most medical schools in developing countries. The author has briefly described bioethics teaching in selected medical schools worldwide.

In Asia there are many hindering factors for starting and strengthening MH programs. These have been briefly described. The literature and art resources used in MH teaching are mainly from a western context. The multiplicity of languages also raises questions. Interdisciplinarity and collaboration between various departments both within and outside the medical school could be difficult.

Patient and illness narratives are being increasingly used in medical education. Selected initiatives are described. The author has also briefly described his experiences with MH modules at two Nepalese medical schools, MCOMS and KISTMC. In the vast majority of medical schools in developing countries MH is not a part of the curriculum. The author feels MH can be started as an elective program and later a case can be made for its inclusion in the curriculum.

CONCLUSION

MH programs are common in developed countries and preliminary evidence seems to suggest that MH has an important role to play in creating more humane doctors. Hard objective evidence however, is lacking and may be difficult to come by. MH programs are not common in developing nations. The author had shown that it is possible to conduct MH programs in a resource limited setting in a developing country. MH programs can be started as elective programs for interested students and a case made for their eventual inclusion in the curriculum.

REFERENCES

Acuna, L. E. (2003). Teaching humanities at the national University of La Plata, Argentina. *Academic Medicine*, *78*, 1024–1027. doi:10.1097/00001888-200310000-00017

Al-Umran, K. U., Al-Shaikh, B. A., Al-Awary, B. H., Al-Rubaish, A. M., & Al-Muhanna, F. A. (2006). Medical ethics and tomorrow's physicians: an aspect of coverage in the formal curriculum. *Medical Teacher*, *28*, 182–184. doi:10.1080/01421590500271365

Andre, J., Brody, H., Fleck, L., Thomason, C. L., & Tomlinson, T. (2003). Ethics, professionalism and humanities at Michigan state University College of human medicine. *Academic Medicine*, *78*, 968–972. doi:10.1097/00001888-200310000-00005

Arnott, R., Bolton, G., Evans, M., Finlay, I., Macnaughton, J., Meakin, R., & Reid, W. (2001). Proposal for an Academic Association for Medical Humanities. *Medical Humanities*, *27*, 104–105. doi:10.1136/mh.27.2.104

Ber, R., & Bar-et, Y. (2003). Faculty of medicine of the Technion-Israel Institute of Technology, humanities in medicine. *Academic Medicine*, *78*, 1071–1072. doi:10.1097/00001888-200310000-00044

Biswas, R., et al. (n.d.). Problem based self-directed life long participatory learning in medical educators and their audience: Reflective lessons learnt from a lecture series. In Patricia F. Geinare (Ed), *Trends in continuing education*. New York: Nova Science Publishers. Retrieved from https://www.novapublishers.com/catalog/product_info.php?products_id=7955

Biswas, R., Dhakal, B., et al. (2003). Medical student narratives for understanding disease and social order in the third world. *Eubios Journal of Asian and International Bioethics (Tokyo)*, *13*, 139-142. Retrieved on December 12, 2009 from http://www.eubios.info/EJ134/ej134h.htm

Blasco, P. G., Moreto, G., & Levites, M. R. (2005). Teaching humanities through opera: leading medical students to reflective attitudes. *Family Medicine*, *37*, 18–20.

Bryan, C. S., & Babelay, A. M. (2009). Building character: a model for reflective practice. *Academic Medicine*, *84*, 1283–1288. doi:10.1097/ACM.0b013e3181b6a79c

Coulehan, J., Belling, C., Williams, P. C., McCrary, S. V., & Vetrano, M. (2003). Human contexts: Medicine in society at Stony Brook University School of Medicine. *Academic Medicine*, *78*, 987–992. doi:10.1097/00001888-200310000-00009

DasGupta, S. (2007). Between stillness and story: lessons of children's illness narratives. *Pediatrics*, *119*, e1384–e1391. doi:10.1542/peds.2006-2619

DasGupta, S., & Charon, R. (2004). Personal illness narratives: using reflective writing to teach empathy. *Academic Medicine*, *79*, 351–356. doi:10.1097/00001888-200404000-00013 del Pozo, P. R., & Fins, J. J. (2005). The globalization of education in medical ethics and humanities: evolving pedagogy at Weill Cornell medical college in Qatar. *Academic Medicine, 80*, 135–140. doi:10.1097/00001888-200502000-00005

Downie, R. S. (1991). Literature and Medicine. *Journal of Medical Ethics, 17*, 93–96, 98. doi:10.1136/jme.17.2.93

Elcin, M., Odabasi, O., Ward, K., Turan, S., Akyiz, C., & Sayek, I. The first medical humanities programme in Turkey. *Medical Education, 40*, 278–282. doi:10.1111/j.1365-2929.2006.02390.x

Eng, K. H. (2000). Can Asians do PBL? *CDTL Brief, 3*, 3–4.

Evans, D. (2001). Imagination and medical education. *Medical Humanities, 27*, 30–34. doi:10.1136/mh.27.1.30

Evans, H. M., & Macnaughton, J. (2004). Should medical humanities be a multidisciplinary or an interdisciplinary study? *Medical Humanities, 30*, 1–4. doi:10.1136/jmh.2004.000143

Evans, M. (2002). Reflection on the humanities in medical education. *Medical Education, 36*, 508–513. doi:10.1046/j.1365-2923.2002.01225.x

Frich, J. C., & Fugelli, P. (2003). Medicine and the arts in the undergraduate medical curriculum at the University of Oslo Faculty of Medicine, Oslo, Norway. *Academic Medicine, 78*, 1036–1038. doi:10.1097/00001888-200310000-00020

Friedman, L. D. (2002). The precarious position of the medical humanities in the medical school curriculum. *Academic Medicine, 77*, 320–322. doi:10.1097/00001888-200204000-00011

Gensini, G. F., Conti, A., Lippi, D., & Conti, A. A. (2005). Full integration of teaching 'medical humanities' in the medical curriculum: the challenge of the Florence medical school. *Medical Principles and Practice, 14*, 64–65. doi:10.1159/000081928

Gordon, J., & Finkelstein, J. (2003). University of Sydney medical humanities program. *Academic Medicine, 78*, 1069–1070. doi:10.1097/00001888-200310000-00042

Gorgulu, R. S., & Dinc, L. (2007). Ethics in Turkish nursing education programs. *Nursing Ethics, 14*, 741–752. doi:10.1177/0969733007082114

Grant, V. J. (2003). University of Auckland faculty of medical and health sciences, medical humanities courses. *Academic Medicine, 78*, 1072–1073. doi:10.1097/00001888-200310000-00045

Greaves, D., & Evans, M. (2000). Medical Humanities. *Medical Humanities, 26*, 1–2. doi:10.1136/mh.26.1.1

Gulpinar, M. A., Akman, M., & User, I. (2009). A course, 'The Human in Medicine', as an example of a preclinical medical humanities program: A summary of 7 years. *Medical Teacher, 21*, 1–8. doi:10.1080/01421590802638014

Hooker, C. (2008). The medical humanities a brief introduction. *Australian Family Physician, 37*, 369–370.

Jones, T., & Verghese, A. (2003). On becoming a humanities curriculum: the center for medical humanities and ethics at the University of Texas health science center at San Antonio. *Academic Medicine, 78*, 1010–1014. doi:10.1097/00001888-200310000-00014

Kidd, M. G., & Connor, J. T. H. (2008). Striving to do good things: teaching humanities in Canadian medical schools. *The Journal of Medical Humanities, 29*, 45–54. doi:10.1007/s10912-007-9049-6

Kirklin, D. (2003). The Centre for Medical Humanities, Royal Free and University College Medical School, London, England. *Academic Medicine, 78*, 1048–1053. doi:10.1097/00001888-200310000-00023

Kopelman, L. M. (1998). Bioethics and humanities: what makes us one field? *The Journal of Medicine and Philosophy, 23*, 356–368. doi:10.1076/jmep.23.4.356.2576

Kumagai, A. K. (2008). A conceptual framework for the use of illness narratives in medical education. *Academic Medicine, 83*, 653–658. doi:10.1097/ACM.0b013e3181782e17

Kumar, N. K. (2006). Bioethics activities in India. *Eastern Mediterranean Health Journal, 12*(Supplement 1), S56–S65.

Lancaster, T., Hart, R., & Gardner, S. (2002). Literature and medicine: evaluating a special study module using the nominal group technique. *Medical Education, 36*, 1071–1076. doi:10.1046/j.1365-2923.2002.01325.x

Larijani, B., Zahedi, F., & Malek-Afzali, H. (2005). Medical ethics in the Islamic republic of Iran. *Eastern Mediterranean Health Journal, 11*, 1061–1072.

Lehmann, L. S., Kasoff, W. S., Koch, P., & Federman, D. D. (2004). A survey of medical ethics education at U.S. and Canadian medical schools. *Academic Medicine, 79*, 682–589. doi:10.1097/00001888-200407000-00015

Levine, R. B., Kern, D. E., & Wright, S. M. (2008). The impact of prompted narrative writing during internship on reflective practice: a qualitative study. *Advances in Health Sciences Education : Theory and Practice, 13*, 723–733. doi:10.1007/s10459-007-9079-x

Macnaughton, J. (2000). The humanities in medical education: context, outcomes and structures. *Medical Humanities, 26*, 23–30. doi:10.1136/mh.26.1.23

Milligan, E., & Woodley, E. (2009). Creative expressive encounters in health ethics education: teaching ethics as relational engagement. *Teaching and Learning in Medicine, 21*, 131–139. doi:10.1080/10401330902791248

Miyasaka, M., Akabayashi, A., Kai, I., & Ohi, G. (1999). An international survey of medical ethics curricula in Asia. *Journal of Medical Ethics, 25*, 514–521. doi:10.1136/jme.25.6.514

Murray, J. (2003). Development of a medical humanities program at Dalhousie University faculty of Medicine, Nova Scotia, Canada, 1992-2003. *Academic Medicine, 78*, 1020–1023. doi:10.1097/00001888-200310000-00016

O'Rourke, M. F. (1999). William Osler: a model for the 21st century? *The Medical Journal of Australia, 171*, 577–579.

Ogur, B., & Hirsh, D. (2009). Learning through longitudinal patient care-narratives from the Harvard Medical School-Cambridge Integrated Clerkship. *Academic Medicine, 84*, 844–850. doi:10.1097/ACM.0b013e3181a85793

Pearson, A. S., McTigue, M. P., & Tarpley, J. L. (2008). Narrative medicine in surgical education. *Journal of Surgical Education, 65*, 99–100. doi:10.1016/j.jsurg.2007.11.008

Peterkin, A. (2008). Medical humanities for what ails us. *Canadian Medical Association Journal, 178*, 648. doi:10.1503/cmaj.071851

Pullman, D., Bethune, C., & Duke, P. (2005). Narrative means to humanistic ends. *Teaching and Learning in Medicine, 17*, 279–284. doi:10.1207/s15328015tlm1703_14

Sammet, K. (2003). University hospital Hamburg-Eppendorf, University of Hamburg, Institute for the history and ethics of medicine. *Academic Medicine, 78*, 1070–1071. doi:10.1097/00001888-200310000-00043

Scott, P. A. (2000). The relationship between the arts and medicine. *Medical Humanities, 26*, 3–8. doi:10.1136/mh.26.1.3

Shankar, P. R. (2007). Conducting a voluntary module: personal experiences. *Journal of Medical Sciences Research, 2*, 55–58.

Shankar, P. R. (2008). A voluntary medical humanities module at the Manipal College of medical sciences, Pokhara, Nepal. *Family Medicine, 40*, 468–470.

Shankar, P. R. (2008a). Medical students and medical teachers learn together: preliminary experiences from Western Nepal. *South East Asian Journal of Medical Education, 2*, 79–82.

Shankar, P. R. (2008b). Using case scenarios and role plays to explore issues of human sexuality. *Education for Health (Abingdon), 20*.

Shankar, P. R. (2008c). Can medical humanities take root in Asia? *Journal of Clinical and Diagnostic Research,* JCDR (published online first 24 Feb 2008).

Shankar, P. R. (2008d). *Medical humanities: sowing the seeds in the Himalayan country of Nepal. Literature, arts and medicine blog.* Posted April 14th, 2008. Retrieved December 8, 2009, from http://medhum.med.nyu.edu/blog/?p=113

Shankar, P. R. (2009). A Voluntary Medical Humanities Module in a Medical College in Western Nepal: Participant feedback. *Teaching and Learning in Medicine, 21*, 248–253. doi:10.1080/10401330903020605

Shankar, P. R. (2009b). Creating and maintaining participant interest in the Medical Humanities. *Literature, art and medicine Blog Posted October 28th, 2009.* Retrieved December 8, 2009, from http://medhum.med.nyu.edu/blog/?p=215

Shankar, P. R. (2009c). Design the shoe according to the foot! *The Clinical Teacher, 6*, 67–68. doi:10.1111/j.1743-498X.2009.00269.x

Shankar, P. R. (2010). Sir Robert Hutchison's petition and the medical humanities. *International Journal of Medical Education, 1*, 2–4. doi:10.5116/ijme.4b8a.fba9

Shankar, P. R., & Piryani, R. M. (2009). Using paintings to explore the Medical Humanities in a Nepalese medical school. *Medical Humanities, 35*, 121–122. doi:10.1136/jmh.2009.002568

Shankar, P. R., & Piryani, R. M. (2009a). English as the language of Medical Humanities learning in Nepal: Our experiences. *The literature, art and medicine blog Posted on 22nd April 2009.* Retrieved December 8, 2009 from http://medhum.med.nyu.edu/blog/?p=175

Shankar, R. (2008e). *Arts and humanities: a neglected aspect of education in South Asia. BMJ Medical Humanities Blog posted on 17th July 2008.* Retrieved December 8, 2009, from http://blogs.bmj.com/medical-humanities/2008/07/17/arts-and-humanities-a-neglected-aspect-of-education-in-south-asia/

Shankar, R. (2009a). Establishing a medical humanities in Nepal with the help of a FAIMER fellowship. *BMJ Medical Humanities blog* posted 7th December 2009. Retrieved December 9, 2009, from http://blogs.bmj.com/medical-humanities/2009/12/07/establishing-a-medical-humanities-in-nepal-with-the-help-of-a-faimer-fellowship-by-ravi-shankar/

Shapiro, J., Coulehan, J., Wear, D., & Montello, M. (2009). Medical Humanities and Their Discontents: Definitions, Critiques, and Implications. *Academic Medicine, 84*, 192–198. doi:10.1097/ACM.0b013e3181938bca

Shapiro, J., Morrison, E. H., & Boker, J. R. (2004). Teaching empathy to first year medical students: Evaluation of an elective literature and medicine course. *Education for Health (Abingdon), 17*, 73–84. doi:10.1080/13576280310001656196

Shapiro, J., & Rucker, L. (2003). Can poetry make better doctors? Teaching the humanities and arts to medical students and residents at the University of California, Irvine, College of Medicine. *Academic Medicine, 78*, 953–957. doi:10.1097/00001888-200310000-00002

Skelton, J. R. (2000). Teaching literature and medicine to medical students, part I: The beginning. *Lancet, 356*, 1920–1922. doi:10.1016/S0140-6736(00)03270-0

Spike, J. P. (2003). Developing a medical humanities concentration in the medical curriculum at the University of Rochester School of medicine and dentistry, Rochester, New York. *Academic Medicine, 78*, 983–986. doi:10.1097/00001888-200310000-00008

Sumathipala, A. (2006). Bioethics in Sri Lanka. *Eastern Mediterranean Health Journal, 12*(1), S73–S79.

Tokuda, Y., Hinohara, S., & Fukui, T. (2008). Introducing a new medical school system into Japan. *Annals of the Academy of Medicine, Singapore, 37*, 800–802.

Tsai, D. J. (2008). Community-oriented curriculum design for medical humanities. *The Kaohsiung Journal of Medical Sciences, 24*, 373–379. doi:10.1016/S1607-551X(08)70135-9

Various authors. (2003). Special theme brief articles: United States. *Academic Medicine, 78*, 1059-68.

Wachtler, C., Lundin, S., & Troein, M. (2006). Humanities for medical students? A qualitative study of a medical humanities curriculum in a medical school program. *BMC Medical Education, 6*, 16. doi:10.1186/1472-6920-6-16

Wang, W. D., & Lue, B. H. (2003). National Taiwan University College of medicine: the design of medical humanities courses for clerkships. *Academic Medicine, 78*, 1073–1074. doi:10.1097/00001888-200310000-00046

Wear, D. (2003). The medical humanities at the northeastern Ohio Universities College of medicine: historical, theoretical, and curricular perspectives. *Academic Medicine, 78*, 997–1000. doi:10.1097/00001888-200310000-00011

Wellbery, C., & Gooch, R. (2005). A web-based multimedia medical humanities curriculum. *Family Medicine, 37*, 165–167.

ADDITIONAL READING

Ars Medica www.utpjournals.com/ars/ars.html

BMJ Group blogs: Medical Humanities http://blogs.bmj.com/medical-humanities/

BMJ Medical Humanities http://mh.bmj.com/

Cell2Soul blog www.cell2soul.typepad.com/

Cell2Soul www.cell2soul.org

Hektoen International A Journal of Medical Humanities www.hektoeninternational.org/

Humane medicine health care www.humane-healthcare.com/

Journal of Medical Humanities www.springer.com/humanities/journal/10912

Literature, art and medicine blog http://medhum.med.nyu.edu/blog/

Medical Humanities http://medhum.med.nyu.edu/links.html

The Pharos www.alphaomegaalpha.org/the_pharos.html

The Yale Journal for Humanities in Medicine www.med.yale.edu/intmed/hummed/yjhm/

UCL Medical Humanities resource database http://www.mhrd.ucl.ac.uk/

Section 2

Chapter 17
The User Driven Learning Environment

Rakesh Biswas
People's College of Medical Sciences, India

Joachim Sturmberg
Monash University and The University of Newcastle, Australia

Carmel M. Martin
Trinity College Dublin, Ireland

ABSTRACT

This chapter is an introduction to user driven learning that initially dwells on features that are unchanged such as the role of collaborative social interactions in human learning and certain aspects that are evolving and helping create a learning transformation through web based technologies. The chapter is interspersed with user driven learning narrative examples taken from the authors' own experience of sharing data over the web to accumulate learning points as well as the experience of a significant population of other web based learners in discussion forums, blogs and other networking sites. This is an attempt to create a background that may help illustrate the evolution of user driven health care, which is another form of user driven learning on the web with particular reference to individual user clinical problem solving, be it initiated by patients, health professionals or other actors in a care giving collaborative network across a web interface.

INTRODUCTION

"Do you think me a learned, well-read man?"
"Certainly," replied Zi-gong, "Aren't you?"
"Not at all," said Confucius.
"I have simply grasped one thread which links
     up the rest"

DOI: 10.4018/978-1-60960-097-6.ch017

(Recounted in Sima Qian (145-ca. 89 BC), "Confucius," in Hu Shi, The Development of Logical Methods in Ancient China, Shanghai: Oriental Book Company, 1922; quoted in Qian 1985:125, in Castells, M. (1996). *The Rise of the Network Society*, Oxford: Blackwell. (p1)

What drives us to learn? Is it our jest for reward in the form of feel good food for thought? We learn anything for these food for thought rewards and like animals in a circus seem to be constantly foraging for it. Learning is not confined to childhood or the classroom, but takes place throughout life and in a range of situations.

Mikael Wiberg in an extensive article on net learning has brought out interesting facets of learning in general. (Wiberg 2007) According to him, what it is to be knowledgeable can be defined either in terms of how much one person has read and learned in isolation, or how knowledgeable a particular person is about different threads to grasp in order to gain access to other peers in different social networks. The latter concept pinpoints the social dimension of learning processes, the social interaction setting, and goes back to a Socratic understanding of knowledge gaining through conversations and argumentations with others.

Traditional libraries that have been often considered temples of learning where silence is valued and protected but they are nothing but isolated learning environments where the single individual has no access to a second opinion from another person, no access to a complementary perspective, or external critique, neither does s/he have any chance to get complementary literature from anyone which might have a different reference library. Given this, there is not much social interaction in this kind of traditional learning environment. (Wiberg 2007)

In modern libraries it is perhaps easier to break past this 'silence' barrier where the library user predominantly browses an electronic information network rather than a paper based disconnected media.

Unfortunately, this advantage of the modern library is under utilized as even systems for online universities, or distance education may not have adequate support or encouragement for social interaction. Most of these systems assume a centralized communication model in which the learning peers (i.e. the students) mostly communicate with one central peer (i.e. a mentor or advisor). This leads in many cases to communication related to the structure rather than the content of an online education and does not support spontaneous, creative social learning processes. (Wiberg 2007)

Learning schools are redirecting the focus from what has been labeled "traditional computer-based learning environments" towards *user-driven learning networks* supported by social internet based applications. The assumption that computer-mediated learning will occur in the classroom, managed by a teacher, is now being challenged, not by schools and educational software developers, but by the consumer growth of personal technologies – [give some examples]. (Sharples 2002)

User driven learning is a form of conversational experiential learning between networked users in web space.

The experiential learning model suggests that learning requires individuals to resolve abilities that are polar opposites, and that the learner must continually choose which set of learning abilities he or she will use in a specific learning situation. In grasping experience some of us perceive new information through experiencing the concrete, tangible, felt qualities of the world, relying on our senses and immersing ourselves in concrete reality. Others tend to perceive, grasp, or take hold of new information through symbolic representation or abstract conceptualization–thinking about, analyzing, or systematically planning, rather than using sensation as a guide. Similarly, in transforming or processing experience some of us tend to carefully watch others who are involved in the experience and reflect on what happens, while others choose to jump right in and start doing things. (Baker 2002)

This chapter is mostly about illustrating how this model is active on web space and what are the lessons that we can grasp to improve it further.

Most of the other chapters would concern human centric user driven learning in health care and at the outset it may be necessary to illustrate this introduction to what essentially constitutes a user driven learning environment in topics other than human centric health care.

Illustrating User Driven Learning for Non Human Centric Human Activities

One of the important uses of user driven learning on the web is to get help on trying to identify an entity be it tangible in the form of an inanimate or animate object or abstract like trying to identify a diagnosis from one's symptoms.

The following query related to a plant in author RB's garden was posted to a google group centered on discussions related to Indian trees.

Query

We have noticed these leaf changes in our queen's crepe myrtle from a potted sapling since Jan 2008

These persist even today although the plant apparently continues to thrive otherwise in a separate location removed from its restrictive pot.

Would be grateful for your comments, suggestions regarding these peculiar changes and remedies.

Rb

Response 1
I notice a couple of leaves having a sort of crumpled appearance. It could be the larvae of some insect on the rear side of the leaves. Sometimes, the moths lay their eggs on the rear portion of the leaves and the larvae build some kind of cocoon around themselves. If that is the case, removing the cocoon should help.

Regards

Yp. kerala, India

Response 2
Hi Rb, Sometimes I've had an occasional deformed leaf, usually caused by either minor insect damage or drought stress as leaves are starting to expand. Again, I wouldn't worry about it at all. Enjoy the color of the new growth!

Regards--

Kg, Florida USA

Response 3
Thanks Kg.

Yes I guess this is a minor problem after all as long as they aren't failing to thrive.

Rb

Response 4
Thanks Yp.

I shall keep that in mind. Rb

Figure 1. Image Apr 18 2008

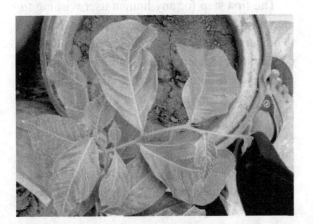

Figure 2. Image Jan 25 2009

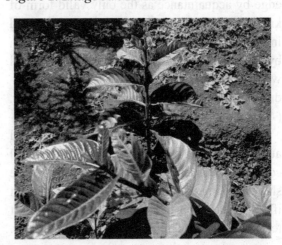

Interpreting Conversational Learning in Health Care

The above illustration of non human centric conversations around health care draws a parallel between what could very well have also been conversations centered around human health as often humans have queries particularly on symptoms that may be harbingers of future illnesses that could become chronic. The initial query posed by the author in the above illustration also demonstrates a possible concern for the mild leaf ill health becoming chronic. However his worries are put to rest by the group.

Learning is a cyclical process (Figure 1) of reflective observation on day-to-day concrete experiences followed by abstract conceptualization and active experimentation at either individual or group levels (Kolb 2000).

Concrete experience corresponds to "knowledge by acquaintance", i.e. direct practical experience (or "Apprehension" in Kolb's terms), as opposed to the *abstract conceptualization* of "knowledge about", i.e. theoretical and may be more comprehensive (or "Comprehension").

This distinction was first made by Aristotle, and has been discussed by epistemologists ever since.

Patients know their illness by direct acquaintance, whereas health professionals know that same illness only through comprehension. In the health care context many people regard knowledge by acquaintance as the only valid form of knowledge, and they distrust the "book-learned information". This is no better illustrated than by the most frequently asked question to social workers from parents: "Do you have any children?" Answer "no", and your credibility is shot. (Atherton 2009)

The objective of learning is geared toward attaining desirable outcomes, and experiential conversational learning helps us to attain these short and long term in a real world context, even if the outcome may be as small as attaining a short term piece of mind related to a clinical problem.

Effective learning involves constructing an understanding integrating new experiences to existing knowledge. (Sharples 2002)

USER DRIVEN APPROACH TO HUMAN TROUBLESHOOTING (CLINICAL PROBLEM SOLVING)

"The soul of medicine is easy to understand. You master the microcosm and the macrocosm and in the end let things happen as it pleases God."
Mephistopheles in Goethe's Faust

To a large extent, present day traditional approaches to medical problem solving is based on principles of troubleshooting where the "human hardware" is visualized as a collection of individual components, and as in hardware trouble shooting, one has to identify the "malfunctioning component" and then either do a component level repair or replace it (one may label this as reductionist but we have decided to ignore labels for now).

Understanding the "malfunctioning component" requires detailed knowledge of its anatomy and its position relative to its neighboring ones. The lack of such detailed knowledge of the anatomy is one of the major impediments for laypeople to understand their own health and disease, as they may not be able to get a visuospatial orientation of what is happening where without this basic understanding.

The first step for any human user wishing to gain a proper grasp of health systems would be to understand "system components" and their connections to each other. Web interfaces offer a multitude of sites displaying atlases of human anatomy that any user is free to browse. Never before, has the human body been so very freely available for public viewing and learning. Gradually in the near future as the secondary school curriculum evolves with our needs, a medical school level knowledge of anatomy may be acquired at a school level (especially as anatomy is not rocket science if one just cares to go through the pictures and read the labels but then one may expect the same with rocket science in a space future).

Once a suitable visuospatial orientation of the human system components is obtained, individual users would have the important task of trying to figure out which components is/are malfunctioning as a first approach to medical problem solving. Ascertaining meaning from symptoms generally does this, for example a cough would indicate an irritation of the bronchial tree, a chest pain may suggest a dysfunction of multiple components in the chest and depending on suitable qualifiers the exact component responsible (be it the heart or a covering of the lung or the esophagus) may be discovered.

Similarly a lot depends on the observational skills of all categories of medical learners/potential users. One has to simply learn to be a patient listener and observer of fellow humans, two of the most important characteristics of a successful medical practitioner

An increased rate of breathing may indicate a lung problem (which could even be secondary to a cardiac cause). Swollen limbs and feet may indicate an excess fluid in the micro layers of the skin and in the same patient sitting up, a pulsating vein at the root of the neck would indicate heart failure causing increased venous pressures leading to venous engorgement in the neck. Further clues to the cause of the heart failure may again be elicited on listening to the heart sounds. A whooshing sound like that of a murmur may indicate a damaged valve and trained ears can identify which valve/s is/are damaged. In modern times most of these clinical observational skills have been supplemented with macro imaging techniques that continues to make remarkable technological strides. The skills of listening to the heart sounds and trying to deduce which valves may be affected is largely getting replaced with being able to visualise the dynamics of the heart at the bedside and soon the traditional stethoscope

would get replaced with the ultrasound scanner that would be incorporated in the mobile pc phone.

It is a pleasure to witness the medical student with a good knowledge of anatomy, learn most of these skills within a period of one year provided he practices these predominantly observational skills. It is interesting to see how category one (lay) users seem to understand the anatomical areas involved once explained in a patient manner particularly with the advent of macro imaging techniques that allow most humans to share and view the human anatomy in X-rays, computerized reconstructions of multidimensional X-rays, Magnetic resonance images etc all without opening the human system box (body).

Further micro level causes may then be ascertained with micro imaging techniques originally initiated with the invention of the microscope and this requires sampling tissue from individual system components that are deduced to be at fault which would even include fluids in and around those components.

APPROACH TO DISEASE CAUSALITY AND ROLE OF CLINICAL DECISION SUPPORT SYSTEMS

Our understanding of disease begins with identifying macro anatomical system component abnormalities (the anatomical and morphological diagnosis) and proceeds further to micro etiologies (the etiologic diagnosis). Etiologies/causes can generally be classified as due to

1. Infections - other microorganisms that look to share the Earth and our body with us and sometimes end up in violence with our own micro cells inside our body.
2. Immunological - our own system cells that police our components misdirect their attack on our own component cells.

3. Congenital - manufacturing defects

4. Trauma - all possible environmental accidents that the human body may be subjected to including surgery.

5. Genetics and epigenetics – the relationship between the DNA building blocks and the environment as expressed in human bodily systems. (Marin-Garcia, Goldenthal & Moe, 2008; Tang & Ho, 2007)

6. Health Determinants – the influence on our health of our socio-economic and political and environmental context.(WHO Commission on Social Determinants of Health, 2008)

More recently these categories have become blurred with the emergence of new knowledge about complex disease system (Strohman, 1995). Previously, our understandings were that gene and environment chemicals, medical interventions, environmental pollutants, interactions and lifestyle choices were the determinants of human health. More recently, epigenetic reprogramming has been recognised as a key determinant of the origins of human disease. Epigenetics is categorized as *"heritable changes in gene expression that do not alter DNA sequences but are mitotically and trans- generationally inheritable. Epigenetic reprogramming is the process by which an organism's genotype interacts with the environment to produce its phenotype and provides a framework for explaining individual variations based, in part, on uniqueness of cells, tissues, or organs despite identical genetic information. The main epigenetic mediators are histone modification, DNA methylation, and non-coding RNAs. They regulate crucial cellular functions and work on developmental plasticity such that exposures to endogenous or exogenous factors during critical periods permanently alter the structure or function of specific organ systems. This may be linked to "adaptive" phenotypes to meet the demands of the later-life* (Marin-Garcia, Goldenthal & Moe, 2008; Tang & Ho, 2007).

Clinical Decision Support Systems

In recent times medical decision-making has been supplemented by electronic clinical decision support systems that have the power to let users' access standard background information according to their requirements.

The user may key in symptoms and observational findings and be presented with possible anatomic and etiologic differential diagnoses that may be suitably narrowed down to a single diagnosis with entry of further qualifiers. Machine learning systems look at raw data and then attempt to hypothesize relationships within the data, and newer learning systems are able to produce quite complex characterizations of those relationships. In other words they attempt to discover humanly understandable concepts. Learning techniques include neural networks, but encompass a large variety of other methods as well, each with their own particular characteristic benefits and difficulties. (Coeira 2003)

However, a clinical decision support system is only as effective as its underlying knowledge base, which changes rapidly as medical science evolves. (Purcell 2005) Sim and colleagues have proposed that the next generation of clinical decision support systems should be not only evidence based, but also "evidence adaptive," with automated and continuous updating to reflect the most recent advances in clinical science and local practice knowledge. (Sims et al 2001) Flexibility in incorporating information from diverse sources and adaptability to varied practice settings are likely to be the quality criteria by which decision support systems are judged in the future (Purcell 2005).

Introduction to User Driven Health Care

Often in day-to-day practice both individual patients and health professionals are in situations where the information available is limited and difficult to apply to a given patient.

A gap between the paucity of what is proved to be effective for selected groups of patients and the infinitely complex clinical decisions required for individual patients has been recently recognized and termed the inferential gap. The breadth of the inferential gap varies according to available knowledge, its relevance to clinical decisions, access to the knowledge (i.e. what the physician actually knows at the time of a clinical decision), the variable ways in which knowledge is interpreted and translated into a decision, the patient's needs and preferences, and a host of other factors.

User driven health care may be defined as, "Improved health care achieved with concerted collaborative learning between multiple users and stakeholders, primarily patients, health professionals and other actors in the care giving collaborative network across a web interface." (Biswas 2008). It needs to be differentiated from the presently more ubiquitous consumer driven health care, which is essentially a strategy for users/consumers to decide how they may pay for their own health care through multiple stakeholders like employers who provide the money and insurance companies who receive the premiums. (Tan 2005)

That said the scope of medical practice is to one of caring, the making of wise decisions in the best interest of the patient (Osler, McWhinney, Fugelli, Sturmberg). The Aristotelian notion of phronesis encompasses more than information, "best available evidence", consensus or guidelines, it results from the conversation between the experts of the experience and the expert in comprehension.

The Individual Clinical Encounter as a Lived Multidimensional Learning Experience in Suffering

As currently conceptualized contemporary medicine cannot adequately accommodate concepts that resist quantitative analysis and therefore cannot logically differentiate complex human beings with natural intelligence from machines with artificial intelligence. Currrent computer based clinical decision support systems suffer from the same limitations. Medicine needs a more robust knowledge based system capable of recognizing patients and clinicians as persons. One that is more likely to be driven by natural intelligence than artificial. A truly person-centered medical epistemology requires a revised conception of medical uncertainty and recognition that "the well proven" clinician–patient interactions represent the essence of the *praxis of medicine.* (Henry 2007)

The clinical encounter is a tremendous learning experience for both the individual patient as well as health professional. This is not a new insight as is evidenced by these two quote from Osler who practiced medicine at a time when none of the present day technological cures were available:

""It is more important to know what patient has a disease, than what disease the patient has." (others have ascribed this quote to Hippocrates)

and

"Carry a small note-book, and never ask a new patient a question without note-book and pencil in hand...Begin early to make a three-fold category - clear cases, doubtful cases and mistakes. And learn to play the game fair, no self-deception, no shrinking from the truth; mercy and consideration for the other man, but none for yourself, upon whom you have to keep an incessant watch. It is only by getting your cases grouped in this way that you can make any real progress in your post-collegiate education; only in this way you gain wisdom with experience." (Osler 1904, 1928)

No one individual in present times may always be comfortable with the opinion of another single individual but would need to synthesize his/her thoughts from an array of information packets delivered by a group of diverse individuals. The diversity of information also allows for understanding and unpacking the multiple dimensions of the clinical encounter. In recent times an alternative to the currently dominant EBM (Evidence based medicine) approach has been proposed that has generated considerable discussion. (Tonelli 2006). This alternative centers on the case at hand and recognizes the value of considering the multiple dimensions in the clinical encounter to aid medical reasoning. The five dimensions identified by Tonelli for sense making of a clinical encounter to optimize medical decision-making are:

- Empirical evidence: derived from clinical research.
- Experiential evidence: derived from personal clinical experience or the clinical experience of others.
- Patho physiologic rationale: based on underlying theories of physiology, disease and healing.
- Patient values and preferences: derived from personal interaction with individual patients.
- System features: including biology, environments, health systems and resource availability, societal and professional values, legal and cultural concerns.

User driven health care has the potential to integrate the experiences of illness, the management of the disease and the social consequences in ways that are transformative. It can create a venue to share the many narratives of a particular individual's disease and illness.

For each and every individual patient who suffers it is possible to electronically document her/his clinical encounter with the entire social network that supports her/his healthcare. This persistent documentation in individual personal health records (PHRs) made accessible to all stakeholders (that include innumerable patients and caregivers) would serve as a valuable learning resource that may enable improved decision-making utilizing sensemaking derived from multiple dimensions of the clinical encounter.

Expanding the Learning Environment

A web-based solution to integrate healthcare E-learning needs could lie in a simple forum model already in use in various web sites using what is loosely termed as web 2.0 technology. In web sites using this technology user-generated tags allow the site to evolve, enabling individual users to conduct more precise searches, make previously unacknowledged associations between facts, and explore a diverse undercurrent of themes to synthesize learning.

It has been recently named Health 2.0 with reference to health care and has been described to be all about Patient Empowered Healthcare whereby patients have the information they need to be able to make rational healthcare decisions. (Shreeve 2007).

However considering that these approaches narrow the gap between the expert and the patient, it is equally important to always consider that patient means sufferer, and that people suffering are not "fully capable" to make "the right decisions"

Each and every human has the capacity and likelihood of performing both roles of caregiver and care seeker (patient) in their lifetimes. The illness experience posts would automatically generate related posts depending on the keyword-tags they use to represent their posts and this would enable every user posting his/her individual experience to go through similar relevant lived experiences of other individuals. This would be a tool delivered remotely, often anonymously, and yet may foster a sense of belonging and intimacy. In this way any individual user feeding input into the net can receive automatic feedback that can grow as individual users for this web based solution grow as they keep feeding their own data regularly. This may function purely on the power of human collaborative intelligence rather than artificial intelligence and yet may prove to be much more efficient.

Each and every individual is the author of his own destiny (as well as his own web log) that reflects his experiential life processes and decisions that can shape his/her future. User driven health care is an attempt to help explore further options to make those decisions

Answering Complex Individual Health Information Needs: Evolution of Medical Knowledge in a Post EBM Framework

Self-organization is the property of well functioning complex adaptive systems that allows the natural relationships among individuals and groups to shape the nature of an evolving knowledge base. (Martin 1998)) Self organization also refers to the adaptive capacity of an individual and their family and social network to sustain healthy living or survival.(Martin & Sturmberg, 2009) The organizational complexity of an individual's interactions with his environment defines the level of his functionality. The more the connections an individual is able to develop and more the complexity of his network the more it may reflect his/her vitality (Biswas 2003). This is even witnessed at a micro level inside the human body where there is a demonstrable withering of neuronal connections and complexity with senescense and a resultant loss of neuronal functionality reflected in overall loss of functionality of aging. (Lipsitz 1992). Quite a few studies demonstrate the relationship between intimacy and health, and how disease survivors who report positive family relationships or access to support groups consistently live longer than those without them. The challenge for us ahead is coupling our traditional focus on monitoring efficiencies with providing deeper human connections to promote sustainable behavior change. (Darsee 2007)

The inscrutably enduring power of the anecdote itself is what incites all our most fearsome defenses. The irony in our growing intolerance of the anecdote is that storytelling is full of lessons

in imagination and invention so beneficial to the creative investigator. (Campo 2006). If only all our daily processes were documented along with the anecdotes generated from them they may yet be a valuable form of evidence. It may not be an impossible dream in this electronic information age.

James Surowiecki in his book "The Wisdom of Crowds," mentions four key qualities that make for collective wisdom. It needs to be diverse, so that people are bringing different pieces of information to the table. It needs to be decentralized, so that no one at the top is dictating the crowd's answer. It needs a way of summarizing people's opinions into one collective verdict. And the people in the crowd need to be independent, so that they pay attention mostly to their own information, and not worrying about what everyone around them thinks.

As a word of caution it is possible to imagine highly profitable and very destructive feedback platforms based on servers in unscrupulous jurisdictions that are driven by advertising from personal litigation lawyers and purveyors of therapeutic snake oil. Avoiding this and achieving the best for citizens will require vision, balance and coordinated effort between all those concerned for the individual user in this new wage of democratized voice. (Hodgkin 2007)

FUTURE DIRECTIONS IN USER DRIVEN LEARNING AND HEALTH CARE:

There is no ready-made theory of personal learning, or coherent set of empirical studies, that we can call on to inform the design of technology to support learning in multiple contexts over long periods of time. Technology would increasingly provide an environment in which conversational learning takes place; one that enables conversations between learners. It shall continue to extend the range of activities and the reach of human discussion, into other worlds through the computer as a means of communication, through phone, email and computer based discussions. (Sharples 2002). The Media could be perceived as active computing systems within which mind-endowed individuals (people and intelligent systems) converse. (Pask 1975).

User driven health care applying multidimensional approaches of persistent clinical encounters and wisdom of crowds has the potential to be transformational in challenging the complex, high cost, institutional approach that typifies health care delivery systems today. The health care industry desperately needs ideas that offer lower costs, higher quality and greater convenience and accessibility. Also relaxing central control will make local trust and strategic health workers feel more engaged in the project (Kmietowicz 2007) While dominant players are focused on preserving business models of expensive care and technology arsenals, user driven innovations promise cheaper and simpler access to virtual clinical encounters thus meeting learning needs of the vast majority of patients who may otherwise suffer simply due to lack of information.

CONCLUSION

User driven learning is a form of conversational experiential learning between networked users in web space. User driven health care may be defined as, "Improved health care achieved with concerted collaborative learning between multiple users and stakeholders, primarily patients, health professionals and other actors in the care giving collaborative network across a web interface." Web based sharing of individual patient and health professional conversations and experiences depending on individual user needs through PC and mobile interfaces would make for better E-learning in health care enabling learners to integrate information and knowledge and practice medicine with additional wisdom.

REFERENCES

Armstrong, E. C. (2004). *Morning POEMs (Patient Oriented Evidence that Matters): Teaching point-of-care, patient focused evidence-based medicine*. Retrieved August 16, 2007, from http://www.fammed.washington.edu/ebp/media/stfm-9-03-morningpoems.doc.

Atherton, J. S. (2009). *Learning and Teaching; Experiential Learning*. Retrieved from http://www.learningandteaching.info/learning/experience.htm

Baker, A., Jensen, P. J., & Kolb, D. A. (2002). *Conversational learning: an experiential approach to knowledge creation*. Westport, CT: Quorum books.

Barnacle, R. (2001). *Phenomenology in education research*. Paper presented at AARE conference, Fremantle

Biswas, R. (2003). Patient networks and their level of complexity as an outcome measure in clinical intervention. *BMJ rapid response to Edwards N, Clinical networks. BMJ (Clinical Research Ed.), 324*, 63.

Biswas, R. (2007a). *User driven health care model to answer present day patient physician needs*. Paper presented at the meeting of the IEEEP2407 working group, London, UK.

Biswas, R., Umakanth, S., Strumberg, J., Martin, C. M., Hande, M., & Nagra, J. S. (2007b). The process of evidence-based medicine and the search for meaning. *Journal of Evaluation in Clinical Practice, 13*, 529–532. doi:10.1111/j.1365-2753.2007.00837.x

Castells, M. (1996). *The Rise of the Network Society*. Oxford: Blackwell.

Christakis, N. A. (2004, Jul 24). Social networks and collateral health effects. *BMJ (Clinical Research Ed.), 329*(7459), 184–185. doi:10.1136/bmj.329.7459.184

Coiera, E. (1997). *Guide to Medical Informatics, the Internet and Telemedicine*. London: Chapman & Hall.

Glasziou, P. (2006). Why is evidence-based medicine important? *Evidence-Based Medicine, 11*, 133–135. doi:10.1136/ebm.11.5.133

Goldberg, M. (1997). Ten rules for the doctor-detective. *Postgraduate Medicine, 101*(2), 23–26.

Henderson, J. V. (1998). Comprehensive, Technology-Based Clinical Education: The Virtual Practicum. *International Journal of Psychiatry in Medicine, 28*(1), 41–79. doi:10.2190/NQEN-KRT8-19GA-R0BV

Henry, S. G., Zaner, R. M., & Dittus, R. S. (2007). Moving Beyond Evidence-Based Medicine. *Academic Medicine, 82*, 292–297. doi:10.1097/ACM.0b013e3180307f6d

Hodgkin, P., Munro, J. (2007). The long tale: public services and Web 2.0. *Consumer policy review, 17*(2): 84-88

Kmietowicz, Z. (2007). MPs "dismayed" at confusion about electronic patient records. *BMJ (Clinical Research Ed.), 335*(7620), 581. doi:10.1136/bmj.39339.414306.DB

Kolb, D. A., Boyatzis, R., & Mainemelis, C. (2000), Experiential learning theory: previous research and new directions. Prepared for R. J. Sternberg and and L. F. Zhang (Eds.), *Perspectives on cognitive learning, and thinking styles*. NJ: Lawrence Erlbaum, 2000.

Lipsitz, L. A., & Goldberger, A. L. (1992). Loss of 'complexity' and aging. Potential applications of fractals and chaos theory to senescence. *Journal of the American Medical Association, 267*, 1806–1809. doi:10.1001/jama.267.13.1806

Marín-García, J., Goldenthal, M. J., & Moe, G. W. (2008). Transcriptional, Proteomic, SNPs, Gene Mapping and Epigenetics Analysis. In *Aging and the Heart* (pp. 417–440). Profiling the Aging Cardiovascular System. doi:10.1007/978-0-387-74072-0_13

Martin, C. (1998). *The care of chronic illness in general practice*. (PhD Thesis) Unpublished Epidemiology and Population Health, Australian National University http://normed.academia.edu/CarmelMartin/Papers/74540/The-Care-of-Chronic-Illness-in-General-Practice, Canberra.

Martin, C., & Sturmberg, J. (2009). Complex adaptive chronic care. *Journal of Evaluation in Clinical Practice, 15*(3), 571–577. doi:10.1111/j.1365-2753.2008.01022.x

Martin, C. M., & Kaufman, T. (2007b). *Glossary of Terms in New Orientations, a Shared Framework: A way forward to adaptive Primary Health Care Systems across Canada: A Discussion Monograph*. Commissioned by the Canadian Association of Community Health Centre Associations, and the Association of Ontario Health Centres (www.cachca.ca)).

Matthews, D. A., Suchman, A. L., & Branch, W. T. (1993). Making "connexions": enhancing the therapeutic potential of patient-clinician relationships. *Annals of Internal Medicine, 118*, 973–977.

Miles, A., Loughlin, M., & Polychronis, A. (2007). Medicine and evidence: knowledge and action in clinical practice. *Journal of Evaluation in Clinical Practice, 13*(4), 481–503. doi:10.1111/j.1365-2753.2007.00923.x

Osler, W. (1904). *Aequanimitas with Other Addresses to Medical Students, Nurses and Practitioners of Medicine*. Philadelphia: The Blakiston Company.

Osler, W. (1928). *The Student Life and Other Essays*. London: Constable.

Pask, G. (1975). Minds and media in education and entertainment: some theoretical comments illustrated by the design and operation of a system for exteriorizing and manipulating individual theses. In Trappl, R., & Pask, G. (Eds.), *Progress in Cybernetics and Systems Research, 4* (pp. 38–50). Washington, London: Hemisphere Publishing Corporation.

Purcell, G. P. (2005). What makes a good clinical decision support system. *British Medical Journal, 330*, 740–741. doi:10.1136/bmj.330.7494.740

Sharples, M. (2002). Disruptive Devices: Mobile Technology for Conversational Learning. *International Journal of Continuing Engineering Education and Lifelong Learning, 12*(5/6), 504–520. doi:10.1504/IJCEELL.2002.002148

Shaughnessy, A. F., Slawson, D. C., & Becker, L. (1998). Clinical jazz: harmonizing clinical experience and evidence-based medicine. *The Journal of Family Practice, 47*, 425–428.

Shreeve, S., Holt, M., & O'Grady, L. (2007). *Health 2.0 Definition*. Retrieved December 2007, from http://health20.org/wiki/Health_2.0_Definition

Sim, I., Gorman, P., Greenes, R. A., Haynes, R. B., Kaplan, B., & Lehmann, H. (2001). Clinical decision support systems for the practice of evidence-based medicine. *Journal of the American Medical Informatics Association, 8*, 527–534.

Smith, R. (1996). What clinical information do doctors' need? *BMJ (Clinical Research Ed.), 313*, 1062–1068.

Stewart, W. F., Shah, N. R., & Selna, M. J. (2007, March/April). Bridging The Inferential Gap: The Electronic Health Record and Clinical Evidence. *Health Affairs, 26*(2), 181–191. doi:10.1377/hlthaff.26.2.w181

Strohman, R. C. (1995). Linear genetics, nonlinear epigenetics: complementary approaches to understanding complex diseases. *Integrative Physiological and Behavioral Science, 30*, 273. doi:10.1007/BF02691601

Sturmberg, J. P. (2007). *The Foundations of Primary Care*. Oxford, UK: Radcliffe Publishing.

Surowiecki, J. P. (2004). *Wisdom of the crowds*. New York: Random house.

Tan, J. (2005). *E-health care information systems*. New York: Wiley Imprint.

Tang, W.-Y., & Ho, S.-M. (2007). Epigenetic reprogramming and imprinting in origins of disease. *Reviews in Endocrine & Metabolic Disorders, 8*(2), 173–182. doi:10.1007/s11154-007-9042-4

Thiagarajan P. (2006). *Platelet disorders, E-medicine from web MD*. Retrieved August 16, 2007, from webmd.com

Tonelli, M. (2006). Integrating evidence into clinical practice: an alternative to evidence-based approaches. *Journal of Evaluation in Clinical Practice, 12*, 248–256. doi:10.1111/j.1365-2753.2004.00551.x

Van de Ven, A. H., & Schomaker, M. S. (2002). Commentary: The Rhetoric of Evidence-Based Medicine. *Health Care Management Review, 27*, 90.

van Manen, M. (1990). *Researching Lived Experience: Human Science for an Action Sensitive Pedagogy*. New York: State University of New York Press.

Weisz, G. (2005). From Medical Counting to Evidence-Based Medicine. In *Body Counts: Medical Quantification in Historical and Sociological Perspectives // La Quantification médicale, perspectives historiques et sociologiques*, (eds), Gérard Jorland, Annick Opinel and George Weisz, McGill-Queens Press, 2005, 377-393.

WHO Commission on Social Determinants of Health. *(2008)*. Closing the gap in a generation: health equity through action on the social determinants of health. Final report of the Commission on Social Determinants of Health. *Geneva.*

Wiberg, M. (2007). Netlearning and Learning through Networks. *Journal of Educational Technology & Society, 10*(4), 49–61.

Zimmerman, P. (2001). *Summary and comment to "Complementary Methodology in Clinical Research - Cognition-based Medicine" - a new book by Helmut Kiene.* New York: Springer Publishers.

Chapter 18
User Driven Learning in Mathematics

Monica Kochar
Pathways World School, India

ABSTRACT

This chapter explores the author's personal journey in teaching math and traces her path from teacher controlled work toward beginning to implement student user driven learning strategies in math. It begins by spelling out the need for different math learning strategies and progresses to illustrate student user output which she has savored over the years. Finally it emphasizes the importance of letting go. She culminates the chapter with an attempt to express the inspiration that directed her journey.

INTRODUCTION

This chapter is a reflection of my 16 year journey in learning to teach math to school children…

My inquiry into a different system of math teaching started when I saw the way some children arrived in my classes with broken self esteem due to their failure in learning the subject.

I felt the need for a different math – The way of joy!

My journey has spanned explorations into 'what works, how and why?' I have worked on instilling skills of math, but focused more on developing a healthy attitude to math and one's

relation with it. I have worked on building in children the 'emotional strength' to face their aptitude as it is. Through this quest, I am approaching a system of math that uses multiple strategies of teaching. This chapter is an accumulation of few of the strategies.

It is working for me!

SYSTEMS THAT FACILITATE SELF DIRECTED LEARNING

User Driven Learning

Am I creating sessions that allow the students to direct their learning?

DOI: 10.4018/978-1-60960-097-6.ch018

Table 1. Instructions to the students with the rubric

Instructions	Rubric

Write a 200 to 300 word piece on information graphs covering the following areas:
    1. What is an information graph?
    2. Who are the people who use it?
    3. How is an information graph better than numerical data?
    4. What is the mathematical composition of a graph?
    5. Collect any 5 information graphs from any source (internet, magazines, newspaper etc). Describe what each represents
	Rubric: 15 marks
	Points 1 to 3:
	Language – 5 marks (to be assessed by the English teacher)
	Point 4:
	Accurate information – 5 marks
	Point 5:
	Accuracy – 5 marks

Using IT

This task was created as individualized work. The students had to research and send me their findings within 40 minutes of class time. I wanted them to understand Information Graphs better. I asked them to use any search engine and research information on Information Graphs. This was the task sheet:

I found that with this method, the students took responsibility of learning in their hands and could direct the pace of their work. It gave them space to learn from their favourite medium – computers - and made math contextual. The only thing I had to watch out for and teach them was surfing correctly using the search engine.

The outcome - They loved it!

90% of work emailed after 40 min.

Choice!

Grade 6 needs an involvement of the creative emotional side a lot along with the intellect. Too much mental work and you lose them! I try to give them as much opportunity to involve their creative self as possible.

At the end of basic Geometry, I asked them to make a presentation using all words learnt. The key was – *present in the form you would love to!*

Some students used a power point, some charts, some wrote definitions and some poems. The important aspect is that 'they had a choice' in the matter. Through this I could not only reinforce Geometry definitions, it also became a fun involvement for the children and I got to see some brilliantly creative work!

IT and Worksheet

This was a typical 'student directed class' for me. All I did was to create a structure for them to work in. They worked very well to learn the concepts. I wanted to use a strategy that allowed me to do a lot of drill without the drudgery leading to boredom. So I turned it into a self study lesson. The students studied using an internet module. Each student worked on his-her computer. The whole work was done in the class.

Instructions to students:

1. Go to the site www.aaamath.com
2. Go to the percentage 'self learning' module

Figure 1. A student's work: poems on the vocabulary

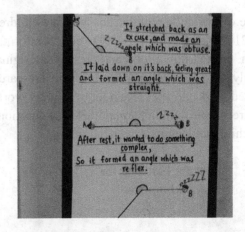

Figure 2. Grade 7 task sheet on the whiteboard

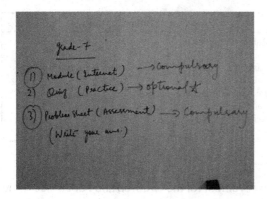

3.   Read and understand each sub concept
4.   Practice few sums using the online quiz
5.   When you are ready, take a worksheet from me (separately on each module)

Hence the students could learn at their own pace and it also reinforced English comprehension skills for them. They decided the time for their assessment on their own, and so were secure!

At the end of the week, a student said, "*Now I understood percentage!*"

I have often organized work in this form, individual or group work. I find that there is a sense of ease in the students when they have a chance to learn at their own pace. The only difficulty is when some students are unable to process the English very well. They need assistance.

Research

One of the skills required for new age children of 21st century is the capacity to collect information, present it in a form and present an original analyses to it. An independently handled research based work! So I involve a lot of it in my work. I direct their thinking around few key questions in child like language:

1.   "What am I looking for?"
2.   "How am I doing it?"

3.   "What did I find?"
4.   "Overall picture"
5.   "The conclusion"

The topic could be any. It could be same for the whole class or different for groups/individuals. I once asked a grade 6 class (divided into groups of 3-4) to decide on a topic of their interest and investigate into it. They took simple topics, but we followed the 5 steps above. At present, a grade 8 child is involved in: "Why were forensic Sciences invented?" I am waiting with baited breath for her results!

The difficult part for them is to come up with an independent conclusion.

(Kyriacou, 1997, page 49) "Another benefit of investigational work is that it can foster creative thinking…to encourage pupils to explore their own ideas"

MULTIPLE INTELLIGENCES (M.I)

How many intelligences do I explore with my lessons?

(Gardner 1993: xxiii) …there exists a multitude of intelligences, quite independent of each other; that each intelligence has its own strengths and constraints.

I experiment with M.I in the classroom. I have created lessons or projects that entail use of *multiple intelligences*.

I have received some fantastic projects from each of the sections! Goose bumps rise on my flesh as I think of them. Some children ooze creativity. This is a great strategy for bringing fun in class, giving an expression to creativity, reinforcing concepts and generating enthusiasm in the children. And when the projects go up on the walls…the classroom is vibrant! It also makes math classes a space where full brain is actively in use, instead of the usual analytical side only.

Here are some examples:

- Make A Magazine - (Problem solving, Linguistics, Visual spatial, Intrapersonal, Logical mathematical) -

  The students are required to create a magazine for sale. They take any topic (fractions, percentage etc) among the ones finished during a term and elucidate it in the magazine. The magazine must contain explanations, applications, pictures, examples and any other information. They also find out the cost of producing the whole magazine and the price to be put if they were to sell it at a percentage profit. The magazine could be in print or soft copy

- Designing A Logo - (Visual spatial, Linguistics, Intrapersonal, Logical mathematical)

  Design a logo representing "My Life as I see it". Justify your logo. Why do you think it represents *you*?

It should have minimum 2 lines of symmetry and rotation symmetry of order 2

Blew me off when I saw this!

- Music - (Musical, Interpersonal, Musical, Intrapersonal, Logical mathematical, Linguistic)

  Pick up a short poem that explains a concept or a rule. You can get enough from the net or the students could make one! Divide the class in groups. Let each group set the poem to music and present it to class. Following the presentation each group has to answer few problems based on the rule, to ensure that it is reinforced. Next time a student needed to remember the rule, he hummed to himself the song and continued the test!

- Art - (Visual, Mathematical, Interpersonal, Logical mathematical)

Create a composition that uses at least 5 different shapes, has 1 line of symmetry on the full A4 page. Colour it/shade it to make an artistic presentation

- Drama - (Kinesthetic, Linguistic, Logical mathematical, Musical, Interpersonal)

  Give the students a short story related to math. An anecdote from the life of a mathematician, story form of a math problem or a logical problem. Each group converts the story to a script and enacts it as a drama. They can add music if they wish!

(Mark Wahl, 1999, page 34) Yes, intuition, movement, color, mystery, feeling, estimation, touch and rhythm all have a place in math learning!

MANAGEMENT SYSTEMS IN CLASS

Does my class have an order that leads to learning or is it chaotic?

"While an inquiry-based classroom allows learners significant freedom to create, chart their own learning, debate, and engage in activities (NRC, 1996, pp12-13), their explorations should be within a structure. The teacher provides this structure with

Figure 4. Art work by a student

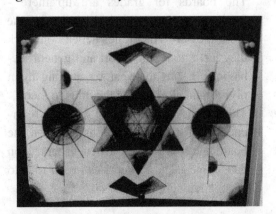

Figure 5. Part of a script penned by a group

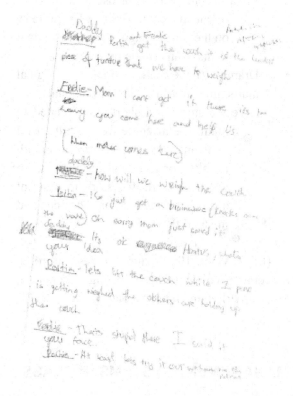

management strategies that help her to create a safe, well-organized, and effective environment where all learners can learn. She orchestrates discussions so that learner participation and thinking are at a high level. She also ensures that learners understand the core content in every lesson."

Some of my systems in class that work very well for me:

- The boards for grades are up there - Students grade themselves daily for the work they do. The grades depend on work they have done, the effort and general behaviour. I start the year by grading them myself and slowly give the onus to them.
- The submission chart is up there for reference - A list of submissions is up on the board and I fill it as and when a submission date comes. The students can refer to it to check their submissions.

- The CW and HW is clearly written on the board - Right in the morning, I reach 10 early; the day's work is put up on the board. Both the CW and HW. That gives the students a focus as soon as they enter the class.
- Of course, anytime it can change as per the spontaneous needs!
- The papers are ready - I *never* have to do last minute running for printing etc. I am very clear as to what I have to do on each day and the required material is ready on my desk…99% of times.
- Portfolios are on the shelf - Every student maintains a portfolio containing all the submitted papers. These are always available in the class for reference.
- The learners know what to expect - "Tell them what you are going to tell them, tell them, and then tell them what you have told them." (Kyriacou, 1997, page 40)
- There is a clear rhythm of work as is evident from the example above*.
- The classroom is filled with students work all over! The boards, my cupboards, walls and the door too.
- Task sheets - Task sheets are given with clear instructions and expectations defined well.
- The feedback is as quick as possible with clear rubrics

This works very well for everyone; but especially for the Special Education Needs children (Special Education Needs or SEN - (Kyriacou, Kris, 2009, page 73) A child has SEN if s/he has a learning difficulty that calls for special educational provision to be made) who lack cohesion and order in their own minds. Organized classes give them a scaffold.

The Physical Space

How does physical space facilitate learning?

Environment of the Class

In Reggio Emilia, a northern Italian town whose early childhood programs are internationally acclaimed, classrooms feature displays of children's work, collections of "found" objects, ample space for supplies (all aesthetically arranged), and clearly designated spaces for large- and small-group activities. Reggio Emilia educators stress the need for a classroom environment that informs and engages the child. They consider the physical environment to be "another teacher." And in the sense that it can motivate children, enhance learning, and reduce behavior problems, environment really is an extra teacher. (n.d. Retrieved on 12th dec 2009 from http://www2.scholastic.com/browse/article.jsp?id=4134.)

I couldn't agree more! For me the classroom has to be *waaarrrmmm* and welcoming. The environment has to motivate them to work and get into the flow of work. My most touching scene is when children walk quietly to the board, looking at their artifacts and smile to themselves. (Humphreys, 1993, page 94) "Belonging is also communicated through photographs and work of students being displayed on classroom walls and school corridors."

Teachers vary greatly on their preferred arrangements, but most agree that the days of 30 desks lined in neat rows and facing the teacher's desk up front are long gone. Instead, some teachers like to arrange desks in cooperative groups of four, while many others prefer a U-shaped configuration, where everyone has a front row seat. (n.d. Retrieved on 12th dec 2009 from http://www2.scholastic.com/browse/article.jsp?id=4134.) I would say let the desk placement be organic! I start with a neat arrangement in the morning, by the end of the day it is chaos, for the number of times it changed during the day. My seating is flexible and need based.

Let the environment be emotionally friendly. Colourful, warm, vibrant. Let there be music sometimes. Allow a bit of tuck (!) once in a while.

Humour, laughter and friendliness. All of this has a positive effect on the cognitive functioning.

"To have the best mental performance and the most efficient pattern of brain activity, you need a match between the type of mood you are in and the type of task you are doing," said Jeremy Gray, Ph.D., a Research Scientist in the Psychology Department in Arts & Sciences and lead author of the study. "This is one of the first studies to really show that performance and brain activity is a product of an equal partnership or marriage between our emotional states and higher cognition." (Everding, Gerry; 2002) (3)

"Some classrooms allow dogs inside to site with children while they read. This practice helps relieve anxiety and better reading scores result" (Everding, Gerry; 2002) (3) I remember my classroom in The Valley School, Bangalore, India. A dog would walk in and sprawl in front of the board. If I tried to remove him, the children would glare! So I had to step around carefully lest I disturb his peace, while I tried to teach the intricacies of higher math to the 12th graders!

The Growth Angle

Are we growing deeper and higher?

Collaborative Learning

I wanted to take a backseat in the class. To simply observe the children. To create a structure where learners are working well, but 'without my interference'. Hence was born the idea of collaborative learning. I wanted the children to experience learning from each other. To discover the power and potential of working together. To feel the thrill on being independent of the teacher. By and large I let them create their groups. But I ensured quietly that each group had 1 person who could help others; children who did not get along were together (☺) and insisted in them to come to me only if they failed as a group to solve something.

Many facets of Collaborative Learning - Snapshots from my classes:

- *CW*-working in small groups to solve a/the problem/s
- *Projects* – to be done collaboratively
- *Peer learning* – 1 on 1 work – each one teach one
- *Teach the class* – 1 student comes to the board and teaches a concept/problem to the whole class
- *Choose the teacher*! – if half the class has 'got it!' and the other has not, each who has not picks a up a teacher among the 'got it!' group and learns

(Pavitra, 1961, page 129) "…team work takes into consideration the need of the child for contact, association and collaboration with other children…social needs."

Attitudes to Learning

I focus a lot on building and nurturing attitudes to learning. What are the attitudes that enhance and support learning? These are my favourite attitudes (I am ever in search of *better*):

- Communication – processing all information and communicating it properly in the solution to any problem. It could also entail defining key terms in a topic.
- Collaboration – learning to work in harmony with peers
- Organization – material and time management.
- Reflection – thinking about the learning, classes and my teaching styles
- Problem solving – well…this is math!
- Information Processing - There are children who can't process information very fast. It is for them that information has to be broken into pieces, the sub components. The ideas have to be broken down and or-

dered again. I of the strategies I use is: with a complete attention and focus, with all the clarity in the mind I have, I speak:
Step 1….
Step 2….
Step 3….

No! I am not spoon-feeding. I am transferring my clarity to their minds. And this transference will happen as far as I can be crystal clear. My tone, facial expression, body language and eyes will all participate in unison to transfer this clarity.

That is when the learner would 'get it'. Fear and incomprehension would return and joy spread over his being. The emotional blocks would open and learning would continue.

It helps if you mark all the steps on the board with a different colour. *Help the child to process the information.*

The Fear Factor

She was 10 when she came to my class…shivering for she feared math more than anything in the world! I started slowly. Letting her do the amount of work she could in the class. Giving her a work of '5 questions a day' for HW. The aim was building her confidence and her math slowly over a period of time. We made a bond

Figure 6. Board work sample for info processing

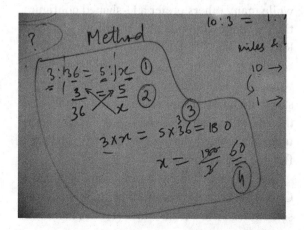

and that led to an increase in her determination to work harder. Then came the projects in the class Based on art, drama, language...*affinity leverage* (Levine, 2002). She resonated with language, her strength. She did a brilliant work of making a math magazine (Figure 3).

The magazine was the turning point for her and she blossomed...attacked math with a frenzy. Then came the best day of our lives when she said, "I do not fear math anymore"..."I want to teach a lesson to the class". And she took a topic 'brackets in algebra' and taught the whole class! A moment imprinted in our lives...

1 on 1 Learning

As he looked at me with soft eyes and said, "How?" I just knew what he needs. I dropped the textbook and pen, took him out to the tiled floor and asked him to walk right-left-up-down till he understood how a vector is created. I did not know during the classes how much he must have felt lost, confusing left with right. A light came in his eyes as he understood. He worked quietly from the text after that for 30 min. It is when you are teaching a child 1 on 1 that all the mysteries are de-mystified. It is then that the blockages in the learning unroll themselves before your eyes. And you can see the entire panorama of the space called the 'child'. You understand the learning style and you know how to face it. 1 on 1 teaching to me is the best space

to unravel the mysterious way children seem to learn. It is here that the best contact is established between the teacher and taught! A relationship where something blossoms. A relation of safety.

Higher Order Thinking-Using Math as a Tool to Work the Mind

(Jones 1995) "In the hands of the ancient Greeks mathematics becomes a systematic body of knowledge rather than a collection of practical techniques. Mathematics is established as a deductive science in which the standard of rigorous demonstration is deductive proof."

Why?
How do you know?
Justify your answer
What is the logic?
Explain your solution

These are some of my favourite questions to ask in class, especially grades 7 and upwards. The fruition of the questions I find in analytical Geometry – Euclid's Geometrical proofs and problem solving based on the theorems.

A beautiful memory wafts in...

Grade 10 math class and a difficult 'Prove this' problem. I divide the class into groups and ask each group to work it out together. 39 children...about 13 groups. I walk around, just observing. The class

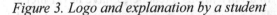

Figure 3. Logo and explanation by a student

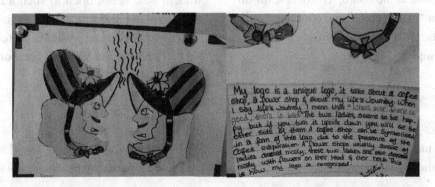

Figure 7. Cover page of the magazine created by the student

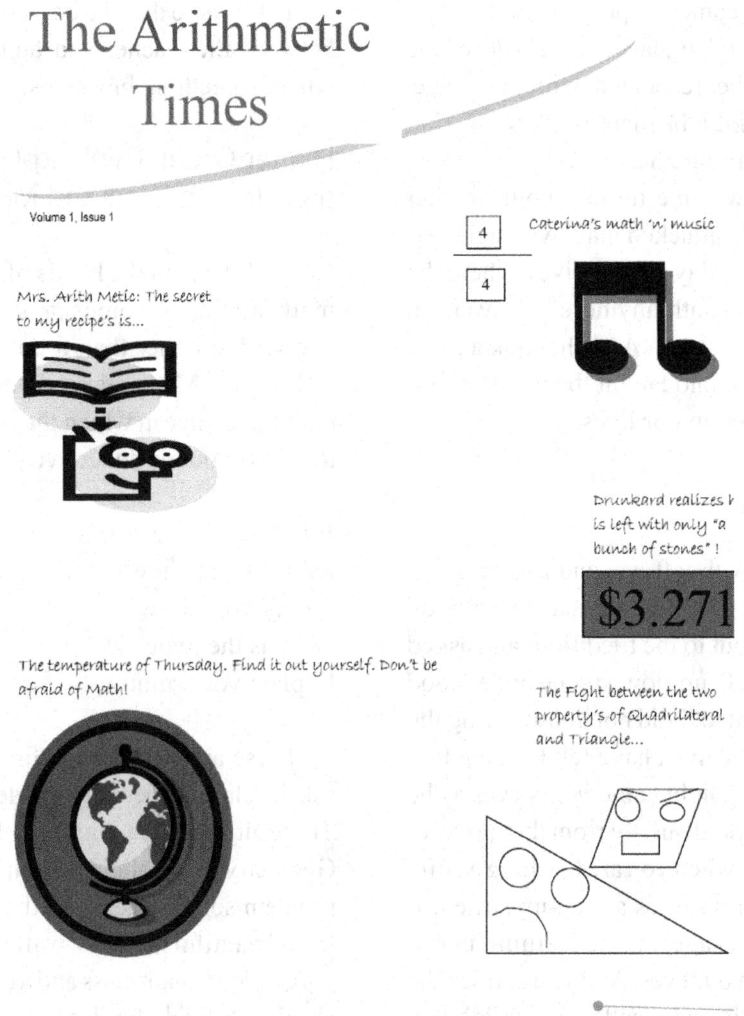

The Arithmetic
Times

Volume 1, Issue 1

Mrs. Arith Metic: The secret
to my recipe's is...

4
4
Caterina's math 'n' music

Drunkard realizes h
is left with only "a
bunch of stones" !

$3.271

The temperature of Thursday. Find it out yourself. Don't be
afraid of Math!

The Fight between the two
property's of Quadrilateral
and Triangle...

is raft with students completely involved. End of 20 min, I get 10 different ways of solving the same problems! One child from each group comes to share the solution at the board. The best solution came from our 'math genius' and contained only 2 steps and one extra construction.

Mesmerizing!

1 to 1 Chat

Nothing works better than pulling a child away from friends and just have a 'man to man' chat. I keep it candid, two-way and stay away from judgments. It is based on facts. I give a complete feedback – nice/not so nice/urrrgh!

In all my life as a teacher, I have never met a student who is not open to such a feedback and who does not show some improvement after it. When we have clear systems of feedback, then we can say that the learner is responsible for the learning that happens!

Grow!

If I don't grow and expand, I will suffocate and die! These are my own personal disciplines:

- Read – expand horizons

  I am always on the go searching for variety of strategies I can bring in the class, new thinking in education, behavioural sciences or classroom management

- Plan

  Learners are very calm and collected when they I know what is expected from them. The clearer your instructions are the calmer and focused the class would be. *The teacher's clarity transfers to the learners.*

  Be 'ready'.

  I spend a lot of time in planning; although I can also give it up on a second's notice and do something new if it is not working. Once I had an idea while I was walking from my table to the board (!) and I dropped all planning and launched into the idea.

- Know yourself

  It is in understanding me that I understand the world better. I believe in it! My quest is as much without as is within. To go deeper and find greater depths and heights of the person I am. My current boss told me once, "Ever since I am watching you, I only see you growing." I am always upgrading my skills as per the need. Every difficulty in the class is an opportunity to grow…

- Networking

  Network with people-colleagues or online. Talk!

- Evaluation through learners

  My best critics are students. Often I stop teaching and have a friendly chat with them on, "So how do you think the classes are going? Any suggestions?" I have also taken feedbacks from them on me as a person, and have found it to be 99% accurate! They know me best. They are generally very honest,

straight and, it always humbles me to see, gentle.

- Professional up-gradation

  Workshops, trainings, conferences, seminars…

- Blogging

  I write a blog (www.teachingmathcreatively. blogspot.com) where I share all the ideas I use in the class. It is very reaffirming when people visit it and leave a comment/suggestion. It is also a good way of collating the data on the universal server!

- Go Google!

  Internet has created an explosion in my mind! There is so much on it to learn. One can easily be on a self–education program.

Getting Attuned To the Children

Relate to the learner. Know him-her. Strike a rapport. (Turnbull, 2007, page 99-100) "…although rapport seems to just happen with some people, the important thing to realize is that it can be created – you can be *creative* in establishing rapport"

Be aware of the 'feedback loop', which Goleman (2006, page 38) defines as "when two people interact face to face, contagion spreads via multiple neural circuits…These systems for emotional contagion traffic in the entire range of feeling, from sadness and anxiety to joy."

Be *sensitized*…Be *present in the moment.*

(Goleman, 2006, page 280) "Socially intelligent leadership starts with being fully present and getting in a synch."

It was the class of 9 special needs children. I introduced the word 'Perpendicular' to them. Suddenly there was palpable tension and fear in the class. I sensed it and there was no way I could have gone ahead with properties. I asked the children to learn to pronounce it loudly. Twist the word in their mouth. Play with it. Sing it. Break it into sounds per-pen-di-cu-lar. Relate it to some

Figure 8. Print screen of author run group at http://mathematics24x7.ning.com

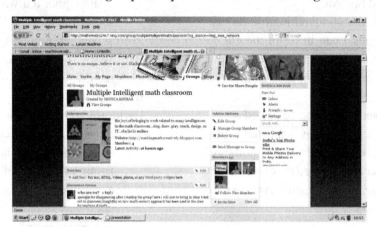

life object. I went on and on and we laughed; till I *sensed* the fear and tension disappearing. Then we went into studying the concept. Feedback loop.

System Creation: The Essence of Teaching

Do I teach or does teaching unfold in the system I create?

And finally I come to THE principle which has been the inspiration and the defining quality to the work that I do. This is where the quest is directed, the search for the elusive…In each of us there is something that seeks an expression and the greatest joy for us is when that something gets a chance to express itself. What is this 'something' and what is that gives it a chance to express? All I know is the feeling when this expression comes is - *Aha!*

Swabhava

Swabhava…is there a word in English for it? One could say it is the *essential self principle* of a person.

A learner-centric education is essentially an education that respects the Swabhava of the learner. Such an educator would never force learning on the learner, rather work on building

variety of strategies/scaffoldings to bring out the highest aptitude of the learner in the subject. The search, I think, is never ending. There is no 'best system of learning.' Each learner is unique and therefore will demand a unique system of learning to unfold his-her highest potential. I deeply respect this uniqueness, and therefore don't have 'Everyone gets an A in the test!' attitude anymore, it progressively withering away as my inquiry progressed. This is the reason I am forever in search of a *better* system, a wider repertoire of strategies and on the road to deepen myself. How can I create systems that help nourish children and their uniqueness?

Figure 9. Students record their Aha! moments in class

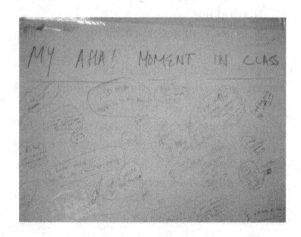

He could never really achieve in the math class. He was always left behind and watched quietly as others outperformed him again and again. Then one day I asked them to write a poem on the topic of the day 'Quadrilateral'. He was the first one to write. And gave a good one! I gave him a hearty pat, aware that this was his moment. I saw him smiling for the first time! Poetry brought out something in him.

There is always a surprise waiting when a project is done in the class. There is always one child who is always quiet in the class and kind of left out, who finds a space to show his prowess and feels happy and connected with the class. Something blossoms!

She never related to math! In fact she started shivering when math started. Till I asked on a day for them to express understanding of their learning in the way they wished. Paragraph, Bullets, Diagrams…etc. Out came her box of colours and she spent the rest of the class creating a visual for her learning.

Something opened in her…the relationship began.

(Cousinet, 1950, page 20-21) "New education…is really a new attitude towards the child. An attitude of understanding and love, and above all an attitude of respect."

Letting Go

Let go…sounds difficult!

But put simply, letting go is a way of accepting one's own limitations in handling the situation. Accepting that, maybe it is not meant to happen now. It is humility. When nothing works…let go. Stop stressing yourself with – 'why can't they learn/behave/write/talk properly….etc…the endless list of learning!' Maybe that will work! ☺

It is not out of defeat that I say this. But out of a conviction. (Cousinet, 1950, page 20-21) "A conviction that the child has within himself, everything that allows a true education, and particularly a ceaseless activity, incessantly revived, in which he is totally engrossed, the activity of a growing being who is continuously developing and to whom for that very reason, our help may be useful, but our direction is not necessary."

Almost At the Beginning of the Journey!

Can I accept that nothing can be taught?

The beginning of the journey is the point of *shift* I make from being a teacher to becoming a facilitator. From being a controller of class, to becoming creator of a space where learning unfolds freely within a fluid system.

I take inspiration from deep teachings on education and systems from the modern international education. The result is my own creative expression! An expression that only waits for that quiet gleam of joy, which comes in the eyes of a student when he-she experiences the thrill of '*aha! I got it*'. My goal is to create space for them to reach *their* best and not the state standard!

The scaffolds I create are as far as possible respectful of the integrality of the learner and her-his process of learning. It invites the mind and emotions both to participate in the exploration. However, behind this scaffold/system is awareness, an acceptance and respect of human life as a process of growth and expansion. The acknowledgement of *svabhava* and an effort to perceive it.

I feel this is the future of education – a new synthesis of deeper teachings and modeling systems from the west. When the fundamental principles of learner-centered approach are understood, assimilated and internalized, each day at school is fresh, new and unpredictable!

REFERENCES

Classroom organization. (n.d.). *Classroom organization: the physical environment*. Retrieved December 12, 2009, from http://www2.scholastic. com/browse/article.jsp?id=4134

Everding, G. (2002). *ReadingModule*. Retrieved December 12, 2009, from http://www.edu-cyber-pg.com/culdesac/ReadingModule/EmotionTies-ToCognitive.html

Gardner, H. E. (1983). *Frames of Mind: The theory of Multiple Intelligences*. New York: Basic Books.

Goleman, D. (2006). *Social Intelligence*. London: Arrow Books.

Humphreys, T. (1993). *A Different kind of Teacher*. Dublin, Ireland: Newleaf, an imprint of Gill and Macmillan limited.

Jones (1995). *A Short History of Rigour in Mathematics*. Retrieved December 12, 2009, from http://www.rbjones.com/rbjpub/maths/math003.htm

Kyriacou, C. (1997). *Effective Teaching in Schools*. London: Nelson Thornes.

Levine, M. (2002). *A Mind at a Time*. New York: Simon and Schuster.

NRC. (1996). *NRC*. Retrieved from http://educationnorthwest.org/webfm_send/203

Sutra (n.d.). *Spiritual-Theosophy Dictionary on Sutra*. Retrieved from http://www.experiencefestival.com/a/Sutra/id/195147

Turnbull, J. (2007). *9 Habits of Highly Effective Teachers*. New York: Continuum International Publishing group

Wahl, M. (1999). *Math for Humans*. Langley, WA: LivnLern Press.

KEY TERMS AND DEFINITIONS

Collaborative Learning: A situation created in classroom where 2 or more children learn together.

Higher Order Thinking: When students think about facts in order to distill, synthesize or conclude, they are engaged in higher order thinking. They are encouraged to distill original conclusions.

Attunement: Becoming aware of the other person. To flow in harmony with the emotions experienced in the person in front of you.

Information Graphs: A chart or a drawing showing relationship between changing things. It presents facts in visual form.

Inquiry Based Learning: A way of teaching where a teacher involves students in the learning process through focusing on questions, problem-solving activities, and the use of critical thinking. It works on higher cognitive thinking.

Multiple Intelligences: A term coined by Howard Gardener. According to him the original definition of intelligence, IQ, is limited and out-dated. He coined the term 'multiple intelligences' and proposed to view individuals through them to see the vaster potential.

Logo: A graphic mark used by organizations to aid instant recognition. Famous example is *Nike*.

Swabhava: A term given by Sri Aurobindo. The essential self principle of an individual. The principle around which life tries to govern itself. The deepest urge in us.

Chapter 19
A User Driven Learning Environment in Botany

J. M. Garg
Independent Researcher, India

Dinesh Valke
Independent Researcher, India

Max Overton
Independent Researcher, Australia

ABSTRACT

This chapter introduces the reader to a sample 'user driven learning environment' created in an online community with a special interest centred on trees and plants. It traces the development of an online learning community through the lived experiences and thoughts of its founding members and also includes conversational learning experiences of other users to illustrate the process of 'user driven learning' in online communities. It illustrates innovative sense making methodologies utilized by group members to create a more meaningful 'User driven learning environment' while simultaneously contributing in a positive way to create information resources at no cost along with creating awareness & scientific temper among members.

INTRODUCTION

The internet enables everyone to communicate with others and have immediate access to information. Globalization of virtually every aspect of our lives, combined with new communication technologies, creates a need and opportunity to engage individuals and groups of learners who are separated in time and/or space, and may come from different cultural backgrounds. (Moisseeva 2007). User driven learning is a form of conversational experiential learning between networked users in web space.

An online learning community is a common place on the Internet that addresses the learning needs of its users through proactive and collaborative partnerships. Through social networking and computer-mediated communication, users work as a community to achieve a shared learn-

DOI: 10.4018/978-1-60960-097-6.ch019

ing objective. Learning objectives may arise out of discussions between participants that reflect personal interests. In an online community, people communicate via textual discussion that may be synchronous or asynchronous. (Online learning community 2009)

User driven online learning communities have been found to function on a few simple principles identified as early as 1998:

1.   Online learning communities are grown, not built.
2.   Online learning communities need leaders.
3.   Personal narrative is vital to online learning communities. (Clarke 1998)

As there are very few illustrations of such user driven learning interactions we present a detailed outline of online community building by users who may have been pushed into a leadership role to answer their own learning requirements.

USER NARRATIVES ON THE PERSONAL NEED FOR LEARNING ON A TOPIC

J.M.Garg has long been interested in the avifauna of India, at first using photography to capture the beauty that lay all around him, and later using the Internet to connect with people that had similar interests. He quickly learned that there was hardly any e-group devoted to photographing, identification, discussion, learning etc. on Indian Flora.

I have been closely associated with e-groups related to identification and discussion on Birds, Butterflies etc. Association with these groups ignited in me a desire to photograph these beautiful creatures that are closely associated with the human beings and to our environment. This resulted in heavily investing my hard-earned money in photographic equipments like camera, lenses, tripod etc., sometimes rather against the wishes of my family. Digital photography has changed the world like never before, as has been done by World Wide Web, e-mails etc. I think e-groups have done something similar which has resulted in better documentation of our Flora and Fauna, our environment and all other aspects which one can think of. It has given the layman a power/tool to do something worthwhile and contribute towards some cause, which hitherto was a preserve of the experts/researchers, who mostly confined themselves in the journals or books and away from the layman.

While being associated with the e-groups related to Birds, Butterflies etc., I felt that there were hardly any groups related to discussion and identification of Indian flora. I was finding it difficult to learn about trees surrounding my place i.e. Kolkata, where I was staying. There are hardly any good books available in the market which a layman can lay hands on, to know even our common plants and trees.

I had a few solo exhibitions in Kolkata mainly focussing on Bird photography and the response from the people was tremendous. Tears still roll down from my eyes when I think of the villager who came to Kolkata for some purpose and entered in my exhibition. He spent about an hour through my various exhibits. When he was going away, I asked him how he felt. He was speechless and after sometime he told me that what he has seen he has no words to describe. I feel myself lucky that I showed something worthwhile to a villager who could not have even imagined such beauty in wildest of his dreams. Going down my memory lane, there are so many examples that I would not go on to write here as that would take this chapter beyond its length.

Impressed by my work of photography, one of my colleagues who had planted hundreds of trees and made the neighbourhood totally green in the past few years decided to photograph and document them and possibly collaborate on some kind of a book. I made lot of trips with him looking for, and photographing different plants and trees in different areas of Kolkata all the while learning about them. He had a book called Trees of Delhi by Sri Pradeep Krishen and on his recommendation I bought a copy for myself. This book was not written by a botanist, most possibly by a layman like me, who with his passion had mastered the trees of Delhi while photographing them also. The book is certainly a masterpiece, layman-friendly written; it impresses both - the layman as well as the expert. This further lit the desire in me to learn more about our trees in Kolkata and wherever I went, this reference helped me identify my trees to a great extent. Though the book is written on Trees of Delhi, it covers the common trees found all over India.

I gradually began to feel that among my friends & elsewhere, there were hardly any discussions on plants and trees; perhaps everybody considered them to be mundane or routine, and not worth photographing and learning about. I wished I could find a few people who were as interested to know more about trees as I was.

Dinesh Valke had a similar problem. He started off posting images on 'Flickr', adding a tag as identification. The problem was, his knowledge of plants was not good enough to label all the images correctly, and identifications like 'pink flower' or 'garden plant' did not really help anybody. He needed a site that involved other people in the identifications so that the sum of their knowledge was greater than any one member's.

My company got acquired by a larger company, there followed the transition time as well as trying time... what kind of job I would land with? While most of my colleagues smoothly blended into newer and similar environment, I was desperately searching my lost work routine. I found Art and Graphics have nothing to do with serious software coding. And I found myself assuring quality of the software product that my company develops... which was not a very difficult job, neither was very interesting. My sanity at stake, I

had to think: where will I get in the world by only being content with software. This was somewhere in December 2006, when finally the devil set up his workshop in my perfectly bored mind... the first tool he purchased was a camera phone, and started his business of capturing potted plants in the company's premises!! The photographs were turning to be useless if it were stored in a private album, or were to be shown to friends without knowing what the plants are!! By then, some of my colleagues may have already given hopes about my new found passion.

That is when the first thought germinated: the need to exhibit the photographs to public, with at the least the name of the plant put as title. Having put some serious efforts for choosing a photo-sharing site on the internet, decided that Flickr is the most ideal and convenient -- that is, from the perspective of searching and retrieving the desired set of photos. Flickr uses the power of "tags"... tag is a word, or some words which are relevant to a context... in Flickr, every photo is "tagged" with relevant set of words. These tags, also known as keywords, need to be relevant: to the context, and to the person who would wish to get to that context. Here is where I got stuck -- how do I get to know the names of plants? Friends and acquaintances were quick to give up on enquiries. Back to internet... and Google was the saviour. Naivity has its own advantages... the words I used for search were as simple as "pink flower", "garden flower" which I would not think of using today. But those words then fetched me results of all sorts, proving beneficial in a special way... I found some of sites showing up regularly, they contained large store of information. Very soon there were more than handful of sites listed as my favourites... and I knew fairly well enough to visit particular site for specific search.

It was during this time I found a site called Flowers of India... the name itself promised me that I my search for a flower's identity may start and end here itself!! I was awed by the collection of flowers, meticulously categorized easing search, I was more surprised to know that the site is run by just two people -- more surprises– Dr. Tabish Qureshi who created and maintains the site is a physicist, and Thingnam Girija who gets more and more new flowers to the site is a psychologist!! This first visit to FOI was one of the turning points in my journey towards wild and beautiful Nature. The urge to go get new plants just got extra strong.

From then, the weekends got priority for experiencing wild life, frequenting the nearby Tungareshwar Wildlife Sanctuary, Yeoor Hills, Sanjay Gandhi National Park, Karnala Bird Sanctuary, became a strong habit. The local folks prove to be good guides, and often point out sights which I would tend to not see. With every other visit, I found that the internet cannot help me identify all the plants that I sighted... one of the chief reasons I discovered: flora endemic to Western Ghats is not much discussed on the internet.

Why is it not much discussed? How does a layman enthusiastic about getting familiar with flora of his / her region get the knowledge? The text books published by Botanical Survey of India are not easily accessible to general public; their contents too would not suit common man's understanding. Two samaritans changed this situation for me to a great extent. Shrikant Ingalhalikar and Isaac Kehimkar released reference books illustrating the wild flora that I was looking for. Yet, this did not dampen the main question, WHY is flora of India not on the internet?

The question must have been strongly looming in many like-minded people... I found it resounding in a Google Group called 'Indiantreepix' which I recently joined... J. M. Garg created this e-Group with the intention of creating awareness of Indian flora, it is a large community of people with varied backgrounds helping in identification and discussion of Indian Flora. Discussion helps me gain relevant knowledge, and provides opportunity to deliver my contributions.

SETTING UP A FORUM FOR USER DRIVEN LEARNING: INITIAL PHASES

J.M.Garg considered the idea of an Internet group dedicated to discussion and identification of Indian trees after getting deeply inspired from 'The Monk who Sold his Ferrari' by Robin Sharma. But he was worried that such a mundane subject would not attract enough people to achieve these ends. People would not only have to join the group, but also participate, offering up pictures of trees for identification and, just as importantly, be prepared to identify other people's pictures and discuss these identifications. The thought of starting a group and then having it fail raced his mind time & again. But thoughts from the book by Robin Sharma (an expert in leadership and personal development), made him think otherwise. He learnt the value of focus, of passion & of helping others, and of a desire for excellence from it. With these attributes, he thought, Indiantreepix could not fail

And so, on a June day in 2007, Indiantreepix Google e-group was born (Figure 1). Indiantreepix is devoted to creating awareness and helping in identification along with discussion on, and documentation of Indian Flora. Posting of photos for identification, discussion and general sharing is solicited, the attachments hopefully illustrating different aspects of the plant. Every species discussed gets included in the Indiantreepix Database, which has now developed into a very useful resource of pictures and information on Indian Flora.

I wrote to different persons and other e-groups for membership and by the end of the month Indiantreepix had around 112 messages, with a membership of around 50 members.

Whenever a message was posted seeking identification or confirmation, I referred the various books I had by then & also the information available on the Net. To my surprise, I was able to help everybody to some extent in the identification

Figure 1. Web shot of Indiantreepix in Google group

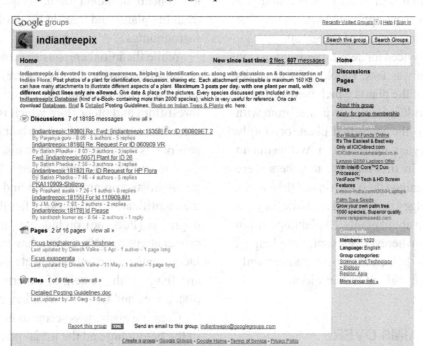

process although at that time there were hardly any experts on the forum. While I helped everybody, the learning points started getting strongly etched in my mind. I started realizing that helping others was possibly one of the best ways to learn. If I had made some mistake, there were always other members who corrected me and I learnt a little more. I think this is the process of learning in an e-group - those who work hard and help others, tend to learn more than those who simply request and depend on others for identifications, discussions, etc. It is a win-win situation for everybody in an e-group.

I remember writing to many people and experts requesting each of them, for becoming a member of Indiantreepix. I used to be disappointed when I would not get any positive response. But my spirit was buoy when I would receive any positive response as it helped me in my quest for helping the members in the identification and discussion of Indian trees.

I continued my efforts by giving almost 2 to 4 hours every day to the group in the form of request-

ing for membership, helping in the identification, posting pictures of the trees that I photographed and processed. Almost 30 to 40 members every month used to get added to Indiantreepix.

In the process I learnt a lot of things; identification was a difficult process for a layman member like me as it required lot of time. I knew I have limitations of time for myself as I could not infringe on the time I would give to my family as well as allow any laxity in performance of my duties. The only way to go ahead was to involve more and more experts, who could help the members in identification with very little of their time. Also, with more membership, there would be more possibilities of a tree or plant getting identified, as some of the lay members could be aware of the plant and may give their feedback. Any member whether a layman or an expert giving substantial time to the group, I would request him or her to be a Moderator / Manager of the group. I need to share the group's powers with others, for them to be an integral part of the group and be passionate about it. They should also feel the stake in the group to give their best. That is how initially, 3 to 4 moderators were appointed within the first few months of the starting of the group.

Whenever my need for helping with discussion or identification was less, I looked for the links on the internet of the plants which were posted. I would then provide information in the forum with relevant links to the identified plant, or simply copy-paste relevant matter from Wikipedia in the mail itself. In this manner, members were benefited and I gained their trust, as all their mails were acknowledged and replied to, while they got new information about plants. Explaining certain botanical terms wherever relevant, with help of Wikipedia links, helped members, and certainly me too, in learning about Indian Flora.

CHANGING AIMS OVER TIME FOR USER DRIVER LEARNING IN BOTANY

Indiantreepix was initially set up as a means of identifying tree species, but it rapidly became apparent that other plants needed to be included. It currently attempts to identify not only Indian trees, but shrubs, herbs, grasses and sedges, cultivated plants and flowers, mosses and liverworts, fungi, and plants not endemic to India. The broadened scope of the group could mean that it appeals to a wider range of people and hopefully will attract experts from taxonomic groups other than Indian trees.

After few months of starting of Indiantreepix, I realised that as far as trees are concerned, their number is very limited and if we have to grow, the scope of the group has to be widened to include discussion on the herbs, shrubs etc. Thus posts on Indian Flora were allowed though some of the members thought it otherwise. Some of the members wanted that posts should be restricted only to the wild flowers/plants but again I allowed posts on Indian flora including those on the garden plants. Is it not that if one has to start

learning about Indian Flora, his quest has to start from the plants and trees in his garden and in his surroundings?

While the initial emphasis seems to be on the common flora as the members were in the learning stage, it has now changed to learning about the forest flora and other flora which is not so common. More and more posts are being received on new plants which have not been discussed earlier.

With more and more experts, botanists and taxonomists joining the group and helping with the identification etc. difficult families like those of grasses (Poeceae), orchids etc., are also getting proper attention. Discussions have also started on identification and other aspects of mushrooms and fungi, with the help of experts in the group. Succulents and Cacti are also being discussed.

Creating awareness seems to be the emphasis in the beginning and the initial phase. The focus now seems to be shifting to photographing, identification and documenting new flora which has not been covered till date.

CONVERSATIONAL PROCESS OF USER DRIVER LEARNING IN BOTANY

This is explained below by quoting a few conversations here from Indiantreepix, which shows how everybody participates & learns in the process:

An example on the tree Ficus Krishnae...

Anoop Rajan: Few days back me and Tejal saw *Ficus Krishnae* at Rani baugh, Bayculla Zoo. Just wanted to ask is it of Indian origin, because someone told me it's not native to India.

J.M.Garg: It has originated in India. Pl. see the link for details: http://toptropicals.com/catalog/uid/Ficus_krishnae.htm

Anoop Ranjan: Thank you for the instant reply with evidence. So I have e-group teacher.

Madhuri Pejaver: I don't know the origin myself. But just a story can it explain Indian origin? Of course, I knew the story, but my doubt, if it has

Indian Origin, why there is only one plant in Jijamata Udyan only? There may be one or two more which I am not aware of, but not many for sure.

Why this plant is not seen commonly around/ not in Mumbai, near Mumbai, in Yeoor forest, in forest area near Bhandup, near Thane, in Nagala block? Because I have visited all these areas with tree lovers but not a single tree of *Ficus Krishnae* is seen. Is it seen at any other place in Maharashtra, in other states? If so let us know. According to me Victoria Garden now known as Jijamata Udyan was built by Britishers as a botanical garden. Hence they must have brought these plants from different areas, nations, continents? It can be a collection of plants. If the plant is indigenous has to get reported from other places from India if not in Mumbai.

Vaishali Kulkarni: I recently saw the *Ficus Krishnae* tree in outskirts of Bangalore, at a place called Vani school, where they have some not so common plants planted round the school area.

Madhuri Pejaver: Is it natural there or planted? If planted from where did they get it? If natural is it only one or more? Let us get information from all on the group. We will be able to understand the distribution of is plant.

Satish Phadke: There is one planted in Garware college campus in Botany Dept., Pune, Maharashtra.

Ulhas Rane: Krishna's Buttercup Tree as it is known is a variety of *Ficus benghalensis* and it is not an independent species. That is why it has to be written as *Ficus benghalensis* var. *krishnae*. Variations in plants happen due to several ecological / environmental reasons and sometimes those variant plants could be cultivated /multiplied retaining their characters / variations. Krishna's Buttercup Tree is such variation which is being cultivated by grafting in many gardens all over India because of unique shape of its leaves and the associated story. Of course, the tree itself also takes a beautiful form like the original plant *Ficus benghalensis*- the Banyan tree. I do not think that this variety multiplies naturally. Since

Ficus benghalensis is indigenous to India, we could also conclude that the variant '*krishnae*' is also indigenous.

Madhuri Pejaver: As you rightly said this might not be breeding naturally, as I have not seen flowers, fruits on this plant as we see on *F. benghalensis*.

Anand Kumar Bhatt: Ficus benghalensis, F. religiosa both are native to India. It can be inferred that *F. benghalensis* var. *krishnae* is also native to India. Ulhas has rightly pointed out the possible reason why it is not widespread.

A.S.Kannan: Most of the Bangaloreans interested in trees would know the large *Ficus krishnae* in the North eastern part of Lalbagh. I have never looked for fruits in the tree, but I will look into it when I visit Lalbagh next time.

J.M.Garg: I have read somewhere, but not getting hand on the book right now. That it was found first at Bot. Gardens, Howrah, Kolkata. At that time after studies, it was considered a separate species. But subsequently, it was seen that normal Banyan (*Ficus benghalensis*) trees grew from its seeds in some of the cases. That is why it was considered as a variety & not a separate species.

A.S.Kannan: If a normal Banyan tree grows from the seeds, it sounds like the manifestation of a recessive gene.

Anand Kumar Bhatt: I have never seen Lalbagh *Ficus krishnae* so I don't know how tall it is. Bose and Choudhury's book says that the tree rarely goes beyond 5 meters, and is propagated through cutting and layering. That explains why it is not endemic in India and is not easily grown from seeds as Banyan and Peepal.

Madhuri Pejaver: It a nice discussion going on. Adding a lot in knowledge. This was needed and I think that's the moto of the group. But Kannan ji, I could not understand the part of role of gene you have written. Can you elaborate it please?

Mahadeswara Swami: I have seen few trees in Karnataka and Tamil Nadu. A few were available in Lalbagh, Bangalore a few years back. I have seen one in Agri-horticulture society, Chennai, long back. But I do not know whether these trees still exist. Perhaps more of these trees may be found in Eastern and North Eastern regions of India, as most of the Ficus trees were originated in this region.

Sushmita Jha: There is at least one *Ficus Krishnae* (planted?) in the Buddha Jayanti Park, Delhi. I have a fallen leaf from that tree.

Tabish: Delhi has lots of Krishna Figs. Almost every large garden (like Lodhi garden) has it.

A.S. Kannan: Before I attempt to answer your question, I must add a disclaimer saying that I am a novice in trees and my opinions come purely from an understanding of how Genetics operates in all organisms! I hope some experts can add better clarity to this. A detailed description of Genetics will be out of place in this group. So I will try to illustrate the outcome here. Assume that the leaf shape (of Krishna's buttercup) is the manifestation of a recessive gene. If this is true, a seed that is a result of cross pollination from a different tree is most likely to grow into a tree with a normal leaf. This is because a normal leaf will be a dominant gene and will override the recessive gene. For the seed to grow into a tree with a buttercup leaf, it should be self-pollinated, or grafted as suggested by most of the folks here. Hope this helps!

A.S. Kannan: I have attached two photographs of *Ficus krishnae* in Lalbagh. One of the photographs shows how the branch touches the ground to grow another tree from there. Yes, with the tendency of the branches to go low and touch

the ground, these trees may not grow more than 5-6 meters.

Kiran Srivastava: True, I have seen one tree in the Delhi Zoo too!

Ushodayan Thampy: The Krishna fig is not mentioned in older Indian Floras- certainly not before 1910. There is a small story behind its identification.

The director of the Royal Botanical Garden at Howrah, David Prain, has brought a branch of the tree by a resident of Calcutta in 1896 who would not say where it came from or how old the tree was. All he revealed was that it grew somewhere close to Calcutta, and the tree is an ordinary banyan tree whose leaves were miraculously transformed into little jars by Lord Rama (or Lord Krishna according to competing legends). He was not able to examine the parent tree.

By 1901, Prain had succeeded in growing 2 specimens in the Botanical garden from cutting. One specimen was planted out in the main collection of the garden and the other he send to Kew garden in London to be grown under glass. And while he was waiting for the plants to grow older and develop their first fig, he sent specimens of the strange leaves to be examined by expert Botanists. One such expert was Dr. C. de Candolle in Geneva.

C. de Candolle studied the pocket leaves closely and likened them to those of pitcher plants. He noticed that this was the kind of pitcher leaf whose outside is made up of the upper surface of the leaf. (In all other cases, it is the underside of the leaf that forms the outside of the pocket.

Figure 2. a) Ficus Krishnae leaf 2 b) Ficus Krishnae leaf and fruit

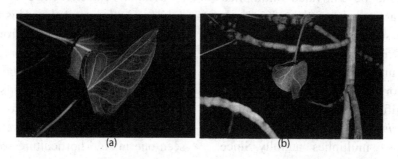

(a)   (b)

But he could not give any reason for this, but said that they might help the tree to retain small quantities of rainwater.

C. de Candolle was faced with a basic question- did these leaves come from a new species of plant? Or were they just strange, anatomical freaks, a chance mutation.

C. de Candolle decided that it was a true natural species in its own right. He would need to examine the figs to confirm this fact, and that might take a few years. In the meantime, he named the plant *Ficus krishnae* and published his findings.

Sometime in the 1930s it slowly became clear that the tree was not really a separate species, but a freakish variety of the banyan. The basis of this discovery was that, if we grow the Krishna fig form a cutting, it will produce pocket leaves identical to the mother plant. But when raised form seed, 90 percent of the seedlings revert to the true banyan form, with only 10 percent retaining the unusual pocket leaves. Botanists call such trees bud-sports, and thay are indeed merely horticultural varieties of some stable species. That's why and how *Ficus krishnae* became *Ficus benghalensis* var. *krishnae*.

This literature is form Trees of Delhi by Pradip Kishen page no. 35. I thought this information will add a good literature to the discussion.

Anand Kumar Bhatt: Thank you, Ushodayan for the info.

Swagat: I have seen one in Hiranandani- Powai (Mumbai). It's planted there.

Madhuri Pejaver: Yes indeed, it's very good information added in discussion. Thanks for the same. When I asked the first question I never thought that we will be able collect such good and informative material. Ushodayan ji's note support information by Ulhas ji. The only point differs that in Ulhas ji's note, he has mentioned that there are no fruits where as in this mail fruit bearing chances are mentioned. Can anybody tell whether fruits are seen on these plants? As I said I have not seen fruits anytime, other mails too support it, somebody is going to look out for

fruits hence forth. Let us see if we notice fruits we will take photos and put on mail. But I feel Ulhas ji must be correct there may not be fruits.

Anand Kumar Bhatt: I think I read somewhere that it has got figs, but if you try to raise plants from the seeds, 90% would revert back to original Bargad and only 10% would be the krishnae. So that probably is the reason why cutting is used for propagation.

Raghu Ananth: Attached some photographs of the Dwarf *Ficus benghalensis* var. *krishnae* from Lalbagh, Bangalore. Photo date: 13 Apr 2008. Looks like, it was fruiting at that time.

Nudrat: *Ficus krishnae* is not considered to be a separate species as it is not mentioned as such in Dr. Almeida's Flora of Maharashtra. The tree at Jijamata Udyan Mumbai does set fruits somewhere between August - October. The fruits are same like those of Ficus benghalensis and the germination pattern of these two trees are identical as I have worked on germination pattern of both these trees. So indeed, *Ficus krishnae* is a var. of *F. benghalensis*.

Madhuri Pejaver: This is really interesting. I think this is the time to visit then Jijamata udyan and see the fruits. Did you find the development of 90% seeds as *F. benghalensis* and 10% as *F. krishnae* as what is explained in previous mails? Do you have any photo taken? If so can you mail it?

Madhuri Pejaver: Here, Raghu ji, in your 2nd photo we can see the fruits. They are like figs as described by some mail. It has really turned out to be a good discussion. Any other information? Every bit is valuable.

V. Tejal: I had seen figs on the tree (*Ficus krishnae*) on our to Jijamata udyan on 10th August 2008. Anoop, could you recollect seeing them too?

Madhuri Pejaver: That is something. Some news. Now, let me see when I get time to visit.

Nita: On a tree trail at Rani Baug, Byculla, Bombay, I spotted figs on the *Ficus krishnae*. I have taken pics. Now let me figure out how to upload them here......

Anand Kumar Bhatt: Somebody earlier had sent pictures. One of them is attached which I had saved.

Learning Points

Detailed learning about *Ficus benghalensis* var. *krishnae*'s ecology, habitat, historical background, distribution, religious importance, treatment a plant as variety or as a species, manifestation of a recessive gene, the problems associated with taxonomic identifications etc. Certainly, the exchange of ideas and information between members of the group does lead to a greater understanding of the problems associated with taxonomic identifications.

Another example concerning the difference between the genera Senna and Cassia:

Dinesh Valke: A large shrub of *Cassia* planted along an avenue near Yeoor Hills, photos taken on 22 AUG 09 (Figure 3). My friend Ajinkya Gadave has already commented in Flickr about this plant to be *Cassia spectabilis*. Please validate ID.

N. S. Dungriyal: Looks like *Cassia glauca*.

Kenneth Greby: I don't believe that this is *Senna spectabilis* (Syn. *S. excelsa, S. carnaval*) due to the flattened seedpods. *S. spectabilis* has roundish to squared (in cross-section) pods with some mucilage present. This looks closer to *S. surattensis*, but I am not positive of that ID.

Yazdi Palia: Could it be *Cassia fistula*? Please check up-

http://en.wikipedia.org/wiki/Golden_Shower_Tree

Dinesh Valke: Yazdi ji, many thanks, but not *Cassia fistula*... Ken, you may be correct. My own first thought matches that of Nayan ji. (I will check later, faintly recollect *S. surattensis* and *C. glauca* are synonymous). Will wait for any further validations?

Tabish: Nayan's ID seems correct to me. *Cassia glauca*, now known as *Senna surattensis*. It has glaucus pinnate leaves, 5-petalled flowers, and flat seedpods up to 20 cm long. The habit also looks right - it is more commonly seen as a shrub.

Gurcharan Singh: Not *Cassia fistula* at least which has distinctive cylindrical long pods. This one seems more probably *C. surratensis*, the only thing that looks different to me is the thin long stalk of pod. The specimens in our garden don't have such long stalks. Leaves and flowers resemble.

Pankaj Oudha: Dear Yazdy, pictures of *Cassia fistula* pods and flowers for your reference.

http://ecoport.org/
ep?SearchType=pdb&PdbID=43989
http://ecoport.org/
ep?SearchType=pdb&PdbID=51252
http://ecoport.org/
ep?SearchType=pdb&PdbID=101448

Nayan Singh: Gurcharan ji, yesterday I id it as *Cassia glauca*, but somehow it is missing in the thread, what do you think about this wild guess?

Figure 3. a) Cassia flower and 3 b) Cassia tree

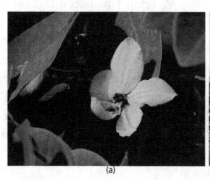
(a)
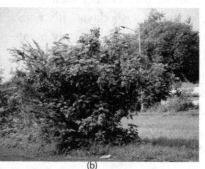
(b)

Nayan Singh: Sorry Gurcharan Singh ji, troubling you, in the other thread of the same topic, I came to know that new name of *Cassia glauca* is *Senna surattensis*, my confusion is now clear.

Satish Pardeshi: It is *Cassia glauca* Lamk., Encyclop. Meth. Bot. 1: 647, 1785; Baker in Hook.f., Fl. Brit. Ind. 2: 265, 1879; Cooke, Fl. Pres. Bombay 1: 453, 1958 (Repr.); Almeida, Fl. Mah. 2: 179, 1998. Synonyms: *Senna sulphurea* (DC. ex Collard) Irwin and Barneby in Mem. New York Bot. Gard. 35(1): 78, 1982; Pradhan et al, Fl. SGNP 244, 2005. *C. surattensis* Burm. f. ssp. *glauca* (Lamk.) K. & S. Larsen, Fl. C.L.V. 18: 102, 1980; Singh et al, Fl. Mah. St. 1: 790, 1996. *C. arborescens* Vahl, Symb. Bot. 3: 56, 1794. *C. sulphurea* DC ex Collad. Hist. Nat. Med. Casses 84, 1816. *Robinia javanica* Burm. f. Fl. Ind. 163, 1768 (non C. javanica L., 1753). *Senna arborescens* Roxb. Fl. Ind. 2: 345, 1832. *C. fastigiata* Vahl. Symb. 3: 57, 1974.

Common names: Karud, Motha-tarved. *C. surattensis* is a synonym of *C. glauca*. The pod with a beak at the other end is one of a diagnosing character very important diagnosing character is All 10 Stamens Are Fertile. Stalked glands present on the rachis at lowermost 2-3 pairs of leaflets. I hope this may clear the doubts about ID.

Dinesh Valke: Many thanks, Satish ji, for validating the ID and providing its specifics. Current accepted name would be *Senna surattensis* (as Tabish has already pointed earlier in this thread). How do we follow current accepted names in India? Is there anybody in India which regulates / maintains such information and knowledge? If there is, does it imply that there would be chance that a species is known by different names across the world, at any given time? Please respond only at your leisure.

Swagat: *'Cassia glauca'* is called 'Motha Tarvad' 'मोठा तरवड' in Marathi. So now, we have to say... *'Senna surattensis'* is called 'Motha Tarvad' 'मोठा तरवड' in Marathi.

Kenneth Greby: I know that most of the shrubby plants (and some of the trees) formerly in Cassia were shifted to *Senna* approximately 10-15 years ago. Some name changes involved simply swapping the genera names; others were not as direct as the example recently discussed. Most of the tree species in *Senna* have rather ill-smelling (when crushed) foliage; I believe all are yellow-flowered. *Cassia* may be pink, red, white, yellow. I'm not certain what other characteristics were used (perhaps DNA) to separate the two genera.

The GRIN listing is generally accepted as the standard for most genera here in the USA. Here is their listing for *Senna*: http://www.ars-grin.gov/cgi-bin/npgs/html/genus.pl?11066 & for Cassia: http://www.ars-grin.gov/cgi-bin/npgs/html/genus.pl?2145

Satish Pardeshi: I say that *Cassia* is preferred over *Senna*. Please visit following link http://www.ars-grin.gov/cgi-bin/npgs/html/taxon.pl?9339. It is the rules and articles of ICBN-International code of Botanical Nomenclature that decides the accepted names of a genus or a species or a family. There are many articles of the code and the plant name which is validly published as on 1 May 1753 were considered valid and correct. However, there were many amendments done- the outcomes were mentioned as code. The latest of which is Vienna 2005. If a plant name or a genus is (not validly) published then that the later name of the same plant or the genus which is validly published (at a later date) is given priority over the previously not validly published name. That's why we have two or more names of same plants.

http://en.wikipedia.org/wiki/International_Code_of_Botanical_Nomenclature

http://www.bgbm.org/iapt/nomenclature/code/default.htm

http://www.bgbm.org/iapt/nomenclature/code/SaintLouis/0000St.Luistitle.htm

Dinesh Valke: Satish ji... thank you very much for the information. NPGS / GRIN and KEW are best suited for me !!!

Gurcharan Singh: Nayan ji, your wild guess was correct in one sense. *Cassia glauca* Lam. and *C. surattensis* Burm.f. are both synonyms of now correctly known *Senna surattensis* (Burm.f.) Irwin & Barneby. At the finer level true surattensis with larger (2-4 inches) leafets in 4-6 pairs, pods 6-8 inches long and known as *Senna surattensis* (Burm.f.) Irwin & Barneby subsp. *surattensis*, whereas *C. glauca* Lam. (*C. glauca* var. *suffruticosa* Koenig in Flora of British India) with 6-9 pair of smaller leaflets (1-2 inches) and smaller pods (3-4 inches. is *Senna surattensis* (Burm.f.) Irwin & Barneby subsp. *sulphurea* (DC. ex Collad) Randell.

And now an interesting one. *C. glauca* Lam. was published in 1789, whereas *C. surattensis* Burm.f. in 1768, and hence latter gets priority when two are treated as same species. At subspecies level, true *surattensis* is subsp. *surattensis* (no authority, as it is automatically created name if we treat *C. glauca* as distinct subspecies-it is autonym). and now you will ask why not to use subsp. *glauca* as name. Well *Cassia glauca* Lam, 1789 and *C. sulphurea* DC. ex Collad., 1816 are synonyms, and hence former is prefered, but when transferred to genus *Senna* (all 10 stamens perfect), *Senna glauca* Roxb., is already used for a different species, and *sulphurea* gets preference. I hope it was not very boring..

Madhuri Pejaver: Not at all boring. Without turning a single page of the book the Botany of 1973 is getting revised for me.

Nayan Singh: Thanks Gurcharan ji. Thanks a lot for your detail and very-very informative note.

J. M. Garg: Thanks, Singh ji, for your efforts, explaining the things in such a simple way. Botany is being enjoyed this way, in contrast to what we felt in school days.

Gurcharan Singh: I think we should follow GRIN for species which are listed (many Indian species are not) and Kew World checklist species (for families which have been completed). For rest we can always develop a consensus.

Learning Points

Detailed learning about difference between species *Senna surattensis* & *Cassia fistula* & between genus *Senna* & *Cassia*. *Senna surattensis*'s ecology, botanical naming system being followed, ICBN-International code of Botanical Nomenclature, importance of GRIN (Germplasm Resources Information Network), Kew World checklist etc.

IMPLEMENTING NEW IDEAS FOR USER DRIVER LEARNING IN BOTANY

Conscious that a large amount of information on Indian Flora was accumulating, J.M.Garg set about creating a Database for the benefit of the group's members. If any plant already in the database came up for discussion again, it would be a simple matter of accessing the Indiantreepix database as it contains information about botanical names, common names, flowering data, earlier 'Indiantreepix' thread links, and other useful links giving relevant information about a particular plant. All the posts made on Indiantreepix were included in the database in the form of a hyper link that could be followed to reveal the information stored previously. The information available in the Database is not just for the layperson though. Details of taxonomic treatments by and for expert botanists are also available. There are many websites available for the dissemination of information and Flickr sites for images, but the Database holds an accumulation of knowledge available to members and is a good example of User Driven learning in Botany. The data collated by the group is not always perfect and depends on the feedback from the members and experts in the group. The data stored in this Database is only as good as its sources, however, and is dependent on feedback from members and experts in the group. As more data is collated and worked into usable information database, it will keep on improving. It is vitally important that the members continue to add information and look at ways of improving the accuracy of the identifications fed into the system.

It was encouraging that just after seven months time, we have graduated more than 250 messages per month. This was possible because of a master stoke, which possibly no other e-group has ever tried/ attended. Why don't I create a database? After all everybody is spending so much of time on the group which in terms of man-hours, will be quite substantial. Why so many man-hours should be wasted? Or why should not so many man-hours result into something substantial, which will help us in our quest of knowing about Indian Flora further. I tried experimenting with this in an Excel sheet and after about a month, I was ready with a database of around 125 plants in March'08, which had already been discussed on 'Indiantreepix' till that time.

Though, it was a time consuming expertise, but its benefits to the members and others were manifold. If any plant was posted/discussed on this forum again, I have to simply copy from the Indiantreepix database and paste it in the mail against the reply as it had botanical names, common names, flowering data, earlier 'Indiantreepix' thread links, other useful links giving relevant information etc. about a plant. If one knows the plant i.e. to say a Bauhinia and he wanted to look for the exact species of Bauhinia, he can look at the different Bauhinia species available in the Indiantreepix Database like Bauhinia acuminata, Bauhinia purpurea, Bauhinia variegata etc. This way 'Indiantreepix Database' became a very good reference for the members in a situation where it was very difficult to find a good book in the market for a layman. All the posts made on Indiantreepix were included in the database in the form of a hyperlink. In the process, we realised

that flowering of lot of trees has been delayed, compared to what is stated in the reference books.

We also realised that one day this database will serve as a good data for the purpose of verification and analysis of the facts on Indian Flora and for the purpose of research etc. It pleased me a lot that hard work and passion of hundreds of members may be leading us to make a substantial contribution to the Indian Flora, though in a small way to start with & without any formal organisation or without spending a penny from anybody's pocket. Appreciation me and other contributors received from others, itself was enough for efforts of different members.

A question comes to everybody's mind why I chose a Database over a website. But I think such works i.e. website etc. are already done by Tabish ji (and host of other websites are also available), while Dinesh ji is doing a similarly wonderful job on Flickr. I, myself, put my images on Wikimedia Commons (which can be used by anybody all over the world without permission as per licence conditions). I am also connecting pictures on Wikipedia- a wonderful collaborative efforts, in which my contributions may be limited, but it has such tremendous value- one can use its contents in a way one likes without taking anybody's permission. We all know net is full of information these days & more & more information is added every day to it. It's just available at a click away on search. I personally feel that doing things which are different & help in matters which other things available can't- it is a better value proposition. Even all discussions on Indiantreepix are searchable & can be seen by anybody. One can manipulate it in a way he wants & use it as per his requirements. Data is not always perfect & depends on the feedback from the members & experts on the group. It always keep on improving as more & more feedback is received & more & more plants get identified.

MEASURING PERFORMANCE/ SUCCESS OF USER DRIVEN LEARNING IN BOTANY

How successful has Indiantreepix been? Looking purely at the number of messages received, interest has grown from an average of 124 messages per month in 2007, to 508 per month in 2008 and 1,291 per month in 2009. The number of messages received does not necessarily reflect the content and efficacy of the site, but it does indicate its popularity – the willingness of people to enter into the spirit of identifying Indian flora. There are now over a thousand members of Indiantreepix, many of them recognized experts in some field of botany.

I knew that the if a group has to grow to make a substantial Impact in the scene of Indian flora, continued efforts is required for increase of the membership including adding more and more experts on the forum. I have to spend time every day where on an average I was writing to around 10 persons individually for becoming the members of Indiantreepix. For this, I have to become the member a lot of other groups which were concerned with nature and various fields like Birds, Butterflies, Insects, Reptiles, and Conservation etc. Some of these were becoming new members while some of the old members may be getting away because of the time constrains or decreasing interest in the subject. Thus, there has always been a churning in the group with some of the old members getting away while new members coming into its fold. The membership of the group has been consistently increasing every month by around 30 to 40 Nos. due to the sustained efforts made by me in a pro-active way. I set a target of 500 members at the end of one year of Indiantreepix. I know it was a very stiff target though not impossible to achieve. Though always came to my mind and in the minds of others that one day we may be exhausted of the new members to whom we can write to become members or of the trees we can discuss in the forum. But it was not

true, but only a fear in my mind and by the end of one year completion of Indiantreepix, I was so happy to see the membership at 450 Nos., though extra-ordinary efforts were required in the process.

There were occasions when we will get some of the very good members with good knowledge of Indian flora and a lot of time to spare to the group. Such occasions result in picking up activity in Indiantreepix. The member of messages received and growth in the group is reflected from the posts per month as per details below:-

June-Dec.'07- around 100-150 messages
Jan.- June'08- around 300- 500 messages
June-Dec.'087- around 600-700 messages
Jan.- June'08- around 1000- 1400 messages

It has moved to a new higher trajectory now with many good experts, who are willing to contribute, joining the group with around 2200 messages in August'09 & more than 1015 members.

MANAGING CONFLICTS AND SENSE MAKING FROM MULTIPLE INPUTS DURING USER DRIVER LEARNING IN BOTANY

J.M.Garg spends time each month inviting new members to join, especially experts from other fields that had an abiding interest in botany and Indian flora. Membership has risen in the last two years to over a thousand, and messaging on-list to an average of seventy a day. Members come from diverse backgrounds and include taxonomists, botanists, doctors, engineers, conservationists, forest officials, NGOs, ecologists, photographers, environmentalists, naturalists, authors, farmers, birders, trekkers, garden lovers, nature lovers, animal lovers etc. There are persons having expertise in different climatic areas of India: Western Himalayas, Central and Eastern Himalayas, Western India, Central India, South India, Tropical East India, each area having its unique climatic conditions and flora. In fact there is hardly a region from which the members are not available. Membership includes a lot of high profile individuals with whom anybody would like to be associated because of their immense contribution in their areas of working. The group now has persons who are deeply passionate about Indian flora and are working on the platform of making Indian flora available on the Internet in the form of write-ups, photographs, local names etc. With such a background, conflicts are inevitable, which Moderators have to manage properly in such a way that it doesn't become a source of acrimony between members.

This is explained below by quoting a few conversations here from Indiantreepix. Gurcharan Singh introduced a group thread that dealt with the use of author names and synonyms for inclusion in Indiantreepix Database. (see Table 1)

The Plant names without author names are sometimes used in general purpose books and text books, not in taxonomic treatments or databases. Whenever these are used without author names, it is understood that there is only one species by that name, or the validly published one. If we apply this logic our names would be written as shown in Table 2.

In all these cases the synonym is of earlier date, and should be used as correct name and not as synonym. We are using them as synonyms because they were named as accepted names in Hooker's Flora of British India, and other Indian Floras, but the indian material was subsequently found to be different species. The citations would be meaningful if properly cited as shown in Table 3.

Table 1.

Gurcharan Singh: Consider these names in our databases:	
Indigofera astragalina	Syn: I. hirsuta
Phyllanthus amaru	Syn: P. nirurii
Ficus microcarpa	Syn: F. retusa
Crateva adansonii	Syn: C.. religiosa
Acalypha lanceolata	Syn: A. indica
Zizyphus mauritiana	Syn: Z. jububa

Table 2.

Indigofera astragalina DC., 1825	Syn: I. hirsuta Linn., 1753
Phyllanthus amarus Schumach., 1827	Syn: P. nirurii Linn., 1753
Ficus microcarpa Linn.f., 1781	Syn: F. retusa Linn., 1753
Crateva adansonii DC., 1824	Syn: C. religiosa G. Forst., 1786
Acalypha lanceolata Willd, 1768	Syn: A. indica Linn., 1753
Zizyphus mauitiana Lamk., 1789	Syn: Z. jujuba Mill, 1789.

Table 3.

Indigofera astragalina DC., 1825	Syn: I. hirsuta Baker (non Linn., 1753)
Phyllanthus amarus Schumach., 1827	Syn: P. nirurii Hook.f. (non Linn., 1753) (however, I don't find any standard publication following this nomenclature. The most usually followed is this one:
Phyllanthus fraternus Webster, 1955	Syn: P. niruri Hook.f. (non Linn.))
Ficus microcarpa Linn.f., 1781	Syn: F. retusa auct. (non Linn., 1753)
Crateva adansonii DC., 1824	Syn: C. religiosa Auct (non G. Forst., 1786)
Acalypha lanceolata Willd, 1768	Syn: A. indica Linn., 1753 (I don't know of any publication which cites A. indica as synonym of A. lanceolata. In case they are synonyms, A. indica should be accepted name, unless it is another case of misidentification with A. indica)
Zizyphus mauitiana Lamk., 1789	Syn: Z. jujuba Lamk. (non Mill, 1768)

Our databases are slowly expanding and should soon become most frequently visited by plant lovers and botanists, and I feel the need for proper representation of data. This can happen only if names of species and authors are properly represented.

It may take some time to correct older records, but at least from now onwards we can decide to include names and synonyms with proper author citation, to make our databases useful to botanists in general and researchers in particular.

This statement was then followed up by an active discussion on the need for proper referencing, and the need for the entries to be kept simple so as to remain comprehensible by non-taxonomy members.

Pankaj Kumar: With due respects to Dr. Gurcharan Singh, For author citations, according to ICBN, it is recommended that abbreviations needs to be followed for authors using following reference (RECOMMENDATION 46A, ICBN): Brummitt, R. K. and C. E. Powell. 1992. Authors of plant names: a list of authors of scientific names of plants, with recommended standard forms of their names, including abbreviations. Royal Botanic Gardens, Kew. There are various editions of this book, which keep updating information with the new author names and their abbreviations. So, Carolus Linnaeus is cited as 'L.' and not as 'Linn.' And Jean-Baptiste Lamarck is cited as 'Lam.' and not as 'Lamk.'. Some of these abbreviations are present at the following site: http://en.wikipedia.org/wiki/List_of_botanists_by_author_abbreviation The latest code of ICBN: Vienna Code is available at the following link for free: http://ibot.sav.sk/icbn/main.htm. I am sending this information just in case members want it to be standardized properly, for use by both taxonomists as well as non-botanists.

Gurcharan Singh: Thanks Pankaj ji for information. We are students all our life, and there is nothing better than learning few things. Nothing to feel apologetic.

Padmini Raghavan: Would it be expecting too much for the site to stay simple and interesting for non-botanists? Or could the more specialised and higher level discussions be put on a different link so as not to intimidate the lay plant-lover? (Just a suggestion, which I hope is taken impartially.)

Pankaj Kumar: Hello All, Giving this site slightly botanical touch will not at all hamper the Botanical understanding of the non-botanical experts!!! It will not at all hamper anyone in anyways. I know people like Tabish who are not at all from a botany background but still I find him better than at least me most of the time. But of course the decision should be accepted by all and not only by me.

Amit Ray: I concur with this opinion. Indiantreepix is tending to get a bit too scientific for me. Please do not get me wrong. I am a lay person with love for photography and nature and that is what has drawn me to this group when Garg ji started it. I do appreciate the help provided by the experts. This is just my opinion - many probably will not agree. Thanks and regards to all of you.

Gurcharan Singh: Amit ji, Padmani ji and other non-botany colleagues, All of us are bound by one thing: Love for photography, love for nature and curiosity to know what plant I have clicked. In that no one is botanist or non-botanist. All of us also want our plant to be identified correctly, and it is here that botanical names come in handy, and they are more meaningful when author name is attached. No garden lover would have missed the common garden flower cornflower. We all also know that it is botanically Centaurea cyanus, but incidentally it is also known as bachelor's button, blue bottle, ragged robin. If you search for blue bottle on the internet, you will reach Centaurea cyanus, Muscari neglectum, species of Gentiana or even an insect Calliphora vomitoria. Safeda for us in Delhi and elsewhere is Eucalyptus spp. but if ask any one from Kashmir for a twig of Safeda, he/she will give you Populus spp. All these problems are not there when using botanical name. Each species will have only one accepted scientific name, known all over the world. You can extract all common names for this plant, not vice versa as indicated above.

And now the names with authors. I will just give you just yesterday's example.Swagat ji (17625) uploaded a photograph which I identified as Atropa acuminata Royle., appropriately known as Indian belladona, a very important medicinal plant common in Himalayas. If you look for its description in Older Indian books you will find it identified as A. belladona Linn., the European bellodona L. which looks totally different (see it on Flowers of India-often cultivated in gardens). So won't you like to know whether your plant is belladona (deadly-nightshade) or Indian bella-dona. Botanically it can be written (as per present practice in Indiantreepix and Flowers of India):

Atropa acuminata	Syn: A. belladona

What is your opinion is it correct? Or else this one is better:

Atropa acuminata Royle	Sy: A. belladona Clarke (non L.)

Make your choice, shortcut and confusion or clarity. Not to forget, many experts here in the group burn midnight oil to see that your plants are correctly identified. A plant sent by me at 1.30 in night was identified by Pankaj ji at 2.15 at night. We can all see the efforts and contributions of Kenneth to see that our plants are correctly identified. All have love for plants and passion for photography.

M. Sundararaman: Dear and respected Dr Gurcharan, You have kindly provided enough excuse for me not to undertake studying about trees and Saplings and their Botanical Names. I am a B.E by Qln and spread tree-planting culture within my limited means of understanding. My

Group of such "Unpads" in the "Friends of Nature" group (including IT/commerce) raise Saplings of "Thespesia populnea", Neem, Pongamia glabra (or pinnata), Cassia fistula, Sterculia....in 1/2 Litre or one-litre milk-sachet and distribute freely to provide more health and environment with the grace of God, the Almighty. However, I would like to be guided whenever it becomes necessary. I really wonder how our friend Sri Garg gets time and energy to moderate his group while in office in an important Portfolio. I am attaching a write-up on my hobby which keeps me healthier at 68 and also the world healthy by more Oxygen and greenery. You can spread this hobby for practice to your friends in the retired life.

Pankaj Oudha: Thanks, Guruchahran ji for your comments. I work with Traditional Healers. They don't have basic modern education. They are not aware whether ovary is superior or infe-rior but still they identify the plants without any mistake. There is no chance of mistake as they have to use it for patients. Small error may lead to the death of patients. They identify plants from distance. I have observed that they have far more information than our standard floras have. They don't use modern scientific names (and methods of quoting it) but still they know much more than the so called experts. Ayurveda is in front of us as example, without modern complexities of modern nomenclature. I feel that along with adopting modern science there is need to learn methods of ancient science specially for plant identification. I show my pictures to Traditional Healers. Without any delay they identify it from picture. They don't ask for pictures of all parts. They identify it even from one or two leaf stage. I feel that we must learn this art of identification, instead of wasting time to "please" the western researchers. Let world follow our system of nomenclature if they want to learn from Indian experiences. Please correct me, if I am wrong.

J.M.Garg: Dear members, I think the discussion will be unending with pros & cons on everything including this topic. I thank all the participants for contributing their frank views on the matter, which only shows how much one cares for this group "Indiantreepix'. Question was only from my side, as I update the database, as below: "........ I don't know how to go about it. It may take me sometime to comprehend the whole thing........." As on date, I will be trying to give Author name along with the Bot. names to be more specific (it hardly complicates anything while adding value to our members) - to start with for new addition to the Database or the plants, where there are chances of confusion (as pointed out by Singh ji for the few species in this thread). May be I get to comprehend the things over time & look for expanding, provided time is available or somebody else takes up the job of updating the database (as it keeps me away from wonderful discussions that take place on this group, helping members with Ids & learning a lot in the process). I close this thread here only & request members not to give any more feedbacks in the matter.

Gurcharan Singh: Dear Sundaram ji, Let me first show my appreciation to know that there is someone older than me in this group. We are separated by four years. I greatly appreciate the great work you are doing. I still remember as child picking up Guchhi (Morchella), Kan dole (Halvella) as two most delicious wild plants (now guchhi with overexploitation, is costlier than gold), which I could remember from childhood (no botany knowledge) and could identify specimens botanically when in M. Sc. In that sense there is no botanist and non-botanist. My mother could identify young plants of Saag, Sarson, belonging to Brassica, whereas many botanists can't do it from even flowering specimens. Yours, mine, my mother and similar cases are isolated ones. We want the progress of whole India, for that information spread is essential, and more important correct one at that, so that we don't spend crores of rupees on importing products from outside. India and Africa are richest areas are floristic diversity, but among poorest in the World, because is paucity of information, and proper exploitation. Let us not just be happy with our heritage. In this world of competition, we have to learn more to compete and progress. I remember once visiting Nainital- on way we stayed in a village. The whole village was out of their homes for 8-10 hours because a holy person had come to give herbal cure for their eyes. When they came back I asked for the plant my host got from the saint. I went out and showed him plants growing in front of his house. It was Eclipta alba, (Bringaaraja in Sanskrit; Bhangra, mochkand in Hindi). There are thousands of such instances in our country. There is need to educate our people, and that is possible, if we know them correctly our self. That has been my objective throughout.

LIMITATIONS/ STRENGTHS OF USER DRIVER LEARNING IN BOTANY

One of the limitations of Indiantreepix as a User Driven learning site for botany is its very strength. It has a wide base of knowledge made up of everyone from botanical experts to persons eager to learn all they can about Indian flora, to people who just like the pictures and can only make general comments about identification. Furthermore, an expert can sometimes get it wrong and a layperson can make a good guess. If there is disagreement about a particular identification, who is to be believed? Is there any way of lending weight to some identifications and politely throwing doubt on others?

Max Overton has suggested a numerical scale by which the information offered up for identification can be judged and one by which the reliability of the persons identifying it can be ascertained. The former scale could be formed along the lines of complete information including a full suite of photos being at the high end of acceptability and a fuzzy photo being at the low end. He suggests a simple scale along these lines shown in Table 4.

Table 4.

Information provided	Acceptability
Photos of all plant parts, habitat, location, soil	5
Some photos, location	4
Some photos, or a single one with location	3
Single photo with general location	2
Photo out of focus, too distant, or too general	1

Table 5.

Knowledge field of member	Reliability for specific identification
The family of the plant to be identified	5
Families related to plant to be identified	4
General group of plants (trees, shrubs, herbs)	3
A good general knowledge of plants	2
A guess at the identification	1

These values could be assigned after posting, by J.M.Garg, and should not cast aspersions on the person asking for the identification. There are many reasons why full information cannot be provided, and it undoubtedly makes identification harder unless an expert can recognise it. An expert need not be someone with a botanical degree; it could be someone who happened to see a very similar plant in a garden.

The reliability of the identifier is the other aspect that needs to be addressed. This is not something that individual members should be concerned about, nor feel affronted if their identification is assigned a low reliability. For instance, if a grass was offered up for identification and three members entered into an argument about the species shown, would it not be more realistic to lend greater weight to the expert in the Poaceae than to the member who loved forest orchids or the one who worked with fruit trees? The next species up for identification may be an orchid and the reliability of those same three members would be reassigned.

Max has suggested a scale along the lines shown in Table 5.

In the example given previously, the member working in the Poaceae would be assigned a reliability record for the grass of 5, but only 3 for the orchid, whereas the orchid enthusiast would be 3 for the grass and 5 for the orchid. The fruit tree expert would be 3 for both species.

Max suggests that J.M.Garg, as controller of the Database, assigns a numerical value for each

identification made, based on the information provided and the knowledge base of the identifier. This does not even have to be published in a message to the members as a whole, but can be held in the database for users. A combination of the two scales may provide a greater range of acceptability, and one can imagine that an identification by an expert in that field based of a full set of information (Rating $5 \times 5 = 25$) would be more reliable than an identification of one fuzzy photo by a layperson making a guess (Rating $1 \times 1 = 1$).

However, J.M.Garg feels that the system suggested by Max is very complicated & difficult to implement in the 'Indiantreepix' environment, where he himself is pressed hard for time. Further useful reliable links are also provided along with 'Indiantreepix' links in the Database, from which one can easily verify the correct identification of a plant or otherwise.

REQUIREMENTS FOR SUCCESS OF USER DRIVEN LEARNING IN BOTANY

Good inspiring leadership, sustained efforts, innovative approach, deep passion for the subject & the welfare of the members is required for any user driven learning to become successful.

Reasons for this astonishing growth?

1. Sustained hard work and devotion of time on regular basis everyday by the Moderators of the group.
2. Sharing power and responsibility among the Moderators/Managers.
3. Due credit being given to Moderators/ Managers along with regular encouragement to them.
4. Putting the man-hours spent by experts and other members on the group to good use in the form of 'Indiantreepix Database'.
5. Working in the scenario where other resources like books and information on Net of Indian flora being deficient or very sketchy.
6. Maintaining gentle and cordial environment among members and experts.
7. Constant Expert's guidance.
8. Good Management & a clear vision
9. Understanding the needs of the members & helping them to the extent possible.

FUTURE DIRECTIONS

Online learning in botany through Indiantreepix has inculcated a feeling of attachment among the members toward the Indian flora. They care more about it as a result of increased knowledge and awareness about it. The group has played a vital role in creating awareness, inculcating a scientific attitude, helping in identification, spreading knowledge and bringing it within reach of a layman, and helping in the documentation of Indian Flora.

Earlier the Flora used to be illustrated with the line drawings but now with the coming of digital photography, things have changed. Books, websites etc. on Flora are more and more illustrated with good quality photographs. 'Indiantreepix' has developed a passionate band of volunteers who will come out to different areas all over India and photograph Indian flora in all its splendour.

'Indiantreepix Database' has become a good resource for having good collection of photographs of hundreds of species although they remain copyright to the members concerned.

Time is not far away that Flora of India and its states will be illustrated with these good photographs. Lot of members were put up this excellent photograph after identification/ confirmation on 'Indiantreepix' at Wikimedia Commons, Flicker, Web shot, Picasa etc. Hundreds of articles on Wikepedia & other sites are now been illustrated from the pictures uploaded by the members on Wikimedia Commons, Flicker etc.

What is of the more important that 'Indiantreepix' has inculcated a feeling of attachment among the members towards the Indian flora. They have started to care more about it and with their increase in knowledge, their passions have also increased. 'Indiantreepix' has played a very vital role in creating awareness, inculcating scientific temper, helping in identification, spreading knowledge, bringing it within reach of a laymen, helping in documentation etc. of Indian Flora.

With activity on the up-swing with more than 2000 messages in August, 2009, it is not far to visualise its impact in the future. All are contributing their own bit in compiling virtual image library of Indian flora. It is not far off when India will be having its own e-flora on the lines of e-flora of China, e-flora of Pakistan etc. The image resource of 'Indiantreepix Database' and other contributions of the members elsewhere, may play a vital role in this. The contributions of 'Indiantreepix' will continue to be felt in the websites, books and other media in one form or the other. This is not to forget the services it is rendering now as mentioned in the 'Contributions' above.

Max states that Indiantreepix as a User driven botanical resource has the opportunity of becoming a premier source of information on Indian flora. He is confident that with an ever-growing enthusiastic membership and a careful consideration of the identifications made through interactive messages and database compilation, this group can make a valuable contribution to the science of Botany within India.

CONCLUSION

This was an illustration of a 'User driven learning environment' created in an online community with a special interest centred on trees and plants. It tried to trace the development of an online learning community through the lived experiences and thoughts of its founding members and also included conversational learning experiences of other users to illustrate the process of 'user driven learning' in online communities. A few points made in some of the conversational threads were directly related to sense making from multiple inputs which illustrates the 'user driven' nature of learning among increasingly connected human users of the web. This entire conversational learning can redefine learning in Botany and an entire textbook could be written in a conversational

manner covering other topics in this as well as other subjects.

REFERENCES

Clark, C. J. (1998). *Let your online learning community grow: 3 design principles for growing successful Email Listervs and online forums in educational settings*. San Diego State University. Retrieved September 14, from http://www.noend-press.com/caleb/olc/3Principles_Online_Comm.pdf

Moisseeva, M. (2007). *Online learning communities and collaborative learning. Institute of International Education, New York*. Retrieved July 21, 2009, from http://www.iienetwork.org/?p=41543.

Wikipedia (2009). *Online learning community*. Retrieved September 14th from http://en.wikipedia.org/wiki/Online_learning_community.

Chapter 20
Online Learning in Discussion Groups:
A Sense–Making Approach[1]

David J. Schaefer
Franciscan University of Steubenville, USA

Brenda Dervin
The Ohio State University, USA

ABSTRACT

Recently, theorists concerned about the democratic quality of electronic group discussions have advocated the incorporation of situational information to facilitate consensus/dissensus activity. In this chapter, we demonstrate the utilization of a discussion group design and analytical process informed by Sense-Making Methodology to highlight the relationship between situational aspects of online dialogue and consensus/dissensus activity. We analyzed 1,360 messages submitted to three pedagogical discussion groups. The postings fell into two broad situational modes: (a) dialogic, which coincided with an outward orientation and a greater number of agreeing/disagreeing micro-practices, and (b) contemplative, which demonstrated more inwardly-focused personalized observations and far fewer agreeing/disagreeing micro-practices. These findings suggest that, counter to received theories advocating the privileging of user-to-user interaction within online discussion groups, both modes appeared to be important for robust communicative activities.

INTRODUCTION:

Situation Movement States and Consensus/Dissensus in Online Public Spheres

As global digital networks began to encircle the globe in the 1970s, researchers developed electronic bulletin board-style discussion groups to facilitate asynchronous dialogue among far-flung colleagues. Over time, systems like USENET, BITNET, The WELL, and others became popular among users (Hiltz and Turoff, 1977/1993; Rheingold, 1993; Schaefer, 1999a). Meanwhile, practitioners within a variety of fields, including education, politics, and health care, increasingly utilized computer mediated

DOI: 10.4018/978-1-60960-097-6.ch020

communication (CMC) to enhance dialogic processes between participants in online forums (see Gurak & Antonijevic, 2008; Kim, Lee, & Guild, 2009; Schaefer & Dervin, 2009). Educators, for example, were optimistic about the use of such systems for the creation of online environments to facilitate democratic discussions among students (Ess, 1996; 2000; 2002; Ess and Cavalier, 1996). Today, a wide array of online discussion systems have been increasingly incorporated into course designs, marketed by companies like Jenzabar, WebCT, SCT, and Facebook.

Within health care, practitioners sought to use CMC in a variety of ways. Forster (2009) noted that, since the 1990s, there had been an explosion in the development of online discussion groups, listservs, and blogs devoted to health care topics. Users scoured the Internet for information on particular diseases, posed questions to health care professionals, and created blogs that chronicled personal experiences with treatments, often obtaining support from other patients, family or friends (Heilferty, 2009). Heilferty (2009) noted that while the majority of online health-related information had been created by medical professionals, the rapid growth of online forms and blogs provided a wealth of user-generated content that proved to be popular among users.

Ironically, however, researchers have also questioned the potential of online discussion groups to facilitate productive dialogues. Recent findings have suggested that such systems often reinforce powerful hegemonies that distort and steer communicative processes. For example, Ess (2002) reported that several international networks had been captured by commercial imperatives that controlled and limited possibilities for the democratic exchange of ideas and discussion. Yates (2001) argued that pedagogical discussion groups were at the mercy of non-democratic practices that seriously hampered the emergence of productive dialogue. Schaefer (2000) identified more than eight control-oriented practices that impeded democratic web discussions, including insider-

outsider labeling and excluding, flaming, abusive moderator practices, etc. Smith, McLaughlin, and Osborne (1998) reported that USENET users often experienced harsh reproachment techniques in response to transgressive behaviors. Qian & Scott (2007) found that bloggers often expressed concern about the negative effects of disclosing personal information online. Within health care, Forster (2009) noted that concerns over the quality of online information "raise[d] questions about the extent and effectiveness of blogs as a means of dialogue among... patients" (p. 24). Kim, Lee, & Guild (2009) pointed out that information seekers needed to actively assess the credibility of online health care information as a guard against potentially erroneous or misleading user-generated content passed around in online forums.

In order to better understand dialogic processes within online public spheres, computer-mediate communication (abbreviated CMC) theorists began to draw upon the theoretical work of German philosopher Jurgen Habermas (see Baynes, 1994; Ess, 1996; 2000; 2002; Herring, 1993; Papacharissi, 2002; Papacharissi, 2004; Rananand, 2003; Sharrock and Button, 1997; Yates, 2001). Habermas (1984) defined an Ideal Speech Situation[2] as one in which all interlocutors presupposed symmetrical structural conditions. Smaling (2000) noted that approximations of ideal speech situations only occurred when participants were made aware of otherwise hidden coercive structures. Thus, theorists have argued that awareness of situational characteristics of CMC is crucial for undistorted communicative action. Ess (2002) argued that proper critique of CMC discussion fora required analysis of "situational empowerment"--the means by which systems tacitly impose structural constraints on users. Brothers (2000) noted that one of the primary limitations of CMC was the lack of appropriate situational information -- circumstantial information surrounding the creation of online content (i.e. what *led* a user to contribute an online posting [e.g., he/she just wanted to kill time, or connect with an admired

person, or vent frustration with a problem, etc.)"--
needed by participants to evaluate the credibility
of others' information.

Despite this current interest in contextual influences in CMC, Hiltz and Turoff (1977/1993)
reported that explicating the nature of situational
variables within CMC environments had been a
key research concern for the past several decades.
For example, in the 1970s, designers of early CMC-
based DELPHI systems incorporated features that
queried users about situational assumptions and
uncertainties in order to contextualize the group
decision-making process. They noted that making
such information explicit generally aided group
decision-making.

In the 1980s, Winograd and Flores (1987)
drew upon speech act theory for similar purposes.
They developed a system called The Coordinator
to facilitate CMC decision-making within organizational contexts. The system asked participants
to identify the illocutionary nature of their speech
act prior to posting their message (e.g., making a
request or promise, making or accepting an offer,
reporting, acknowledging). They concluded that
rather than facilitating decision-making, asking
participants to identify such acts at the start of
the process often irritated users, thus impeding
communicative action.

In the 1990s, perhaps as a result of the impact
of the oft-cited Coordinator findings, researchers
shied away from further explication of situational
variables in CMC research. More typically, situations were simply defined as (a) task/problem
contexts faced by users in CMC studies (e.g.,
requiring users to engage in team-writing or
research projects; see Broome and Chen, 1992;
Chidambaram, Bostrom, and Wynne, 1990;
Sproull and Kiesler, 1991; Straus, 1996;) or (b)
media conditions imposed on research subjects
in quasi-experimental designs (e.g., comparing
performance in CMC and Face-to-Face [FtF]
groups, exploring the impact of anonymity; see
Valacich, Dennis, and Nunamaker, 1992; Poole,

Holmes, Watson, and DeSanctis, 1993; Walther,
1992; Whitworth, Gallupe, and McQueen, 2000).

Typically, CMC researchers explored how
groups could reach consensus (and avoid dissensus) within empirical online contexts. Consensus-
making and/or dissensus-avoiding were chiefly
operationalized as static dependent variables
occurring at the conclusion of an online discussion (Gallupe & McKeen, 1990; Hollingshead,
McGrath, & O'Connor, 1993; Mabrito, 1992;
Olaniran, 1994; Valacich, George, Nunamaker,
& Vogel, 1994; Rice, 1980).

However, as argued by Carter (1988; 1991;
2003), Dervin (2003a; 2003b), and others, one
of the reasons why researchers have been unable
to more fully understand how communicative
processes impede or facilitate the development
of productive online dialogues is because many
of their investigative designs are inadequate for
illuminating the complexities of dialogic practice
as situated process. Rather, current models are
often based upon outmoded transmission/linear
flow models that obscure complex communicative processes (Forman-Wernet, 2003). Thus, few
studies have been conducted that actually explore
the relationship between grounded situational
variables and agreeing/disagreeing processes in
CMC environments.

In order to develop situationally oriented con-
sensus/dissensus research, we needed a methodology that would allow us to focus on the time-space
situated communicative *actings* or *energizings*
that constituted dialogue in online discussion
groups. Toward this end, we drew upon Sense-
Making Methodology (Dervin, 2003a) and the
communication-as-procedure framework (Dervin
and Clark, 2003) as part of an ongoing research
project designed to more fully illuminate how
communicative processes actually facilitate or
impede the development of democratic practices
within pedagogical discussion groups (see Schaefer, 2001; Schaefer & Dervin, 2001; Schaefer &
Dervin, 2003; Schaefer & Dervin, 2009).

SENSE-MAKING METHODOLOGY:

Reconceptualizing Online Dialogue as Verbings

Heavily influenced by Carter (2003), Sense-Making Methodology (Dervin, 1984; Dervin & Foreman-Wernet, 2003) provides both metatheoretical and empirical frameworks for explicating dialogic processes within online discussion groups. In development since the mid-1970s, Sense- Making Methodology posits as its core premise the gappiness/discontinuity of reality, which mandates human agents to continually bridge (and unbridge) gaps via time-space situated cognitive, behavioral, emotional, or spiritual practices[3]. In essence, these practices are communicative behavings that constitute the *hows* of communicating – the *verbings* by which individuals make and unmake sense as they move through time-space, confront gaps, and so on. As suggested by this approach, such theorizing mandates a shift in focus from *communicative nouns* (descriptions of senders, receivers, media, effects, etc.) to *communicative verbs* – behavioral processes by which humans make and unmake bridges over gaps.

Sense-Making Methodology's focus on time, space, movement, and gap is represented by a multi-dimensional gap-bridging metaphor as illustrated in Figure 1. The metaphor mandates that researchers explore six key gap-bridging dimensions: (a) contexts – the social/cultural contexts within which human communicators operate; (b) situations -- time-space anchored moments where agents find themselves blocked, stopped, or hindered; (c) gaps -- the questions, confusions, and muddles agents experience; (d) bridges -- the cognitive/emotive/spiritual procedures agents use to construct/deconstruct sense over gaps; (e) verbings – the communicative actings or energizings by which these procedures are actualized, and (f) outcomes/uses -- the helps/hindrances agents receive or avoid within communicative situations

Methodologically, the Sense-Making approach provides multiple sets of tools to study communication along any of the dimensions. For example, to study situations, researchers can focus on the situation movement states experienced by

Figure 1. Sense-making methodology's central metaphor (Note: Graphic used with permission from Dervin, Foreman-Wernet, and Lauterbach (2003))

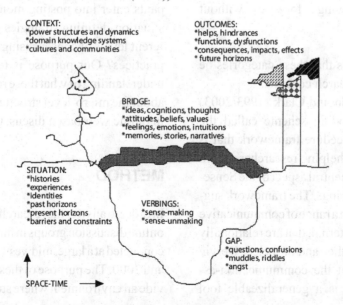

CONTEXT:
*power structures and dynamics
*domain knowledge systems
*cultures and communities

OUTCOMES:
*helps, hindrances
*functions, dysfunctions
*consequences, impacts, effects
* future horizons

BRIDGE:
*ideas, cognitions, thoughts
*attitudes, beliefs, values
*feelings, emotions, intuitions
*memories, stories, narratives

SITUATION:
*histories
*experiences
*identities
*past horizons
*present horizons
*barriers and constraints

VERBINGS:
*sense-making
*sense-unmaking

GAP:
*questions, confusions
*muddles, riddles
*angst

SPACE-TIME →

humans as they move through time-space. Specifically, this focus taps "the different qualitative ways in which [a] respondent see his or her movement through time-space blocked" (Dervin, 2003c, p. 260). For example, Dervin (2003c, p. 262) provides a useful coding list of various situation movement states. These include:

- *Decision* -- deciding between multiple roads in order to continue;
- *Problematic* – feeling impelled along an unwanted road;
- *Spin-out* – feeling lost while trying to progress down a road
- *Wash-out* – feeling that the road has suddenly disappeared;
- *Barrier* – feeling blocked from the road one wishes to travel down;
- *Being Led* – following someone else down a road;
- *Waiting* – standing on the road in anticipation of a specific event;
- *Passing Time* – waiting on the road without expecting any particular events;
- *Out to Lunch* – disconnecting from one's surroundings, experiences;
- *Observing* – watching the activities of others; and
- *Moving* – moving forward without observing.

Dervin recommends that these categories be tailored to specific research contexts.

Additionally, Dervin and Clark (1993/2003) posit an additional coding scheme called the communication-as-procedure framework that is particularly useful for helping researchers zoom in on perhaps the most central aspect of the Sense-Making metaphor: verbings. The framework suggests that humans utilize a range of communicative actions, internal and external, that are relationally oriented towards self, other, and/or society. Dervin and Clark suggest that the communication-as-procedure framework is a generalizeable tool

for conceptualizing verbing analytics; they offer multiple verbings as exemplars but suggest that researchers develop their own taxonomies tailored to individual research designs. Hence, by mapping and studying the verbings utilized by online discussion group participants, we can begin to (a) explicate the relationships between the dynamic communicative practices that constitute these environments and (b) identify potential sources of distortions that could hamper the development of effective online dialogue.

In previous research (e.g., Schaefer, 2001; Schaefer & Dervin, 2001; and Schaefer & Dervin, 2003; Schaefer & Dervin, 2009) we reported the development of a verbing template and codebook specifically designed for the analysis of online dialogues and demonstrated its usefulness for identifying potentially distortive communicative practices -- in particular, the tendency of online participants to become locked into dialogic patterns that somewhat limit their ability to learn and grow.

In the present study, we zoom in on the situation-defining strategies employed by online participants and their relationship to the consensus/dissensus verbing practices that are a primary focus in CMC and electronic public sphere research. We ask one central question: When online participants enter into posting moments with different situation-defining strategies do they exhibit different levels of consensusing/dissensusing micro practices? Our purpose is to tease out a better understanding of what these relationships suggest about the micro-level structural conditions found in online web-based discussion groups.

METHOD

In order to answer the research question, we hosted online discussion groups in three ten-week courses conducted at a large, midwestern university in 1999 and 2000. The purpose of these groups was to provide an environment where students could engage in online dialogue to develop an enhanced understanding of multiple and competing perspectives on course-related topics (e.g., racism [affirmative action; reverse racism; slavery reparations] and popular/elite forms of media and culture [coverage of the Columbine High School massacre, gender-based stereotyping, media influence]), a typical approach in online public sphere research (see Ess, 2000; 2002; Watanabe, 2007). Academic discussion groups were selected for analysis because, following Dewey (1916/1966), Ess (2000), and Ess and Cavalier (1996), we argued that public educational institutions play a primary role in fostering the dialogic skills necessary for citizens to reach consensus in public spheres. Further, educational CMC researchers have increasingly drawn upon Habermasian discourse ethics in their research designs (e.g., Englund, 2000; Ess, 2000; Lakeland, 1993; Lehmann-Rommel, 2000). We received human subjects review clearance before proceeding with the data collection phase.

Overall, 124 participants contributed 1,360 messages over a thirty week period (approximately 45 messages per week). Students came from many states in the U.S. and several foreign countries. As was typical for this university, the students' basic demographics were 55% (n=68) female and 45% (n=56) male; 80% Caucasian (n=95) and 20% (n=24) other ethnicities; and 97% (n=113) in their 20s and 3% (n=4) 30 years of age or older. Their socio-economic characteristics were more diverse. They reported their family heads-of-household as being roughly 14% (n=16) blue collar, 21% (n=28) white collar, 33% (n=38) middle management, and 32% (n=35) professional[4]. It should be noted, however, that participation in our research was optional; students received extra credit and were free to withdraw their consent at any time without penalty (none chose to do so). The groups were not moderated by the instructor; rather, participants (a) proposed topics for discussion, (b) were free to comment on postings made by others, and could (c) edit their own entries as needed (e.g., to fix typos, make clarifications, etc.).

Following the mandates of the communication-as-procedure framework with its focus on communicative micro-moments, the unit of analysis was defined as the individual posting, reconceptualized as a time-space bound posting *moment*[5]; interactive aspects of each posting *moment* were captured through the coding of consensusing and dissensusing tactics, as addressed below.

The goal for this study was to explore the relationship between the situation-defining strategies selected by users and the micro-moment consensusing/dissensusing verbings that occurred within the postings. The situation-defining strategies selected for this study were provided to the participants as part of the posting entry form; users chose one of eight (first course) or nine (second and third courses) situation movement state indicators to identify the purpose of their posting. Following the advice of Dervin (2003) to tailor Sense-Making-based taxonomies to individual research contexts, the set of situation-defining strategies were modified based upon two key sources: preliminary analysis of postings contributed to a pilot discussion group conducted in 1997 and warrants from previous CMC research. Thus, ten situation movement state indicators were selected for inclusion on the posting-entry form[6]. These included:

- *Praising others*
- *Relating similar experiences*
- *Seeing connections*
- *Seeing contests*
- *Sharing pleasure, achievements, insights* (first course only)
- *Sharing pleasure, achievements* (second and third courses only)
- *Sharing achievements, insights* (second and third courses only)
- *Sharing struggles, barriers*
- *Asking questions*
- *Asking for help* (first course only)

These situational choices were provided as clickable interface "doorways" without further explanation to the participants. Users were simply instructed to click on the choice they felt most closely matched their communicative goals when submitting their posting.

Once the data had been collected, frequencies were computed for these indicators and the verbing coding commenced. This step utilized a customized template inspired both by Dervin and Clark's (2003) communication-as-procedure framework and previous CMC/dialogic research literatures. The codebook was tested for intracoder and intercoder reliability; all codes were found to have reliability coefficients of.80 or higher using the percentage of agreement between coders, adjusted for chance agreement (Krippendorf, 1980; Miles and Huberman, 1994). Postings across all classes were combined into a single data corpus in order to facilitate the focus on the constellations of communicative verbings occurring within individual posting moments.

For purposes of the analysis presented in this chapter, we focused on two verbing categories that emerged from the codings:

(a) *Consensusings* -- agreeings/accordings with other participants' observations, perspectives, or discussions:

  ◦   *I am commenting on something that someone said in class. She was speaking about "The Politics Of Race" and she said that all black people in Los Angeles cannot be judged on the LA riots. I absolutely agree with that.* ("ogea")

(b) *Dissensusings* -- disagreeings or discordings with the observations, perspectives, or discussions of other participants:

  ◦   First of all, I felt that sunshine's bash on students that go out was a little too harsh ("Lucy")

A posting was coded as a "yes" if any single statement in the posting exhibited consensusings or dissensusings; it was coded as a "no" if it did not include these verbings. Upon examination of the verbing frequencies, we collapsed the consensusing and dissensusing categories into a single variable to facilitate analysis, allowing us to focus on whether a posting either exhibited or eschewed public sphere style discussion and debate, coded either as consensusings/dissensusings or no consensusings/dissensusings. In previous research (Schaefer & Dervin, 2003; 2009), we found much larger differences in postings accounted for when comparing consensusing and dissensusing practices together as a single group against non-consensusing/dissensusing postings, suggesting that both agreeing and disagreeing are two sides of the same dialogic practice[7]. Additionally, since our primary purpose was a comparison of the prevalence of consensusing/dissensusing micro-practices across posting moments – and since the Sense-Making metaphor suggested that humans communicate within situational contexts -- we used the ten different situational movement state indicators as predictors of the presence or absence of the consensusings/dissensusings, which were conceptualized as the criterion variables.

RESULTS

In the following sections, we first examine the descriptive results for (a) the prevalence of situation-defining strategies across all of the postings (the "doors" by which participants entered into the posting moment) and (b) the extent to which postings also exhibited consensusing/dissensusing verbings.

Figure 1 displays the frequency results for the situation-defining strategies -- i.e. the situation movement states by which users entered each posting moment. Across the 1360 posting moments, we found that six doors captured 87% of all posting moments with roughly equal dispersion -- 13% to 15%. These six were, from highest use to lower use, seeing connections (15.2%), relating similar experiences (15.2%), sharing pleasure, achievements (15.1%), sharing insights, ideas (14.8%), sharing struggles, barriers (13.5%), and praising others (13.2%). The three "doors" which received less attention included seeing contests (5.1%); asking questions (4.3%); and seeing causes/outcomes (2.5%).

We were not surprised by the relatively even spread of use of the situation-defining strategies used by the participants, which represented both self-relating-to-self and self-relating-to-others situation states (which we will refer to by the shorthand terms *self-self* and *self-others*). Drawing upon the classic conceptual distinction between *intrapersonal* and *interpersonal* communication (see Fisher, 1978), the former might be described more as focused on *meaning-making*; the latter more on *meaning-sharing*, although it was clear from the results that many postings generally

mixed both modes. What was instructive was that the three least-used doors were suggestive of the deepest struggles aimed at meaning-making: seeing contests, seeing causes/ outcomes, and asking questions. This confirmed prior work (Schaefer & Dervin, 2003; Schaefer & Dervin, 2009), which found that online discussions could be used to allow participants to examine themselves, their lives, and their connections to society. However, these results suggested that some sort of intervention may be required to facilitate this potential, since these strategies were among the least-selected situational indicators.

Figure 3 portrays the consensusing/dissensusing verbing activity coded in the postings. As illustrated in Figure 3, 56.9% of the postings featured consensusing/ dissensusing verbings, while 43.1% did not, indicating that participants were more likely to engage in agreeing/according or disagreeing/discording tactics when composing their postings.

Figure 2. Percentages of user-selected situational movement state indicators

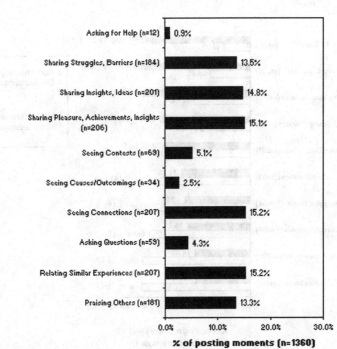

Figure 3. Percentages of consensusing/dissensusing criterion verbings

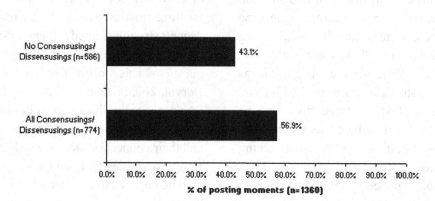

For example, in one typical posting, "Lock" asserted: "*Like I said I just completely agree with what [name removed] said and think that we must focus on the children but then we can not forget about the adults that raise these kids*"; in another, "Carmen" took issue with comments made by another participant: "*She also claims that the black players are on the ground looking up to the white*

players. I definitely disagree with her entire argument."

The importance of focusing on consensusing/ dissensusing in this study, however, is not their mere presence but rather how the use of these practices differed when participants entered their online posting moments with different situation-defining strategies. This focus is the subject of the data presented in Figure 4.

Figure 4. Percentages of situational indicator selection when consensusing/dissensusings are present or absent

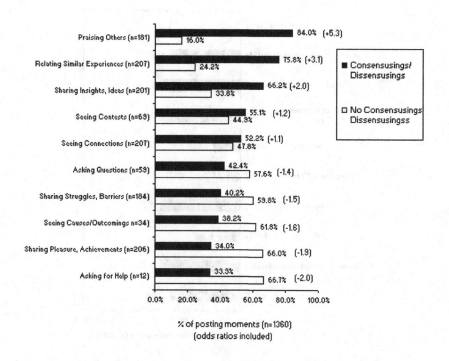

Figure 4 directly addressed our research question -- how user selection of situation movement state indicators (i.e., entry "doors") related to the occurrence of consensusing/ dissensusing micro-practices within the posting moments. The focus of our analysis was on which situation movement states related to proportionately more agreeing/disagreeing activity. As illustrated in Figure 4, the situational indicators provided strong evidence that the selection of different situational indicators led to differences in consensusing/ dissensusing activity. For example, "praising others" was five times more likely (84% of 181 posting moments with an odds ratio of 5.3[8]) to feature consensusing/

dissensusing activity. Looking at other strong situational indicators, "relating similar experiences" was 3.1 times more likely (75.6% of 207 posting moments) and "sharing insights, ideas" was 2.0 times more likely (66.2% of 201 postings) to exhibit consensusing/dissensusing activity. Additionally, "seeing contests" was 1.2 times more likely (55.1% of the 69 postings), and "seeing connections" was 1.1 times more likely (52.2% of 207 postings) to feature consensusing/dissensusing activity in the postings.

Conversely, the remaining situation movement state indicators were less likely to exhibit consensusing/dissensusing activity in the postings. "Asking for help" was 2.0 times less likely to feature consensusing/dissensusing activity (66.7% of 12 postings), "sharing pleasure, achievements" was 1.9 times less likely (66.0% of 206 postings), "seeing causes/outcomes" was 1.6 times less likely (61.6% of 34 postings), "sharing struggles, barriers" was 1.5 times less likely (59.8% of 164 postings), and "asking questions" was 1.4 times less likely (57.6% of 59 postings) to exhibit consensusing/dissensusing activity in the postings.

By reexamining the doorways through the lens of Dervin's (2003c) situational taxonomy discussed earlier, some interesting patterns emerged. First, the postings that were most likely to exhibit consensusings/dissensusings tended to illustrate two key situational states: (a) "being led" – e.g., relating similar experiences, praising others (e.g. comments that acknowledged the influence of others: "*I appreciate [Marcel]'s honesty and willingness to share. This allowed me to be more honest with myself*" [Pandora]) -- and (b) "observing" -- e.g., sharing insight/ideas, seeing contests, and seeing connections. Second, although postings that were less likely to feature consensusings/dissensusings also featured one (a)"observing" situational state -- seeing causes/outcomes – these postings more generally related to three other situational states: (b) "barriers/gaps" – e.g., asking questions, sharing struggles/barriers; (c) "moving" -- e.g., sharing, pleasure/achievements; and (d) "decision" – e.g., asking for help.

Hence, these findings suggest that there were two predominant communicative modes utilized when participants posted to the discussion groups: (a) dialogic, where participants were situationally more focused on relating to others (self-to-other) – e.g., sharing similar experiences praising others, sharing insights/ideas -- and (b) contemplative, where participants were more situationally focused on self-understanding (self-to-self) – e.g., asking for help, sharing pleasure/achievements, seeing causes/outcomes, sharing struggles/barriers, and asking questions.

Both modes, of course, involved posting to an online discussion group – hence potentially talking with others and sharing. But the teleological purpose of each mode was very different. For dialogic postings, participants were turned outward and there seemed to be little meaning-making struggle and much agreeing/disagreeing in their communicatings; for contemplative postings, participants were turned inward, engaging in an introspective form of communicating. In the contemplative mode, participants could use the online discussion as a means of self-therapy where they used the online experience for meaning-making or, in the Frierean (1970) sense, as a kind of talking cure or means of conscientizing.

The two modes of communicating that we identified in the current project -- dialogic and contemplative -- could be observed by skimming the data corpus. For example, the dialogic mode was clearly observed in the following thread. Here, "Pandora" chose the "Praising Others" situation-movement-state doorway when posting the following message:

I wanted to thank [Marcel] for being so honest about the emotional struggle she felt when conducting her own personal sense-making interview....I am currently trying to work on my personal interview. At first I believed I didn't remember anything racist occuring [sic] from me, to me, or observed by me. As I sat down a couple nights ago, I was flooded with many memories for all three categories. It was a very powerful and emotional experience for me. I realized then that maybe I was just trying to actively forget....I appreciate [Marcel]'s honesty and willingness to share. This allowed me to be more honest with myself. I didn't feel ashamed that I too was very emotional. I think our society has become emotionless. Knowing that another person was personally moved by this experience helped me to be more honest with myse lf.

"Carolina" then responded to this posting by selecting the "Relating Similar Experiences" situation movement state:

I would also like to thank [Marcel], not only for insight, but also for her telling the class how to conduct these self interviews. I was not sure exactly how to go about starting this assignment until [Marcel] explained that it took her quite some time to start hers, and the best way to do it is to just sit down and brainstorm about all the experiences one has had with racism. .... This connected to my life because I, like Pandora, was not quite sure if I have had any racial experiences within my life .....The impact which this had on my life is that once I sat down and began to think about my

past, I realized that my life was full of instances dealing with racism. [Marcel] showed me that if one just sits down and thinks about ones' childhood, that experiences dealing with racism are more likely to present themselves.

In these two messages, the self-others relationally oriented situation movement states of "Praising Others" and "Relating Similar Experiences" accompanied postings that actively agreed/ accorded with other participants in the discussion, in essence, forming community structures through the employment of consensus/dissensus bridge-building practices.

In contrast, the contemplative mode often demonstrated a different emphasis by eschewing consensus/dissensus verbing practices, as illustrated in the following posting by "Larry." Here, Larry selected the "Sharing Struggles, Barriers" situation movement state:

I would like to share a racist experience that I recently had. I went to [local] Mall this past summer and I went to [department store1] in search of cosemetics [sic] that I usually buy there. Not at this particular [department store1] but others. The associate informed me that they did noy carry a black cosmetic line there at [mall]. I was shocked....I was just surprised that this brand new mall was not equipped with a black cosmetic line in the [department store1] store. All the other [department store1] carried it....It would have helped if they had carried at least one black cosmetic line. I think this is a racial issue.

The same sort of communicative step-takings could be observed in a posting by "Piatti," who also grappled with racial barriers. S/he, too, selected the "Sharing Struggles, Barriers" situation movement state:

After I read "Resisting Temptation", I really got confused. I never thought Asian American in the U.S is "Exotic pets" of White American. I really did not understand what the author wanted to say over this article. All what I can catch is that there is very deep and stiff Gap between among minorities in this society. ....I went to L.A to visit my friend. Since he did not have a car, we had to get a taxicab. When we went to taxi stop, one African American driver picked my bag and brings into his trunk. At that moment, my friend was shouting at driver, "We are not going to use your cab" I was so embarrassed about his behavior. After that happened, we got Chinese taxi driver. I asked him why he did that to African American driver, he said that "Here in L.A, black and yellow do not get along". He had very bad experience with couple black folks who mugged him. After he got mugged, he prolongated [sic] his thought about African American to others.....As we can see from this, one small incident makes that people judge and categorize whole ethnic group. I bet that African American also hate Korean in LA. Is that media working on this, or white government perpetuates both minorities? We have to think carefully about this incidence. If both African American and Asian American can exchange some of culture and working together for their community, they can make some resolution for next generation Why they hate each other? Is every individual has a certain reason to hate each other?. I do not think so..... What we have to do right now is making some channels to communicate each other. What we have to do is listening. Let's listen carefully, we can solve any kind of problems in the world

In this case, the self-self-oriented contemplative struggle that was recounted *without* recourse to consensusings/dissensusings provided space for a moment of conscientizing: the participant recounted an unpleasant experience that led her/him to contemplate action to change an unjust social system – often touted as the goal of a Habermasian-style public sphere.

In sum, the selection of a situation movement state indicator -- i.e. the poster's choice of a situation defining strategy -- appeared to foreground

contextual information that (a) mapped onto the general presence or absence of agree-disagree micropractices and (b) signaled the utilization of a dialogic or contemplative mode within the postings, with "being led" and "observing"-style situations tending to be more dialogic while "moving," "struggling with barriers," and "decision"-style situations were more contemplative. Hence, this finding suggests the importance of examining time-space contexts when analyzing communicative processes within online groups.

CONCLUSION

As online discussion groups continue to be adopted for use within a variety of environments, including health-care, theorists have become increasingly concerned about the democratic quality of discussions that occur within electronic contexts. In particular, recent publications have urged the development of methods by which contextual information can be incorporated into the design of electronic public spheres in order to improve the robustness of online dialogue.

In this chapter, we have demonstrated the utilization of a Sense-Making informed discussion group design and analytical process to facilitate understanding of the time-space bound nature of online dialogue. Our findings suggest that online postings generally fell into two broad modes: (a) *contemplative*, an introspective-style characterized by low levels of consensusing/dissensusing activity with a focus on barrier/gap, movement, and decision states; and (b) *dialogic*, a relational mode characterized by a high level of consensusing/ dissensusing and an emphasis on the states of being led and observing.

Counter to many of the received theories about the need to privilege user-to-user interaction within online discussion groups, these findings suggest that both modes – dialogic and contemplative – appear to be important for robust dialogue within online public spheres, even though the latter does not necessary accompany consensusing/dissensusing activity, the assumed *telos* of such a sphere. Choosing *not* to engage fellow participants in agreeing-disagreeing tactics appeared to open up structural spaces for participants to voice their own beliefs and sentiments outside of a judgment-oriented, consensus-dissensus context, albeit with an always-present but sometimes silent audience.

In particular, this finding sheds theoretical light applicable to the sense-making processes at work in health-related online forums and blogs where users typically focus on their own experiences related to particular diseases. Previous research (Forster, 2009; Gurak & Antonijevic, 2008; Heilferty, 2009; Kim, Lee, and Guild, 2009) has suggested that such postings often alternate between contemplative, narrative-style accounts of users' daily experiences and dialogic interactions designed to solicit online support or alternative perspectives. In particular, Forster (2009) noted that while many health-care-related blog posts were characterized by "very little feedback" (p. 24) – serving, essentially, as *contemplative* moments, *dialogic* sentiments also emerged: "40% of posts acknowledge the presence of the online community and often in terms of thankfulness" (p. 24).

As a result of our study reported here, we argue that the incorporation of Sense-Making Methodology's situation movement state elements directly into the design of online discussion groups positively enhances the democratic quality of dialogue among participants by promoting both publicly-oriented and personally-oriented micro-practices. In particular, facilitating personally-oriented practices -- and the associated meaning-creating activity that accompany them -- within a public sphere may loosen the grip that dialogically manifested group hegemonic practices (e.g., flaming, boundary-defining and enforcing) appear to have on discussion group designs.

Of course, the findings in this chapter are limited in scope – representing data and conclusions drawn from one set of pedagogical discussion groups. Additional study of more discussion groups – including those found in newsgroups, blogs, or other online contexts -- is needed to verify and amplify these findings. However, we believe these findings warrant additional study and suggest important directions for designers seeking to enhance the democratic quality of online discussions: whenever possible, incorporate situational/contextual characteristics into the interface. Our findings suggest that the democratic quality and robustness of online dialogue may be enhanced as a result.

REFERENCES

Baynes, K. (1994). Communicative ethics, the public sphere, and communication media. *Critical Studies in Mass Communication, 11*, 315–326. doi:10.1080/15295039409366908

Berelson, B. (1952). *Content analysis in communication research*. NY: Hafner.

Blalock, H. (1979). *Social statistics*. New York: McGraw-Hill.

Broome, B., & Chen, M. (1992). Guidelines for computer-assisted group problem solving: Meeting the challenges of complex issues. *Small Group Research, 23*(2), 216–236. doi:10.1177/1046496492232005

Brothers, R. (2000). The computer-mediated public sphere and the cosmopolitan ideal. *Ethics and Information Technology, 2*, 91–98. doi:10.1023/A:1010073319706

Carter, R. (2003). Communication: a harder science. Dervin, B., Chaffee, S., and Foreman-Wernet, L. (Eds). *Communication, a different kind of horse race: Essays honoring Richard F. Carter* (pp. 369-376). Cresskill, NJ: Hampton.

Carter, R. F. (1988). On paradigmatic productivity. In B. Dervin, L. Grossberg, B. O'Keefe, & E. Wartella (eds.), *Paradigm strategies in communication: Vol 1 Issues* (pp. 144-147). Beverly Hills, CA: Sage, 144-147.

Carter, R. F. (1991). Comparative analysis, theory, and cross-cultural communication. *Communication Theory, 1*(2), 151–158. doi:10.1111/j.1468-2885.1991.tb00011.x

Chidambaram, L., Bostrom, R., & Wynne, B. (1990). A longitudinal study of the impact of group decision support systems on group development. *Journal of Management Information Systems, 7*(3), 7–25.

Dervin, B. (1983). *An overview of sense-making research: Concepts, methods, and results to date.* Presented at International Communication Association annual meeting, Dallas, May, 1983.

Dervin, B. (2003a). Chaos, order, and Sense-Making: a proposed theory for information design. In Dervin, B., & Forman-Wernet, L. (Eds.), *Sense-Making methodology reader* (pp. 325–340). Cresskill, NJ: Hampton. (Original work published 1999)

Dervin, B. (2003b). Information← → Democracy. In Dervin, B., & Forman-Wernet, L. (Eds.), *Sense-Making methodology reader* (pp. 73–100). Cresskill, NJ: Hampton. (Original work published 1999)

Dervin, B. (2003c). A theoretic perspective and research approach for generating research helpful to communication practice. In Dervin, B., & Forman-Wernet, L. (Eds.), *Sense-Making methodology reader* (pp. 251–268). Cresskill, NJ: Hampton. (Original work published 2001)

Dervin, B., & Clark, K. (2003). Communication and Democracy: Mandate for procedural invention. In Dervin, B., & Forman-Wernet, L. (Eds.), *Sense-Making methodology reader* (pp. 165–193). Cresskill, NJ: Hampton. (Original work published 1993)

Dervin, B., Forman-Wernet, L., & Lauterbach, E. (Eds.). (2003). *Sense-Making methodology reader.* Cresskill, NJ: Hampton.

Dervin, B., & Schaefer, D. (2003). Peopling the public sphere. In Dervin, B., & Forman-Wernet, L. (Eds.), *Sense-Making methodology reader* (pp. 341–347). Cresskill, NJ: Hampton. (Original work published 1999)

Dewey, J. (1966). *Democracy and education.* New York: Free Press. (Original work published 1916)

Englund, T. (2000). Rethinking democracy and education: Towards an education of deliberative citizens. *Journal of Curriculum Studies, 32*(2), 305–313. doi:10.1080/002202700182772

Ess, C. (1996). The political computer: Democracy, CMC, and Habermas. In Ess, C. (Ed.), *Philosophical perspectives on computer-mediated communication.* Albany, NY: SUNY Press.

Ess, C. (2000). Wag the dog? Online conferencing and teaching. *Computers and the Humanities, 34,* 297–309. doi:10.1023/A:1002075505432

Ess, C. (2002). Computer-mediated colonization, the renaissance, and educational imperatives for an intercultural global village. *Ethics and Information Technology, 4,* 11–22. doi:10.1023/A:1015227723904

Ess, C., & Cavalier, R. (1996). Does the Internet democratize? Philosophical dialogue on-line as a microcosm/case study. (Unpublished paper). Retrieved from http://www.lcl.cmu.edu/CAAE/Home/Forum/report.html

Fisher, B. (1978). *Perspectives on human communication.* New York: Macmillan.

Forman-Wernet, L. (2003). Rethinking communication: Introducing the Sense-Making methodology. In Dervin, B., & Forman-Wernet, L. (Eds.), *Sense-Making methodology reader* (pp. 3–16). Cresskill, NJ: Hampton.

Foster, L. (2009). *Expression of coping with cancer: A content analysis of 'Blog for a Cure.'* Paper presented at the International Communication Association annual meeting, Chicago, IL, May 2009.

Friere, P. (1970). *Pedagogy of the oppressed.* New York: Seabury Press.

Gallupe, R., & McKeen, J. (1990). Enhancing computer-mediated communication: An experimental investigation into the use of a group decision support system for face-to-face versus remote meetings. *Information & Management, 18,* 1–13. doi:10.1016/0378-7206(90)90059-Q

Glantz, S. (2002). *Primer of biostatistics.* New York: McGraw-Hill.

Gurak, L., & Antonijevic, S. (2008). The psychology of blogging: You, me, and everyone in between. *The American Behavioral Scientist, 52*(1), 60–68. doi:10.1177/0002764208321341

Habermas, J. (1984). The theory of communicative action: *Vol. 1. Reason and the rationalization of society.* Boston: Beacon.

Heilferty, C. (2009). Toward a theory of online communication in illness: Concept analysis of illness blogs. *Journal of Advanced Nursing, 65*(7), 1539–1547. doi:10.1111/j.1365-2648.2009.04996.x

Herring, S. (1993). Gender and democracy in computer-mediated communication, *Electronic Journal of Communication, 3* (2).

Hiltz, S., & Turoff, M. (1993). *The network nation.* Cambridge, MA: MIT. (Original work published 1977)

Hollingshead, A., McGrath, J., & O'Connor, K. (1993). Group task performance and communication technology: A longitudinal study of computer-mediated versus face-to-face work groups. *Small Group Research, 24*(3), 307–333. doi:10.1177/1046496493243003

Kerlinger, F. (1986). *Foundations of behavioral research.* New York: Holt, Rinehart, and Winston.

Kim, J., Lee, S., & Guild, J. (2009). *Healthy communication: Mere communication effect on managing chronic health problems.* Paper presented at the International Communication Association annual meeting, Chicago, IL, May 2009.

Krippendorff, K. (1980). *Content analysis.* Newbury Park, CA: SAGE.

Lakeland, P. (1993). Preserving the lifeworld, restoring the public sphere, renewing higher education. *Cross Currents, 43*(4), 488–502.

Lehmann-Rommel, R. (2000). The renewal of Dewey - Trends in the nineties. *Studies in Philosophy and Education, 19,* 187–218. doi:10.1007/BF02764159

Lyytinen, K., & Ngwenyama, O. (1999). Sharrock and Button... and much ado about nothing. *Computer Supported Cooperative Work, 8,* 285–293. doi:10.1023/A:1008720609782

Mabrito, M. (1992). Real-time computer network collaboration: Case studies of business writing students. *Journal of Business and Technical Communication, 6*(3), 316–336. doi:10.1177/1050651992006003003

Miles, M., & Huberman, A. (1994). *Qualitative data analysis.* Thousand Oaks, CA: SAGE.

Ngwenyama, O., & Lyytinen, K. (1997). Groupware environments as action constitutive resources: a social action framework for analyzing groupware technologies. *Computer Supported Cooperative Work, 6,* 71–93. doi:10.1023/A:1008600220584

Olaniran, B. (1994). Group performance in computer-mediated and face-to-face communication media. *Management Communication Quarterly, 7*(3), 256–281. doi:10.1177/0893318994007003002

Papacharissi, Z. (2002). The virtual sphere: The internet as a public sphere. *New Media & Society, 4*(1), 9–27. doi:10.1177/14614440222226244

Papacharissi, Z. (2004). Democracy online: Civility, politeness, and the democratic potential of online political discussion groups. *New Media & Society, 6*(2), 259–283. doi:10.1177/1461444804041444

Poole, M., Holmes, M., Watson, R., & DeSanctis, G. (1993). Group decision support systems and group communication. *Communication Research, 20*(2), 176–213. doi:10.1177/009365093020002002

Qian, H., & Scott, C. (2007). Anonymity and self-disclosure on weblogs. *Journal of Computer-Mediated Communication, 12*(4), 1428–1451. doi:10.1111/j.1083-6101.2007.00380.x

Rananand, P. (2003). Internet and democracy in Thailand. In Banerjee, I. (Ed.), *Rhetoric and reality: The Internet challenge for democracy in Asia.* Singapore: Times Media.

Rheingold, H. (1993). *Virtual community.* New York: Harper Perennial.

Schaefer, D. (1999a). From community to community-ing. *Electronic Journal of Communication, 9* (2, 3, 4).

Schaefer, D. (1999b). *Sense-making design for web sites: Cyber-possibilities for an electronic public sphere.* Paper presented at the session "Methodology between the cracks: Sense-Making as exemplar," International Communication Association 49th Annual Conference, San Francisco, CA, May 27, 1999.

Schaefer, D. (2000). *Rethinking Electronic Public Spheres: Beyond Consensus/Dissensus.* Paper presented at the conference "Social Justice, Peace, and International Conflict Resolution: Civic Discourse beyond the Millennium," Rochester Institute of Technology, Rochester, NY, July 20-22, 2000.

Schaefer, D. (2001). *Dynamics of electronic public spheres: Verbing online participation.* (Doctoral Dissertation, The Ohio State University, Columbus, OH, U.S.A.).

Schaefer, D., & Dervin, B. (2001). *Dialoguing in electronic public spheres: Reconceptualizing participation as verbing micro-practices.* Paper presented at the sixth annual Rochester Intercultural Conference "The Intercultural World and the Digital Connection," Rochester Institute of Technology, Rochester, NY, July 19-21, 2001.

Schaefer, D., & Dervin, B. (2003). *The constitution and distortion of electronic public spheres: A conceptual and empirical rethinking of online communication outcomes as verbing micro-practices.* Paper presented at the International Communication Association annual meeting, San Diego, CA, May 23- 27, 2003.

Schaefer, D., & Dervin, B. (2009). From the dialogic to the contemplative: A conceptual and empirical rethinking of online communication outcomes as verbing micropractices. *Ethics and Information Technology, 11*(4), 265–278. doi:10.1007/s10676-009-9206-x

Schneider, S. (1997). *Expanding the public sphere through computer-mediated communications: Political discussion about abortion in a Usenet news group.* (Doctoral Dissertation, Massachusetts Institute of Technology, 1997).

Sharrock, W., & Button, G. (1997). On the relevance of Habermas' theory of communicative action for CSCW. *Computer Supported Cooperative Work, 6,* 369–389. doi:10.1023/A:1008644224566

Smaling, A. (2000). What kind of dialogue should paradigm-dialogues be? *Quality & Quantity, 34,* 51–63. doi:10.1023/A:1004747524463

Smith, C., McLaughlin, M., & Osborne, K. (1998). From terminal ineptitude to virtual sociopathy: how conduct is regulated on Usenet. In Sudweeks, F., McLaughlin, M., & Rafaeli, S. (Eds.), *Network and Netplay.* Menlo Park, CA: AAAI/MIT Press.

Sproull, L., & Kiesler, S. (1991). *Connections: New ways of working in the networked organization*. Cambridge, MA: MIT.

Straus, S. (1996). Getting a clue: The effects of communication media and information distribution on participation and performance in computer-mediated and face-to-face groups. *Small Group Research, 27*(1), 115–142. doi:10.1177/1046496496271006

Valacich, J., Dennis, A., & Nunamaker, J. (1992). Group size and anonymity effects on computer-mediated idea generation. *Small Group Research, 23*(1), 49–73. doi:10.1177/1046496492231004

Valacich, J., George, J., Nunamaker, J., & Vogel, D. (1994). Physical proximity effects on computer-media group idea generation. *Small Group Research, 25*(1), 83–104. doi:10.1177/1046496494251006

Walther, J. (1992). Interpersonal effects in computer-mediated interaction: A relational perspective. *Communication Research, 19*(1), 52–90. doi:10.1177/009365092019001003

Watanabe, M. (2007). Conflict and intolerance in a web community: Effects of a system integrating dialogues and monologues. *Journal of Computer-Mediated Communication, 12*(3), 1020–1042. doi:10.1111/j.1083-6101.2007.00361.x

Whitworth, B., Gallupe, B., & McQueen, R. (2000). A cognitive three-process model of computer-mediated group interaction. *Group Decision and Negotiation, 9*, 431–456. doi:10.1023/A:1008780324737

Winograd, T., & Flores, R. (1987). *Understanding computers and cognition*. Reading, MA: Addison-Wesley.

Yates, S. (2001). Gender, language and CMC for education. *Learning and Instruction, 11*, 21–34. doi:10.1016/S0959-4752(00)00012-8

Yin, R. (1989). *Case study research*. Newbury Park, CA: SAGE.

ENDNOTES

[1] A refereed version of this chapter entitled Online discussion groups, situation movement states, and dialogic quality: The potential for democratic electronic public spheres was presented at the International Communication Association Annual Meeting, New York, NY, May 28th, 2005.

[2] Although Habermas himself has critiqued his own usage of this concept, it has proven to be theoretically robust and useful for CMC researchers. See Brothers, 2000; Ess, 1996; Herrin, 1993; Lyytinen and Ngwenyama, 1999; Ngwenyama, and Lyytinen, 1997; Sharrock and Button, 1997.

[3] For an extended overview of the development and application of Sense-Making Methodology, see Dervin, Forman-Wernet, and Lauterbach (2003).

[4] As part of their course participation, all students were required to post a minimum number of messages to the web-based discussion groups. Our goal was to neutralize the usual inequalities in participation levels – often reported as a problem in CMC research (e.g., Herring, 1993; Schneider, 1997; Yates, 2001) -- in order to give our attention to structural micro-practices its sternest test. Statistical analysis yielded no significant differences for the average number of postings for each demographic grouping; the F-tests for one-way analyses of variance were all not significant.

[5] Fixing the case/unit of analysis as the individual posting moment -- although somewhat controversial within traditional quantitative social science research (see Kerlinger, 1986) -- follows a strong content-analytic tradition

in communication scholarship (e.g., Berelson, 1952; Krippendorf, 1980; Miles and Huberman, 1994; Yin, 1989) and has been effectively utilized in prior CMC research (e.g., Schneider, 1997; Forster, 2009).

6   Due to minor adjustments to the interface, participants in the first class had eight options to chose from while those in the second class had nine. Additional discussion of the design of these situational doorways can be found in Schaefer, 1999b.

7   Overall, 43.1% (n=586) of the postings did not feature consensusings and dissensusings, while 56.9% (n=774) did. Of the latter, only 6.9% featured dissensusings by themselves, while 93.1% featured solo consensusings (63.7%) or a combination of consensusings and dissensusings (27.9%), prompting our decision to collapse consensusing/dissensusing into a single variable.

8   Odds ratios are non-parametric statistics typically employed in biostatistics (Glantz, 2002). We opted to use this approach due to the drastically uneven *n*s in our comparative groups since odds ratios are "invariant with respect to the relative numbers of cases that appear in each column (or row), a property that gives [them] an advantage over measures of association which do depend on... marginal distributions...." (Blalock, 1979, p. 312).

Chapter 21
Unlearning and Relearning in Online Health Education

Suptendra Nath Sarbadhikari
CAL2CAL Institute, India

ABSTRACT

This chapter discusses the role of integrating medical education with medical practice through online collaborative learning among the various stakeholders involved with healthcare education and practice. It elaborates the discussion with examples of information needs and information-seeking behaviors of patients and physicians. The role of the Internet (infrastructure), and especially the WWW (applications and content), is elucidated with respect to the concepts of online collaborative learning as applied to medical education and practice where the emphasis is on user driven healthcare.

"Data is a campfire around which organizations huddle for heat and light. The irony is in the fact that neither the heat nor the light yields a solution. The solution emerges out of the huddling (i.e., through the organizational interaction in a discussion forum)". -Ontario Ministry of Health and Long-Term Care, anonymous. Quoted in: http:// www.unmc.edu/Community/ruralmeded/quotes_ groups_rural_medical_ed.htm

"We are evolving from the information age, focused on mass consumption, into the conceptual age, one fuelled by innovation." – Robert Kelly in

Creative Expression Creative Education: http:// www.temerondetselig.com/Creative%20Expression%20Creative%20Education.htm

INTRODUCTION

User driven healthcare is defined as "Improved health care achieved with concerted collaborative learning between multiple users and stakeholders, primarily patients, health professionals and other actors in the care giving collaborative network across a web interface." (Biswas *et al.*, 2008).

In this chapter I would try to discuss some of the applications and prospects of online collabora-

DOI: 10.4018/978-1-60960-097-6.ch021

tive learning for user driven health care. At the beginning let us look at some of the studies trying to integrate medical education with practice.

We begin with the perspective from the Southern hemisphere. From Australia, Van Der Meyden (2007) states that the fulfillment of general practice as a major provider of medical education remains an exciting and challenging task — and its realization may well mean a continuing renaissance of general practice in countries. In a similar project, summative evaluation will be done when the University of New South Wales, Australia's new program graduates work in the existing health care system. It is proposed that they will be followed up to see whether they apply the public health values in their practice (Klinken Whelan and Black, 2007).

In the Northern hemisphere, Canadian medical educators believe that educational programming must be offered with content beyond the provision of medical knowledge and skills. Non-clinical physician, patient and system related issues must be addressed in educational programming to support optimum physician performance and better healthcare outcomes (Lynn and Bluman, 2009).

Globally, medical informatics can play a vital role in integrating medical practice with education (Sarbadhikari 2005). To cite an example, there has been team based learning collaborative like: http://www.tlcollaborative.org/ that is a group of health professions educators dedicated to using team-based learning to further medical and allied health education. Another such example is: http://therapeuticseducation.org/

Although Wikipedia is the mother of all wikis, emerging specialized wikis like Medpedia: http://www.medpedia.com/ and WikiDoc: http://www.wikidoc.org/ as well as informative portals like Medline Plus: http://medlineplus.gov/ are gradually dislodging the practicing physician as an information source.

Open source communities like Mirth and user driven healthcare forums like Mediscuss: http://www.mediscuss.org/ are a few steps in such direction.

On the other hand, Anderson *et al* (2008) discusses learning based on patient case reviews. They conclude that patient case reviews initiate reflective processes providing feedback about performance in real life situations. Family physicians are in favor of patient case reviews as a learning method, because it embraces the complexities they encounter in their daily practice and is based on personal experiences.

Biswas *et al* (2009) have discussed the role of open health information management for developing a novel, adaptable mixed-platform for supporting health care informational needs. Their platform enables clients (patient users) requiring healthcare to enter an unstructured but detailed account of their day-to-day health informational requirements that may be structured into a lifetime electronic health record.

While integrating medical education with medical practice is one aspect, using online collaborative learning to achieve that is another aspect. The aim of this chapter is to analyze the role of online collaborative learning in the backdrop of user driven healthcare. Therefore, more stress will be given on discussing the efforts that are underway to fruitfully harness the potentials of online collaborative learning. The "users" in this scenario include both the care givers (physicians) as well as the care seekers (patients).

The next section deals with the Internet and the Web, followed by a section on the some examples of online collaborative learning for user driven healthcare. The concluding section focuses on the future prospects.

THE INTERNET AND THE WORLD WIDE WEB

The *Internet* or the *Net* is a "Network of (computer) networks". It is the global data communications backbone, *i.e.*, the hardware and software infrastructure, that provides connectivity between resources or services and the users of such facilities. In contrast, the *WWW(World Wide Web)* or commonly alluded to as the *Web*, is one of the services communicated via the Internet. It is a collection of interconnected documents and other resources, linked by symbolic hyperlinks, which are reference or navigation elements in a document to another section of the same document or to another document that may be on or part of a (different) domain and URLs (Uniform Resource Locators).

"*Web-based*" and "*online*" are now virtually synonymous terms since even where the "online" connectivity is through LAN, many of the applications are routed through the "Net"!

Google – is perhaps the most widely used tool in the WWW! It is a *search engine* designed to search for information there. Information may consist of web pages, images and other types of files. Google does not store any information in its site but points towards other sites that may offer the information relevant to the search phrase.

Incidentally, Google does not have access to a vast majority (perhaps more than 80%) of pages in the WWW, since they belong to the deep Web (also called Deepnet, the invisible Web, or the hidden Web) and is not part of the surface Web, which is indexed by most search engines.

However, there is no guarantee that a "Googled" site is providing authentic information. Especially in the healthcare domain this can mean the difference between life and death! There have been some efforts to endorse the authenticity of sites catering healthcare information.

Health on the Net Foundation (HON) is a not-for-profit organization founded under the auspices of the Geneva Ministry of Health and based in Geneva, Switzerland. This came about following the gathering of 60 of the world's foremost experts on telemedicine to discuss the growing concerns over the unequal quality of online health information. The mission of the foundation is to guide the growing community of healthcare consumers

and providers on the World Wide Web to sound, reliable medical information and expertise. In this way, HON seeks to contribute to improved health care through patient empowerment and better informed health professionals. HON Foundation issued a *code of conduct* (HONcode: http://www. hon.ch/HONcode/Conduct.html) for medical and health Web sites to address reliability and usefulness of medical information on the Internet. HONcode is not designed to rate the veracity of the information provided by a Web site. Rather, the code only states that the site holds to the standards, so that readers can know the source and purpose of the medical information presented.

It is interesting to note how the Web has transformed with time. Historically speaking, there has never been any "Web 1.0", but the Web has evolved into "Web 2.0" and "Web 3.0".

Web 2.0 is a term coined by Tim O'Reilly that describes the trend in the use of WWW technology and web design that aims to enhance creativity, information sharing, and, most notably, collaboration among users (social web dealing with data). These concepts have led to the development and evolution of web-based communities and various hosted services. To exemplify, social-networking sites (*e.g.*, Orkut and Facebook); wikis (*e.g.*, Wikipedia and Citizendium); and blogs (*e.g*, Twitter) are all too familiar now.

Boulos et al (2006) had mentioned the Web 2.0 applications like wikis, blogs and podcasts as a new generation of Web-based tools for virtual collaborative clinical practice and education. Giustini (2006) has found that RSS feeds, podcasts and search tools are being used by physicians, medical pupils and patients. Sandars and Haythornthwaite (2007) have shown how podcasts can be used on the move to increase total available educational time.

While Crespo (2007) has discussed some public health applications through Web 2.0, Tan and Ng (2006) had made headlines globally by showing the role of "Googling" for diagnostics.

Ferguson (2007) found that patients have different patterns of usage depending on if they are newly diagnosed or managing a severe long-term illness. Frost et al (2008) showed that disease-specific communities for patients with rare conditions aggregate data on treatments, symptoms, and outcomes to improve their decision making ability and carry out scientific research such as observational trials

The Economist newspaper reported in 2007 that among the User generated content in certain support groups only 6% of information is factually wrong and that only 3% reported that online advice had caused serious harm.

Another similar sounding term is "Health 2.0".

Health 2.0: http://www.health2con.com/ (and the closely related concept of *Medicine 2.0*: http://www.medicine20congress.com/ocs/index.php/med/med2009) are terms representing the possibilities between health care, eHealth and Web 2.0. They describe the fact that all, whether professionals or patients, can share information on the Internet about health and medical conditions. Health 2.0 also maintains a wiki: http://health20.org/wiki/Main_Page

The formal definition of Medicine 2.0 (Eysenbach 2008) is "Medicine 2.0 applications, services and tools are Web-based services for health care consumers, caregivers, patients, health professionals, and biomedical researchers that use Web 2.0 technologies as well as semantic web and virtual reality tools, to enable and facilitate specifically social networking, participation, apomediation (means that there are agents – *i.e.*, people or tools which stand by: http://p2pfoundation.net/Apomediation), collaboration, and openness within and between these user groups."

Apo is derived from the Latin for "stand by" and mediate comes from the Latin *mediare* to "be in the middle". Apomediation describes the fact that when one accesses information on the Internet, one keeps out the middlemen (like own doctor or an insurance salesman), and allows one to go directly to the source of information, even if it is not a formal "expert" (apomediary or apomediator) source. The information may come from a professional, or it may come from someone considered to be more of a peer.

Hughes *et al.* (2009) however, argue that four major tensions are represented in the literature on Health/Medicine 2.0: viz., (a) lack of clear definitions; (b) issues around the loss of control over information that doctors perceive; (c) safety and the dangers of inaccurate information; and (d) issues of ownership and privacy.

From Web 2.0 to Web 3.0 has been a journey of adding a dimensionality.

Web 3.0, a phrase coined by John Markoff of the New York Times in 2006, refers to a supposed third generation of Internet (3GI)–based services that collectively comprise what might be called "the intelligent Web"— such as those using semantic web, microformats, natural language search, data-mining, machine learning, recommendation agents, and artificial intelligence technologies — which emphasize machine-facilitated understanding of information (rather documents) in order to provide a more productive and intuitive user experience.

All these are not without their shares of problems. While the connectivity becomes more and more accessible and affordable, problems of communications and cultural differences do not seem to be lessened. *Interoperability* is a property referring to the ability of diverse systems and organizations to work together (inter-operate). The driving force of interoperability is to create suitable standards. Though there are many "*standards*", often there are too many for comfort. A considerable amount of juggling may be necessary to integrate the various components and modalities involved in effectively delivering user-driven healthcare.

Another major problem in establishing online interactions is lack of basic infrastructure like electricity and telecommunications in a substantial part of the world barring a few developed countries. Many parts of Europe are not as "well-connected" as North America. Nevertheless, many countries in Africa are not even aware of what is "connectivity".

In the next section we try to explore some of the applications of online collaborative learning for user driven healthcare.

ONLINE COLLABORATIVE LEARNING FOR USER DRIVEN HEALTHCARE

We shall try to see how online learning operates in the healthcare domain – among physicians / medical educators; and also between patients and physicians.

We begin with the concept of online networking among medical teachers.

In India, some (700 odd, as on July 2009) of the medical educators in different medical schools have formed an e-group: MEU_India. There, in the month of February 2009, the topic of "Medical education networking" was discussed and the transcripts: Medical-Education-Networking-Week-1-Transcript.pdf and Medical-Education-

Networking-Summary.pdf are available at http://groups.google.com/group/meu_india/files?hl=en

The topic was discussed under four weekly sub-heads of:

1. What is medical education networking and why do we need it? SWOT Analysis
2. Types of networking - Departmental, Institutional, Regional, National and International; Social and Professional; Face to face and Virtual (Web-based)
3. Experiences on the preparation, success and failure of networking among all the participants
4. Strategies (personnel and timeframe) to ensure efficient Networking; Summary and Conclusions

The gist emerging from the discussions was that successful networks – where useful information is exchanged cordially – usually have as members highly motivated and dedicated persons. Contrastingly, the not-so-successful mailing lists (electronic networks) usually have mostly disinterested members among them. Practical issues

Figure 1. Screenshot of MEU India group

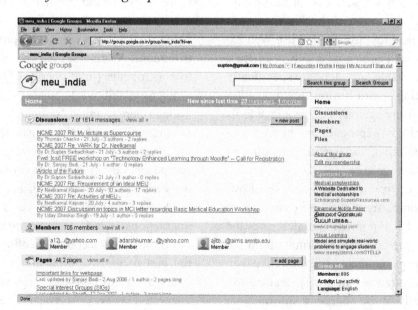

like lack of adequate time management and lack of suitable access to the Internet only compound the problems.

For successful and sustainable online interactions, mentoring is often necessary. Online mentoring can transcend time and space barriers. A summary of discussions in another online forum of the PSG-FAIMER South Asia Regional Institute is available free at:

- http://psg-faimer-2007.wikispaces.com/ file/view/Mentoring-ML-Web-Report-Supten.pdf

Both the examples presented above reflect peer-to-peer learning among medical educators. The insights gained by sharing of the collective wisdom go a long way in sensitizing the educators to the need of modifications in ways medical education is effectively imparted. Further, better educated and communicative medical educators are more likely to encourage and mentor better qualified future medical educators.

Now let us look at an actual conversation (with minimal editing of social niceties in the mail responses) that had taken place at the aforementioned MEU-India group during a three-day period (from July 06 to July 09, 2009). The debate was on whether to include "*e-learning*" in the core curriculum for faculty development programs (FDPs). The Medical Council of India (MCI) had prescribed a draft syllabus for such workshops but has not included e-learning in it. This was not a pre-planned flow of ideas but had arisen spontaneously following an announcement about the FDP proposals by the MCI.

Conversation

Supten (me): I strongly second Dr. (B.V.) Adkoli's view that "We can't escape from emphasizing e-learning and motivating the teachers to learn how to cope up with the information, and obsolescence of technology. The designing of posters,

digitizing and effective presentations also need to be addressed."

In fact this age is called as an age of "Information Explosion" and most of us feel at sea as to how to cope with that. I'd like to quote Dr. Joseph Ana - the Mentor of BMJ West Africa edition in this matter:

- "subjecting health information to some test of veracity and utility before mass release
- filtering the information before mass release
- spreading the skills for appraising information as widely as possible, especially in this era of world-wide-web. That way the end-receiver / user can very quickly discern not-so-useful information and avoid / discard it.
- publishing quality assurance of websites or other sources of health information may also help end-receivers / users to know which ones to rely on"

Of course Health on the Net Foundation does have the HONcode: http://www.hon.ch/

However, the art and science of filtering information is a bare necessity in this information age, especially in an information-intensive domain like medical education and research.

TS (Dr. Tejinder Singh): For faculty development basic course, we already have suggestions to include e learning, managerial skills, statistical methods, research methodology, writing papers etc. – all in a 3 day course.

This is not to belittle the importance of any such suggestion but this obviously is not possible. The feasible option in my humble opinion is to have a basic menu useful for all and then have a number of 'side dishes' in the form of 'electives' or focused courses, which people can take depending on their interest.

This reminds me of a study by McLeod et al, ABC of pedagogy for medical teachers, published in 2003 in Medical Education. The authors proposed that just as you have to learn ABC before you can learn the language, same way, there is a collection of basic issues, which have to be learnt before you can go on to become an expert in ME (something, which Neelkamal said in her poetic style- that you learn alphabets, after which some go on to stop after reading how to learn and some go to writing poems, depending on inclination). Based on this assumption, they proposed a list of topics- developed after using a Delphi technique— which are a must for FD programs.

Can we work to develop ABC of medical education for Indian medical teachers?

Supten: There is a saying that tomorrow's doctors are taught by today's teachers with yesterday's curriculum.

Let us take the example of the recent pandemic of swine flu:

1. WHO Pandemic alert: http://www.who.int/ csr/disease/avian_influenza/phase/en/
2. Current situation of the pandemic: http:// www.who.int/csr/disease/swineflu/en/

Has it reached the textbooks yet?

Is not the disease a real threat?

Do the doctors / medical educators and students need not know anything about it?

If the answer to the first question is "NO", and the second "YES", should we say "NO" to the third question?

If not, then how can the necessary knowledge be gathered if the medical educators are not aware of the need for "Information Filtering" from the Internet?

Of course, the organizations like the WHO, CDC, and the various national governments will issue hard copies of necessary guidelines - but will that ever be possible in real time as on the Net?

Therefore, if this aspect does not come within the "ABCs" of medical education in India, are we not encouraging out datedness and detachment from ground reality?

The above example is not an aberration. Even when various Professional Societies release various guidelines for categorizing / managing diseases, it often takes a few years to reach the textbooks.

As an aside, I would like to quote Prof. Vinay Kumar - the present primary author of Robbin's Pathology. In a recent Conference he predicted that very soon the print media will hardly have any existence and if we do not learn the basics of e-learning, we may carry on teaching yesterday's textbooks.

Onkar (Dr. Onkar Singh): Yes, it is very true that tomorrow's doctors are taught by today's teachers with yesterday's curriculum. So, we must look into the ABC of medical education for Indian medical teachers and I strongly recommend this. Thank you very much for encouraging e-learning.

Sanjay (Dr. Sanjay Bedi): There has to a balance between what is practical and what is ideal. The latter has no end. But we have start somewhere and that is ABC, the bare grassroots of Medical Education. Once we have a foundation ready we can can think of building a skyscraper over it and that too one storey at a time. I agree with TS Sir that we have to start with ABC of Indian Medical Education. As far as Swine flu example those who need to know, know it in sufficient details, A bit out of context here.

Supten: Thanks Sanjay for your comments. Way back in 1995 I had written a Guest Editorial for the Journal of the Indian Medical Association (JIMA): Sarbadhikari SN. Medical informatics-- are the doctors ready? J Indian Med Assoc. 1995 May;93(5):165-6.

I cannot say that a lot has changed over these 14 years as far as attitude towards medical informatics is concerned.

In 2004, I had written an article: Sarbadhikari SN. Basic medical science education must include medical informatics. Indian J Physiol Pharmacol. 2004 Oct;48(4):395-408. I am attaching this article with this mail.

There have been numerous studies on the information seeking behavior of the patients and the physicians and the effect on their relations. I am attaching a couple of relevant articles.

Now in urban India many patients first look up for relevant information from the Net and confront the doctor with the information from there. If the doctors/medical educators and students are not aware how to judge the authenticity of the sites how will they gain rapport with the patient?

Moreover, even friends and relatives will often come with questions (raised by web-based information) to clarify their doubts on issues directly related to their health.

Learning how to optimally tap the (medical education and research) resources from the Net is something to be learnt - firstly by all medical educators - so that they can transfer the knowledge to the students.

TS: Thanks for the elaborate reply. Broadly, FD consists of many activities- professional development and content expertise being one of them- but for all practical purposes within our context, when we talk of FD, our focus is mainly on the educational aspect. You have given me the answer in your last line - the teachers have to transfer the knowledge to the students and it is this competency that we are trying to develop. They still have to formulate learning objectives (related to e learning), deliver the content and assess for their learning.

Content expertise is a different matter altogether with a different approach, audience and logistics. We do not include laparoscopy in FD programs nor do we include PET. We depend heavily on the principle of transfer of learning, meaning that if we have taught the faculty, how to impart skills and how to assess for those skills, they will be able to use this knowledge in variety of settings.

I am somehow not able to connect to your argument regarding swine flu- because it is a very elastic argument, which can be stretched to any limit. We can argue for including software and

hardware courses also because computers can crash and so on.

We need to build the core skills of faculty in this process- specific content can always be delivered in various expert forums.

Supten: I am not saying that all medical educators should know how to develop their subject-specific course content electronically.

However, each and every teacher MUST know how to separate the wheat from the chaff from the vast information (that is essential for learning) available on the Internet.

We should also be able to teach the teachers and students how to identify authentic resources on the World Wide Web (WWW). This is essential because when the patients and / or students confront us with some information from the Net, if we cannot justify why the source is not a trusted one, we would be appearing as confused.

If a patient asks questions through email and we do not reply to that properly or at all, the patient may think that we are simply ignoring.

I repeat - I believe that everyone should be aware of how to optimally tap the rich and up-to-date educational resources on the Net.

In other words, if we cannot be uploaders (knowledge generators and disseminators), we should be judicious downloaders (knowledge users).

I gave the example of the swine flu pandemic because it is a matter of urgency albeit it is yet to reach the textbooks. In other words - should we totally ignore teaching anything that is not in a textbook? We must get authentic information (that is why I cited only WHO sources) and disseminate the information to the students as well. For that we also need to know how to ensure authentic information.

Same things will stand for the various guidelines published by the different Professional Societies for classifying and managing various disorders specific to the disciplines. Usually these are published in journals (and in most of the cases such articles are accessible online free) and we should be able to access and incorporate them in our teaching even before the textbooks can print those guidelines in the subsequent editions.

Therefore, my point of discussion is not at all discipline-specific (like laparoscopic surgery or fMRI) but more like learning how to utilize best a new source of information - the WWW - to impart better education in all disciplines.

Navneet (Dr. Navneet Kaur): I was just trying to comprehend the context of this discussion. As I understand, we are discussing the ABC of medical education in reference to the MCI recommended workshop on Basic workshop in ME technologies. I think the Day 2 of workshop on media in medical education will be very incomplete without an introduction to e-learning (which is more relevant than discussing OHP, flip charts etc). And how far a medical educator goes into e-learning can be a matter of individual choice (as has already been suggested by you).

Even the disadvantage of excessive use of technology in ME should be highlighted so that young teachers do not underestimate the importance of core competence required to be a good teacher.

Adkoli: Thanks to a good debate going on.

I don't think there is much of difference in what TS and Supten are saying; only the emphasis is different. TS is emphasizing on the role of "learning how to learn" while Supten is stressing the need for every medical faculty to be familiar with the "e-learning, information retrieval and IT" as a core skill in a futuristic perspective.

Having accepted the premises that we broadly agree with the scheme suggested by the MCI, we can press the GO button to let the FDPs take off in the present format. However, I appreciate the value additions voiced by Supten and others relating to the e-learning which is a key for future developments. I foresee two important tasks to be taken up simultaneously.

1. A database/directory of all medical educators along with the profile of individual members starting with this network (it has already exceeded 600) need to be hosted on a web-site. Since this

started with NCME forum, this can be the nucleus. AIIMS group (Yogesh Kumar) can take up the task of designing such a database with inputs from Drs Rita Sood, Supten, Sanjay, Avinash, TS and others willing to contribute time/effort).

2. The second task is Content generation and dissemination. A Resource page containing all the books, articles, modules, manuals, workbooks, PowerPoint, in FD can be categorized, and made accessible (on password) to all the members and visitors of the site. We also need to merge or cross link with other resources like projects and web-discussions, irrespective of whether it belongs to NTTC, FAIMER or other sources. This should be done in a spirit of mutual reciprocation and cooperation (though initially one is likely to have reservation in sharing one's hard earned presentations, with time, this fear will be demystified).

While the first task can start immediately, the second one is more challenging and requires continuous inputs from all MEUs, FAIMER centers, NTTCs and research community in general. These tasks coupled with other networking activities which we have stressed time again (starting on-line journals, short term and long term fellowships/ degrees, organization of annual meetings / workshops, and even informal "Gup-Shups" (chitchat) during professional meets!) would definitely strengthen the network and give impetus to the development of scholarship and field of medical education in India, a much cherished dream of one and all.

Rakesh (Dr. Rakesh Biswas): Thanks Dr Adkoli. This initiative would in effect be a first step toward 'learning how to learn' through e-learning (and other learning formats).

Supten: Thank you for reconciling the apparently divergent views!

I am willing to spare my time and efforts for the first activity as necessary.

For the second, I would like to point out to a couple of Archives that were the follow-ups of the monthly discussions led by Saira at PSG-FRI.

1. Assessment: http://assessment.psgfaimer. googlepages.com/
2. Educational Research: http://sites.google. com/site/mededucationalresearch/Home

Similar Archives are also available from CMCL-FRI:

3. http://cmcl.faimer.googlepages.com/ resources

The above conversation is an excellent example of how apparently divergent views can be integrated positively if the intent is there. While the debate had started with whether to include e-learning in the core curriculum for FDPs for medical educators, ultimately a substantial number of the participants (all medical educators from India) joined the bandwagon favoring e-learning as a core skill. This was the effect of arguments based on published papers as well as due to the sharing of personal experiences.

Now I shall share some of my experience with the students also.

Figures 2-5: Screenshots of discussion forums of my online health informatics course

In the above examples (Figures 2-5), there is a pattern of fellow students (peers) trying to help the other students. The interactions in the Figure 2 are from a different batch than that from the Figures 3-5. In the second instance the students – being from other parts of the world – had actually exchanged ideas while I was offline (and asleep). The next morning when I saw their exchanges, I congratulated them and also added a few other pertinent issues and pointed to a few more resources available on the Web. Had the students not interacted in this way, the others (silently observing students) too would not have gained further insights that came out only through this form of collaborative asynchronous learning.

Next, we glance at a few selected papers that explicitly discuss the effects of the Internet on the patients and the physicians.

Pena-Purcell (2008) explores the role of a particular race *viz.*, Hispanics' utilization of health resources on the Net. This study found out lower Internet health information seeking among His-

Figure 2. A student referring to a useful site helping to understand the module

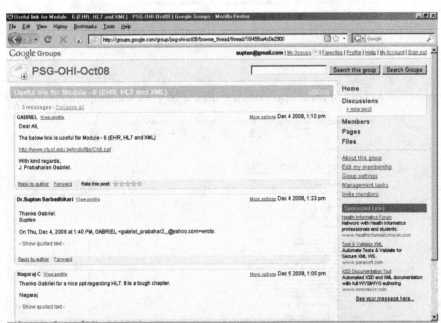

Figure 3. A student asking a question related to the just uploaded study materials

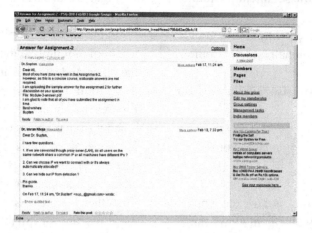

Figure 4. Another student replying to the question raised by the fellow student

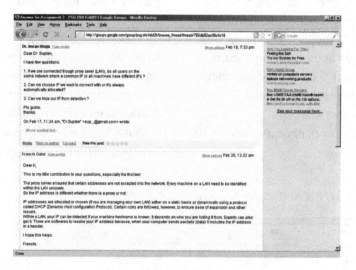

Figure 5. My response to both of them appreciating their efforts in sharing the knowledge

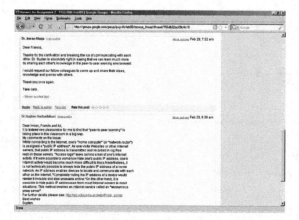

panics than non-Hispanic whites thus providing further evidence of differences in Internet health information seeking among Hispanics and non-Hispanic whites. The author feels that cultural discordance may be a possible explanation for Hispanics' view that the Internet negatively impacts physician-patient relationships. The author suggests that strategies to increase Hispanics' access to Internet health information will likely help them become empowered and educated consumers, potentially having a favorable impact on health outcomes. This may be extrapolated to other patient populations as well and research aimed at exploring such preferences may go a long way in enhancing collaborative learning among patients and physicians.

Liu *et al* (2008) discuss the effects of patient (individual) and community characteristics in determining the communications with the physicians. They found that the sizable variation in bypass rates among their sample of Critical Access Hospital service areas suggests that strategies to reduce bypass behavior should be directed at the local community or facility level. Changing rural residents' perception of their local care, helping them gain a better understanding of the function of primary care, and increasing the number of Primary Care Physicians (PCPs) might help hospitals retain patients and rural communities stay healthy.

Iverson *et al* (2008) discuss the impact Internet use and change in behavior between patients and the physicians. In their study they saw that about 58% of the (patient) respondents reported using the Internet to find health information. About 55% of them reported a change in the way they think about their health as a result of that information. Further, about 46% of these individuals reported making subsequent health-related behavioral changes. The authors conclude that albeit many concerns have been expressed about resulting changes in patient-physician dynamics, online information gathering has the potential to foster

greater patient engagement in health maintenance and care.

While Hay *et al* (2008) describes the Internet-information seeking behavior of new rheumatology patients, Diaz et al (2005) had explored the information-seeking guidance of patients from their doctors. In the first study, the authors conclude that the majority of patients research their conditions online prior to initial appointments, but are unlikely to discuss that research with physicians even though discussion is related to higher satisfaction. Physicians may want to consider strategies for enabling communication about online research.

Diaz et al (2005), on the other hand, had earlier stated that Primary care physicians should recognize that many patients would like guidance as they turn to the Internet for medical information. Physicians can utilize quality assessment tools and existing resources that facilitate referring patients to authoritative, commercial-free, patient-oriented medical information on the Internet.

Then again, Gonzalez-Gonzalez *et al*; (2007) explore the Information Needs and Information-Seeking Behavior of Primary Care Physicians working in settings where consultations are of short duration. Here the PCPs have time to answer only one out of five of their questions. The authors argue that better methods are needed to provide answers to questions that arise in office practice in settings where average consultation time is less than ten minutes.

Bennett *et al* (2005) had earlier compared the information–seeking behavior of physicians belonging to different specialties. They found that Family physicians consider the Internet important to the practice of medicine, and the majority uses it regularly. Their searches differ from colleagues in other specialties with a focus on direct patient care questions. Almost half of family physicians use hand held computers, most often for drug reference.

There have been quite a few studies trying to plot the web-relations between the patients and the physicians. Grazi (2006) says that Web consulting is a powerful tool for patients and health professionals that emerged owing to physician communication problems. Nevertheless, the Internet is still pushing physicians toward a reconsideration of the principles of medical ethics and a reevaluation of rules and regulations to deal with these new communication methods.

Anand et al (2005) find that email exchanges between the parents of pediatric patients and their pediatricians seem to be different from those generated by the telephone, with more emails related to medical versus administrative issues and more resulting in office visits. Approximately one out of four exchanges result in multiple emails back and forth between parent and provider. Parents who have actually exchanged emails with their providers overwhelmingly endorse it, although they are reluctant to pay for it.

Foy and Earls (2005), on the other hand, stress on the need for developing a community consensus to diagnose and manage ADHD patients. This has to involve all the stakeholders including school personnel, physicians, school nurses, and mental health professionals.

Biswas et al (2009) have proposed that learning for the health professional could be organized into health professional e-portfolios linking the health professional with his/her patient records. A patient could look up the range of cases his/her health professional has come across corroborated and validated by the network and decide if this particular health professional has handled a similar case with a similar initial illness trajectory.

All the studies mentioned above exemplify how online collaborative learning can go on among peers (medical educators; patients) or among bigger groups including both the healthcare seekers and the healthcare providers. Moreover, the processes may be further intertwined such that knowledge gained from a particular community (of either patients or physicians or both) can be quickly shared among all the other groups that may have stakes in such findings.

Another step beyond static informative websites and emails is that of the virtual learning environment.

Second Life (SL) is a virtual world that allows patients to interact in a 3D environment with peers and healthcare providers. Watson *et al* (2008) present a framework that demonstrates how applications within SL can be constructed to meet the needs of patients with diabetes mellitus, allowing them to attend group visits, learn more about lifestyle changes, and foster a sense of support and emotional well-being. They believe that this experiential approach to education may prove more engaging, and therefore successful, than existing strategies.

FUTURE PROSPECTS

The rate at which technology is advancing, it is futile or perhaps even foolish to try to predict what the future holds in store for us!

I (Sarbadhikari 2008) had written about how to develop good e-learning courses. Later on this was modified as a lecture and uploaded at the Supercourse: http://www.pitt.edu/~super1/lecture/lec35331/index.htm. This can be done for student (UG and PG) as also for patient education. Further, patient posts may be encouraged and that can lead to further educational discussions in a deidentified manner. Innovative ideas should be encouraged and tested in the model of user driven healthcare. Of course, the infrastructural availability to all the users will decide how much of this will be achievable and how much will remain in the domain of science fiction.

McGrath et al (2006) had found that the lack of cohesion across health and education sections and national and state jurisdictions in Australia is counterproductive to effective national policies in medical education and training. They had also recommended that all prevocational positions should be designed and structured to ensure that service; training, teaching and research are appropriately balanced. Further, they have stressed on the need for health education research to ensure this. This sort of an approach will be essential for all other countries as well.

Certainly health education researchers can focus on studying the impacts of patient inputs (both face-to-face and online) on medical education and practice.

To conclude, online collaborative learning is very likely to integrate medical education and practice through user driven healthcare in the near future.

REFERENCES

Anand, S. G. (2005). A Content Analysis of E-mail Communication Between Primary Care Providers and Parents. *Pediatrics, 115*, 1283–1288. doi:10.1542/peds.2004-1297

Andersen, R. S. (2008). Learning based on patient case reviews: an interview study. *BMC Medical Education, 8*, 43. doi:10.1186/1472-6920-8-43

Bennett, N. L. (2005). Family physicians' information seeking behaviors: A survey comparison with other specialties. *BMC Medical Informatics and Decision Making, 5*, 9. Retrieved from http://www.biomedcentral.com/content/pdf/1472-6947-5-9.pdf. doi:10.1186/1472-6947-5-9

Biswas, R. (2009). Open Information Management in User-Driven Healthcare. In Niiranen, S. (Eds.), *Open Information Management: Applications of Interconnectivity and Collaboration*. Hershey, PA: Information Science Reference.

Biswas, R., Martin, C., Sturmberg, J., Shankar, R., & Umakanth, S., Shanker, & Kasthuri A. S. (2008). User driven health care - Answering multidimensional information needs in individual patients utilizing post EBM approaches: A conceptual model. *Journal of Evaluation in Clinical Practice, 14*, 742–749. doi:10.1111/j.1365-2753.2008.00998.x

Boulos, M. G. K., Maramba, I., & Wheeler, S. (2006). Wikis, blogs and podcasts: a new generation of Web-based tools for virtual collaborative clinical practice and education, *BMC Medical Education, 6*, 41. Retrieved from http://www.biomedcentral.com/content/pdf/1472-6920-6-41.pdf

Crespo, R. (2007). Virtual community health promotion. *Preventing Chronic Disease, 4*, A75.

Diaz, J. A. (2005). Brief Report: What Types of Internet Guidance Do Patients Want from Their Physicians? *Journal of General Internal Medicine, 20*, 683–685. doi:10.1111/j.1525-1497.2005.0115.x

Eysenbach, G. (2008). Medicine 2.0: Social Networking, Collaboration, Participation, Apomediation, and Openness. *Journal of Medical Internet Research, 10*, e22. Retrieved from http://www.jmir.org/2008/3/e22/. doi:10.2196/jmir.1030

Ferguson, T. (2007). *ePatients white paper*. Retrieved July 24, 2009 from http://www.e-patients.net/e-Patients_White_Paper.pdf

Foy, J. M., & Earls, M. F. (2005). A Process for Developing Community Consensus Regarding the Diagnosis and Management of Attention-Deficit/Hyperactivity Disorder. *Pediatrics, 115*, e97–e104.

Frost, J. H., Massagli, M. P., Wicks, P., & Heywood, J. (2008). How the social web supports patient experimentation with a new therapy: The demand for patient-controlled and patient-centered informatics. *AMIA... Annual Symposium Proceedings / AMIA Symposium. AMIA Symposium, 6*, 217–221.

Giustini, D. (2006). How Web 2.0 is changing medicine [Editorial]. *British Medical Journal, 333*, 1283–1284. doi:10.1136/bmj.39062.555405.80

Gonzalez-Gonzalez, A. I. (2007). Information Needs and Information-Seeking Behavior of Primary Care Physicians. *Annals of Family Medicine*, *5*, 345–352. doi:10.1370/afm.681

Grazi, G. L. (2006). Web Relationships Between Physicians and Individuals Seeking Information on Hepatopancreatobiliary Diseases. *Archives of Surgery*, *141*, 1176–1182. doi:10.1001/archsurg.141.12.1176

Hay, M. C. (2008). Prepared Patients: Internet Information Seeking by New Rheumatology Patients *Arthritis & Rheumatism (. Arthritis Care and Research*, *59*, 575–582. doi:10.1002/art.23533

Hughes, B., Joshi, I., & Wareham, J. (2008). Health 2.0 and Medicine 2.0: Tensions and Controversies in the Field. *Journal of Medical Internet Research*, *10*, e23. Retrieved from http://www.jmir.org/2008/3/e23/. doi:10.2196/jmir.1056

Iverson, S. A., Howard, K. B., & Penney, B. K. (2008). Impact of Internet Use on Health-Related Behaviors and the Patient-Physician Relationship: A Survey-Based Study and Review. *The Journal of the American Osteopathic Association*, *108*, 699–711.

Klinken, W. A., & Black, D. (2007). Integrating Public Health and Medicine: First Steps in a New Curriculum. *Education for Health* 7 (online), 122. Retrieved from http://www.educationforhealth.net/articles/subviewnew.asp?ArticleID=122

Liu, J. (2008). Bypass of Local Primary Care in Rural Counties: Effect of Patient and Community Characteristics. *Annals of Family Medicine*, *6*, 124–130. doi:10.1370/afm.794

Lynn, B., & Bluman, B. (2009). It Takes More than Medical Knowledge and Skills. Retrieved July 24, 2009, from http://www.university-cme.ca/canada/editorial.php?show_id=5&lang=en

McGrath, B. P. (2006). Lack of integration of medical education in Australia: the need for change. *The Medical Journal of Australia*, *184*, 346–348. Retrieved from http://www.mja.com.au/public/issues/184_07_030406/mcg10993_fm.pdf.

Medsphere and Webreach. (n.d.). *Medsphere and Webreach*. Retrieved from http://www.medsphere.com/press/20080701

Mirth (n.d.). *Mirth*. Retrieved from http://www.mirthcorp.com/community/overview; http://www.mirthcorp.com/archives/2085

Pena-Purcell, N. (2008). Hispanics' use of Internet health information: an exploratory study. *Journal of the Medical Library Association: JMLA*, *96*, 101–107. doi:10.3163/1536-5050.96.2.101

Sandars, J., & Haythornthwaite, C. (2007). New horizons for e-learning in medical education: ecological and Web 2.0 perspectives. *Medical Teacher*, *29*, 307–310. doi:10.1080/01421590601176406

Sarbadhikari, S. N. (2005). The State of Medical Informatics in India: A Roadmap for optimal organization. *Journal of Medical Systems*, *29*, 125–141. doi:10.1007/s10916-005-3001-y

Sarbadhikari, S. N. (2008). How to design an effective e-learning course for medical education. *Indian Journal of Medical Informatics*, *3*(1). Retrieved from http://ijmi.org/index.php/ijmi/article/view/y08i1a3/15.

Tan, H., & Ng, J. H. K. (2006). Googling for a diagnosis—use of Google as a diagnostic aid: Internet based study. *British Medical Journal*, *333*, 1143–1145. doi:10.1136/bmj.39003.640567.AE

The Economist. (2007). *Health 2.0: Technology and society: Is the outbreak of cancer videos, bulimia blogs and other forms of "user generated" medical information a healthy trend?* The Economist, September 6: 73-74

User driven healthcare innovation (n.d.). *User driven healthcare innovation*. Retrieved from http://www.pervasivehealthcare.dk/projects/index.php#13

User driven test beds at Lombardi, Italy (n.d.). *User driven test beds at Lombardi, Italy*. Retrieved from http://www.remine-project.eu/index.php?option=com_content&task=view&id=12&Itemid=36

Van Der Weyden, M. B. (2007). Expanding primary care-based medical education: a renaissance of general practice? *The Medical Journal of Australia, 187*, 66–67. Retrieved from http://www.mja.com.au/public/issues/187_02_160707/van10686_fm.html.

Watson, A. J. (2008). Brave New Worlds: How Virtual Environments Can Augment Traditional Care in the Management of Diabetes. *Journal of Diabetes Science and Technology, 2*, 697–702.

Wikipedia (n.d.). *List of open source healthcare software*. Retrieved July 24, 2009 from http://en.wikipedia.org/wiki/List_of_open_source_healthcare_software.

Chapter 22
Developing Community Ontologies in User Driven Healthcare

Jane Fitzpatrick
University of the West of England, UK

Willie Ako
University of Bristol, UK

ABSTRACT

In developing equitable health systems, the World Health Organisation (2005) advocates strengthening the repository of social science research to inform policy decisions affecting health care. The players include the patient, family and community members and health care professionals. This requires a genuine engagement with community perspective on health issues. This chapter examines how health care professionals can engage in understanding user perspectives in order to develop effective health care policies and programs. This case study explores how involving an indigenous community enabled them to develop an effective health promotion and malaria prevention initiative in a remote rural community in PNG It draws on participant narratives to explore user perspectives and understandings of the health impact of a focused health promotion and malaria prevention initiative. It illustrates that poverty dominates their health experiences. The chapter illustrates how the development of a collaborative empowerment approach to research can have a significant impact on the strategies members of indigenous communities can develop in order to optimise their health experiences. It argues that in order to develop effective approaches to health care policy and design health needs to be appreciated in the context of lived experiences of those affected.

INTRODUCTION

This chapter examines how health care professionals can work with a range of stakeholders in designing and delivering health care focused on service user needs. There are many theories about how individuals and communities can be encouraged to change their behaviours in order to improve their health status. However, many do not address the context and situated belief systems of the individual and the community that they live in. If the reference frames of the individual and

DOI: 10.4018/978-1-60960-097-6.ch022

or community are not addressed this may impact dramatically on the efficacy and effectiveness of health improvement and treatment initiatives. This chapter explores how health care professionals can engage in dialogue with stakeholders that respects the legitimacy of all perceptions and belief systems of health and illness. It examines how health care professionals can engage in understanding user perspectives in order to develop effective health care policies and programs. It argues that this type of approach will enable us to develop effective partnerships in designing and implementing user focused approaches to healthcare.

The chapter draws on the literature in developing partnership approaches to health service design and delivery. In order to explore the issues in context it reviews a case study that explores the experience of a small research project, conducted with members of the Kewapi language group in Papua New Guinea. It draws on participant narratives to explore user perspectives and understandings of the health impact of a focused health promotion and malaria prevention initiative.

BACKGROUND

Case Study Context in Papua New Guinea

There are over 800 language groups in Papua New Guinea each have separate cultures and traditions. The research discussed in this chapter emerged from discussions with members of the Kewapi language group who live in an urban settlement in Port Moresby the capital city. It was extended to develop an insecticide treated bed net (ITN) initiative in the Batri villages in the Southern Highlands of Papua New Guinea.

Simms (2002) attests that people populating urban settlements in PNG survive in difficult circumstances. They live in poor housing and have limited access to basic amenities. Water is supplied via a standpipe which may serve up to

50 people and this may be cut off for days with no replacement available to them. They have no mains electricity and so live by natural light and candle light and by cooking on wood fires or on a primus stove. They have no access to refrigerators and have to shop for fresh food on a daily basis. Fifteen people made up of three immediate family units may live in a tiny dwelling of about 35 square meters. They share their water source and latrine with up to 40 other people living within a very small area.

Professor Simms (2002) affirms that settlement communities in PNG are poor places where basic amenities are scarce. He also asserts that they have a reputation for being violent areas where health workers are reluctant to enter. He comments on the abject poverty and extreme difficulties people face in coping with illness in such conditions. In a similar vein, the Voluntary Services Overseas (VSO) policy documents (VSO, 1999) state that it does not place volunteers in Port Moresby, since it is perceived to have problems with law and order. These conditions contribute to a range of debilitating conditions such as diarrhoea and malnutrition. In addition, the tropical climate means that diseases such as malaria, dengue fever, and tropical ulcers thrive.

Thus, members of the Kewapi language group face a myriad of health issues due to the context in which they live their lives. Poverty dominates their health experiences. The environment that they live in are poor; the standard of shelter basic at best. They have limited access to clean water and sanitation. Lack of skills of the population mean that work is hard to find; lack of gainful employment means that some resort to misuse of alcohol. This in turn leads to violence.

Neito et al. (1999) argue that research projects that intend to affect the health status of indigenous communities must involve members in their design and operationalisation in order for programs to be effective and sustainable. This case study explores how involving an indigenous community enabled them to develop an effective health promotion and malaria prevention initiative in a remote rural community in PNG..

This study was designed to examine if and how an empowerment approach to research might translate into the PNG context and enable members of the community to recognise, explore and address health issues facing them in their urban and rural environments. It sought to address the power dynamics within the research process, including within the community, and facilitate an inclusive research approach..

In order to engage with the members of the community it was imperative that the research team identified with the context of the lived reality of the participants. This process is described below.

DEVELOPING USER ONTOLOGIES

What Are Ontologies?

Ontology concerns the nature of 'reality'. In the context of knowledge sharing, however, it refers to the *specification of a conceptualization*. In exploring health issues a common ontology identifies the vocabulary and assumptions shared by the parties engaging in discussion. Gruber (1995) argues that there is an underlying assumption that language is used in a consistent and coherent manner. It is recognised that different stakeholders hold different knowledge bases and that each knows things that others do not. It is not a requirement that all the possible questions need to be answered. In this case study the members of the community share a wealth of indigenous knowledge. They also know about the realities of surviving in a settlement with poor resources. The study sought to enable members of the research project to engage with these realities and consider ways of optimising the lived health experience of the participants. In engaging with this mission, it was decided to adopt a research approach with a stated political aim and to evaluate its transference into a developing world context.

DEVELOPING ONTOLOGIES WITHIN AN EMPOWERMENT RESEARCH APPROACH

Empowerment Research

Some scholars perceive empowerment research as a form of action research (Sturt 1999). Holter and Schwarts-Barcott (1993) describe three types of action research in their typology:

- The *technical collaborative* in which the researcher has the predetermined agenda
- The *mutual collaboration* approach which involves the researcher and participants identifying problems together, followed by mutually agreed action cycles
- The *enhancement* approach which begins by working collaboratively from the outset. It also takes the process further to affect the collective consciousness.

Boultier et al., (1997) extends this typology beyond the enhancement approach suggesting that empowering approaches to action research are within the domain of the conflict resolution.

Within the paradigm of empowerment research, it is imperative that the research team and members of the research population develop a shared understanding of the mission and intention of the research. The research becomes a collaborative project in which stakeholders contribute to the design, implementation and analysis of the data in order to find new ways forward in addressing the community's health issues. Within this context, the language used is explored and examined in order to develop shared meanings. This includes contributing to and affirming the conduct of the study the data and the interpretation of the findings.

It is important that participants also develop a respectful dialogue and shared understanding with members of their community. This includes enabling members of the community to develop a shared understanding with their peers.

Peer Learning

Studies suggest that peer learning enhances individual's understanding of health behaviours. Several authors suggest that this is the case when addressing sensitive issues such as sexual health issues (Adamchack 2006; Green et al 1999; Louk 2009). In addition, it appears to be successful when working with at risk communities such as disadvantaged groups or displaced persons (Peersman et al, 2001). However, as already noted with EBM, Crossley and Holmes (2001) argue that educational policies developed in industrialized countries are often adopted in developing countries without a review of their applicability to this context.

The study began in 2004. During a three-month period, members of the community met with researchers to negotiate a series of workshops on health related topics. The second evaluative phase of the project was conducted over a four month period in 2005. The study draws on the public health agendas focused on the prevention of communicable diseases articulated in the Papua New Guinean Health Strategy published by the PNG Department of Health (PNG DoH, 200;, WHO, 2002,2004). It sought to enable participants to

begin to recognise and find ways of managing some of the concerns facing them as members of their community and as Papua New Guineans. The project was extended into a malaria prevention initiative with the extended families of the community living in the villages they originate from in the Southern Highlands.

Erima is a settlement area situated near Jackson's International airport, 11 kilometres from Port Moresby, the capital of Papua New Guinea. Papua New Guinea, the second largest island in the world, after Greenland, lies south of the equator, North East of Queensland in Australia.

Papua New Guinea became an independent country whilst maintaining membership of the British Commonwealth in 1975. It was liberated from partial occupation by the Japanese by the Australians in 1945, it then became a United Nations trusteeship, administered by Australia. Following this Australia was granted limited home rule in 1951. Autonomy in internal affairs came nine years later, and in September 1975, Papua New Guinea achieved complete independence from Australia (Ako, 2002; Infoplease, 2005).

The Executive Board of the United Nations Development Programme (Executive Board

Figure 1.

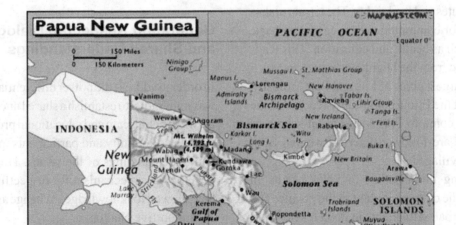

313

UNDP; (2002) reports that it is a young nation that grapples with major development problems. It is beset with major health problems and there is a lack of access to basic education and other services. The UNDP observes that there is a decline in living standards in PNG and vulnerable groups such as young women and disadvantaged populations are most at risk. Australian Aid for International Development (AusAID) one of the major aid donors, sponsored by the Australian government, suggests that earlier gains in health and education are in danger of being eroded (AusAID, 2004).

Papua New Guinea is a country of rich diversity. It is believed, that humans first came to live in Papua New Guinea over 50,000 years ago. They are thought to have arrived as a result of island hopping across the Indonesian archipelago from Asia. There is evidence of gardening from 9,000 years ago. This makes Papua New Guineans amongst, if not the oldest farmers in the world (Tree, 1996).

The peoples of Papua New Guinea speak over 800 indigenous languages. These language groups developed from the difficult terrain and each attest separate traditions and cultures. People can identify closely with a tight family grouping. Papua New Guineans attest that this tribal identity can result in ferocious fights over issues such as family disputes and land rights. The terrain makes it difficult for communities to access even basic services such as health and education. This leads many people from the Highlands region to gravitate to the largest cities of Lae and Port Moresby. Members of the Erima community report that the single men come to Port Moresby in search of work. They are followed later by women from their home village.

Increasing urbanisation in PNG results in changes in the cultural context of the people. The growth of urban settlements in PNG results from the urban drift as people try to seek work. People in remote areas of the country perceive that education is more accessible in urban centres. This provides another incentive to move to urban areas.

There were several issues affecting the design of the project. These included

- The cultural context of the study,
- Negotiation of the themes for discussion,
- The development of networks to establish and sustain the project at the national, regional, university and field level.

This context raised several questions including:

1. Was it possible to respond to the communities' request for information to optimise their health experiences?
2. Was it possible to undertake a project which would be meaningful to the residents of the community and which might enable them to make a difference to their lived health experience?
3. Could we find a way of sharing ideas that enables members of the community and research team to explore their understandings of health issues in order to develop an effective health promotion and treatment strategy.

POWER DIFFERENTIALS:

Generating Respectful Dialogue and Shared Understandings

In order to address the power differentials in situ, it was imperative to establish a shared understanding between health care and educational professionals and the community and participants' perspective and understandings of the issues. This involved developing a mechanism for respectful dialogue that allowed for knowledge exchange and reciprocal supportive challenge.

The researchers established a conversational dialogue with the participants in order to generate new ideas and establish a forum for authenticating the emerging data. This mirrored the type of dialogue used in the traditional Southern Highlands Council of Elders forum, held by members of the community. The conversations were challenging and made both researchers and participants review their perspectives on their contexts and health initiatives.

The Process of Dialogue

The researchers and participants brought different knowledge to the dialogue about their contexts and health issues in situ. The researchers had knowledge of health promotion and factors impacting on public health workers and their professional expertise. The participants had indigenous knowledge, and lived experience of their contexts in the village and the settlement.

From the outset, it was important to recognise and respect the stakeholders including community members and the research team. Setting the agenda to explore these understandings in order to bring about changes to improve health experiences were important aspects of the research relationship. The process of developing a shared language and understanding of issues in context involved working with elders from the language group fluent in English Pidgin and Kewapi in developing a conversational forum for discussion. These key people have knowledge of the cultural norms and of the system of tribal discussions used in the villages.

In order to develop an inclusive approach with members of vernacular communities, Lim (2003) argues that communication needs of participants and researchers must be addressed. This includes both interpretation and capturing other media such as oral histories and visual clues. In order to capture the language needs of the project both translation and interactive teaching strategies were used to stimulate discussion.

The model of engagement adopted emphasised that the relevance, timing, venue content and style of delivery should match the cultural experience of the participants. From the outset, members of the community living in the settlement appreciated that the research came to them in their physical space. The initial project took place in 'our front yard'. This meant that the researchers had a direct appreciation of the physical situation in which the people live their lives.

Members of the community stated that they had had no opportunity for discussing health related topics with a health professional in their home setting. Health care professionals fear the settlement areas and rarely if ever conduct outreach clinics in these areas. The participants shared concerns that they often felt belittled when they attend the clinic or hospital. They welcomed this opportunity to share discussions in a forum within their own environment. Participants made comments such as:

No one comes to our place. You have come and seen what it is like to live here

You have brought ideas about things we can do to make things a bit better

You really try and understand about our culture and the ways we do things

You respect our views

You have also worked in a way that we can all understand. You speak English and we can translate into Pidgin and Kewapi so everyone can take part. Dr. T came with you and he can speak Pidgin and Dr. A he speaks our language, so if people are not as good in English they have been able to take part.

The researchers have attempted to engage in the context and with the lived experience of members of the community. The workshops were conducted in situ with the people in their 'Front Yard' and the topics were negotiated following extensive reviews of the contemporary public health agendas and public concerns expressed in the national newspapers. This attempt to develop a genuine understanding of their experiences seems to have had a positive impact on the development of the project. The commitment to enabling everyone to participate was also an important factor.

During the first phase of the research in 2004 the workshop topics were identified from the PNG Department of Health strategic aims and modified in negotiation with members of the community. Thus, they focused on topics that were perceived to be relevant to members of the community. They focused on:

- Malaria and Tuberculosis
- Respiratory conditions
- Pain management
- Healthy Eating
- First aid and minor illnesses
- Family Planning
- Recap and evaluation and action plan

Drawing on the work done in the first phase of the project in 2004 the topics were extended, at the request of the community, to focus on First Aid. The topics of the workshops conducted in 2005 therefore included immediate first aid for:

- Heat stroke and heat exhaustion
- Small cuts and abrasions
- Minor burns and scalds
- Preventing infection in wounds, and
- Networking to develop community development initiatives

The initial research sought to explore if and how a collaborative empowerment approach to health education would affect the participants lived experiences. The sessions were as interactive as possible. So that everyone could take part in the discussions, translation took place throughout the discussions. The discussions were augmented with resources such as stories from community members, photographs, pictures from books, commodities such as items needed for a simple First Aid kit, from the local shops and simulation of some of the issues. Where flip charts were used to capture some of the issues Dr. Jane the lead researcher attempted crude drawings as well as using simple vocabulary. These provoked a lot of humour since they put her drawing skills to the test! However, these attempts were seen as a good way to be inclusive. Indeed members of the community later reported that they were not used to people drawing pictures to explain things. They stated that the use of visual cues such as items available in the context and from the local shops, illustrations from their childrens' school books and naïve drawings done by the research team, enabled people to engage with the discussion more actively since they clarified their understanding.

The emerging process of developing shared meanings is captured in the diagram of Figure 3.

Figure 2. Example of diagram used to explore the life cycle of the Malaria Parasite reproduced with permission from Fitzpatrick 2006 in CONNECT

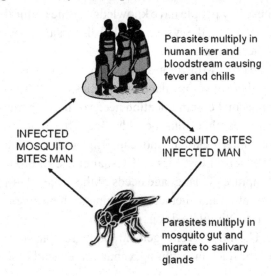

Figure 3. The process of developing shared meanings

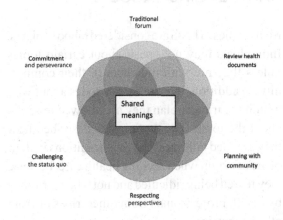

UNCOVERING AND MEDIATING TRADITIONAL BELIEFS

In order to develop effective health initiatives, which are relevant and effective in the local context it is imperative to explore and mediate the local belief systems of the community. The model of engagement in which respect for the views of all concerned was an overt commitment enabled members of the community to explore with the research team their hidden understandings of health.

Makundi et al (2006) report that developing effective malaria prevention and treatment programs in Tanzania, capturing the traditional perspectives on health and drawing on the expertise of traditional healers, was beneficial to strategic development. Neito et al (1999) argue that failure to engage with communities in exploring their belief systems and subsequently enabling them to transform their understanding in order to complement their traditional remedies will compromise malaria prevention strategies.

SORCERY:

Implications for Developing Effective Health Strategies

The forum for dialogue developed in this project allowed members of the community to share their traditional beliefs about health and illness. Sorcery continues as a belief system that informs the way in which the people respond to illness and disease. This is a major consideration in developing effective health strategies in PNG.

Boulton–Lewis et al. (2002) report that there is evidence to suggest that Western and non-Western views of health differ dramatically in the way they are constructed. The dominant mode of thought in Western biomedicine defines health as the absence of disease. In contrast in non-Western societies health is associated with an integration of mind and body. Fabrega (1997) refers to the 'village level societies' where it is believed that sickness occurs because of victimisation by another within the group. Health then becomes the domain of the 'protohealer' for relief of symptoms or healing of the condition. The emphasis of healing is on the resolution of social or moral ambiguity rather than on the relief of physical symptoms. Williams (1998) notes that this belief is reflected in PNG society where traditional healers currently continue to practice.

These extracts from Boulton-Lewis et al's (2002:12) study illustrates the PNG person's beliefs that suggest sickness depends on relationships and spirit influences:

At home people might be jealous and they might do puri puri (magic spell or spirits) ... it will affect you to be sick so you have to live in a good relationship with others. It can start from an argument or somebody stealing a girl from a clan. They have to go and settle it like go and pay the right price. Like give food and pigs. If you don't solve it you will get sick. This is to do with relationships.

and

When you are washing, the evil spirits that live in there (the creek) well if the spirits are not happy that will make you cautious

In PNG there a range of traditional health beliefs that inform the way that people understand their health experiences. Sorcery is perceived to be a key medium that affects the person's wellbeing. If someone feels unwell or sustains an injury this is attributed to some misdeed they have done to another person. In his study of the Imyan worlds of Irian Jaya, the Indonesian part of the island, Timmer (2000) reports similar beliefs. He explores how people believe that coughing is linked to the past behaviour of the person. Therefore, if the person behaves better then the illness will respond. This is significant since for example in the treatment of TB, a prevalent disease in PNG which requires long term treatment with drugs, the patient may feel significantly better two weeks into the treatment. The belief that it is one's behaviour that is affecting how one feels, rather than the drug, mitigates against the person completing their treatment regime. A volunteer perspective, by a doctor with VSO (1999), suggests that the people may also get ambiguous messages from doctors from other countries. This volunteer reports his frustration in providing health care for people with illnesses, such as carcinoma of the mouth. He was unable to treat this condition, and resorted to sending the patient to the traditional healer. The rationale the doctor gave for this decision is not made explicit. Did he admit there would be treatment available elsewhere or does he lead the patient to believe that this is the most appropriate treatment for the condition? What is clear is that the lack of facilities and reliance on traditional healers leads to a conflict between perceptions of appropriate health care.

APPRECIATING AND CHALLENGING TABOO'S

Many topics in PNG are considered taboo subjects. Individuals may not speak about certain topics unless they are with members of their community. In addition, there are strict codes about who within the tribe or clan they are allowed to speak about the topic. The participants described how they avoided talking about their traditions in their place of origin when seeking health care, because they feared being ridiculed and not taken seriously by health professionals from other tribes or from other countries.

The nature of taboos in PNG is diverse. Some are specific to particular language groups whilst others may straddle a number of cultural groups. For example, sexual health is a taboo subject in many PNG communities. However, the participants wanted to learn about things that would help them in their environment and context. During discussions about malaria and its effects on maternal and child health a member of the community asked if they could have a discussion about family planning. Other participants affirmed this request. This was surprising, since the literature and the advisors to the project had affirmed that family planning is a taboo subject. This request was framed within the context of general health and the cultural transition being experienced by members of the community:

Can we talk about family planning in one session. Many women get sick when they are pregnant. Also when we have many children it is difficult to make sure we have money to look after them properly to feed them and send them to schools can we talk about this

During one session participants shared their traditional ways of communicating with their children about their cultural norms:

In the village traditionally men lived in the long-men house and women lived with the children in small houses. The men take the responsibility to speak with the boys about family planning and women speak with the girls

Unlike in the village setting, where men and women lived in separate dwellings, in the urban context, a family of two parents and six children may share a living space of two meters by three. The gender divide is therefore less evident within this spatial context. This contributes to different contexts in sharing conversation and advice about cultural issues.

Therefore, in response to the statement about who advises the boys and girls about cultural norms the lead researcher asked;

But how do you live here? It seems as if you live with the father and mother and the children live with you together. So who now takes the responsibility to talk about these things? Have you found a new way to talk about these things? If it isn't part of your traditional way of speaking between man and woman then how do you address the issues?

This question provoked a lot of discussion about how members of the community can find a way to discuss such topics. They began to realise that the older generation, who had grown up in the village, were making assumptions about how much their young people know of the cultural traditions of their village in the Southern Highlands. They recognised that the young people born in Port Moresby were not being exposed to the type of discussion held in the village setting and therefore were not aware of the tribal codes of conduct expected of them.

It was unusual for such discussions to take place with so many of the community including men, women and children. The project was designed to be as inclusive as possible. The research was conducted with a colleague who is an elder with from the Kewapi language group. The team

were undertaking the study at the invitation of community members The lead researcher, who was female, had made a commitment to learning as much as possible about PNG society before starting the project. She is a public health nurse and has extensive experience of working with diverse groups in the UK. Te presence of a woman leading the dialogue may have had an impact on the way members of the community engaged with the conversations that took place. It is usual of men to take the lead in the traditional forum for discussion. However, education also awards status to the member of the tribe..The members of the community appreciated this commitment and felt that their context and cultural traditions were being respected and affirmed whilst they were considering the implications these have for living in the twenty first century. This enabled them to share issues that they would not usually air.

One participant reported:

We are able to tell you about sorcery. We don't usually tell outside our community. Health care workers laugh at us. You understand that we have traditions that we respect and help us to think about new ways of looking at them.

EXTENDING SHARED UNDERSTANDINGS TO THE VILLAGE COMMUNITY

The commitment to sharing understandings extended to a ITN bed net initiative conducted in the Batri villages. A two-way radio was used to develop the initiative. This included dialogue about the experience of malaria in the village, the need to attain data about the prevalence and morbidity related to malaria in the villages and the demographic profile of the population. Members of the research team, the language group living in Port Moresby and those living in the isolated rural villages networked to put together a bid for ITN bed nets to the British High Commission.

In compiling the bid the stakeholders brought together data from the national data sets and form local sources such as elders detailed registers of the local demographics and aid post statistics.

Documentary evidence and Public health documents revealed the following profile of malaria in PNG.

- Malaria is the second most significant cause of death in PNG (Save the Children Fund 2003)
- In 1994, 47% of the population of two villages in PNG were positive for the plasmodium falciparum parasite, the most dangerous form of malaria (Felger et al. 1994)
- In 2005, Mueller et al's studied eleven villages between 1,400 and 1,700 meters above sea level.
- Following the 2002 rainy season, 53% had symptoms of malaria.
- 6-10 fold increase in parasite prevalence compared with previous studies
- 12 fold increase in enlarged spleens

The members of the community were able to inform the background data by providing information held at the local aid post.

In a population of Population 1.400

- 5 people per year were dying of cerebral malaria
- 39 people per month reporting to the aid post with
- Acute malaria
- Chronic Malaria
- Fevers, lethargy etc
- Anaemia

Malaria and its complications were also contributing to post partum haemorrhage and maternal death. The combined information was used to inform a bid to the British High commission for 400 WHO approved ITN bed nets.

Local knowledge also illustrated how, when malaria hit the village it affects all of the members of the community as this quote illustrates.

When malaria comes everyone is affected. Mothers are ill and cannot look after the children. There is no one to bring water or to tend the gardens so everyone becomes very sick.

The forum for distribution of the ITN bed nets and instruction about their care and maintenance was located on the Batri airstrip. Members of the village congregated on the air strip. They built a podium from bush materials so that everyone would be able to see the speaker and appreciate the formal distribution of the bed nets. The bed nets were presented by roll call to the senior female member of the household.

The researcher from the 'Erima empowerment research project', who is also a member of the language group, travelled with the bed nets and stayed in the village and conducted a series of discussions with village elders who had agreed to coordinate passing on information to the community who numbered 1500. The focus was to reinforce the efficacy of using bed nets in malaria prevention and to share information about the care and maintenance of the bed nets.

It was apparent during the process of discussion that the participants understanding of malaria and its impact on their community is mediated by traditional beliefs. For example some people believe that sickness comes because of bad feelings between or within the tribe. Since there is no school or medical aid post in the village the people do not have the opportunity to consider other reasons for illness.

Carrasquilla (2001) describes similar findings in his study of an ecosystem approach to malaria prevention in Colombia. In his study, he found that health sector leadership was limited and that community participation was non-existent. He found that women in Columbia are the main actors in developing health promotion activities in both rural and urban areas. In the PNG context there were a range of factors impinging on the

Table 1. Diagram of factors affecting the community living in the village drawing on Layder's research map

		Papua New Guinea Rural context
history	Context	**Macro Social forms of organisation** **Traditional Society spiritual beliefs, gender dynamics, living in 'open' spaces** **Mediated by missionary influence and** **Western Colonial Powers'** **Diverse Tribes in urban area** **Sense of remoteness lack of opportunity to access health and education**
	Setting	**Intermediate Social Organisation** **Living in a rural community** **Community networks support living in hostile terrain** **Perceived lack of opportunity to access employment, education and health Care**
	Situated Activity	**Social activity** **Remote location Social relationship** **Networks reflect the need to establish kinship networks.** **Bride price is still practised** **Focus on everyday survival. gardens, hunting**
	Self	**Self Identity and Individual's Social Experience** **Individuals belong to a tribal group responsibilities are to the tribe** **Gender roles** **Focus on daily activities for survival**

development of an effective health promotion and malaria prevention initiative as outlined in Table 1.

Traditionally resources are distributed to the male elders of the community. In this instance, the research team and members of the community living in the settlement and in the villages had many conversations why women and children were to receive the bed nets this initiative. This involved extensive discussion about cultural norms and the need to develop a strategy to target the members most at risk of profound complications of malaria. This reorientation of beliefs about the position of women can be challenging since it confronts some basic understandings of societal norms within the tribe. To sustain the dialogue and develop a shared understanding requires commitment perseverance by all those involved.

IMPACT OF SHARING KNOWLEDGE AND DEVELOPING NETWORKS

The development of a collaborative empowerment approach to this research project has had significant impact on the strategies members of

this community are developing to optimise their health experiences. The participants in this study have gained confidence in addressing individual and local health needs. They now take responsibility for various aspects of their lives. For example, they keep small first aid kits developed in the first phase of the project topped up. This prevents the children getting infected cuts since they have equipment to treat them immediately to hand. They have also decided to share this idea with visitors coming from their village in the Highlands. One of the women living in the settlement takes the responsibility to take the women visiting from the village to the supermarket and they then make up similar basic first aid kits to take home with them.

Engagement with the process of developing the bid and deploying the ITN bed nets to the Batri villages has led to a sense of empowerment in the wider networked community. This ownership has led to very effective use of the mosquito nets. This has resulted in a rapid decline in malaria related illness in the area. Participants in Erima commented:

Your coming here and working with us in our place has made us think. It was important that you came and saw how we live and try to understand our ways and culture. We now realise we cannot wait for people to come. We can make changes ourselves. It is difficult but it can be done. Last year when you came many of the 'boys' didn't have work, but this year they have nearly all got something. For example, they are working as security guards or if they have other skills they are driving or working as offsiders (fare collectors on the local buses). It is important that they are working and feel they can contribute to the community.

The malaria prevention initiative has also had a dramatic impact and improved the quality of life in the remote village in PNG. It has prevented members of the community experiencing malaria to the extent that it ends in a critical event that in the past would ultimately result in death. In February 2006 a member of the village reported:

Since you sent the mosquito nets to the village we have had no deaths and we have not had to send anyone to hospital. It shows that malaria was a significant illness in our community. We are so grateful that you and the British High Commissioner have been able to think of us and help us. Fitzpatrick 2006:22

ISSUES CONTROVERSIES PROBLEMS

Scientific enquiry demands that researchers adopt an approach to which satisfies demands for rigour in engaging with the process of enquiry. These demands range from adopting a research methodology which addresses the question whilst adhering to conventions on research design and modes of analysis and ethical conduct.

Within the landscape of research there is a plethora of methodologies The literature on health care research grades this into various hierarchies. These suggest that Randomised Control Trials aspire to the 'gold standard' in research. However if we consider that there is a continuum in research there emerges a profile of research approaches which are fit for purpose with reference to the topic of enquiry. Greenlaugh and Russel (2007) challenge the assumption that generalisable truths from population driven evidence can be transposed into the experience of the individual. They assert that one must not lose sight of the need for an interpretative framework to inform the decision in applying research evidence.

With the spectrum of research enquiry the researchers intention will have an impact on the choice of approach (Hanney et al 2009). Whilst some will emphasise reliability and generisability others will foreground validity and affirmation of the participants perspectives. Each serves to contribute insights into the development of health care policy and practice.

The development of inclusive user focused initiatives is complex and time consuming. It requires equitable commitment and shared responsibility that can be difficult to achieve. In the context described here there can be a dependency culture. This has come about as a result of prior experience of donor initiatives which embedded a paternalistic attitude to indigenous peoples.

Other agencies may have other perspectives on working with communities and these must be acknowledged and explored. In order to develop effective approaches to health care policy and design health needs need to be appreciated in the context of lived experiences of those affected.

A perception of a genuine engagement with the community can open up the possibility of discussion with the community about how members of the community can affect their health experiences. This involves an affirmation of traditional belief systems and a commitment to working with members of the community to explore the context in which they have evolved. This can then lead to a discussion about the emergence of a different context in which alternative explanations and practices can emerge. This approach is however fraught with a range of ethical dilemmas in developing trust, inclusiveness and respectful dialogue.

INTERNATIONAL TO CONTEXT SPECIFIC AGENDAS: CONTROLLED VERSUS REAL WORLD APPLICATION

In contemporary health care settings, agendas of evidence based practice (EBP) and efficiency and effectiveness of clinical care are paramount. An underlying concern is the efficacy and cost effectiveness of care and treatment options. A key question being asked is does research address the dynamics of user engagement with treatment? For example, if a drug has been developed in a controlled study in which the selected research population have been invited to participate are the findings transferable to other populations who do not conform to the selection criteria?

In Sackett's original definition of EBM in 1996 he describes it as:

Conscientious and judicious use of current best evidence from clinical care research in the management of individual patients. Sackett et al 1996

In his later edition he refines this definition and states that EBM is:

The integration of best research evidence with clinical expertise and patient values. Sackett et al 2000

There are various challenges in meeting these criteria since decision-making does not occur in a vacuum. As Tilburt (2008) observes there are a number of factors which impact on the process including:-

- research evidence,
- the clinical state and
- circumstances,

He asserts that the outcome is also dependent on the patient's preferences and actions.

In this analysis there is an implicit assumption that the term 'research' refers to biomedical, clinical or 'basic' research.

Tilburt (2008) extends this analysis to suggest that in institutional and public health contexts decision makers need to take account of the organisational constraints the context of the decision and the population values of the stakeholders. However a limited definition of research confined within the 'biomedical' frame of reference continues to permeate the discussion.

SOLUTIONS IN THE WIDER HEALTH CONTEXT

In developing equitable health systems, the World Health Organisation (2005) advocates strengthening the repository of social science research to inform policy decisions affecting health care. This change in emphasis allows us to consider what other types of research can offer in enabling us to develop health promotion and treatment strate-

Figure 4.

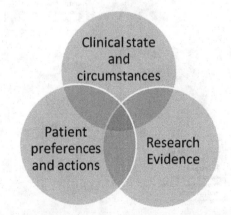

gies which will enable communities to optimise their health experiences. The cycle of EBM then extends to take account of factors such as societal and organisational issues. This also allows us to explore the dynamics of knowledge resources and networks held by the stakeholders involved in health policy design and implementation.

The diagram shown in Figure 5 illustrates the dynamic interplay between the stakeholders in decision making in health care practice. The players include the patient, family and community members and health care professionals. Their views are mediated by a range of factors including the societal and organisational context combined with access to knowledge resources and networks.

CONCLUSION

As the USA National Working Party on Evidence Based Care reports (2009), study designs often do not address the cultural and ethnicity of the health care population. They therefore draw conclusions about the effectiveness of a treatment without full information about the cultural norms of the population. This could result in care or treatment that draws wrong or harmful conclusions about

Figure 5. Extended dynamic model of Evidence Based Practice (authors model)

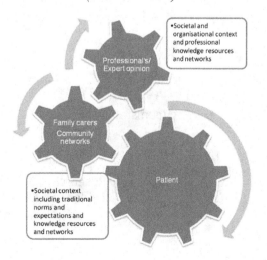

its suitability for culturally diverse populations, children, older adults and those with multiple health conditions. The research is conducted in controlled rather than real world settings. If we are to address these shortcomings, it is important to find ways of developing a range of research approaches which will enable us to develop our knowledge and evidence base in order to enable us to engage with individuals and communities effectively.

This will involve the development of comparative research in defining key questions and research methodologies that are inclusive of the consumer of health policies and products. For example, it will involve the development of approaches that:

- Involve patients/consumers and representative organizations measure consumer-focused endpoints, such as quality of life measures and functionality.
- Include patients/consumers on pre-clinical and post-market review panels within government regulatory bodies to ensure critical assessment of research and pinpoint goals and outcomes of importance to real-world patients.
- Provide incentives for research organizations to demonstrate methods for including patient/consumer perspectives.
- Ref NWG on EBP (2008)

The study described above demonstrates that with commitment to shared understandings and respect for differing perspectives communities living in adverse conditions can and do improve their health experiences. However this requires a move away from a donor mentality towards genuine partnership and reciprocal dialogue (Ako 2002; Ako and Fitzpatrick 2007). This is in contrast to expectations of top-down policy design and implementation. This requires a genuine engagement with community perspective on health issues. It requires a reframing of the issues to considering health rather than disease process. In addition, it implies that recruitment of and commitment to working with 'hard to reach' communities must become a real in developing world contexts like PNG.

REFERENCES

Adamchak, S. E. (2006). Youth Peer Education in Reproductive Health and HIV and AIDS: Progress, Process and Programming for the Future Youth Issues Paper 7. *Family Health International, Youthnet program*, Arlington, VA.

Ako, W. Y. (2002). *Factors Affecting the Formulation and Implementation of the 1993 Educational Reforms in Papua New Guinea. Doctoral Thesis*. Bristol: The University of Bristol

Ako, W.Y., & Fitzpatrick, J. (2007, June). Empowering the Initiation of a malaria prevention strategy to combat malaria in Papua New Guinea. *Rural and Remote Health*.

AusAID. (2004). *Country Programs: Papua New Guinea*. Retrieved September 22, 2004, from http://www.ausaid.gov.au/country/papua.cfm

Boultier, M., Mason, R., & Rootman, I. (1997). Community action and reflective practice in health promotion research. *Health Promotion International, 12*(1), 60–78.

Bouton-Lewis, G., & Lewis, D. (2002). Conceptions of Health held by Aborigional, Torres Strait Islander and Papua New Guinean Health Science Students. *Close Up 2 H Higher Education Conference*. University of Lancaster.

Carrasquilla, G. (2001) Cad. Suide Publica, Rio de Jeniro 17. *Suplemento,* 171-179.

Crossley, M., & Holmes, K. (2001). Challenges for educational research. interantional partnerships and capacity building in small states. *Oxford Review of Education, 27*(3), 395–409. doi:10.1080/03054980120067429

Executive Board of the United Nations Development Programme and the United Nations Populations Fund. (2002). *Country Co-operations Frameworks and Related Matters: Country Programme Outline for Papua New Guinea (2003-2007)* New York: UN

Fabrega, H. (1997). Historical and cultural foundations of health behaviour. In Gochman, D. S. (Ed.), *Handbook for Health Behaviour Research1 Personal and Social Determinants*. New York: Plenum Press.

Felger, I., Tavul, L., Kabintik, S., Marshall, V., Genton, B., Alpers, M., & Beck, H. P. (1994). Plasmodium falciparum: extensive polymorphism in merozoite surface antigen 2 alleles in an area with endemic malaria in Papua New Guinea. *Experimental Parasitology, 79*(2), 106–116. doi:10.1006/expr.1994.1070

Fitzpatrick (2007). Malaria: promoting awareness and prevention of a critical crisis in a remote area of Papua New Guinea through community involvement. 2006 Volume 5 Number Global connections *CONNECT The World of Critical Care Nursing* 2006 5 1 22

Green, L. W., & Kreuter, M. W. (1999). *Health promotion planning: An educational and ecological approach* (3rd ed.). Mountain View, CA: Mayfield.

Greenlaugh, T andd Russel J2009 Evidence-BasedPolicymaking *a critique Perspectives in Biology and Medicine, 52*(2), 304–18 Baltimore, MD: The Johns Hopkins University Press

Gruber, T. R. (1993) What is an Ontology? Toward principles for the design of ontologies used for knowledge sharing. Presented at the Padua workshop on Formal Ontology, March 1993, later published in *International Journal of Human-Computer Studies, 43*(4-5), 907-928.

Hanney, S. R., Gonzalez-Block, M. A., Buxton, M. J., & Kogan, M. (2003). The utilisation of health research in policy-making: concepts, examples and methods of assessment. *Health Research Policy and Systems*, 2003.

Holter, I. M., & Scwartz-Barcott, D. (1993). Action research: What is it? How has it been used and how can it be used in nursing? *Journal of Advanced Nursing, 18*, 208–304. doi:10.1046/j.1365-2648.1993.18020298.x

Holter, I. M., & Scwartz-Barcott, D. (1993). Action research: What is it? How has it been used and how can it be used in nursing? *Journal of Advanced Nursing, 18*, 208–304. doi:10.1046/j.1365-2648.1993.18020298.x

Infoplease (2005) *Infoplease.* Retrieved April 21, 2005, from http://www.infoplease.com/ipa/A0107875.html

Layder, D. (1994). *New Strategies in Social Research.* Cambridge, UK: Cambridge Polity Press.

Lim, R. (2003) *Outside the classroom: Oral and visual research methods applied in vernacular settlements.* Conference Proceedings, International Conference on Integrating Teaching with Research and Practice in the Built Environment. Wadham College Oxford.

Louk, W. (2009). Peters, H., Gerjo Kok, Geert T. M., Ten Dam, Goof J Buijs, & Theo G. W. M. Paulussen(2009) Effective elements of school health promotion across behavioral domains: a systematic review of reviews. *BMC Public Health, 9*, 182. Published online 2009 June 12. doi:.doi:10.1186/1471-2458-9-182

Makundi, E. A., Malebo, H. M., Mhame, P., Kitua, A. y., & Warsame, M. (2006). Role of Traditional Healers in the management of severe malaria among children below five years of age: The case of Kilosa and Handeni Districs in Tanzania. *Malaria Journal, 5*, 58. http://www.malariajounal.com/contents/5/1/58. doi:10.1186/1475-2875-5-58

Mueller, I. (2005). Namuigi, P., Kundi, J., Ivivi, R. Tandrapah, T., and Bjorge, S. Epidemic Malaria in the Highlands of Paua New Guinea. *American Journal of Tropical Medicine, 72*, 554–560.

Neito, T., Mendez, F., & Carrasquilla, G. (1999). Knowledge Beliefs and practices relevant for malaria control in an endemic urban area of the Columbian Pacific. *Social Science & Medicine, 49*, 601–609. doi:10.1016/S0277-9536(99)00134-3

Peersman, G., Flores, S., Zee, A., & Eke, A. (2001) Interventions for preventing HIV in young people in Low Income countries, *The Cochrane Database of Systematic Reviews,* The Cochrane Library. http://www.cochrane.org/colloquia/abstracts/capetown/capetownPD11.html

PNG DoH. (2001). *National Health Plan 2001-2010.* Port Moresby: Department of Health, Government of Papua New Guinea.

Sackett, D.L. Strauss, S.E. Richardson, W. S. Rosenderg, W.and Haynes, R.B. *Evidence Based Medicine How to Practice and Teach EBM*, 2nd Edition Edinburgh Churchill Livingstone

Sackett, D. L., Rosenberg, W. M., Gray, J. A., Haynes, R. B., & Richardson, W. S. (1996). Evidence based medicine: what it is and what it isn't. *British Medical Journal, 312*, 71–72.

Save the Children. (2003). Papua New Guinea: Training volunteers to improve community health. Retrieved from http://www.savethechildren.net/new_zealand/what_we_do/our_projects/papua_new_guinea.html

Simms, P. A. (2002) Papua New Guinea needs law and order above all. *British Medical Journal.* 2002 325:914-915 (26 October)

Sturt, J. (1999). Placing empowerment research within an action research typology. *Journal of Advanced Nursing, 30*(5), 1057–1063. doi:10.1046/j.1365-2648.1999.01202.x

The National Working Group on Evidence-Based Health Care. (2008). Advancing the Evidence of Experience: Practical Issues for Patient/Consumer Inclusion http://www.evidencebasedhealthcare. org/index.cfm?objectid=80363086-1372-4D20-C8275AD1BBB7C263

Tilburt, J. C. (2008). Evidence bsed medicine beyond the bedside: keeping an eye on the context. *Journal of Evaluation in Clinical Practice, 14*, 721–725. doi:10.1111/j.1365-2753.2008.00948.x

Timmer, J. (2000). *Living Within Intricate Futures: Order and Confusion in Imjan Worlds*. Holland: Centre for Pacific and Asian Studies.

Tree, I. (1996). *Island in the Clouds*. London: Lonely Planet.

VSO. (1999). *Country Profile PNG*. Retrieved April 5, 2005, from http://vsocanada.ca/attachments/papua_new_guinea.pdf

WHO. (2002). *Core Health Indicators for Papua New Guinea*. Retrieved from http://www3.who. int/whosis/country/compare.cfm?country=PNG &indicator=strMortChildMale2002,strMortChil dFemale2002&language=english

WHO. (2004). *Roll Mack Malaria Partnership*. Retrieved from http://www.rbm.who.int/cgi-bin/ rbm/rbmportal/custom/rbm/home.do

WHO. (2005). Priorities to take forward the health equity policy agenda WHO Task Force on Research priorities for equity in health. *Bulletin of the World Health Organization*, 12.

Williams, C. (1998) Mysticism Medicine Papua New Guinea. *Wellbeing magazine, 71*, 50-57

Chapter 23
Psychiatric Illness and Personal Narrative:
Implications for Social Networking in the Information Age

Edward Kim
Robert Wood Johnson Medical School, USA

ABSTRACT

Psychiatric illness is perhaps the richest and most challenging narrative for consumers to develop because core symptoms of disease may distort perceptual and interpretative brain functions. These distortions may fragment and disrupt personal narratives of wellness, illness, and recovery. Advances in psychopharmacology enable better management of core symptoms, while evidence-based psychotherapies help consumers manage residual symptoms and reduce relapse risk. So-called recovery-oriented treatments that focus on improving functioning and success in life, relationships, and work enable consumers to pursue goals that are not limited to managing their disease. These advances in the management of psychiatric illness create opportunities and needs for greater social awareness and integration. As Internet access becomes more common among all strata of societies, the use of the Web-based social networking may accelerate the development of new models of recovery. Social networking may expand the consumer's understanding of their past and present through web-based shared discussions with other consumers and professionals. Online psychiatric-related activity generally falls into several categories related to information acquisition, treatment facilitation, and social networking. Professional and consumer education are available on the Internet, though the quality of information may be variable depending on whether or not the material undergoes scientific review. Virtual communities (VCs) may range from professional communities of practice to peer-based support networks comprised of consumers alone or consumers and professionals. The tension between confidentiality and transparency, and the potential for deception due to anonymity are ethical challenges that must be addressed as VCs and social networking evolve in health care.

DOI: 10.4018/978-1-60960-097-6.ch023

INTRODUCTION

Historical Perspectives on Psychiatric Illness

Psychiatric illness is frequently stigmatized in many multiple cultures in ways that lead to alienation from mainstream social networks and even the healthcare system. The Institute of Medicine (2006) identified stigma as a major factor in the isolation of mental health services from mainstream medicine. The unique combination of stigma, fragmentation of service delivery and conditions that affect cognition and judgment pose major barriers to consumer-driven treatment. Nevertheless, these challenges do not diminish the need for individualized, recovery-oriented treatment (Rogers et al, 2008).

Evolution of Psychiatric Treatment

The conceptualization and treatment of psychiatric illness evolved during the 18th century Enlightenment. The so-called "moral treatment" of psychiatric illness that emerged engaged patients in productive physical and vocational activity designed to promote a sense of accomplishment and well-being (Taubes 1998). The absence of pharmacological therapies to reduce the severity and recurrence of psychiatric illness limited treatment options to environmental and social therapies. Treatment facilities evolved into semi-autonomous communities that shielded patients from the social and environmental stresses that often precipitated relapses. A core assumption was that work in itself was therapeutic because it provided patients with an experience of self-efficacy and self-worth. The social dimensions of therapeutic communities also provided a sense of belonging and engagement, though patients needed accommodations for their varying degrees of comfort with social interactions. Further understanding of the psychological and social dimensions of psychiatric illness led

to the development of therapeutic interventions to improve consumers' ability to cope with and self-manage certain elements of their disorders, with varying success.

Biological Psychiatry

The emergence of psychotropic medications to modulate psychiatric symptoms reduced patient dependence on environmental interventions and enabled a broader spectrum of patients to benefit from psychosocial therapies (Ban, 2001). These early psychotropic medications facilitated the de-institutionalization of thousands of consumers who had been confined to residing in psychiatric facilities. The opportunity for fuller integration into society was challenged by the continuing vulnerability to relapse that might be induced by medication non-adherence, the natural course of disease, and psychosocial stresses (Klerman, 1977).

The Mind-Brain Challenge in Psychiatric Treatment

Psychiatric illnesses may impair the very functions needed to process, integrate, and organize an effective help-seeking response. These subtle neurocognitive deficits may reduce their ability to process non-verbal social cues, organize and process complex social interactions independent of acute or residual psychiatric symptoms (Lysaker and Buck, 2007; McDermott and Ebmeier, 2009; Wingo, Harvey and Baldessarini, 2009). Such deficits may present barriers to collaboration with concerned significant others and treatment providers, and may lead to a negative spiral of increasingly polarized interactions. The experience of hospitalization disrupts an individual's educational, social, and vocational path and can be experienced as losses of identity. The effective clinician will understand not only the diagnostic significance of the symptoms, but also the effects of such symptoms on the individual's experience of themselves, their relationships, and their role in life.

Psychiatric Treatment and Shared Narrative

Effective treatment planning emerges when consumer and provider collaborate to form a shared narrative of the disease (Charon 2001). The consumer is an experiential expert in that no one has better knowledge of their current symptoms, when they started, and their current narrative, from early development to recent precipitating events. The clinician brings expert knowledge to help clarify the diagnosis, which will lead to a range of treatment options and provide prognostic considerations. Having studied or cared for patients across the full cycle of illness and recovery, the clinician also has a general framework for helping set expectations of the work ahead. With this expertise the provider may anticipate decisions, challenges, and opportunities the patient has not yet experienced. Through meaningful dialogue the consumer-clinician team establishes a common understanding of the current situation, then proceeds to negotiate the potential options. This dialogue, which creates a new reality for both patient and clinician, is common to all medical practice. However, in psychiatric practice the narrative may be less readily intelligible due to perceptual and cognitive distortions that are part of the clinical presentation of illness.

Historically, user-driven mental health services are among the earliest manifestations of shared narrative in medicine. The clubhouse model is based on peer-to-peer counseling that focuses on strengths and life goals rather than symptoms and treatment goals (Herman et al, 2005). Evolution of the model has led to multiple variations; some continue a strictly consumer-based model, while others have fully integrated traditional clinical services into a recovery-based model.

The integrated models provide consumers with evidence-based pharmacological treatments and psychotherapies, while providing access to a social network of peers committed to mutual success in life. Peer mentors demonstrate the possibility of success and may be a source of hope and motivation. They can describe how and why they made certain choices, describe lessons learned from less effective choices, and provide emotional support for the mentored consumer on the process of effective decision making.

Mind vs. Brain, Self vs. Other

This brief summary of the evolution of psychiatric treatment describes the migration from a social to a neurobiological model of psychiatric illness; these are complementary rather than mutually exclusive. While research evidence strongly supports a neurobiological model for psychiatric health and illness, the brain is an open system that can be modified by interactions with the environment. This supports the importance of psychosocial interventions that may include formal psychotherapy, social skills training, and peer to peer interactions.

Social Networking as Shared Narrative

Building on this historical foundation, social networking may expand the consumer's understanding of their past and present through web-based shared discussions with other consumers and professionals. In many ways this models the clinical dialogue, in which seemingly disconnected fragments of experience are woven into a coherent, intelligible narrative that helps orient the consumer to their current situation. Under the best of circumstances, social networking may accelerate treatment and recovery by helping consumers understand the nature of their condition, the potential future available to them, and their role and responsibility in crafting that future. Such insights typically occur through psychoeducational processes in group or one on one sessions. Open networking within communities of consumers may bypass this limitation by exposing the consumer to numerous narratives of others at different points in their journey.

The Internet and Psychiatric Treatment

Given the rapid commoditization of information technology, the Internet is widely accessible in developed nations to virtually all socioeconomic strata through public libraries and personal subscriptions. Online psychiatric-related activity generally falls into several categories related to information acquisition, treatment facilitation, and social networking.

Professional Education

The Internet has been used for quite some time as a medium from continuing professional education of psychiatric professionals. Many programs with relevance to prescribing practices are sponsored by pharmaceutical companies. However, they are required to have complete autonomy from influence of the sponsor. Such resources provide important information regarding the appropriate use of psychotropic medications in ways that may or may not be consistent with the manufacturer's package insert, but are supported by scientific evidence. Web-based resources may include text-based or streaming media as well as live/archived webcasts that may be accessed in real time or asynchronously. These sites are peer-reviewed and often have editorial advisory boards consisting of prominent medical experts. The reliability of the content is therefore quite high. However, the ability to interact and share best practices is limited unless there is an audience response component to the program.

Consumer Information

Consumer-directed information often focuses on increasing patient and caregiver understanding of the illness process, the process of care, and treatment alternatives. The goal of such information is to increase the overall health literacy of the consumer community. Such information is often available on provider websites in order to provide professionals with convenient informational resources to print and distribute to their patients. Professional organizations will subject consumer information to rigorous scientific review to ensure accuracy, and will also ensure that the information is intelligible and avoids the use of technical jargon. Other sources of information include consumer websites, which may have scientific advisory boards to ensure medical accuracy of the information. Discussion boards may or may not be moderated by professionals to ensure accuracy, and provide the added benefit of interaction, allowing consumers to interact with one another and/or professionals to exchange information, experiences, and perspectives. However, the challenge of such a format is to balance accuracy and freedom of expression. Unmoderated discussion boards or personal websites without scientific review may be more likely to disseminate inaccurate information.

Research on the quality of mental health information on the Internet has yielded variable results. Szumilas and Kutcher (2009) reviewed selected Canadian websites for information on risk factors for youth suicide. They found that only 44% of the statements regarding risk factors were supported by scientific evidence. Compared with government websites, nonprofit organization websites were more likely and personal or media websites were less likely to have a positive "evidence-based rating". Griffiths and Christensen (2000) reviewed 21 frequently accessed websites on depression, finding that the overall quality of information was poor and frequently did not cite scientific references to support their claims. Ipser et al (2007) reviewed 67 websites identified through Google, Yahoo, and MSN search engines for information on anxiety disorders. They found that the quality of the information ranged from poor to moderate, again with claims frequently not supported by scientific citations. On the other hand, Morel et al (2008) reviewed 34 sites with information on bipolar disorder, finding that the overall content quality to be good.

Virtual Communities

Virtual communities (VCs) may range from professional communities of practice to peer-based support networks comprised of consumers alone or consumers and professionals. Demiris (2006) describes the diffusion of VCs in healthcare, and describes professional uses such as care coordination, research, disease management and peer support. Information technology may lead to better resource allocation and more informed clinical decisionmaking by promoting more effective interactions through the availability of live or asynchronous interactions distributed across space and time. Peer to peer interactions may provide patients and caregivers with vital support by eliminating geographical barriers. Eysenback et al (2004) conducted a systematic review of published literature on outcomes of VCs, which included electronic peer support groups. Of note, most of the studies incorporated complex interventions in which peer to peer support was a component. Of the 6 pure peer to peer interventions, 3 of which addressed depression as an outcome, there was insufficient evidence to claim that such interventions were effective.

A potential risk of social networking is that consumers may overwhelmed by the sheer volume of information available. As discussed previously, cognitive deficits and psychiatric symptoms may present challenges to effective integration of available information. Another risk is that consumers may be misled by incomplete or biased informa-

tion, or even victimized by predatory individuals. Still others may promote products or services that offer no evidence-based benefit to consumers.

Ethical Considerations in Social Networking

The tension between confidentiality and transparency, and the potential for deception due to anonymity are challenges that must be addressed as VCs evolve in health care (Demiris 2006). Social networking between professionals and consumers raise require additional consideration. While there is no absolute prohibition, most professional societies recognize that client-provider social relationships may adversely influence the objectivity of the professional, leading to suboptimal treatment processes and outcomes. Moreover, social intimacy may confound a provider-patient relationship, leading to potentially unprofessional and unethical romantic or business relationships. The professional mandate of transparency and fiduciary responsibility to the patient may be more challenging if clinicians and patients extend their interactions beyond the confines of the treatment relationships. Professionals are no less tempted than others by the convenience and anonymity of the Internet. Therefore direct social networking with consumers may preclude providing professional services with "friends" or "connections". Social networking may or may not be an effective means of matching consumers and providers. Many questions remain to be answered on this area.

CONCLUSION

Psychiatric illness is perhaps the richest and most challenging narrative for consumers to develop because core symptoms of disease may distort perceptual and interpretative brain functions. These distortions may fragment and disrupt personal narratives of wellness, illness, and recovery. Advances in psychopharmacology enable better management of core symptoms, while evidence-based psychotherapies help consumers manage residual symptoms and reduce relapse risk. So-called recovery-oriented treatments that focus on improving functioning and success in life, relationships, and work enable consumers to pursue goals that are not limited to managing their disease. These advances in the management of psychiatric illness create opportunities and needs for greater social awareness and integration. As Internet access becomes more common among all strata of societies, the use of the Web-based social networking may accelerate the development of new models of recovery. Since many professionals use social networking as a means of business generation, i.e. LinkedIn and Plaxo, this raises questions regarding whether connections found through these means can be converted to client-professional relationships. It seems that sites that have as their specific aims the matching of consumer-provider relationships might have the greatest likelihood of creating greater value than risk, while the non-specificity of general social networking sites may pose greater risks due to the ambiguous nature of the networking process.

The evolution of social networking for psychiatric consumers warrants further study in order to answer several questions, namely:

- In what ways do social networking processes influence adaptive and maladaptive peer to peer consumer engagement?
- How does social networking affect consumer health literacy, assertiveness with treatment providers, and shared decision making?
- How does social networking affect consumer adherence to treatment regimens?
- What is the impact of social networking between consumers and providers? Does it enhance engagement? Does it create problematic boundary violations?
- What, if any, moderation of social networking processes provides the optimal

benefit to users? Is moderation by mental health professionals qualitatively different from moderation by consumers?

Answering these questions should provide the field with a better understanding of the effective use of Web-based social networking to assist consumer adaptation and recovery.

REFERENCES

Ban, T. (2001). Pharmacotherapy of mental illness– a historical analysis. *Progress in Neuro-Psychopharmacology & Biological Psychiatry*, *25*, 667–694. doi:10.1016/S0278-5846(01)00160-9

Charon, R. (2001). Narrative medicine: a model for empathy, reflection, profession, and trust. *Journal of the American Medical Association*, *286*, 1897–1902. doi:10.1001/jama.286.15.1897

Demiris, G. (2006). The diffusion of virtual communities in health care: Concepts and challenges. *Patient Education and Counseling*, *62*, 178–188. doi:10.1016/j.pec.2005.10.003

Eysenbach, G., Power, J., & Englesakis, M. (2004). Health related virtual communities and electronic support groups: systematic review of the effects of online peer to peer interactions. *British Medical Journal*, *328*, 1166–1171. doi:10.1136/bmj.328.7449.1166

Griffitsh, K. M., & Christensen, H. (2000). Quality of web based information on treatment of depression: cross sectional survey. *British Medical Journal*, *32*, 1511–1515. doi:10.1136/bmj.321.7275.1511

Herman, S. E., & Onaga, E., Pernice-Duca Fet al. (2005). Sense of community in clubhouse programs: member and staff concepts. *American Journal of Community Psychology*, *36*, 343–356. doi:10.1007/s10464-005-8630-2

Institute of Medicine. (2008). *Improving the Quality of Health Care for Mental and Substance-Use Conditions.* Washington, DC: National Academies Press.

Ipser, J. C., Dewing, S., & Stein, D. F. (2007). A systematic review of the quality of information on the treatment of anxiety disorders on the Internet. *Current Psychiatry Reports, 9,* 303–309. doi:10.1007/s11920-007-0037-3

Klerman, G. (1977). Better but not well: social and ethical issues in the deinstitutionalization of the mentally ill. *Schizophrenia Bulletin, 3,* 617–631.

Lysaker, P. H., & Buck, K. D. (2007). Neurocognitive deficits as a barrier to psychosocial function in schizophrenia: effects on learning, coping, & self-concept. *Journal of Psychosocial Nursing and Mental Health Services, 45,* 24–30.

McDermott, L. M., & Ebmeier, K. P. (2009). A meta-analysis of depression severity and cognitive function. *Journal of Affective Disorders, 119,* 1–8. doi:10.1016/j.jad.2009.04.022

Morel, V., Chatton, A., & Cochand, S. (2008). Quality of web-based information on bipolar disorder. *Journal of Affective Disorders, 110,* 265–269. doi:10.1016/j.jad.2008.01.007

Rogers, J. A., Vergare, M. J., Baron, R. C., & Salzer, M. S. (2007). Barriers to recovery and recommendations for change: the Pennsylvania consensus conference on psychiatry's role. *Psychiatric Services (Washington, D.C.), 58,* 1119–1123. doi:10.1176/appi.ps.58.8.1119

Szumilas, M., & Kutcher, S. (2009). Teen suicidal information on the Internet: a systematic analysis of quality. *Canadian Journal of Psychiatry, 54,* 596–604.

Taubes, T. (1998). Healthy avenues of the mind": psychological theory building and the influence of religion during the era of moral treatment. *The American Journal of Psychiatry, 155,* 1001–1008.

Wingo, A. P., Harvey, P. D., & Baldessarini, R. J. (2009). Neurocognitive impairment in bipolar disorder patients: functional implications. *Bipolar Disorders, 11,* 113–125. doi:10.1111/j.1399-5618.2009.00665.x

Chapter 24

The Gap between What is Knowable and What We Do in Clinical Practice

Maartje H.J. Swennen
University Medical Centre Utrecht, The Netherlands

ABSTRACT

Evidence-based Medicine (EBM) is a tool that aims to bring science and medicine together by enabling doctors to integrate the latest best evidence with their clinical expertise and the individual patient's wishes and needs. However, EBM has both strong supporters and antagonists and is confronted with many barriers that impede uptake of the best evidence by doctors. To date, it remains poorly understood why doctors, do, and do not, incorporate high quality evidence into their routine practice. I will take you down the road of how I became more and more intrigued by all the challenges that EBM faces. In addition, I will explain to you how I hope to contribute to closing the gap between what is knowable using EBM methods and what we do.

INTRODUCTION

This chapter takes you through the rationale behind and my own reflections on why I became involved in research on the implementation of Evidence-based Medicine (EBM). For this, I have partly rewritten a joint paper on EBM into a first person narrative. The original paper is accepted for publication by the Journal of Evaluation in Clinical Practice (Swennen, Van der Heijden, Blijham, & Kalkman, in press). This chapter adds a more

comprehensive description of what EBM aims at and why. In addition, it includes my thoughts and feelings at each step of my learning process.

I would not have been able to initiate or continue my research without the support of Dr. Geert van der Heijden, Professor Geert Blijham, Professor Yolanda van der Graaf and Professor Cor Kalkman; all having the University Medical Centre Utrecht (The Netherlands) as their (primary) affiliation. This means that in this chapter 'I' often will reflect 'we'.

First, I will provide you with some information about my background. I graduated from Medical

DOI: 10.4018/978-1-60960-097-6.ch024

School at the Utrecht University (The Netherlands) in 2002 without ever having heard of EBM. (Nowadays, the curriculum of my Medical School comprises EBM). After Medical School I decided not to start my residency in Internal Medicine, because I felt I had to protect myself against the emotional burden of me wanting to become an oncologist. For me, being an oncologist would be all about providing the best care to patients, and pay even more attention to the ones that could not be cured. Hence, after much deliberation I chose to work for the Executive Board of the University Medical Centre Utrecht and became a non-practicing doctor. This allowed me to work on the crossroads of management and doctors, and inspired me to try to bring management and doctors together by solving misunderstandings that impeded collaboration. The Executive Board offered the opportunity to do an MSc on Healthcare Management, and so it happened that late 2003 I *first* heard about EBM during this MSc. I could not believe that until then I had been completely unfamiliar with EBM. During all my medical lectures and internships I never questioned to which extent the knowledge and skills I was taught were (or were not) evidence-based. I fully trusted the teachers, i.e. experienced doctors, to be right, just like my fellow students did. In other words, I was blind to whether the advice received from the teachers was authoritative (evidence-based) or merely authoritarian (opinion-based). So, for me, this was quite an eye-opener. Hence, I decided to do my Master Thesis on the implementation of EBM. This Master Thesis resulted in the joint publication and gradually evolved in my PhD-fellowship and an academic training in Clinical Epidemiology. My research and this chapter are about my aspiration to help doctors getting the evidence into practice.

So, I am a supporter of EBM, in that it concerns both Evidence and clinical Expertise to be crucial: The evidence only becomes valuable when clinical expertise guides its proper use in clinical practice. Therefore, I think the name EBM

and some reporting (in science and teaching) are rather unfortunate, because of their focus on the evidence part. It is completely understandable that this still causes many medical students and doctors to conclude that EBM is decontextualized from real life clinical practice; or is all about certainty; or that clinical expertise is considered less important.

I believe that all doctors want the best for their patients, and therefore deserve further help to become better able to actually do so. In time I hope my PhD fellowship will render helpful solutions that will enable and inspire doctors to further improve patient care.

What Does Evidence-Based Medicine Imply for Medical Decision Making?

Doctors are expected to complement their clinical expertise with findings of research and to take into account the needs and wishes of individual patients. EBM aims to integrate the current best research evidence in a conscientious, explicit, and judicious manner with clinicians' expertise and patients' unique values and circumstances (see also following list) (Guyatt & Rennie, 2002; Straus, Richardson, Glasziou, & Haynes, 2005).

Explanation of key elements of the chosen definition for EBM:

- Best research evidence is considered to be valid and clinically relevant research.
- Clinical expertise refers to the ability to use clinical skills and past experience to rapidly identify each patient's unique health state and diagnosis, their individual risks and benefits of potential interventions, and their personal circumstances and expectations.
- Patient values comprise the unique preferences, concerns and expectations each patient brings to a clinical encounter and

which must be integrated into clinical decisions if they are to serve the patient.

- Patient circumstances refer to their individual clinical state and the clinical setting.

How to even begin trying to reach such a complex aim? For starters, the full-blown practice of EBM is transformed into a continuous cycle of five steps, which are described in detail by Straus et al (2005). In the following list you will only find a short summary of these five steps. Separating evidence from judgment should be considered core academic skills (G. van der Heijden, December 11, 2009).

Description of the five EBM steps:

1. asking answerable clinical questions,
2. finding current best evidence,
3. critical appraisal of the evidence for its validity and clinical relevance,
4. integrating the critical appraisal with doctors' clinical expertise and patients' values and circumstances, and
5. evaluating the four steps for their effectiveness and efficiency.

I agree with Straus et al (2005) that EBM should hold into account the frequency in which conditions are encountered in clinical practice. For conditions doctors encounter every day, doctors need to be completely up-to-date and very sure about what they are doing. Hence, for frequent conditions doctors need to apply at least the first four steps above. For conditions doctors encounter less often, doctors are allowed to conserve their time by seeking out critical appraisals already performed by others (i.e. skipping step 3). For the problems doctors are likely to encounter very infrequently, they mostly 'blindly' seek, accept, and replicate the recommendations they receive from authorities in the relevant branch of medicine. In addition, as evidence is continuously generated, Straus et al also rightly state that EBM implies continuous, self-directed lifelong learning. By not regarding knowledge with humility and by denying uncertainty and curiosity, doctors risk becoming dangerously out of date and immune of self-improvement and advances in medicine.

Unwarranted Variation of Clinical Practice

I consider EBM to be an important tool for medical decision making, because increased use should result in more appropriate healthcare for both individuals and populations. Despite more than 20 years of worldwide efforts to progress EBM, the gap between available and applied evidence remains substantial (Asch et al, 2006; Fisher, Bynum, & Skinner, 2009; Fisher et al, 2003a, 2003b; Grol, 2001; Mangione-Smith et al, 2007; McGlynn et al, 2003; Schuster, McGlynn, & Brook, 1998; Sirovich, Gallagher, Wennberg, & Fisher, 2008).

This gap is visible through unwarranted variation in clinical practice: When similar people, that is, patients with the same medically relevant characteristics, are not treated in a similar manner, then the question is raised if this variation is justified. It was shown that interventions that were likely to be beneficial were not being incorporated into clinical practice and also interventions which were of dubious value or even known to be harmful persisted. Evidence of these variations in medical practice suggests the possibility of inappropriate servicing, wasting of resources and even actual harm to patients. An example of underuse of effective care comes from the US Dartmouth Atlas Project: in many hospital referral regions in 2001, less than 50% of Medicare enrollees with diabetes had eye examinations every two years; in the 'best' regions about 75% of enrollees had them. In addition, depending on the region, from 10% to 70% of Medicare enrollees with diabetes did receive annual blood screening tests of their blood sugar and lipid levels, both of which are important predictors of serious adverse clinical outcomes (e.g. blindness and limb amputation).

So, similar patients (i.e. diabetics) did not receive similar basic care. Of course, there can be good reasons for doctors to purposively decide not to apply the evidence to particular patients (e.g. co-morbidity, side-effects of medication), but this does not fully explain the wide variation observed in clinical practice (Dartmouth Atlas Project, 2007).

As a consequence, appropriateness of care is questioned (Brook, 2009; Burge et al, 2006), and the benefits of healthcare are likely to be suboptimal. Whilst EBM is not necessarily about lower costs, individual and societal costs are arguably higher than would otherwise be the case if high quality evidence was routinely incorporated into routine care (Health Economics Research Group RAND Europe, 2008).

By now, you might think: How could this be? Isn't it obvious that doctors should make evidence-based decisions? To the public and the patients, this is a natural expectation. To doctors, it is a very complex aspiration.

In fact, the advance of EBM was a response to several factors which shook the confidently held view that modern scientific medicine was rational, empirical and founded on a solid research base (Muir Gray, 2001).

The affected confidence in the quality of care increased demands for openness and objectivity of medical decisions. There was also a growing awareness of the limitations of many of the traditional sources of advice and guidance in which doctors placed their trust (e.g. personal clinical experience, expert opinion, tradition and pathophysiology).

The Gap between What is Knowable and What We Do

I wondered why it is so difficult to implement EBM. Is it because doctors think EBM to be a tool that adds to the complexity of clinical practice, instead of reducing it? And is this because the EBM movement did not fully acknowledge the complexity of routine clinical practice, medical decision making and change?

Many barriers to practicing EBM have been described (e.g. Bryar et al, 2003; Cabana et al, 1999; DeLisa, Jain, Kirshblum, & Christodoulou, 1999; Grol, 1997; Grol & Grimshaw, 2003; Haynes, Devereaux, & Guyatt, 2002; McAlister, Graham, Karr, & Laupacis, 1999; McNeill, 2001; Melnyk, 2002; Newman, Papadopoulos, & Sigsworth, 1998; Retsas, 2000; Sackett, Rosenberg, Gray, Haynes, & Richardson, 1996; Straus & McAlister, 2000). Yet, I still did not understand their underlying mechanisms and their interrelations. For example, "lack of time" is the most often reported barrier in the literature. It however may also be a manifestation of other underlying barriers, such as inefficient workflow, lack of necessary facilities, reluctance to change one's trusted routines, or fear of reprisal from skeptical colleagues. Second, although attempts have been made to classify the barriers, a comprehensive approach to their classification is lacking. A current and often used taxonomy (Bryar et al; Grol & Grimshaw) comprises five classes: (1) the individual professional, (2) the team, (3) the organization or environment, (4) the evidence itself, and (5) the patient. A taxonomy needs to be unambiguous and allow for consistent classification, but barriers have been inconsistently classified. For instance, Bryar et al considered "lack of time" to be the most important individual barrier, while Retsas identified "lack of time" as the most important organizational barrier. Third, the current taxonomy of five classes does not reflect a chronological sequence which complicates prioritizing barriers. This impedes the identification of the sequence of conditions needed to improve the practice of EBM. Fourth, the current taxonomy is too limited to classify barriers relating to personal barriers and interpersonal barriers. Personal barriers include attitude and motivation (i.e. willingness), as well as knowledge and skills (i.e. ability). Interpersonal barriers relate to work setting such as culture, collaboration and facilitation (i.e. circumstances).

Most of these personal and interpersonal barriers have a time dependent nature and are probably related to career stage.

The Potential Impact of Differences among Doctors

Just like each patient is unique, each doctor is unique too. In routine clinical practice doctors categorize patients into groups with similar medical characteristics. This creates order and structure in their medical decision making. I wondered if I could translate this principle to my research: Could I categorize doctors into groups, each with a specific set of personal and interpersonal barriers as to how they view and use EBM?

To my knowledge there are no prior studies that have compared different groups of doctors to explore the impact of differences in career stage and work setting on barriers to practicing EBM. In a questionnaire study among Canadian internists, McAlister et al (1999) found that incorporating EBM into practice cannot be predicted by demographic or practice-related factors. A questionnaire study among residents and staff within the Department of Physical Medicine and Rehabilitation in New Jersey by DeLisa et al (1999) revealed that residents reported better information technology skills while staff reported better skills for practicing EBM. At the same time residents showed more interest in training in EBM. In addition, two qualitative studies showed that residents perceived specific barriers for applying EBM, such as lack of mentorship and fear of reprisal from skeptical faculty. The first, by Bhandari et al (2003), used focus groups and individual interviews among Canadian surgical residents, and the second, by Green and Ruff (2005), performed focus groups among Yale residents in a university-based primary care internal medicine program.

These studies proffered the hypothesis that differences among doctors in career stage and work setting could influence their barriers perceived. Therefore, I studied whether differences

in career stage and work setting have an effect on the ability and willingness to practice EBM and on the barriers as perceived by anesthesiologists to do so. In addition, I explored a comprehensive theoretical framework for the unambiguous and consistent classification of barriers.

METHOD

"Not everything that counts, can be counted". (Albert Einstein, 1879-1955)

I wanted to reveal if, how and why doctors of diverse career stages and work settings differed in how they perceived and used EBM in their routine clinical practice. For this, I would also need to gain understanding of the doctors' views that are situated below the surface of the overt barriers to practicing EBM.

Qualitative Study Design

I decided to interview doctors of diverse career stages and work settings. In The Netherlands this means that the Medical Research Involving Human Subjects Act (WMO) does not apply, as was confirmed by the Medical Ethics Review Committee (METC) of the university hospital. So, I was allowed to start with the research. I used purposive sampling of anesthesiologists of diverse career stages in two different departments of Anesthesiology in the Netherlands. I collected data in individual semi-structured interviews. The interview transcripts were analyzed using a grounded theory approach, i.e. inductive theory development based on analysis of qualitative data (Creswell, 2003).

Study Setting

I recruited participants from two departments of Anesthesiology to which I had easy access. One was in a university hospital and one in a general hospital (Table 1). Prior document study confirmed the expected differences in work setting. The university hospital had a hierarchical structure, where the divisions each comprised several departments. A management team of medical and non-medical professionals was integrally responsible for patient care, education, research and the financial budget of a division. In contrast, the general hospital was organized in discipline-specific, self-employed groups of medical consultants. The non-medical professional managers had separate facilitative and coordinating tasks. At the time of study, about twenty times as many residents (40 versus 2) and over three times as many anesthesiologists (43 versus 13) were working in the department of Anesthesiology in the university hospital compared with the general hospital. This university department had a longstanding, i.e. 45 years, resident training program, while the anesthesiologists in the general hospital only had begun involved in training of residents a few months prior to the study. In the Netherlands it takes five years specialization training to qualify as anesthesiologist.

Study Participants

I defined three career stages: (a) residents, (b) consultant anesthesiologists and (c) senior anesthesiologists. Residents were in their five years of specialization training. I defined consultants as having at least ten years of clinical experience after qualifying as anesthesiologist. Seniors were

consultants with significant additional leadership tasks, such as presiding over the division or department, the research program, or the resident training program. Apart from being a study participant the chair of each department was asked to assist in the purposive sampling from their departments (Table 1). I randomly selected study participants from the shortlist of residents, consultants and seniors provided by the chair of each department. None of the department members invited declined to participate. Participants did not receive a fee for their study participation.

Interview Procedures

I performed all interviews. Being a medically qualified senior policy advisor without clinical responsibilities, I understood the concepts of medicine, practicing EBM and implementation. In addition, I had to acknowledge the fact that although I was in favor of EBM, I was not allowed to let my personal opinions influence the participants in any way. Based on a literature review, I identified barriers to practice EBM prior to the interviews. I searched PubMed up to May 2004 using the following search filter: ("evidence-based medicine" OR "evidence-based practice" OR "clinical practice guidelines") AND ("barriers" OR "implementation"). I used the resulting overview of the identified barriers to outline the interview schedule.

Table 1. Characteristics of involved hospitals and study participants (n = 12)

	University hospital (n=7)	General hospital (n=5)
Number of employees **Employment arrangement of doctors**	10,000 Salaried academics	2,700 Autonomous practice on self-employed basis
Beds **Complexity of surgery**	1,042 High (tertiary centre)	559 Moderate (secondary centre)
Study Participants (n = 12) **Residents (n = 4)** **Consultants (n = 4)** **Seniors (n = 4)**	2 out of 40; 1 second-year (female) and 1 last-year (female) 2 out of 33 (one female, one male) 3 out of 3 (male)	2 out of 2; 1 first-year (male) and 1 last-year (female) 2 out of 7 (male) 1 out of 1 (male)

Design of semi-structured interviews with open question approach:

- Introduction to purpose of interview
- Definition of EBM and evidence (check of frame of reference[1-2])
- Perceived gap between existing and applied evidence
- Perceived barriers to practice EBM (list of barriers from literature review as aid for interviews[17-29])
- Prioritizing the barriers perceived as most important
- Possible solutions suggested for their most important barriers

I followed the same procedure for all interviews: They were performed face-to-face in a protected setting. At the start of the interview, I explained the purpose and approach to management and analysis of interview data to the participants and explicitly guaranteed confidentiality of the interviews. I encouraged each participant to speak freely about his or her personal views on EBM and perceived barriers for practicing EBM. With permission of the participants I tape-recorded and verbatim transcribed the interviews, each lasting for at least one hour. The interview schedule comprised open questions (i.e. no response codes) to enable respondents to give their opinion in full. In addition, I used the interview schedule flexibly at appropriate opportunities to allow me to probe for responses, clarify any ambiguities, and to enable respondents to raise other relevant issues not covered by the interview schedule. At the start of each interview, I checked the frame of reference by asking each participant to define EBM and evidence; I matched their definition with mine in case of deviation. Then, I examined the perceived gap between evidence and practice to obtain a first clue on the doctors' perceived level of urgency for practicing EBM. I used the interview schedule most flexibly during the questioning of the barriers perceived for practicing EBM to reflect

the participants' various perceptions and their underlying mechanisms. Then, I asked participants which barriers they considered most important to encourage the participants' contemplation on the interview so far and to find clues why some barriers were considered more important than others. Questioning possible solutions for each participant's most important barriers was used as a positive roundup of the interview.

Data saturation was achieved after the completion of twelve interviews, meaning that performing more interviews in the two settings would probably not render new insights. Hence the final sample comprised the twelve participants originally included.

Qualitative Data Analysis

The twelve interviews comprised over 800 minutes of recorded time (245 pages of transcript). How was I going to analyze this huge amount of qualitative data? At that point I had no prior experience with qualitative data analysis and I had no software available to structure and facilitate the analysis. So, at first I felt quite lost on how to go from here. What proved to be very helpful was that I performed semi-structured interviews. This allowed me to organize the data according to the topic list and the detailed list of barriers. I started by coding the interview quotes. Then, I tabulated and ranked the quotes according to the interview schedule (Textbox 3) and the list of barriers. Additions to this interview schedule were made based on new information derived from the interview data. I identified data patterns within and between each interview transcript using the conventional taxonomy of barriers to practice EBM: (1) the individual professional, (2) the team, (3) the organization or environment, (4) the evidence itself, and (5) the patient (Bryar et al, 2003; Grol & Grimshaw, 2003). The tables were combined by career stages and departments to facilitate the comparison within and between career stages and departments.

Through attempts to classify the resulting coded interview data, an alternative taxonomy for the barriers to practice EBM unfolded: a sequential order of the barriers. In addition to the group discussions two papers inspired the process of reclassification of the barriers. First, the Sicily Statement provided guidance based on the formal logic of empirical (bio)medical research (Dawes et al, 2005).[33] Second, a paper by Glasziou and Haynes placed the five EBM steps (Textbox 2) into a broader context. They described seven stages that reflect the paths from research to improved health outcomes. In particular, they focused on describing the 'leaky evidence pipeline' showing that much knowledge is lost before it ever reaches the patient (Glasziou & Haynes, 2005).

My proposed taxonomy describes sequentially the ten steps taken by an individual clinician before he or she is able to utilize evidence in practice. The model considers this process to be a joint responsibility: The doctor will not be able to successfully meet these ten steps without full support of colleagues and management. I used this alternative ten-conditions-model to report my findings (see Figure 1 in the Results section).

I documented the strategies for coding and interpretation of data in Microsoft Word to prevent selective perception and biased interpretation. My notes were subsequently independently verified by two senior researcher supervisors. Difficulties with interpretation and coding and a random selection were reviewed by the supervisors. The

Figure 1. Ten-conditions-model for barriers for EBM

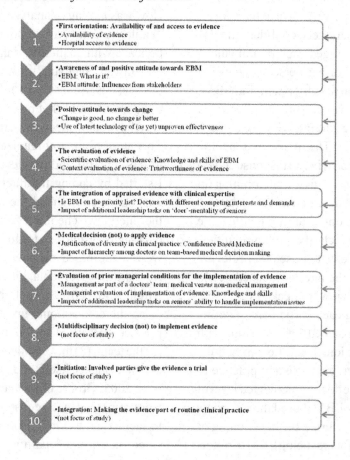

final coding was based on full agreement after discussion of discrepancies.

Sherlock Holmes and the Mystery of the Research Data

As you just read the Methods section, you could have concluded that the data analysis was rather straightforward. This can only be concluded in hindsight, when all the pieces of the puzzle have fallen into place. In real life, you have to be aware that the data analysis in qualitative research often is an incremental process that brings you back and forth between the data and your interpretation of these data. Coding, tabulating and ranking the interview quotes is just the beginning. The true research concerns continuous reflection and explicit definition of surpassing themes, their interrelations and their implications for EBM. My Master Thesis was completed in 2004, but it was not until 2009 that my interpretation of the data fell into place with accumulated knowledge from diverse sources. It took so long partly because it was not until the end of 2008 that I resumed the research fulltime, and partly also because sometimes it just takes time before true inspiration hits you: it is like being a very persistent Sherlock Holmes.

RESULTS

"There is always a better strategy than the one you have; you just haven't thought of it yet". (Pitman, 2003)

At some point, I presumed the analysis of data was completed, so I decided to write a research paper to get my results published. However, as it turned out the analysis was not completed: The proposed taxonomy evolved from seven steps in my Master Thesis (finished in 2004) to ten steps (Swennen et al, in press). This implies that every time I adjusted the proposed taxonomy I had to reanalyze my data. Another challenge was if and

how to use quotes. I really wanted to facilitate the reader to identify with the interviewees. I also felt I needed quotes to underpin my findings. Using quotes is not an obvious choice, as this significantly makes your word count go up which in turn challenges the standards of journals on maximum word counts. I even tried to write two papers to cut down the number of words: One paper on the finding that differences among doctors created different barriers for EBM (using themes), the other on the proposed taxonomy. As it turned out, this was not a good option either, as I was not satisfied with how I had to present the barriers in the first paper. So, only gradually I found a way to combine both findings into one paper. And, of course, each time I tried to report my findings differently, I had to repeat parts of the data analysis. So Sherlock Holmes kept up the good work.

Let the Doctors Speak

In the next part of the chapter I would like to provide a platform for the doctors that I interviewed. All were very willing to provide their honest opinions. I would like you to be open-minded: try to look through the doctors' eyes to gain understanding in their way of thinking and working.

Participants acknowledged a gap between available and applied evidence, and confirmed most barriers to implementation of EBM. These barriers were classified according to the proposed taxonomy (Figure 1).

Condition 1: First orientation: Availability of and access to evidence
For EBM to be possible, evidence must exist (or can be generated). In addition, available evidence has to be accessible to doctors to create the opportunity for use in practice.

1A. Limited evidence available. Evidence in Anesthesiology does exist, although good quality evidence based on large randomized-controlled trials is scarce. For most of the recommendations in the guidelines of the Netherlands Society of Anesthesiology the strength of the evidence can be considered low. For example, a senior stated: *"I think the amount of solid evidence in anesthesiology is still very limited, compared to other medical disciplines."*

1B. Limited hospital access to evidence. All participants had access to the evidence available, although in both hospitals access to internet facilities was not optimal; few computers were available and there was a significant distance between the operating theatres and an Internet-enabled computer.

Condition 2: Awareness of and positive attitude towards EBM
Doctors' use of EBM is unlikely if the concept of EBM is unknown, is misunderstood and/or condemned.

2A. EBM: What is it? All participants declared knowing the concept of EBM, but this contrasted with the definitions given: One senior used Sackett's definition. Most participants defined EBM one-sided as *"practicing medicine based on scientific evidence"*, not mentioning its integration with clinical expertise and patients' values. One resident described EBM as if it meant 'experience based': *"Doing things purely based on experience."* I explained 'my' definition of EBM after participants had given theirs.[1] Non-medical management (i.e. managers not being doctors) was considered to have no or little familiarity with EBM, especially in the general hospital: *"I think the [non-medical] management does not know much about EBM. The managers in this [general] hospital are not doctors and that implies many shortcomings where it concerns EBM and related subjects"* (consultant).

2B. EBM attitude: Influences from stakeholders. Participants had an overall positive association about the concept of EBM itself. However, consultants were suspicious about the potential abuse of EBM by 'others' which could reduce professional autonomy. In particular, they expressed a lack of confidence in non-medical management: *"As long as the evidence does not cost money, management supports it heartily. But as soon as it turns out to cost money, they start to tone down the solidness of the evidence, if you know what I mean."* They also did not trust lawyers, because they *"don't know medicine; they only know letters on paper, the protocols and guidelines. So, if you decide to deviate from the protocol and something goes wrong, you immediately have a problem."* In contrast, residents and seniors stated that guidelines and protocols leave sufficient space for well-founded deviation and were less worried about litigation. A resident said *"I think that you are free to deviate from a protocol, as long as you have good reasons to do so."* A senior pointed out: *"From my experience as an expert witness, a lot has changed in the past ten to fifteen years. At that time many testimonies were based on expert opinion, which made it easy for lawyers to pick the expert that was in their corner. EBM has made the testimonies more objective and well-founded, leading to more consistent statements. As a result, EBM should reduce fear of lawsuits as it can counteract subjective medical testimonies."* Their opinion about health insurance companies was ambivalent: On the one hand they were considered a means for getting new (expensive) effective care into clinical practice and to rightfully claim good quality for each euro spent: *"We don't all go to work in a Rolls Royce, because that is the best car."* On the other hand, they feared that health insurance companies would interpret guidelines as 'the way to do things', forcing doctors to help patients in a way they can't always support. A consultant philosophized that *"perhaps my suspicions have more to do with change than that there really is a problem. Two generations ago there were no guidelines at all... Some doctors miss that sense of freedom of having one's own practice and being* *one's own boss ... But times have changed, in ways that are not always pleasant, yet understandable."*

Condition 3: Positive attitude towards change
A prerequisite for EBM is lifelong learning through continuous critical introspection of weighing one's own ideas and practice against ever-advancing scientific insights. This means that clinicians must be willing and able to change their ideas and practice during their whole career.

3A. Change is good, no change is better. Participants considered resistance to change to be a significant barrier: It takes guts and energy to unchain practice-proven habits because of intuitive and/or technical areas of tension. Residents mainly associated resistance to change with 'older age': *"I am very positive about something I learnt here. ... But the staff in [x] is, of course, not going to listen to me. ... They are very conservative. I think for many older doctors it's all a matter of habit, so they will not teach new things to residents either."* Consultants attributed resistance to change essentially to 'personality traits': *"When doctors have passed the age of 60 they won't change anymore, but beneath this age it's all a matter of character."* One senior stated that both a doctor's career phase and personality influenced one's ability to change: *"Residents don't have critical introspection, but you have to see them in the career phase they are in: They are focused on acquiring knowledge and skills and placing these into a broader, practical context. Among staff you can distinguish two groups; people who apply critical introspection, considering it to be part of being a good doctor, and people who just don't. This has all to do with someone's personality."* All participants acknowledged the gap between evidence and practice, thereby implicitly acknowledging the need for change. However, residents and consultants showed little sense of urgency to change as they were satisfied with their *own* present practice. Seniors being involved

in change management learned that in the end *"change hurts, is always difficult. ... People tend to continue trusted routines and use all kinds of excuses for doing so. As I get older, I increasingly realize that there are just a few people who are really willing to change."*

3B. Use of latest technology of (as yet) unproven effectiveness. In contrast, some participants acknowledged a desire to work with latest technology and medicines, even though there might be no evidence for improved patient outcomes. Participants attributed this desire to convenience (*"Sometimes they think the new drug is easier to work with"* – senior), to the ambition of doctors (*"When there are new means, your ambition obliges you to use them"* – consultant), and to marketing strategies of the pharmaceutical industry (*"Everybody wants the newest stuff. The industry uses very strong marketing, including improper tactics like gifts and nights out. ... For example, there was very strong evidence to use [drug x]; it appeared to be effective and relatively cheap, but anesthesiologists lost all interest as soon as a highly promoted new drug was launched. It still intrigues me."* – senior)

Condition 4; The evaluation of evidence
Doctors must be able to answer any clinical question they might have with the best evidence available. This requires competencies in asking answerable questions, searching for evidence, critically appraising the evidence found and translating this evidence to individual patients.

4A. Scientific evaluation of evidence: Knowledge and skills of EBM. All participants first learned about EBM after graduation, even the residents who graduated in the late 1990s or early in the new millennium, and this was true for graduates of different medical schools. Seniors considered themselves capable of practicing EBM without overestimating their qualifications. For example, *"I am no novice [being a research profes-*

sor and having attended EBM-courses]. I would say my critical appraisal skills are above average ..., but I do not belong to the top. ... I am not as good as professor X [who is a research professor and a clinical epidemiologist]." In contrast, whereas some residents and consultants considered themselves having insufficient knowledge and skills of EBM, others seemed to overestimate their capabilities. For instance, the resident who originally defined EBM as 'experience-based medicine' stated: *"Finding, selecting and critically appraising the literature has become rather easy. ... I never got any supervision in learning EBM, but received plenty of feedback after presentations."* A consultant assumed that he was capable to critically appraise evidence after reading a small manual: *"Recently our national Journal of Medicine published a manual of how to appraise scientific literature. I tore it out and pinned it up, so now I know how it works."*

4B. Context evaluation of evidence: Trustworthiness of evidence. The participants distinguished validity of evidence from its trustworthiness. The latter was considered more important. For example, their Netherlands Society of Anesthesiology enjoyed great reputation and support among the participants because of the perceived trustworthiness and democratic structure of their Society: *"I think that anesthesiologists and residents find the Netherlands Society of Anesthesiology very useful. ... All anesthesiologists have influence on new guidelines. You share your arguments and in the end policies are finalized with a majority of votes."* (– resident) This caused them to trust their Society guidelines, despite the low strength of evidence to support most recommendations. Doubts about trustworthiness which were voiced included suspicion of a potential financial conflict of interest with the pharmaceutical industry that reduced the scientific integrity of guideline authors (*"Some guidelines originate from certain groups ... that consist of certain people that are influenced by certain industries ... in a way that you think, 'this cannot be*

good'." – consultant) or of researchers (*"One of the things I worry about is publication bias. That mainly articles with positive results are published and that most drug research is performed by financially strong pharmaceutical companies that are developing new drugs. There are many old, cheap drugs around that merit study, but when I want to perform research with these drugs I am unable to secure funding."* – senior)

Condition 5: The integration of appraised evidence with clinical expertise

Clinicians should build well-founded opinions about the evaluated evidence and relate the new data to their own clinical expertise.

5A. Is EBM on the priority list?: Doctors with different competing interests and demands. Residents and consultants showed little sense of urgency to integrate evidence with their clinical expertise. They considered themselves and their colleagues primarily 'doers', meaning they relied more on experience than on evidence, when engaged in clinical practice: *"In anesthesiology everything is urgent. You have to go on and you immediately see the effects of your actions. ... So if you are not a 'doer', you have a bad life."* Some participants contrasted anesthesiology ('doers') with internal medicine ('thinkers'). A resident stated: *"I am capable to make fast decisions. Besides, if I am only studying I get bored very easily. ... It is terrible to sift through every detail like internists do."* A senior related this 'doer' mode to EBM-use of anesthesiologists and surgeons: *"EBM still has a long way to go in my profession. ... Anesthesiologists have an immense inclination to consider our profession to be very practical, just like surgeons do. Days are filled with doing things."*

A senior who co-organized local postgraduate EBM training for residents complained: *"The attendance is just too low."* Residents acknowledged this: *"Our attendance varies. We are of course located on all departments, also during shifts. ... So you can't always attend. ... Our enthusiasm varies. Well, everybody is interested, but not everybody feels like 'I need to know it now'.*" Residents felt overwhelmed by all the new knowledge and skills they had to acquire. A coping strategy for the young anesthesiologist was 'tell me how today and why tomorrow': "*It is not that I analyze literature to check if what I am doing is actually the right thing to do. It is more that staff teaches me on the job ('see one, do one') and then I use it in the way I was taught.*" In addition, residents worked with many bosses (i.e. staff), who often had their own preferred ways of doing things. The hierarchical dependence of residents on their bosses put pressure on adapting their work procedures to the boss concerned: "*At the start of your residency it is a great challenge to match the right needle with each boss that supervises you at that moment.*" In conclusion, for residents the question 'what boss does what and how?' was dominant over 'what boss does best?' Likewise, staff was taught on the job when they were residents in the same way as they now trained their own residents ('see one, do one, teach one').

5B. Impact of additional leadership tasks on 'doer'-mentality of seniors. Interestingly, seniors stated that their additional leadership tasks had transformed them from a 'doer' (jumping into action) into a combined 'doer-thinker' (reasoned action, sometimes termed meta-cognition). For example; "*I always was an absolute doer, but in my role as manager I learnt that immediate actions are not always the most effective way. Although I am still a doer, I also became a thinker.*" New responsibilities triggered the need for critical reflection on their own and on their colleagues' clinical performances: "*In the old days I didn't realize that my EBM knowledge and skills were insufficient. ... Although my EBM capabilities improved, I try to gather the EBM experts able and critical enough to provide input for decisions that I have doubts about.*" All seniors stated they weighed (new) evidence against their clinical practice, and encouraged residents and consultants

to do the same (as was confirmed by them, for example a resident stated: "*Senior X really is a leading figure in research and his enthusiasm for research reflects on our ward.*")

Condition 6: Medical decision to apply or not to apply evidence

The consequent *medical* decision process to adopt or not adopt evidence in practice involves the clinicians and the multidisciplinary team in which he or she works (effectiveness, patient safety) and patients (patient values) (Institute of Medicine, 2001).

6A. Justification of diversity in clinical practice: Confidence Based Medicine. Residents in the general hospital noticed little similarity and consensus among anesthesiologists in their clinical routines. According to a resident, the consultants in the general hospital were unaware of this variation: "*In the general hospital the anesthesiologists all practice differently. If they work in such various ways, you would expect them to have good reasons to do so ... but they have not. ... They do not even know that their practices are that different. ... In the university hospital the practices are more similar ... and when their practice appears to deviate from what I have seen so far, they almost apologize for it and start explaining why their practice is probably different than that of their colleagues.*" Residents expressed ambiguous feelings about 'similarity versus variety' of clinical practice. On the one hand they welcomed the chance to encounter a wide range of practices: "*I now have the chance to learn different practices in a safe manner and in the end you will derive your own practice. That is why I think it to be of great value that many different bosses each work in varying ways.*" On the other hand they felt uncomfortable when having to satisfy the specific preferences of each consultant. Seniors strived for medical consensus, but struggled with "*the inclination of in fact all medical disciplines to cover up the lack of consensus.*" Consultants admitted to justify continuing one's own practice by maintaining that 'many roads lead to Rome', for example: "*Your gut feeling gets stronger as your clinical expertise builds up. Then, if a guideline's advice contradicts with your conviction, it's like working against your own nature. ... And I have to admit, as I get older, my intuition proves to be right more often.*"

6B. Impact of hierarchy among doctors on team-based medical decision making. The absence of a formal hierarchical structure among doctors in the general hospital set hurdles for team-based medical decision-making, according to the local senior; "*In a partnership of self-employed consultants everybody is considered equal. Each partnership has a chairman, but this person is not able to decide and say 'tomorrow we all are going to work like X.' I think that a hierarchical structure is an advantage for doctors working in a university hospital.*" Indeed in the academic hospital the hierarchical structure seemed to facilitate medical decision making, but the larger number of anesthesiologists working there created greater challenges to get everybody to agree with and adhere to protocols. The head of the academic department put a lot of effort in involving staff in protocol development to create broad support: "*Mandate is given to a few staff members who consider the specific clinical area of interest as their focus. These staff members then submit a concept protocol to be discussed in the staff meeting [where all anesthesiologists have to attend], and most of the times colleagues accept it unquestioningly and will adhere to it. This is going much better now than five years ago. ... it is also clear to residents to what protocols they have to adhere.*"

Condition 7: Evaluation of prior managerial conditions for the implementation of evidence
Implementation of evidence involves health economic issues, and also timeliness and accessibility (Institute of Medicine, 2001). Clinicians should analyze these elements in conjunction with management and payers to determine local use of new technologies.

7A. Management as part of a doctors' team: medical versus non-medical management. All participants considered doctors to be the most important party involved in dealing with issues concerning the implementation of evidence. When participants were asked to mention other involved parties, neither residents nor consultants mentioned 'management'. This could be because of their interpretations of 'medical management' (i.e. seniors) and 'non-medical management' (i.e. managers not being doctors). Interviews showed that the seniors were considered as one of the medical 'tribe' and their status of 'primus inter pares' was acknowledged. For example, the first-year resident already stated that "*the medical profession considers the doctors that participate in the management more as 'theirs' than as 'the management'.*" In contrast, as pointed out earlier, the opinions of particularly consultants about non-medical management were unfavorable: "*Especially our financial manager has a thankless task, as many doctors consider her as the 'evil mind' who unjustly blocks changes that doctors believe to be important*" (– senior). As a consequence, the impact of management on residents and consultants was stronger when managers had a medical background. On the other hand, the absence of a structural collaboration between medical and managerial experts in the general hospital had a negative impact on integrating medical and managerial forces to solve implementation issues.

7B. Managerial evaluation of implementation of evidence: Knowledge and skills. Only seniors seemed able to evaluate the prior managerial conditions that are relevant for implementing evidence (as will be described in section 7C). Residents had neither knowledge nor skills regarding implementation processes and felt ignorant about all its aspects, as reflected by the following examples; "*I have the feeling that implementation more befalls me than that I am* *actually involved or have influence on the process. It all happens at staff level"* and *"I think money is important, but the big picture is beyond me."* In addition, seniors also doubted the implementation knowledge and skills of the consultants; *"Many anesthesiologists do not have a clear view of all the organizational consequences that come with implementing evidence."* When asked which managerial issues they believed to impede the implementation of evidence at this stage, residents mainly mentioned inadequate communication. Other participants mentioned factors like lack of assistance by management, lack of time (pressure to produce), lack of personnel and finances, lack of direct control on actual implementation behavior, lack of hierarchy among doctors (only in the general hospital), inadequate logistics and computer-associated technology, and the lack of incentives. Except for 'inadequate communication', all these factors were seen as relying on 'others' to do a better or different job and not on the doctors' own efforts.

7C. Impact of additional leadership tasks on seniors' ability to handle implementation issues. The leadership tasks broadened the seniors' view on clinical practice as being part of a hospital where both medical and managerial issues require attention. For example, they showed understanding for the role of financial management concerning the economic choices made in the implementation of EBM; *"Doctors don't realize that the financial manager has to take into account more factors than just what doctors want."* Still, seniors felt that their managerial tasks were sometimes hard to reconcile with their professional loyalty: Especially in the academic hospital, where seniors had formal obligations to both their management team (including managers who were not doctors) and their colleagues, extra pressure was put on the seniors' ability to weigh and reconcile conflicting claims: *"Sometimes you feel like you are in splits, but you have to make both ends meet in the management team. [...] Sometimes this means you have to explain to doctors that, for*

the time being, we will not be able to implement something they want."

Condition 8: Decision to implement evidence or not

The summary of the evidence comprises all quality aspects: effectiveness, patient safety, patient values, efficiency, timeliness and accessibility (Institute of Medicine, 2001). Not only the multidisciplinary team but also other stakeholders, notably the public and patients who are the potential recipients of the health care technology, should be engaged. This enables a comprehensive approach for decision making to determine the 'go' or 'no go' signal for implementation of the evidence involved.

As pointed out earlier, results suggested that the organizational structure of the academic hospital offered better opportunities for this multidisciplinary approach. My study did not comprise the implementation stage itself (step 9) nor its integration (step 10).

Condition 9: Initiation: involved parties give the evidence a trial

A shared 'go' for implementation includes a formal agreement to support the process with all efforts necessary and a clear division of responsibilities. At this stage there will be persuasion rather than enforced cooperation of parties involved. Additionally, discussion will have anticipated both the medical and managerial implications of the implementation process.

Condition 10: Integration; making the evidence part of routine clinical practice

Through continuous evaluation and implementation of evidence, the final result is durable improvement of quality of care to individual patients.

DISCUSSION

In this study the doctors' career stage had an impact on their perceptions and use of EBM methods (principles and tactics): residents, consultants and seniors met different barriers (Table 2). Seniors provided support for the use of EBM methods in routine clinical practice.

Doing vs. Thinking

Exploration of underlying mechanisms for the barriers revealed that the 'doer' mode contrasted with the 'thinker' mode needed for applying the EBM methods. How should I interpret this finding that emerged from the data? For example, did this finding specifically apply to anesthesiologists (and surgeons), or did it fit into a broader context? I could not find anything in the medical or EBM literature. So, I started exploring literature in

psychology and behavioral economics to find an answer. It was then that scientific work from Simon (1947, 1982) caught my attention. He stated that this 'doer' mode is the dominant human approach to decision making in daily life. People can know neither all possible choices nor the consequences of known choices because their rational capabilities are bounded. Applying this to doctors, it is impossible to read and remember every possible fact relevant to the diagnosis and management of patients in their medical specialty, and even if it were possible knowing more does not necessarily improve decision making – because of bounded rationality. In general, people satisfice, i.e. they are often content with the trusted plausible judgment that quickly comes to their mind.

In my experience research further improves through discussing your thoughts with other people. Together with Geert van der Heijden, my co-supervisor, I attended an international confer-

Table 2. Linking career stages to doctors' barriers for EBM

Conditions 1 – 10	Residents	Consultants	Seniors
Condition 1: Availability of and access to evidence	*No differences found between career stages*		
Condition 2: Doctors' EBM attitude	Positive	Positive; but fear of autonomy loss through abuse of EBM by 'others'	Positive
Condition 3: Doctors' attitude to change	Barrier related to age; Little willingness to change oneself	Barrier related to character; Little willingness to change oneself	Barrier related to age and character; High willingness to change oneself
Condition 4: Doctors' EBM capabilities	Limited	Limited	Capable
Condition 5: Doctors' weighing of evidence and expertise	Doer Evidence < Expertise How > Why Hierarchical dependence	Doer Evidence < Expertise	Doer – Thinker Evidence = Expertise
Condition 6: Doctors' decision to (not) apply evidence	See one, do one; Ambivalence towards the need for consensus	Confidence Based Medicine; No need for consensus	Evidence Based Medicine; Strive for consensus
Condition 7: Doctors' acknowledgment of management; and doctors' managerial capabilities	High impact medical management; Low impact non-medical management; Incapable	High impact medical management; Low impact non-medical management; Incapable	High impact medical management; High impact non-medical management; Capable
Conditions 8 – 10	*Our study did not focus on these steps*		

ence in October 2009: the 6th Evidence-based Health Care International Conference in Sicily. It was here that two people (Neal Maskrey and Michael Power) draw my attention to Kahneman's work (2002). Maskrey, Hutchinson, & Underhill (2009) translated Kahneman's work to the world of medicine. At the conference Maskrey chaired a theme group on 'How to make decisions better' that I attended. This inspired me as we immediately understood what the other was talking about and we shared the opinion that Simon's and Kahneman's work offered important clues for improving medical decision making. So, back home, I studied Kahneman's and related work (Gigerenzer, 2008; Maskrey et al) that partly elaborated on Simon's work (1947, 1982): In behavioral economics the 'doer' mode is called "system 1 processing", where decisions and judgments are based on perception and intuitive thinking. System 1 enables humans to make fast and automatic decisions based on pattern recognition. Some of the most highly skilled cognitive activities are intuitive, for example playing chess at the master level. Translating this to clinical practice, we all can relate to the experienced doctors who are respected for their clinical expertise. But system 1 also has its problems. Using short cuts, heuristics and mindlines is comfortable and helpful in clinical decision making, but cognitive biases are lurking, in particular in the absence of reflective thinking. What if the heuristic or mindline a clinician has constructed is faulty or has become obsolete? This is where the 'thinker' mode or "system 2 processing" comes in, which is based on reasoning. EBM relates to this system 2 approach – it implies detailed analysis of all the evidence and the available options. In contrast to the system 1 approach that is fast and relatively effortless, system 2 requires effort and is purposeful.

"He who learns from others, but does not think for himself, is lost! He who thinks for himself, but does not learn from others, is in great danger!" (Confucius, 551-479 BC)

What does this system 1 and 2 learning imply for routine clinical practice? In my opinion, it is okay that most doctors rely on their clinical expertise (system 1), conditioned they regularly check for cognitive biases (system 2): *Are my clinical routines (still) correct?* I believe the challenge in medical decision making is to reflect on heuristics and mindlines when appropriate, and to be willing and able to change one's decision making accordingly. This offers protection for clinicians and patients against cognitively biased decisions. In other words we need to find out when and how doctors could best calibrate their system 1 processing with system 2 processing.

This is actually what the EBM community means by continuous, self-directed lifelong learning to reduce the doctors' risk of becoming dangerously out of date and immune of self-improvement and advances in medicine (Straus et al, 2005). For this doctors would need to learn to practice reflective thinking during their decisions on both diagnosis and patient management.

People make mistakes, with and without EBM. If EBM includes reflective thinking and lifelong learning, it also is about learning from mistakes. I believe in the importance of combining the practical learning (clinical expertise) with the theoretical learning (EBM). For instance, I know that the anesthesiology department in the university hospital has regular 'complication meetings' in which all anesthesiologists and residents have to participate. In these meetings doctors reflect on their clinical practice by discussing complications or mistakes and the lessons learned. In doing so, they underpin their reflections with (lack of) evidence and discuss how to deal with the remaining uncertainties. I realize that EBM often still is a standalone activity, but these complication meetings show the integration of expertise and evidence is possible.

Still, at times, in a medical emergency or clinical setting such as an operating theatre where many decisions may need to be made sequentially in a short time frame, rapid system 1 decisions may be superior to slower system 2 decisions even though they have less risk of cognitive bias.

Residents, that eventually showed to have very little prior knowledge on EBM, were trained on the job in the 'doer' mode by consultants by passing on their 'confidence based' clinical practice routines. In my opinion, this teaching on the job is entirely valid educationally providing there is in-built, objective and recorded assessment of competence, but there ought to be an EBM approach to, say, the selection of medicines used by anesthesiologists. This could also be objectively assessed as part of the specialization training program.

Active involvement of seniors in applying EBM methods could be crucial in the guidance of both residents and consultants. Through additional leadership tasks seniors seemed to have gone beyond the 'doer' mode. By addressing their 'thinker' mode these tasks taught seniors to consider both medical and managerial issues of a hospital and thereby put clinical practice into a broader policy perspective. Therefore seniors could be strong role models in applying EBM methods because of their impact on colleagues through their hierarchical and/or 'primus inter pares' position.

The Impact of Differences in Setting

Application of EBM methods is expected to have an impact on decision making in patient management by teams. Differences in setting and the organizational context of the general hospital complicated the use of EBM methods. The absence of a formal hierarchy among doctors introduced hurdles for medical decision making by teams. In addition, limited collaboration between doctors and non-medical management posed medical and managerial hurdles for the use of EBM methods; it reduced the opportunities to implement EBM methods.

Doing the Right Things for the Right People: The Impact of Differences among Doctors

Differences in doctors' characteristics have an impact on decisions in patient care. For instance, the Dartmouth Atlas Project found that the large differences in U.S. regional spending are almost entirely explained by unwarranted variation in doctors' behavior leading to differences in volume of health care services provided to similar patients (Dartmouth Atlas Project, 2007; Fisher et al, 2003a, 2003b, 2009; Sirovich et al, 2008).

The above and my findings would also imply that the US and Dutch licensing requirements for continuing medical education do not sufficiently make doctors change their own trusted routines into new evidence- based routines. The results of this study indicate we need a better understanding of how differences among doctors in attitude and behavior result in differential use of EBM and hence different clinical decisions.

The data show it may be possible to categorize doctors according to a specific set of barriers for EBM, which eventually have an impact on decisions taken. This subgrouping seems to apply to the relationship between career stage, work setting and medical discipline.

Doing Things Right: Prioritizing Barriers

An important finding was the ten-conditions-model, which evolved from sequencing the reported barriers. This approach helps to determine in which order the barriers have to be dealt with to reach the goal of implementation of high quality evidence into clinical practice, continuous improvement of clinical performance and hence of the quality of individual patient care. The ten-conditions-model could help in classifying doctors among disciplines to their career stage and work setting. This may support structuring the EBM implementation process by identifying priorities to overcome their specific barriers for implementation of EBM methods.

REFLECTIONS ON THE STUDY DESIGN

In my in-depth qualitative study using a small purposive sample, my aim was to lower the threshold to speak freely and not influence the responses by using private settings and guaranteeing confidentiality. The interviews allowed me to use the literature review in the exploration of opinions and experiences of participants with using EBM methods. During the semi-structured interviews, I avoided a pre-set order of topics. Instead, I used a topic check list derived from the literature for checking the coverage of all topics in interview.

Group interviews, as an alternative approach, would have enabled me to include more participants, to arrange more than one meeting per group and to study interactions within and between doctors. At this stage, however, I preferred to secure 'free speech' of individual participants to gather rich data about the barriers perceived and the underlying mechanisms involved. The small sample size and qualitative design does neither allow me to conclude that these are the only relationships seen in subgroups of doctors, nor to generalize my findings to anesthesiology in general, to other medical disciplines or to other settings.

But my findings justify further exploration of the extent and impact of differences among doctors, career stage and work settings in anesthesiology and other medical specialties on the use of EBM methods.

My findings offer a new dimension to the conventional approach of promoting the use of EBM in clinical practice: Triage of doctors to their specific barriers could facilitate doing the right things with the right people. Prioritizing the barriers could help doing things right more often.

"To the individual who devotes his/her life to science, nothing can give more happiness than when the results immediately find practical application. There are not two sciences. There are science and the application of science, and these two are linked as the fruit is to the tree." Louis Pasteur (1871)

I feel that I am now working on the crossroads of science and medicine, and I hope my research will contribute to a closer collaboration between these two worlds. Both science and medicine are crucial for good quality medical decision making. Medical research is only valuable when used by doctors, and doctors will not have to re-invent the wheel if they have access to scientific knowledge. The next phase of the research program is to substantiate my findings and translate these into a generalisable framework. I would like to invite you to elaborate on or to argue against my findings and arguments for triage of doctors and prioritizing the barriers.

ACKNOWLEDGMENT

First, I would like to thank the following colleagues:

Dr. Geert van der Heijden, being my co-supervisor, for his continuing support throughout my research; Professor Geert Blijham, former President of the University Medical Centre Utrecht, for offering me the opportunity of a PhD-fellowship and for allowing me much freedom concerning the what and how of my PhD-work; Professor Yolanda van der Graaf and Professor Cor Kalkman for their support, being my supervisors.

I am also much obliged to Neal Maskrey, Director of Evidence-based Therapeutics, National Prescribing Centre, Liverpool, UK for his inspiring and valuable feedback on the research and on the original paper.

Finally, I would like to thank Professor Rakesh Biswas for the opportunity to publish this adapted paper as a chapter in his book.

REFERENCES

Asch, S. M., Kerr, E. A., Keesey, J., Adams, J. L., Setodji, C. M., Malik, S., & McGlynn, E. A. (2006). Who is at greatest risk for receiving poor-quality health care? *The New England Journal of Medicine, 354*(11), 1147–1156. doi:10.1056/NEJMsa044464

Bhandari, M., Montori, V., Devereaux, P. J., Dosanjh, S., Sprague, S., & Guyatt, G. H. (2003). Challenges to the practice of evidence-based medicine during residents' surgical training: a qualitative study using grounded theory. *Academic Medicine, 78*(11), 1183–1190. doi:10.1097/00001888-200311000-00022

Brook, R. H. (2009). Assessing the appropriateness of Care, its time has come. *Journal of the American Medical Association, 302*(9), 997–998. doi:10.1001/jama.2009.1279

Bryar, R. M., Closs, S. J., Baum, G., Cooke, J., Griffiths, J., & Hostick, T. (2003). Yorkshire BARRIERS project. *International Journal of Nursing Studies, 40*(1), 73–84. doi:10.1016/S0020-7489(02)00039-1

Burge, P., Devlin, N., Appleby, J., Gallo, F., Nason, E., & Ling, T. (2006). *Understanding Patients' Choices at the Point of Referral*. Santa Monica: RAND Corporation.

Cabana, M. D., Rand, C. S., Powe, N. R., Wu, A. W., Wilson, M. H., Abboud, P. A. C., & Rubin, H. R. (1999). Why don't physicians follow clinical practice guidelines? A framework for improvement. *Journal of the American Medical Association, 282*(15), 1458–1465. doi:10.1001/jama.282.15.1458

Creswell, J. W. (2003). *Research design. Qualitative, quantitative and mixed methods approaches*. Thousand Oaks, CA: Sage publications.

Dartmouth Atlas Project. (2007). *Effective care. A Dartmouth Atlas Project Topic Brief*. Retrieved from http://www.dartmouthatlas.org/topics/effective_care.pdf

Dawes, M., Summerskill, W., Glasziou, P., Cartabellotta, A., Martin, J., & Hopayian, K. (2005). Sicily statement on evidence-based practice. *BMC Medical Education, 5*, 1. doi:10.1186/1472-6920-5-1

DeLisa, J. A., Jain, S. S., Kirshblum, S., & Christodoulou, C. (1999). Evidence-based medicine in physiatry: the experience of one department's faculty and trainees. *American Journal of Physical Medicine & Rehabilitation, 78*(3), 228–232. doi:10.1097/00002060-199905000-00008

Fisher, E. S., Bynum, J. P., & Skinner, J. S. (2009). Slowing the growth of health care costs – Lessons from regional variation. *The New England Journal of Medicine, 360*(9), 849–852. doi:10.1056/NEJMp0809794

Fisher, E. S., Wennberg, D. E., Stukel, T. A., Gottlieb, D. J., Lucas, F. L., & Pinder, E. L. (2003a). The implications of regional variations in Medicare spending. Part 1: the content, quality, and accessibility of care. *Annals of Internal Medicine, 138*(4), 273–287.

Fisher, E. S., Wennberg, D. E., Stukel, T. A., Gottlieb, D. J., Lucas, F. L., & Pinder, E. L. (2003b). The implications of regional variations in Medicare spending. Part 2: health outcomes and satisfaction with care. *Annals of Internal Medicine, 138*(4), 288–298.

Gigerenzer, G. (2008). *Gut feelings: short cuts to better decision making*. London: Penguin.

Glasziou, P., & Haynes, B. (2005). The paths from research to improved health outcomes. *ACP Journal Club, 142*, A8–A10.

Green, M. L., & Ruff, T. R. (2005). Why do residents fail to answer their clinical questions? A qualitative study of barriers to practicing evidence-based medicine. *Academic Medicine, 80*(2), 176–182. doi:10.1097/00001888-200502000-00016

Grol, R. (1997). Personal paper. Beliefs and evidence in changing clinical practice. *British Medical Journal, 315*(7150), 418–421.

Grol, R. (2001). Successes and failures in the implementation of evidence based guidelines for clinical practice. *Medical Care, 39*(8Suppl 2), 1146–1154. doi:10.1097/00005650-200108002-00003

Grol, R., & Grimshaw, J. (2003). From best evidence to best practice: effective implementation of change in patients' care. *Lancet, 362*(9391), 1225–1230. doi:10.1016/S0140-6736(03)14546-1

Guyatt, G., & Rennie, D. (Eds.). (2002). *Users' guides to the medical literature. A manual for evidence-based clinical practice*. Chicago, IL: AMA Press.

Haynes, R. B., Devereaux, P. J., & Guyatt, G. H. (2002). Physicians' and patients' choices in evidence based practice. Evidence does not make decisions, people do. *British Medical Journal, 321*(7350), 1350. doi:10.1136/bmj.324.7350.1350

Health Economics Research Group, Office of Health Economics, RAND Europe. (2008). *Medical Research: What's it worth? Estimating the economic benefits from medical research in the UK*. London: UK Evaluation Forum.

Institute of Medicine. (2001). *Crossing the Quality Chasm: A New Health System for the Twenty-first Century*. Washington: National Academy Press.

Kahneman, D. (2002). *Maps of Bounded Rationality: a perspective on intuitive judgment and choice*. Stockholm: Noble Prize Lecture.

Mangione-Smith, R., DeCristofaro, A. H., Setodji, C. M., Keesey, J., Klein, D. J., Adams, M. A., & McGlynn, E. A. (2007). The quality of ambulatory care delivered to children in the United States. *The New England Journal of Medicine, 357*(15), 1515–1523. doi:10.1056/NEJMsa064637

Maskrey, N., Hutchinson, A., & Underhill, J. (2009). Getting a better grip on research: the comfort of opinion. *InnovAiT, 2*(11), 679–686. doi:10.1093/innovait/inp085

McAlister, F. A., Graham, I., Karr, G. W., & Laupacis, A. (1999). Evidence-based medicine and the practicing clinician. *Journal of General Internal Medicine, 14*(4), 236–242. doi:10.1046/j.1525-1497.1999.00323.x

McGlynn, E. A., Asch, S. M., Adams, J., Keesey, J., Hicks, J., DeCristofaro, A., & Kerr, E. A. (2003). The quality of care delivered to adults in the United States. *The New England Journal of Medicine, 348*(26), 2635–2645. doi:10.1056/NEJMsa022615

McNeill, B. J. (2001). Shattuck Lecture -- Hidden barriers to improvement in the quality of care. *The New England Journal of Medicine, 345*(22), 1612–1620. doi:10.1056/NEJMsa011810

Melnyk, B. M. (2002). Strategies for overcoming barriers in implementing evidence based practice. *Paediatric Nursing, 28*(2), 159–161.

Muir Gray, J. (2001). Evidence-based medicine for professionals. In Edwards, A., & Elwyn, G. (Eds.), *Evidence-based patient choice; inevitable or impossible?* Oxford: Oxford University Press.

Newman, M., Papadopoulos, I., & Sigsworth, J. (1998). Barriers to evidence-based practice. *Intensive & Critical Care Nursing, 14*(5), 231–238. doi:10.1016/S0964-3397(98)80634-4

Pasteur, L. (1871). Revue Scientifique.

Pitman, B. (2003). Leading for Value. *Harvard Business Review*, (Apr): 41–46.

Retsas, A. S. (2000). Barriers to using research evidence in nursing practice. *Journal of Advanced Nursing*, *31*(3), 599–606. doi:10.1046/j.1365-2648.2000.01315.x

Sackett, D. L., Rosenberg, W. M., Gray, J. A., Haynes, R. B., & Richardson, W. S. (1996). Evidence based medicine: what it is and what it isn't. *British Medical Journal*, *312*(7023), 71–72.

Schuster, M. A., McGlynn, E. A., & Brook, R. H. (1998). How good is the quality of health care in the United States? *The Milbank Quarterly*, *76*(4), 517–563. doi:10.1111/1468-0009.00105

Simon, H. A. (1947). *Administrative behaviour: a study of decision-making processes in administrative organisations*. New York: The Free press.

Simon, H. A. (1982). *Models of bounded rationality*. Vols 1 and 2. Cambridge and London, respectively: MIT press.

Sirovich, B., Gallagher, P. M., Wennberg, D. E., & Fisher, E. S. (2008). Discretionary decision making by primary care physicians and the cost of U.S. health care. *Health Affairs*, *27*(3), 813–823.. doi:10.1377/hlthaff.27.3.813

Straus, S. E., & McAlister, F. A. (2000). Evidence-based medicine: a commentary on common criticisms. *Canadian Medical Association Journal*, *163*(7), 837–841.

Straus, S. E., Richardson, W. S., Glasziou, P., & Haynes, R. B. (2005). *Evidence-based medicine: how to practice and teach EBM*. Edinburgh: Churchill Livingstone.

Swennen, M. H. J., van der Heijden, G. J. M. G., Blijham, G. H., & Kalkman, C. J. (in press). Career stage and work setting create different barriers for Evidence-based Medicine. *Journal of Evaluation in Clinical Practice*.

Chapter 25
Healthcare Narratives and Self–Care Stories:
Developing a User–Driven Taxonomy for Adults with Cystic Fibrosis

Daz Greenop
Liverpool John Moores University, UK

Sheila Glenn
Liverpool John Moores University, UK

Martin Walshaw
Liverpool Heart and Chest Hospital NHS Trust, UK

Martin Ledson
Liverpool Heart and Chest Hospital NHS Trust, UK

ABSTRACT

The aim of this chapter is to explore how a group of adults with cystic fibrosis (N=40) manage and account for self-care. By focussing on the development of character and plot, narrative analysis will illustrate how distinct patient identities may be constructed and performed as participants defend and justify their preferred self-care practices. These stories do not, however, always fit with the prevailing master narratives on which healthcare is often premised. Drawing on exemplars of 5 distinct types of storytelling an alternative user-driven taxonomy will be suggested which not only recognizes a range of self-care practices but also affirms their legitimacy beyond the horizons of mainstream biomedicine[1].

INTRODUCTION

Cystic Fibrosis (CF) is the UK's most common inherited genetic disorder. It is a multi-organ disease affecting the lungs and digestive system by clogging them with thick sticky mucus resulting

in infections and inflammation that make it hard to breathe and digest food (CF Trust, 2006). Until recently the majority of people with CF were not expected to reach adulthood but improvements in diagnosis and treatment mean that there are in fact now more adults than children living with the condition in developed countries. With adulthood

DOI: 10.4018/978-1-60960-097-6.ch025

however, self-care becomes increasingly complex and costly as patients seek to manage the (often) competing demands of body and society.

According to Best Practice Guidance in the UK, 'self-care is all about individuals taking responsibility for their own health and well-being. This includes: staying fit and healthy, both physically and mentally; taking action to prevent illness and accidents; the better use of medicines; treatment of minor ailments and better care of long term conditions' (Department of Health, 2006). Self-care is not just the responsibility of the 'ill', therefore, but incorporates maintaining health and managing risks more generally. While *everybody* is expected to conform to these 'universal self-care requisites' (Orem 2001) however, if people with CF were to do so it would most likely have serious consequences. That is, because of the high energy demands of their bodies and the malabsorption of nutrients, most people with CF need to eat copious high calorie foods, which, along with regular intensive physical activity, is in fact the opposite of what is normally recommended or expected for most other adults, especially females (Willis, Miller & Wyn, 2001; Stark, Jelalian, McGrath, & Mackner, 2001; CF Trust 2006). For people with CF therefore, 'universal self care requisites' are complicated as diet and physical activity can in fact deviate significantly from healthy norms. Orem's (2001) 'health deviation self care' by way of contrast refers to disease specific activity which, for people with CF, typically includes both medical and behavioural treatments such as daily chest physiotherapy, continuous antibiotics, enzymes and inhaled bronchodilators. These together with regular intensive interventions needed to manage exacerbations make for an unusually demanding self-care regimen.

Given the extensive and often contradictory requirements to both comply to medical prescriptions and conform to societal expectations it is unsurprising that few people with CF do all of their treatment all of the time (Kettler, 2002). There

are many well documented reasons for this and the most significant appears to be forgetfulness (Pfeffer, Pfeffer, & Hodson, 2003; Arias Llorente, Garcia, & Diaz Martin, 2008). The unpleasantness of the treatment, degree of infringement on their lives and embarrassment are also significant factors (Abbot, Dodd, Bilton, & Webb, 1994; Conway, Pond, Hamnet, & Watson, 1996; Gotz & Gotz, 2000; D'Angelo & Lask, 2001; Arias Llorente *et al.*, 2008). These observations, of course, require more systematic consideration and this chapter will demonstrate how a narrative approach can help both challenge the existing order and construct an alternative pluralistic framework of understanding. The self-care stories presented here may or may not fit with the master narratives of healthcare, but we must at least start to recognise their legitimacy if patients are to be respected and a truly user-driven approach is to succeed.

BACKGROUND

This research grew out of a concern that prevailing healthcare models tend to draw from a limited range of experiential evidence and, as a result, silence patient voices that do not fit within mainstream discourses of health and illness. This is perhaps most clearly seen in the research, practice and conceptualisation of compliance which is not only one-dimensional but, at its very heart, also contains the assumption that 'doctor knows best'. Consequently, non-compliance to prescribed regimens has often been regarded as irrational, maladaptive and morally reprehensible as researchers, practitioners and even patients themselves talk about 'failing' to comply (Broom & Whittaker, 2004). The corrective concept of concordance (RPSGB, 1997; DH, 2001) goes some way to addressing this imbalance suggesting, rather, that self-care regimens should be based on a negotiation between equal partners. Caution needs to be exercised, however, as even a two-dimensional concordant encounter is only one aspect of daily negotiations many adults with CF must undertake to achieve a health-life balance – whether at work, at play or at home. Using 5 exemplars, varieties of self-care styles will be explored and connected with a *range* of preferred patient identities through which some participants described and defended themselves as compliant and some as concordant. For others, however, neither model fitted their stories which might be better described as conformant. That is, while they seldom completed their medical regimens, *behavioural* aspects of treatment were regularly and routinely undertaken through 'healthy living' and not usually with CF in mind. Of course not everybody actively self-cares and 2 more marginal groups of participants, for very different reasons, appeared to take little or no direct responsibility for their health.

METHOD

Fifty participants were purposively selected for this study to provide a socially and clinically diverse sample but ten of these dropped out. The interviews consisted of a mixture of closed, semi-structured and open questions intended, firstly, to try and establish routine practices and then, secondly, to explore disruptions to these. The responses from interviewees demonstrate that people are creative storytellers and the master narratives CF patients are often expected to take up are not slavishly reiterated but may be revised and rejected in dialogue with others. Whether specific or general, real or imagined it is in relation to other that diverse patient identities were constructed, performed and defended. It is not simply different *characters* that could be discerned during interviewing, however, but different *plots* too – even if not everybody had a personal self-care story to tell. By focussing on the development of character and plot, narrative

analysis shows how different participants justified their preferred self-care practices. These 'stories' do not, however, always fit with the prevailing 'master narratives' on which healthcare is often premised. Drawing on a variety of responses to the imperative to self-care an alternative user-driven taxonomy is developed here and re-presented in a single exploratory framework.

RESULTS & ANALYSIS

Robinson (1990) and others, describe certain *stable narratives* which lack the kind of structure we might expect because they are 'uncomplicated' by illness and its treatment. While the development of 'plot' might be difficult to discern in such accounts their resemblance to medical case histories, Robinson (1990, p.1178) suggests, indicates that 'the code and culture of biomedicine is the key to unlock their evaluative meaning'. In contrast to these, *chaos narratives* feed on the sense that no-one is in control. In these accounts, Frank (1995, p.97) notes, 'the modernist bulwark of remedy, progress, and professionalism cracks to reveal vulnerability, futility, and impotence'. It was indeed noticeable during analysis that the more compliant participants purported to be, the more stable and uneventful their interviews became and the more non-compliant they claimed to be the more unstable and eventful they appeared. It is at these extremities – what Frank refers to as the 'control-chaos continuum' – that self-care finds no place in participants' accounts of health and life. These accounts are not so much self-stories as stories about *others* (whether highly supportive or highly unsupportive) and seem to be indicative of high levels of 'outsidership' (described here as 'dependence' and 'independence' respectively). Between these 2 sets of outliers preferred styles of self-care, along with some important adaptive processes, can be more readily discerned:

Figure 1. Preferred styles of self-care

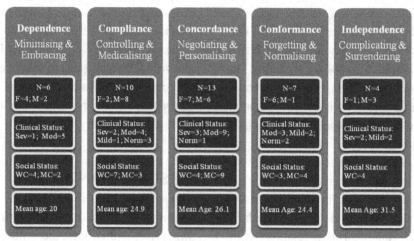

Note: Clinical Status is classified by the Cystic Fibrosis Trust (2000) as: Severe (FEV1 less than 40% predicted); Moderate (FEV1 40-69% predicted); Mild (FEV1 70-89% predicted); Normal (FEV1 greater than 90% predicted). Social Status is based on the British Registrar General's classification system but simplified here as 'middle class' (I-II) and 'working class' (III-V).

Dependence: Stable Narratives and the 'Lazy Patient'

As already indicated, there was a distinct lack of drama in some of the interviews with participants (N=6) in this research. It is tempting to overlook or ignore such accounts as atypical 'outliers' but, like everybody else, these participants too need to be heard. There was conspicuously little resistance (and a good deal of apathy) towards CF and its treatment in these narratives both from patients themselves and those on whom they depend for care. Reflective exegesis suggests, however, that their dependency is not so much on professional medical support but informal and particularly familial support. Nevertheless the implicit 'audience' in these stable narratives appears to be 'a biomedical interpreter and guide' (Robinson, 1990 p.1178) and so their dependence upon the care of others often gives the *impression* of hyper-compliance. Informal carers in particular are invariably presented as supportive and even heroic, while other characters, if not indifferent, still regard them sympathetically as worthy recipients of charity. This positive regard is both unearned and unconditional so participants have little problem either accepting help or adminis-

tering medications in public – in principle if not in practice. This 'care free' detachment from the demands of body and society that these participants presented not only means that they not only become dependent on others for care but can also freely pursue secondary gains or other fulfilments outside the world work and its rewards (Radley, 1994). Unsurprisingly, therefore, the enjoyment of leisure (shopping, relaxing, travel, etc) was one of the few interests to emerge from these interviews while their dependency on others was almost invariably rationalised and indeed justified in terms of 'laziness', relaxing or taking it easy. That said, both of the male participants (M=2/6) additionally indicated other goals as Simon*, for example, wishes to become a driving instructor and Wil\liam* wants to move into his own property. Interestingly both of these also indicated a desire to become more active in their self-care (see below) but neither, as yet, has taken any practical steps towards this.

Exemplar 1: Simon

Simon is a clinically moderate 18 year-old and works part-time at the checkout in a large supermarket. His parents have recently divorced and his older sister who also has CF (not interviewed) lives with their mother while Simon moved into a 2 bedroom council house with their father who is unemployed. He still does Simon's physiotherapy twice a day while his girlfriend makes sure Simon has his tablets and nebulisers before he goes to bed and, he added, she 'tries to look after me'. Simon's mother has just got a job at 'some place in an office' but also remains influential. Despite his declining health and plentiful support, Simon stays up late and sleeps through the day because, he stated, 'It's just the way I am'. As we began to talk about physical activity, however, Simon's usually stable narrative started to become more complicated. Just prior to the following dialogue he stated that he enjoys driving around in his car with friends:

I: What other things do you do then?
P: Just go places and that. My mum's just sent away for a gym card so I've got to go there now.
I: And is that free?
P: You have to pay for it…
I: How much is it?
P: I don't know, she pays it.
I: Are you going to use it?
P: Yeah, definitely.
I: And, uh, it sounds like that might be something your mum's kind of initiated…
P: Yeah, she has, she knows I've gone lazy. Since I've been in [hospital] though it's been alright with that exercise bike [pointing] and that. I've been doing 10 miles a day on that, so, it's just once it's there I'll do it.
I: Have you got anything like that at home?
P: No.
I: Have you ever had or do you plan to get an exercise plan?
P: Yeah my dad's getting a treadmill for the house.
I: Right okay, you're full-on then, aren't you?
P: I know yeah.

It is clear from the above extract how involved both parents have remained, despite the divorce,

as Simon answers 2 questions about what *he* has done with statements about what *his parents* have done on his behalf. Simon's mother has sent for (and paid for) gym membership, and his dad is getting a treadmill. His developing story is not all about them, therefore, but the exercise he is *planning* to do, albeit under duress. Interestingly, the other male in this group used exactly the same strategy while the 4 females simply enjoyed being 'ladies of leisure' (as one participant put it). For a working class male like Simon, however, 'laziness' is more likely to be regarded as failure as an 'active subject' (Whitehead, 2002; Howson, 2004). Simon, or perhaps more accurately *his mother*, therefore regards his laziness as problematic and so, again, he is keen to point out what he *can* do ('I've been doing 10 miles a day') on the exercise bike while in hospital. This strategy continued as we talked:

I: Is there a difference between the physical activities you do, or don't do, including the *physio* and exercise or whatever, and what you're advised to do?
P: No, yeah they just say…they try and make you do a lot of exercise and that, because there's all sorts of different things I can do, I just don't do it.
I: Mm, what do you put that down to?
P: I don't know, laziness probably.
I: Laziness. Do you think it's important? It sounds like you do.
P: Yeah, it is. I've only just, like, really noticed how much it is…
I: … Do you think you'll be able to maintain a new health regime?
P: Yeah, once I get in to the gym and that…
I: Do you ever talk to the *physios* about *physio* or exercise?
P: No not really. I just do what they say like. They used to say try and go to the gym and that. I just said I couldn't be bothered.
I: And that ended the conversation?
P: Yeah.

I: How important is physical activity do you think?

P: Very. It clears your chest and that. I reckon that's why my blows might be down now. Coz I always used to do a lot and I was 60s and 70s and it's starting to take effect. It's gone down.

Simon's initial response to the first question perhaps displays a conflict of desires and expectations ('No, yeah…'). His narrative is similarly ambiguous as he both 'do[es] what they say' and just '[can't] be bothered'. Either way, and again this is characteristic of all participants in this group, Simon does not *talk* to his exercise therapist (or other health professionals) about the issue. It is simply his prerogative to do as he pleases and no further justification is required. So, while his usual passive acquiescence may facilitate passive *medical* compliance, here, it militates against active *behavioural* compliance as he resists requests to 'do a lot of exercise' even though he can. Physical activity is increasingly regarded as central to the management of cystic fibrosis but none of the 6 participants in this group engaged in it. Simon (and also William) is however starting to recognise its importance and this is the real complication to his usually stable narrative. It is not, however, yet *his* story only something expected of him by others – including the interviewer. It is, of course, unclear whether Simon has the capacity to become physically active but he indicates, even if only to satisfy the interviewer, that he has the desire. Like all 'Lazy Patients' interviewed, therefore, Simon's dependency, is presented as a lifestyle choice rather than the result of incapacity so, even without the necessary social and material (including bodily) resources required to be an active subject, he can still draw on available, though clearly limited, discourses to construct a possible or 'virtual' world in which he is capable of so much more.

Compliance: Restitution Stories and the 'Faithful Patient'

Faithful Patients (N=10) actively complied with both medical and behavioural aspects of their regimens – even when the benefits of this was not apparent. In contrast with participants in the previous section, they also tended to present CF *negatively*. That is, far from enhancing the self, illness was regarded as destructive force in their lives – diminishing the self, as Charmaz (1983) and others since have also observed. By resisting the negative images of helplessness and dependence that are often associated with illness and disability, however, participants were also able to construct *other* personally and socially valued identities beyond CF even if these were constantly under threat by CF. The 'diminished self' was not, therefore, the universal experience of these participants as 4 in particular appeared to have *always* been compliant and indeed achieved and maintained new and valued social identities in adulthood. So while CF continued to be evaluated negatively it did not dominate their entire narratives but, rather, was overcome - often against the expectations of others. These participants in particular presented themselves as 'supernormal' (see also Gjengedal, Rustoen, Wahl & Hanesta, 2003), managing to meet the demands of both body and society without compromising either and with little or no need for help from others. Rather, their faith in medicine and fortitude in life meant that clinical expertise and not 'charity' was required. The purpose of the 'supernormal identity' is, according to Yoshida (1993, p.226), for patients to prove that they are 'no worse off than other people' and, indeed, they were sometimes better off. For these participants therefore the signs and symptoms of CF are always carefully and sometimes creatively concealed from all around – including friends and family. Indeed all problems tended to be minimized out of fear of being found lacking in some respect.

Of those who felt they had been found lacking (N=6/10), rather than continue to participate in social life, they withdrew to focus on looking after themselves. Both groups of Faithful Patients' normal narratives of restitution were interrupted by complications which were expressed in terms of 'disappointment', but they never remained 'sad stories' as their faith in restitution promised not only curtailment of the disease and its destructive effects but also a life worth living – even if only by focussing on 'survival'.

Exemplar 2: Olivia*

Olivia is a 30 year old single parent. She is clinically severe and recently moved in with her parents, not so they can look after her but so they can look after her son while she looks after herself. Echoing several other participants in this group, Olivia stated, '...the routine you get in to in the morning, it just becomes your life, you don't have to like it'. She was diagnosed at the age of 21 and did not accept it for several years. This was compounded still further by the premature birth of her son which led to her own self-neglect. Olivia is in fact the only participant in this group who has (had) *open* disagreements with the doctors (though this was regarding coming in to hospital for intensive intravenous treatment [IVs] rather than her *daily* regimen) but she relents, she said, 'Coz they do know better than you, no matter what you say, they know better'. Olivia has just been asked how their disagreements about coming in to hospital for intensive treatment are resolved:

P: He lets me not come in for 2 weeks but my mum says 'at the end of the day [Consultant Physician] knows what he's talking about' so my mum totally trusts him. I had a blood clot once and my face had all swelled up, my whole body, and um, like everyone was panicking and [Consultant Physician] said 'She's breathing isn't she? What's your problem? Don't panic'. So my mum says

now, she knows, as soon as he panics, she panics [laughs]. You know, my lips were blue, my face was like 3 times as big and he's like [softly] *'She's breathing, you know, so it's alright'*. So she's got that trust. Because it is hard, you know, when you first accept CF at 21, you know, death and things like that but they'll help you face it, you know, there's no panic. Nothing's going to happen. Do you know what I mean?

I: And in terms of the daily management of CF, does the doctor's advice play any part in that?

P: As I say, at first I just wouldn't listen to them. [Consultant Physician] just said 'go and see a counsellor, sort your head out, go the gym and you'll feel much better' and I'm like 'no, I'm sick, that won't help' but I've learnt that, yeah, they are right. And I have been the gym and I do feel better. So I'm feeling sorry for myself and they're like 'just get on with it'. At the minute, it's not quite working as I want. I'm still sleeping in the afternoons but eventually I will get better and I will be able to fight the colds off I think.

The hero of Olivia's two stories is her physician who is, from the outset, in control: *letting* her stay at home for an extra 2 weeks. Indeed Olivia's first story clearly sets out to show, not once but twice, why he has earned her trust or at least why her *mother* (who here plays a supporting rather central role) trusts him. It is, moreover, not just her physician's clinical expertise that is extolled but, in the second telling at least, his reassuring manner in a time of crisis. Her mother, to whom we presumably owe this story, is therefore impressed and reassured and so is Olivia. Indeed, she concludes, it gives her hope even in the face of death. She did, after all, live to tell the tale and, perhaps, tells the tale to live. Olivia's second story is necessarily more complicated as it involves her *active* compliance to her doctor's advice when he is not (physically) around to take control, though his encouragement to 'just get on with it' seems to be perpetually ringing in Olivia's ears. As Olivia, like other Faithful Patients, does not like asking for (informal) help when at home, however, this means that *she* must take some responsibility for her health, which indeed she did, again proving her doctors right and herself 'faithful'. For Olivia, however, (for unknown reasons) 'it's not quite working' and she is once again feeling sorry for herself. Indeed, the call to 'just get on with it' now sounds less helpful as with no-one to blame but herself, she simply becomes dejected. The attributions of faith and fortitude that Faithful Patients performed in their stories cannot, therefore, be taken for granted but as Radley (1994, p.159) points out and Olivia demonstrates, she must earn it again and again through her efforts to 'go on as well as possible'. It is, indeed, just a blip as Olivia keeps faith with the restitution narrative she has now made her own, re-assuring herself that she will, eventually, get better and once again take up the fight against CF.

Concordance: Quest Stories and the 'Expert Patient'

Explication of the interview texts suggests that concordant participants (N=13) are *communicative* body listeners. That is, they not only listen to their own unique bodies but also enter into dialogue with other bodies – professional or otherwise. The opinions of others, however, are invariably (or at least preferably) subordinated to their own expertise. Indeed, while these Expert Patients understand their own unique needs, others generally do not so they are often in conflict with them. This requires negotiation skills that may persuade or educate others (which may include CF professionals), though, where these do not succeed, at times it may also include joking or even ignoring them. But whatever strategies are employed, little appears to get in the way of their personally tailored self-care goals or, indeed, any other goals they may have. The narratives

performed during interviewing are therefore progressive success stories that (typically) draw upon multiple discourses as they seamlessly and often conspicuously integrated self-care into their daily lives.

According to Frank (1995) quest stories may take two forms. For 4 participants this entailed 'conversion' through which patients have come to accept CF positively and 'growth' for those 9 others who have always (positively) accepted their CF status (see also Crossley *nee*Davies, 1997; Crossley, 2000). For the former, (all of whom came from unskilled working class families) the focus of their narratives is their own transformation while for the latter their main concern is the transformation of others – through challenging and overcoming opposition. Indeed, one of the central features of the Quest is that narrators seem uniquely willing (and usually able) to manipulate potentially discrediting labels and definitions in social situations so that others' reactions will not be negative. Not every encounter with unsympathetic others was, however, so clearly successful, as Sandra* (below), illustrates.

Exemplar 3: Sandra

Sandra is a 20 year old female who comes from a traditional working class background. She lives alone, has done some part-time casual work in the past, enjoys designing and making clothing and hopes to have children in the future. Sandra is clinically severe and, she has just stated, has CF Related Diabetes (CFRD):

I: And, it's kind of connected, but would you take your insulin and enzymes in public?
P: I'll have my enzymes in public because they just go down dead quick and it could be any tablets, everyone takes tablets. My insulin, it depends where, I won't do it in a restaurant. There's certain places if we've got a booth and there's only me and [Boyfriend], I'll do

it there. But if there's a load of us, I don't, some people are put off, some people don't like needles and the thought of them going in, so I'll always go the bathroom and do it then. And if people can see it, I don't like doing it anyway because I get a bit embarrassed. Coz they'll say, 'Are you diabetic'? And I'll say, 'Yeah'. And they'll say, 'How come you're drinking wine? How come you can have so much sugars'? And I don't explain it very well, I just say, 'Oh it's a different kind of diabetes that I've got'. And they don't understand. They look at you funny and, I don't know, 'O shut up, don't ask' so it's just easier for me to just do it in the toilet [yeah]. Unless I'm with like my real mates that know, like, that have been brought up with me and know everything… [expectorates nonchalantly into a plastic cup] …I think it's harder to explain the diabetes than it is to explain anything else. Coz I don't really understand it myself. I just know that I've got to have it and that we don't produce enough insulin but try and explain to someone else, is, like, they ask too many questions and I think I'm just better off not saying anything.

Sandra's initial (direct) response to the question is not very story-like i.e. taking enzymes in public is basically unproblematic. This could have been the end of the matter (and for several participants it was) but by *voluntarily* introducing a complication (suggesting that while taking enzymes is not problematic insulin is), Sandra herself opens a dialogue and establishes from the outset that she is open and communicative. She is, moreover, kind and considerate so her *silence* is justified on the grounds that 'some people don't like needles'. Her narrative therefore not only develops a twist but is told as a personal quest in which her concealment is done for the benefit of others. It is not just for others, however, as Sandra also concedes becoming 'a bit embarrassed' but this is not, as

with some, because she feels discredited by her illness, rather, it is because she cannot *explain* it and does not want her lack of *knowledge* to be exposed. CFRD is indeed managed very differently to other types of diabetes (e.g. *allowing* the copious consumption of wine and sugars) and thus Sandra risks being *mis*labelled as reckless and incompetent. She is therefore 'better off not saying anything' and safeguarding her creditability as an expert self-carer.

There are, of course, many possible layers of meaning in Sandra's story but her own explanation of her behaviour is itself informative as she clearly distinguishes between *complementing others* (her boyfriend and *real* mates) who 'know everything' and therefore understand; and *opposing others* who do not know her and, therefore, *mis*understand. While Sandra's concealment and silence threatens to undermine her quest, however, with remarkable skill and dexterity she somehow manages to successfully navigate her way through the minefield of opposing and complementing forces and finishes 'better off'. Indeed, *because* of her silence everybody seems to gain something in this quest. Everybody except the interviewer, that is, as this normally kind and considerate person coughed and spat without so much as an 'excuse me'. It is difficult to say whether Sandra's expectoration was intended or not as a hospital setting can absolve patients from the usual expectation to control the signs and signals of illness (Kelly & Field, 1996). Given the immediate narrative context, however, perhaps she is in fact re-asserting control of the interview situation which almost undermined her expertise. What *is* certain is that the interviewer was taken off guard, if not altogether shocked, by the possibility that this young *female* could be so 'inconsiderate'. Indeed, perhaps this was the point that in her quest Sandra has in fact transcended the limitations and expectations imposed on her. She is neither compliant nor conformant but in complete control of her message to others (including the interviewer) and not the other way around.

Conformance: Normalising Stories and the 'Healthy Patient'

It has often been observed that people with chronic illnesses experience 'health within illness' as indeed people with CF have also been observed to do (e.g. Lowton & Gabe, 2003) but this particular group of participants seemed to experience 'illness within health'. Their stories therefore have a very simple plot which Sparks and Smyth (2006, p.56) helpfully capture: 'Yesterday I was healthy, today I'm sick, but tomorrow I'll be healthy again'. Such accounts are therefore often told from the point of view of *health* and so should be analysed that way rather than as expressions of 'denial' (Blaxter, 2004). This is particularly pertinent when considering early onset conditions such as CF which may, additionally, only occasionally (and barely noticeably) manifest itself – as appears to be the case with several of these 'healthy patients'. That is not to say that these accounts are without complication. For three participants in particular this was through the shock of being diagnosed with CFRD but for two others it was a more gradual (and no less troubling) decline in health. In either case, like Crossley's (*nee*Davies, 1997; Crossley, 2000) 'normalising' participants, they never let it 'ruin' their plans for the future. So, Charlotte* is planning to have children, Christine* applied to join the army and now wants to become a policewoman, while Carol* (below) wants to become a teacher or actress, and so on. Indeed, no compromises ever seem to have been made as they invariably return (or expect to return) to life as 'normal'. Crossley refers to her (similar) participants as 'doers' rather than 'thinkers' and these Healthy Patients not only seldom think about their illness but are always doing things for others – sometimes to their own detriment. They are, without exception, 'good citizens' so rather than an emphasis on personal rights, therefore, as Crossley also noted, a strong sense of moral obligation and responsibility towards others becomes

evident. These others are, moreover, invariably healthy peers and so because their frames of reference were almost exclusively non-CF people, participants were also much more likely to feel different compared to others even if they themselves are clinically normal. That is, they may have CF but they are invariably 'healthy CFs', as several participants indeed put it, making use of more general cultural discourses to make sense of their lives as people *minimally affected* by CF even if sometimes this was clearly not the case.

Exemplar 4: Carol

Carol is a clinically moderate student from a professional middle class family. She is currently on a year's sabbatical from college (but still plans to become a stage actress). For now at least, she is trying to focus on her health. All 40 interviews were started with the same request to describe a *typical* routine. In several instances, however, participants began with an *ideal* routine, what is *expected* of them and it is only through further questioning that the extent of their non-compliance becomes apparent. In Carol's case this did not take long as she continuously mispronounced her medications and laughed nervously. Still oblivious to her impending disclosure, the interviewer asked:

I: ...does your routine ever change significantly?
P: Yeah, a lot of the time, like, I've been totally out of routine and I've, like, just stopped taking any medication coz it's really hard to get back into a routine again.
I: And how long might that go on for?
P: Like at one point I was not taking my medication for about a year. It was like just on and off, I'd take things when I remember but like for quite a few years I haven't like taken, you know stuff properly really. I'll have periods when I'll start taking it again properly but it only lasts a few weeks.
I: When was that?

P: It's really been the last…since I was 16, it's when I had my GCSEs that I really slacked everything off.

I: And how was your health during that time?

P: Well, I was in hospital a lot having IVs coz when I take all my treatment I'm really quite well for a CF and, um, but it's only when I don't take my treatment that I have to go in [to hospital].

Carol's relief is almost palpable as she ceases to perform the role of compliant patient and starts to tell *her* story. Indeed she swiftly and successively moves from simply being *out of routine* to not taking her medication for *about a year*, then *quite a few years*, to, finally, *since I was 16* in as many sentences. But not only is Carol's non-compliance chronic and extensive, it has, as far as she is concerned, a direct effect on her health. That is, unlike other Healthy Patients who remain infection free when *not* doing their treatment, Carol is 'quite well for a CF' only when doing it. The problem is, of course, she seldom does 'all' of her treatment, or at least all of it 'properly' and invariably ends up in hospital – for which she alone is to blame. This, it turned out, became something of a theme as the following brief exchange illustrates:

I: How important is the medication in terms of managing your health, do you think?

P: Like, *a hundred percent important really* [laughing]. If I take all my medication, I'm, like, really well and don't show any symptoms of CF but when I don't take it I can make myself really, really ill.

I: Can you possibly tell me about a time when you have managed your medication well?

P: Yeah, there is days when, um like, I'll write my routine down but I have to get up at like 6 o' clock in the morning to fit it all in so I think that's one of the reasons why it's so hard.

Like other people in this group, Carol takes great care with her diet and tries to exercise regularly. Unlike most others, however, this is now insufficient as when she does not do her (medical) treatment she gets *worse* and her non-compliance is *the only reason* why this happens. Indeed because *she* 'fails' to get better we can see how this Healthy Patient becomes reconstituted as a 'bad' patient – which she demonstrated through-out the rest of the interview. It is not surprising that Carol fails. Carol's ideal routine was worked out in great detail but it means getting up at 6 and, she later added, going to bed at ten and taking medicines 4 times a day and doing physiotherapy, which 'is what really lets me down'. She is, it seems, not just being set up but setting herself up to fail. For Carol, the promises of biomedicine while providing hope that she can get better also induce guilt and blame when she does not. Still, either way, this seems preferable to the alternative reality - that she is in fact no longer the 'healthy CF' she once was. That the least compliant patients sometimes put most faith in the healing powers of medicine perhaps appears counter intuitive. But, in buying into its restitutional promises, it may be suggested that their non-compliance, somewhat perversely, actually functions to maintain a normal, 'healthy' identity. Medical regimens, as is often pointed out, serve to remind people that all is not well. However, non-compliance, under the restitutional discourses of biomedicine, keeps the promise and therefore the hope that recovery is always possible – even if only at some future point of need.

Independence: Chaos narratives and the 'Difficult Patient'

Like Healthy Patients, these radically non-compliant participants are opposed on all sides and their illness and the need and/or expectation to self-care exist only at the periphery of their accounts. This is not, however, because they are able to remain 'healthy' and find themselves through 'normal' valued activities but, rather, because they are 'sick' and lose themselves in their many problems. Like Healthy Patients, therefore, their illness is unlegitimated but, unlike them, their entire existences are without purpose as their illness 'spoils' their lives but their lives 'spoil' their illness. Angry at all who come into contact with them, these participants are not just Difficult Patients but also discredited *persons*. Isolated, alone and misunderstood these 'outsiders' are at the other (extreme) end of the control-chaos continuum already described (Frank, 1995). This is perhaps most evident in the unstable structure and circular direction of these anti-narratives as participants move from one complication to another without respite or resolution, as these Difficult Patients tell story after story of rejection and humiliation. Indeed their rejection of medical intervention, however eloquently it is expressed, appears to have been precipitated by their own exclusion from society itself. For the two younger (and relatively clinically healthy) participants, in particular, this appears to have little to do with their illness *per se*. Given their complex circumstances, it is not always clear how much of their difficulty is due to their illness, its denial or other stressors. It is perhaps not important to delineate between such things but, most likely, it seems to be a combination of factors. However, their problems have to first be recognised before they can be addressed but nobody seems to listen or, when they do, simply trivialise or ignore them altogether.

Exemplar 5: Kenneth*

Like Olivia (earlier) Kenneth was diagnosed as an adult. Both of his parents were 'labourers', as Kenneth also was, and when he was younger (and undiagnosed) they 'didn't know what to do' with him 'but I knew or at least my body did' he added. Whether at home or in hospital nobody, even now, knows what to do with Kenneth so, his wife politely disregards his coughing fits while the doctors (below) are equally removed from events as fate takes control of his life. Kenneth therefore rejects any possibility of help but feels that his life hangs by a thread. Before the following episode,

which took place several years ago, Kenneth had been talking about other people with CF who on paper *seem* healthier than he is but are, in reality, 'iller'. He has just tentatively suggested that health is perhaps a state of mind:

I: Do you think it is a state of mind?

P: I don't know, I'd like to think so. But having said that, there's a fear that if I lose that state of mind I could be, you know, 'Goodnight Vienna'. Because I actually remember [CF Consultant's Name], do you know [Name]?

I: Yeah, yeah.

P: I heard him leaving my room once, in the very early days, and he said... I had a bout of pneumonia, now every one's terrified of pneumonia, I've had pneumonia 5 times, um, and it's never killed me yet. Um, he was leaving my room and as he was walking out, I can't remember who he was talking to, he said, 'I don't tend to worry about [Kenneth] much, he just bounces right back'. Um, and I know I've always done that. I know that when I'm seriously ill, virtually in a coma, I just wake up and say 'Christ I'm starving' and I've done that. It was actually around the time I'd been [overseas place]; I near died of heart failure. There was two of us, I'd been [abroad] and the other girl had been [overseas place] the same week, we both had the same problem and unfortunately she died. Now I was very ill, they had me on a heart monitor and I literally woke up and went:

'Ah my God I could eat a horse'

And they said, 'Do you want something?'

I said, 'Yeah'

They said, 'What do you want?'

I said, 'Can I have a cooked *breckie*?'

'Yeah, could you manage one?'

'Yeah I could murder it' [laughs].

The last time [Name] saw me I was dying, I had a nurse around me 24 hours round the clock. The next day I woke up eating my cooked *breckie*. I was out within 3 days and I was seriously, seriously ill. Well he actually said to me, 'Another 24 hours and you would've been dead'. Um, three days after admission and I was discharged and I went straight back to work. So hopefully, in some ways, it might be a mental thing, I don't know. But, um, it's a thing, if it is, I hope I don't lose it, coz I could end up like the other patients.

Although Kenneth carefully sets the stage for the dramatic telling of his near death experience, his story is anti-climactic: he simply gets better and gets on, somewhat comically, with his banal existence. That is, there is no moralising, no character development and little to be learnt about him, his relationships or the world around. Again, and above all, no one appears to be in control. This time, interestingly, the CF physician, a different one to the previous account, seems to concur with Kenneth and indeed legitimates what the entire narrative sets out to prove, that Kenneth 'just bounces right back'. That is, survival is a matter of chance rather than choice, so Kenneth is reluctant to pin his hopes on his own mental resolve (or indeed anybody else's) which, as he cautions in his opening and closing statements, may be lost at any moment. Kenneth accepts the extreme contingency of life with CF. He survived and for no apparent reason another patient didn't. There is nothing that can be done about that and indeed there is nothing to be learned from that other than, perhaps, that he cannot rely on anyone, not even himself. Kenneth is beyond help.

It is with some justification that Kenneth and other Difficult Patients feel beyond the reach of others. A subclass of older people with CF has been created who, like Philoctetes, 'are abandoned on their islands to live long' but, asks Bryan Doerries (classical scholar and director of the Philoctetes Project), 'have we risen to the challenge of taking emotional care of them?' (*The New York Times* March 6, 2007). Of course even Philoctetes was promised healing from the gods whereas for these Difficult Patients the failure

not only of biomedicine, but all who try to help them live purposefully, means that a sense of exile and abandonment prevail. Indeed, there remains a background voice, beyond this world, which still speaks of the possibility of transcending the chaos through 'self-sacrifice' so that dying rather than living becomes their chief end.

Like 'Lazy Patients', Difficult Patients take little personal responsibility for their health, but instead *become* dependent on professional support during times of crisis – which can be inordinately expensive. Regardless of current budgetary constraints, however, it is imperative not to regard these patients merely as a 'drain on resources'. As the distinctive social histories of Difficult Patients in this study make clear, it is certainly not entirely their fault that they bounce back and forth from one crisis to another. While these participants cannot always be accommodated by mainstream interventions, however, as with Lazy Patients, they can at least be met on their terms. Something as small and simple as a random telephone call, for example, could have profound implications particularly if it involves person-centred conversation (rather than patient-centred 'care'). Visiting them at home with a new resolve to listen to their old grievances all over again may also go some way to recovering long-lost trust. Whatever action is taken, it needs to be done sensitively and without ignoring, accusing or trivialising their problems which is, perhaps, the very reason why they now exist in chaos. This acknowledgement of them as persons with problems rather than simply problem patients may even provide them with a way out of the endless cycles of disappointment and disillusionment and start to rebuild their lives.

LIMITATIONS OF THE RESEARCH AND FUTURE DIRECTIONS

One important intention of this study was to provide a diverse range of perspectives but this also meant that participants were difficult to follow-up. As a result, they were unable to collaborate further or comment on emerging findings. It is not therefore being suggested that these interpretations are in any way final or definitive - just one step in an on-going dialogue. This research was also undertaken in the UK which has its own unique social history and classification which was drawn upon both in selecting participants and analysis. Inequality is, however, universal and while other societies may not be divided along these lines it remains imperative for researchers and practitioners to capture structural inequalities as appropriately as possible for any given context – particularly as healthcare *everywhere* is dominated by privileged professionals. It is, indeed, also necessary to explore the plurality of (possible) professional responses to these self-care stories which too remain under developed and under researched.

CONCLUSION

The aim in this chapter has been to explore the tension and complication between these self-care stories and healthcare narratives. Human experi-

ence is, however, infinitely varied so the modes of making sense of it are limited and at times even inadequate – particularly when bodies 'fail' or are 'failed' by others. Even diseased bodies may, of course, also 'succeed' in this world, sometimes unexpectedly, but in either case the primary challenge for patients is to re-ascribe meaning to the illness experience and to reformulate their place in the world by becoming other (Crossley, 1999; Fox & Ward, 2006; Fox & Ward, 2008). Indeed at least 12 participants in this study appeared to shift position at some point in their life suggesting not only the possibility of change but also tentative links between these distinct patient identities:

Any attempt at classifying self-care will, of course, always be unsatisfactory even when self-ascribed. In particular the designations 'Lazy' and 'Difficult', though clearly (and often literally) performed by patients when justifying self-care inactivity, still carry pejorative connotations. Never-the-less, these were preferable to the dwindling range of alternatives and so could still be used positively and perhaps subversively by participants themselves to defend and even proclaim their marginal status - in much the same way as

Figure 2. A user-driven taxonomy of self-care

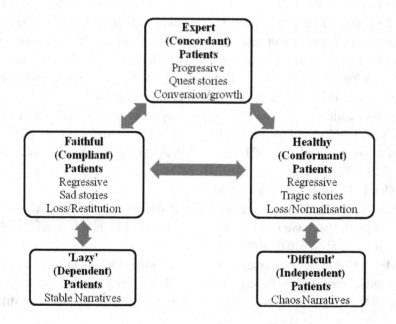

'queer' theorists have also observed. Other more acceptable designations (i.e. 'Faithful', 'Expert' and 'Healthy'), while more clearly connected with mainstream discourses should not be regarded as identical with them but, rather, as with marginal accounts, emerge from a complex interaction between patients, others (including the interviewer) and the generalised other. For this particular group of 40 patients in this particular hospital, there was in fact broad recognition of both compliant 'faithful' patients and concordant 'expert' patients. What appears to be more problematic, however, is when patients become separated from CF services through forgetfulness, laziness and/or other difficulties.

Wherever an individual may (or may not) be located in this proposed taxonomy, it is imperative not to impose one style of self-care on somebody who prefers and practices another. Rather, a fusion of horizons is needed by which researchers and practitioners may become more responsive and receptive to a wider range of patient preferences and needs - especially those who position themselves oppositionally to them. To achieve this it is necessary to look beyond the master narratives of healthcare (what is expected) and hear what patients are saying is realistically possible. Only then will we be able to recognise individual self-care practices and offer support in a manner that validates patients' stories rather than invalidates or 'fails' them. The failure, perhaps, is with medicine itself and those who do not question its master status.

REFERENCES

Abbot, J., Dodd, M., Bilton, D., & Webb, A. K. (1994). Treatment Compliance in Adults with Cystic Fibrosis. *Thorax, 49*(2), 115–120. doi:10.1136/thx.49.2.115

Abbott, J., Dodd, M., Gee, L., & Webb, K. (2001). Ways of coping with cystic fibrosis: implications for treatment adherence. *Disability and Rehabilitation, 23*(8), 315–324. doi:10.1080/09638280010004171

Arias Llorente, R. P., Garcia, C. B., & Diaz Martin, J. J. (2008). Treatment compliance in children and adults with cystic fibrosis. *Journal of Cystic Fibrosis, 7*, 359–367. doi:10.1016/j.jcf.2008.01.003

Ballard, K. (2004). Compliance and concordance. In Gabe, J., Bury, M., & Elston, M. A., *eds.* (2004). *Key Concepts in Medical Sociology* pp.107-112. London: Sage.

Blaxter, M. (2004). Life narratives, health and identity. In Kelleher, D., & Leavey, G. *eds.* (2004). *Identity and Health* pp.170-199. London: Routledge.

Broom, D., & Whittaker, A. (2004). Controlling diabetes, controlling diabetics: moral language in the management of diabetes type 2. *Social Science & Medicine, 58*(11), 2371–2382. doi:10.1016/j.socscimed.2003.09.002

Bury, M., & Taylor, D. (2008). Towards a theory of care transition: from medical dominance to managed consumerism. *Social Theory & Health, 6*, 201–219. doi:10.1057/sth.2008.9

Charmaz, K. (1983). Loss of self: a fundamental form of suffering in the chronically ill. *Sociology of Health & Illness, 5*(2), 168–195. doi:10.1111/1467-9566.ep10491512

Conway, S. P., Pond, M. N., Hamnet, T., & Watson, A. (1996). Compliance with Treatment in Adult Patients with Cystic Fibrosis. *Thorax, 51*, 29–33. doi:10.1136/thx.51.1.29

Crossley, M. L. (1999). Making sense of HIV infection: discourse and adaptation to life with a long term HIV positive diagnosis. *Health, 3*(1), 96–119.

Crossley, M. L. (2000). *Introducing Narrative Psychology: Self, Trauma and the Cronstruction of Meaning*. Buckingham: Open University Press.

Czarniawska, B. (2004). *Narratives in Social Science Research*. London: Sage.

D'Angelo, S. L., & Lask, B. (2001). Approaches to Problems of Adherence. In Bluebond-Langner, A., Lask, B., & Angst, D. B. *eds.* (2001). *Psychosocial Aspects of Cystic Fibrosis* pp.361-79. London: Arnold.

Davies, M. L. (1997). Shattered assumptions: Time and the experience of long-term HIV positivity. *Social Science & Medicine, 44*(5), 561–571. doi:10.1016/S0277-9536(96)00177-3

Department of Health. (2001). *The Expert Patient: A New Approach to Disease Management for the 21st Century*. London: HMSO.

Department of Health. (2006). Supporting people with long term conditions to self care – A guide to developing local strategies and good practice. Available at: http://www.dh.gov.uk/prod_consum_dh/groups/dh_digitalassets/@dh/@en/documents/digitalasset/dh_4130868.pdf.

Donaghy, B. (2004). Supplementary prescribing in cystic fibrosis: responding to an acute exacerbation. *Nurse Prescribing, 2*(2), 84–88.

Field, D., & Kelly, M. P. (2003). Chronic Illness and Physical Disability. In Taylor, S. & Field, D. Eds. (2003 3ʳᵈ edn) *Sociology of Health & Health Care* pp. 117-136. Oxford: Blackwell.

Fox, N., & Ward, K. (2006). Health identities: from expert patient to resisting consumer. *Health, 10*(4), 461–479.

Fox, N. J., & Ward, K. J. (2008). What are health identities and how may we study them? *Sociology of Health & Illness, 30*(7), 1007–1021. doi:10.1111/j.1467-9566.2008.01093.x

Frank, A. W. (1995). *The Wounded Story Teller: Body, Illness and Ethics*. Chicago: The University of Chicago Press.

Gjengedal, E., Rustoen, T., Wahl, A. K., & Hanesta, B. R. (2003). Growing up and living with cystic fibrosis: everyday life and encounters with the health care and social services--a qualitative study. *ANS. Advances in Nursing Science, 26*(2), 149–159.

Gotz, I., & Gotz, M. (2000). Cystic Fibrosis: psychological issues. *Paediatric Respiratory Reviews, 1*(2), 121–127. doi:10.1053/prrv.2000.0033

Howson, A. (2004). *The Body in Society*. Cambridge: Polity Press.

Lowton, K., & Gabe, J. (2003). Life on a Slippery Slope: Perceptions of Health in Adults with Cystic Fibrosis. *Sociology of Health & Illness, 25*(4), 289–319. doi:10.1111/1467-9566.00348

Lutfey, K. (2005). On practices of 'good doctoring': reconsidering the relationship between provider roles and patient adherence. *Sociology of Health & Illness, 27*(4), 421–447. doi:10.1111/j.1467-9566.2005.00450.x

Orem, D. E. (2001). *Nursing: Concepts of practice* (6th ed.). St. Louis, MO: Mosby.

Pfeffer, P. E., Pfeffer, J. M., & Hodson, M. E. (2003). The Psychosocial and Psychiatric Side of Cystic Fibrosis in Adolescents and Adults. *Journal of Cystic Fibrosis, 2*, 61–68. doi:10.1016/S1569-1993(03)00020-1

Radley, A. (1994). *Making Sense of Illness: The Social Psychology of Health & Illness*. London: Sage.

Robinson, I. (1990). Personal narratives, social careers and medical courses: Analysing life trajectories in autobiographies of people with multiple sclerosis. *Social Science & Medicine, 30*(11), 1173–1186. doi:10.1016/0277-9536(90)90257-S

Royal Pharmaceutical Society of Great Britain. (1997). *From Compliance to Concordance: Achieving Shared Goals in Medicine Taking.* Published Jointly by RPSGB and Merck Sharp & Dome.

Sparkes, A. C., & Smith, B. M. (2006). When narratives matter: men, sport, and spinal cord injury. In Rapport, F., & Wainwright, P. eds. (2006). *The Self in Health and Illness* pp.53-67. Abingdon: Radcliffe Publishing Ltd.

Stark, L. J., Jelalian, E., McGrath, A. N., & Mackner, L. (2001). Behavioural Approaches to Cystic Fibrosis: Applications to Feeding and Eating. In *Bluebond-Langner, A., Lask, B., & Angst, D. B. (2001). Psychosocial Aspects of Cystic Fibrosis* (pp. 348–360). London: Arnold.

The New York Times (March 6, 2007). The Difficult Patient, a Problem Old as History (or Older) by Abigail Zuger.

CF Trust (2000) *Growing Older with CF: A Handbook for Adults.* Published jointly by the Cystic Fibrosis Trust and Solvay Healthcare Limited.

Trust, C. F. (May 2006). *The Facts: An Introduction to Cystic Fibrosis.* Available at: http://www.cftrust.org.uk/aboutcf/publications/booklets/The_Facts_0506.pdf

Whitehead, S. M. (2002). *Men and Masculinities.* Cambridge, MA: Polity.

Willis, E., Miller, R., & Wyn, J. (2001). Gendered embodiment and survival for young people with cystic fibrosis. *Social Science & Medicine, 53*(9), 1163–1174. doi:10.1016/S0277-9536(00)00416-0

Yoshida, K. K. (1993). Reshaping of self: a pendular reconstruction of self and identity among adults with traumatic spinal cord injury'. *Sociology of Health & Illness, 15*(2), 217–245. doi:10.1111/1467-9566.ep11346888

ADDITIONAL READING

Baker, L. K., & Denyes, M. J. (2008). Predictors of Self-Care in Adolescents With Cystic Fibrosis: A Test of Orem's Theories of Self-Care and Self-Care Deficit. *Journal of Pediatric Nursing, 23*(1), 37–48. doi:10.1016/j.pedn.2007.07.008

Bauman, Z. (2004). *Identity.* Cambridge, UK: Polity Press.

Bury, M. (2007). Self-care and the English National Health Service. *Journal of Health Services Research & Policy, 12*(2), 65–66. doi:10.1258/135581907780279530

Conrad, P. (1985). The Meaning of Medications: Another Look at Compliance. In Conrad, P. ed (2005 7th edn) *The Sociology of Health & Illness: Critical Perspectives* pp.150-61. New York: Worth Publishers.

Frank, A. W. (2000). Illness and Autobiographical Work: Dialogue as Narrative Destabilization. *Qualitative Sociology, 23*(1), 135–156. doi:10.1023/A:1005411818318

Frank, A. W. (2005). What Is Dialogical Research and Why Should We Do It? *Qualitative Health Research, 15*(7), 964–974. doi:10.1177/1049732305279078

Friedson, E. (1970). The Social Organization of Illness. In Bury, M. & Gabe, J. eds (2004). *The Sociology of Health and Illness: A Reader* pp.177-184. London: Routledge.

Gadamer, H.-G. (1996). *The Enigma of Health.* Stanford: Stanford University Press.

Hyden, L.-C. (1997). Illness and Narrative. *Sociology of Health & Illness, 19*(1), 48–69.

Kinsella, E. A. (2006). Constructions of self: ethical overtones in surprising locations. In Rapport, F., & Wainwright, P. eds (2006). *The Self in Health and Illness* pp.21-31. Abingdon: Radcliffe Publishing Ltd.

Lowton, K. (2004). Only when I Cough? Adults' Disclosure of Cystic Fibrosis. *Qualitative Health Research, 14*(2), 167–186. doi:10.1177/1049732303260675

Lowton, K., & Ballard, K. (2006). Adult cystic fibrosis patients' experiences of primary care consultations: A qualitative study. *The British Journal of General Practice, 56*(528), 518–525.

Marinker, M. (2003). Not to be taken as directed. *British Medical Journal, 326*, 348–349. doi:10.1136/bmj.326.7385.348

Marinker, M. (2004). From Compliance to Concordance: A Personal View. In Bond, C. *ed* (2004). *Concordance: A Partnership in Medicine Taking* pp.1-7. London: Pharmaceutical Press.

McCracken, M. J., & Angst, D. B. (2001). Self-care in Cystic Fibrosis. In Bluebond-Langner, A., Lask, B., & Angst, D. B., *eds*. (2001). *Psychosocial Aspects of Cystic Fibrosis* pp.255-267. London: Arnold.

Mishler, E. G. (1986). *Research Interviewing: Context and Narrative*. Cambridge: Harvard University Press.

Mykhalovskiy, E., McCoy, L., & Bresalier, M. (2004). Compliance/Adherence, HIV and the Critique of Medical Power. *Social Theory & Health, 2*, 315–340. doi:10.1057/palgrave.sth.8700037

Orbach, S. (2009). *Bodies*. London: Profile Books Ltd.

Parsons, T. (1975). The sick role and the role of the physician reconsidered. *The Milbank Memorial Fund Quarterly. Health and Society, 53*(3), 257–278. doi:10.2307/3349493

Paterson, B. (2001). Myth of Empowerment in Chronic Illness. *Journal of Advanced Nursing, 34*(5), 574–581. doi:10.1046/j.1365-2648.2001.01786.x

Raoul, V., Canam, C., Henderson, A. D., & Paterson, C. (2007). Making Sense of Disease, Disability & Trauma: Normative & Disruptive Stories. In Raoul, V., Canam, C., Henderson, A. D., & Paterson, C. eds (2007). *Unfitting Stories: Narrative approaches to disease, disability & trauma* pp.3-11. Waterloo, ON: Wilfred Laurier University Press.

Riessman, C. K. (2003). Performing Identities in Illness Narrative: Masculinity and Multiple Sclerosis. *Qualitative Health, 3*(1), 5–33.

Riessman, C. K. (2008). *Narrative Methods for the Human Sciences*. London: Sage.

Schidlow, D. V. (2004). 'Maintaining the horizontal line': Early intervention and prevention of CF lung disease. *Journal of Cystic Fibrosis, 3*, 63–66. doi:10.1016/j.jcf.2004.05.044

The New Yorker Annals of Medicine. (December 6, 2004). The Bell Curve: What happens when patients find out how good their doctors really are? By Atul Gawande.

Turner, B. S. (1995). *Medical Power and Social Knowledge* (2nd ed.). London: Sage.

Williams, G. (1984). The genesis of chronic illness: narrative re-construction. *Sociology of Health & Illness, 6*(2), 175–200. doi:10.1111/1467-9566.ep10778250

Williams, G. H. (2000). Knowledgeable narratives. *Anthropology & Medicine, 7*(1), 135–140. doi:10.1080/136484700109395

Williams, S. J. (2005). Parsons revisited: from the sick role to…? *Health, 9*(2), 123–144.

Willis, E., Miller, R., & Wyn, J. (2001). Gendered Embodiment and Survival for Young People with Cystic Fibrosis. *Social Science & Medicine, 53*, 1163–1174. doi:10.1016/S0277-9536(00)00416-0

Ziguras, C. (2004). *Self-care – Embodiment, Personal Autonomy and the Shaping of Consciousness*. London: Routledge.

Zola, I. K. (1972). Medicine as an Institution of Social Control. In Conrad, P. *ed* (2005 7ᵗʰ edn). *The Sociology of Health & Illness: Critical Perspectives* pp.432-42. New York: Worth Publishers.

KEY TERMS AND DEFINITIONS

Chaos: The experience of disorder and meaninglessness.

Compliance: The medicalisation of self-care in everyday life by prioritising prescriptions given by health professionals.

Concordance: The negotiation of self-care in everyday life in partnership with others.

Conformance: The normalisation of self-care in everyday life by prioritising socially acceptable practices and activities.

Quest: The promise, pursuit or practice of personal growth and development.

Restitution: The promise, pursuit or practice of healing or the amelioration of physical suffering.

ENDNOTE

[1] The study was approved by Liverpool John Moores University and the local research ethics committee (Ref: 04/Q1505/148). Informed consent was given by all participants and their names have been altered throughout to protect their identity. All such changes have been marked with an asterisk upon first use of the pseudonym.

Chapter 26
Patients with a Spinal Cord Injury Inform and Co-Construct Services at a Spinal Cord Rehabilitation Unit

Susan Sliedrecht
Auckland Spinal Rehabilitation Unit, New Zealand

Elmarie Kotzé
University of Waikato, New Zealand

ABSTRACT

This chapter reports on a qualitative research project which explored patients' experiences of counselling and which provided the impetus for changes to be incorporated in the rehabilitation and health care provided at a spinal cord rehabilitation unit in Auckland, New Zealand. Navigating different landscapes of meaning, philosophies, ideas and practices from approaches such as the relationship-centred model and narrative medicine developed into a collaborative meaning-making partnership between the patient team and the multidisciplinary team that further shaped practices of doing reasonable hope together.

INTRODUCTION

Different models of medical health care to patients and their families have been developed in the quest for optimal and successful provision of service, care and patient satisfaction. There have been a number of shifts in medicine with regard to the models used to shape practitioners' relationships and interactions with their patients. These medical and biomedical practices and approaches regarding what is in the best interests of patients were initially informed by a philosophy that patients should not be burdened with making decisions about their care. The aim was to ease the burden for patients by letting the doctor, who was believed to have exclusive specialist knowledge in this field, make the decisions. However, in recent years, doctors have increasingly been invited to discuss treatment options, including benefits and risks, with patients and their families. These models include the medical model, the bio-psychosocial model (McDaniel, Hepworth, & Doherty, 1992), the integrated care model (World Health Organisa-

DOI: 10.4018/978-1-60960-097-6.ch026

tion, 2001), the relationship-centred model (Beach, Inui, & the Relationship-Centered Care Research Network, 2006; Frankel & Quill, 2005), a narrative approach to health psychology (Murray, 2009) and narrative medicine (Charon, 2006). All these models offer varying positions and responsibilities to health practitioners, the multi-disciplinary team, the patient and his/her family.

This chapter draws on a qualitative research study carried out at the Auckland Spinal Rehabilitation Unit in New Zealand (hereafter called the Spinal Unit). Results from the study and ongoing patient feed-back were used to shape and re-plan certain services. The chapter shows how different landscapes of meaning, philosophies, ideas and practices from approaches such as the relationship-centred model and narrative medicine developed into a collaborative meaning-making partnership between the patient team and the multidisciplinary team that further shaped practices of doing reasonable hope together. Reasonable hope directs attention to what is within reach and it softens the polarities between hope and despair. It maintains that the future is open, influentiable and influenciable and it accommodates contradiction and despair (Weingarten, 2009).

BACKGROUND

The Spinal Unit offers services to in-patients and outpatients. The medical multi-disciplinary team consists of doctors, nurses, physiotherapists, occupational therapists, dieticians, nutritionists, pharmacists, social workers and counsellors. Patients are admitted to the Spinal Unit once they are medically stable and ready for active rehabilitation, usually about four to eight weeks after they were injured, depending on the waiting list at the unit.

The Spinal Unit aims to work in a partnership relationship with patients. This partnership relationship was informed and co-constructed by the findings from the research study and patient feed-back. Negotiating a partnership that speaks

of respect for multiple perspectives and collaboration as described in this chapter will draw on positioning theory and post structuralist definitions of agency.

Providing health care services poses different challenges for both the multidisciplinary team and the patient team (members of a patient's support team can include caregivers, friends and family). The health professionals' purpose at the Spinal Unit is to enable patients to be as independent in their activities for daily living as possible and live a quality life. Quality of life depends on a person's subjective evaluation of the degree to which his/her most important needs, goals and wishes are fulfilled (Frisch, 2006). Independence may be gained through equipment, for example, a wheelchair, or through learning about personal care so that patients can direct others to assist them. Independence can also be gained through education about aspects of the patient's body that may have changed and/or through managing the psychological and emotional adjustments that result from a spinal cord injury. The discourse of what "independence" might look like in the lives of patients with spinal cord injuries becomes a site of deconstruction, questioning and is being held up for review. The process of negotiating new meaning of "independent" may open the possibility of a spectrum of dependencies, independence and interdependence. Health care professionals of the Spinal Unit are committed to working alongside patients to provide the best possible spectrum of service to patients in assisting them with this challenge.

The medical team and the patient team are differently positioned in this: while health care professionals are committed to using their knowledge and skills in the service of patient care, they exercise a choice about whether or not to work at the unit. Patients and families are committed to a healing rehabilitation journey frequently filled with uncertainty, challenges and possible disappointments, and do not experience a similar sense of agency. Agency is defined as participating in the "conversations that produce the meanings of one's life" (Drewery, 2005, p. 315) or the ability to act on the world by resisting, subverting or holding up for review the discourses that shape one's life (Davies, 1991). For patients with an illness, agency means not remaining passive, but a sense that one can make personal choices in dealing with illness and the healthcare system. Agency is a sense of activism about one's own life in the face of all that is uncertain (Mc Daniel et al., 2005, p.6).

Both the multidisciplinary team and the patient team bring various knowledges to the process that are valued differently. Both teams may come up against their own vulnerabilities, limitations in their knowledge and skills, and may face a range of experiences, such as pain, discomfort, frustration, uncertainties and distrust, and may respond with a range of emotions, such as joy, hope, despair or sadness. These responses can push the boundaries of what is possible and often test the partnership between the medical team and the patient team.

Unless actively attended to, power and knowledge resides with the dominant group. Therefore in the light of the above scenario the following questions emerged: How can the partnership between the multidisciplinary team and the patient team be negotiated on an ongoing basis, paying particular attention to collaborative meaning-making (Beach et al., 2006), working towards discursive power and wisdom (Paré, 2002) and "sharing treatment-relevant power" (Williams, Frankel, Campbell, & Deci, 2000, p. 80)? How can this partnership provide significant opportunities for all to experience agency and care some or most of the time? What relationship practices make such a partnership possible?

One step in investigating how this negotiated relationship practices could be produced was a qualitative research project at the Spinal Unit (Sliedrecht, 2007). Former patients were interviewed to reflect on the quality of counselling service they had experienced during their in-patient stay. Their voices plus ongoing discus-

sions with patients gave Susan the opportunity to re-shape, re-plan and re-focus the counselling service. However, the research and subsequent conversations also resulted in changes in other aspects of the medical service provided to patients and their families which included:

- Collaborative and caring relationship with health professionals.
- Incorporating families as decision-makers and supporters in the treatment plans.
- Flexible and multiple ways of speaking grief and loss.
- Learn more about sex, intimacy and spinal cord injury.

Each of these aspects will be discussed separately.

COLLABORATIVE AND CARING RELATIONSHIPS BETWEEN HEALTH PROFESSIONALS, PATIENTS AND THEIR FAMILIES

Collaboration and Care with Health Professionals

The personal experiences of professionals or health care professionals influence and shape their practice (Frank, 1991, 1995, 2001; Weingarten, 2001). The vignette below had a significant influence on the life of one of the researchers, Susan:

No personal experience has had such a profound impact on shaping my (Susan's) professional practice as my own engagement with the healthcare system at the age of twenty-one when my mother was diagnosed with lung cancer. ...the doctors made the assessment that the cancer was too far progressed and they were not going to remove the cancerous growth.

The only medical information that we received as a family was "we opened you up and it was too far gone to do anything, so we closed you up again." This information was given to my mother, who in turn told my father and myself and my two siblings. There was no family meeting, no further discussions from the doctors with regard to her prognosis, no negotiations or discussions with any of the medical team about treatment options or lack thereof – that was the extent of the information.

Mc Daniel, Campbell, Hepworth, and Lorenz (2005) refer to the approach according to which medical practitioners share only limited medical facts with a patient as being informed by a biomedical model of patient care. Such a model accounts for illness in terms of biochemical factors without considering the social or psychological dimensions of people's lives. The unspoken message in this for the family was that the doctors were the experts and holders of medical knowledge and the family was not called on to contribute to or be involved in any of the decision making. Collaborative meaning making was not offered. The knowledge domain was claimed by the medical professionals, while the family was positioned with no or minimal speaking rights, without agency – a sense that one can make personal choices in dealing with illness and the healthcare system (Mc Daniel et al., 2005, p.6).

This way of sharing information silenced the family. The family could not see any bridge to walk across to talk about matters of life and death with their mother or the medical team. Frank (1995, p. 55) emphasises the importance, for ill people to tell and retell their story in the context of listeners who care and who contribute in their unique way. Chaos illness stories are uncomfortable to tell or to listen to and their uncomfortable quality is all the more reason they have to be told. This telling and re-telling assists people in making meaning of their unique life circumstances. If not told and listened to, the interrupted voice remains silenced, and the opportunity for meaning making is hindered.

Youngson (2008), a practising anaesthetist and founder of the Centre for Compassion in Healthcare, emphasises that practices in medical care such as those described above are not satisfactory to many doctors either. Early in his career, he perceived himself as the master of technical excellence, but eventually realised that he preferred what he calls "a renewal of humanity and compassion" (p.2) and came to realize that patients could become his teachers. In his opening address at the 2008 Australian and New Zealand Spinal Cord Society Conference, he shared a story about a patient named Jessie who came to him with an "appalling catalogue of medical complaints" but with an indomitable spirit. Jessie was a high-risk patient with complex medical problems. Youngson explained the potential risks of the operation that Jessie needed and that the risk could be reduced if Jesse had a blood transfusion. Jessie declined the blood transfusion, as she was a Jehovah's Witness:

[Jessie said:] "I'm sorry it makes it more difficult for you but I'll just have to take my chances." In a moving gesture, she took my hand in hers. "Robin, I put my faith in you. I know you'll do the best job you can and God will be watching over you." (Youngson, 2008:p.3)

The experience of having a patient reach out to him in care and other similar experiences with patients taught him about interconnection and interdependence. He related how the shift came about:

...I conceived of the doctor-patient relationship as a one way street. I was the highly trained doctor, the expert, the person with authority and control. Caring was a one-way process. I cared for patients and I determined the process and the agenda. Patients didn't care for me. They were grateful, of course, they took my advice and they did what I told them. But somehow, Jessie [the patient mentioned above] turned the tables on me. She was the one caring for me and supporting me

in my difficulties. The relationship had become a two-way process.

Another important lesson that Youngson (2008) learnt from his patients is what was previously invisible when he adopted the position of the holder of knowledge: humanity. Stepping aside from professional and expert roles, a small mo(ve)ment (Davies et al., 2006) of caring became available – care being given and care being received, as Jesse interrupted the binary thinking about caregiver and care-receiver – instead, a "caring solidarity" (Sevenhuijsen, 1998, p. 147) became possible.

Jim[1]*, a patient at the Spinal Unit, is an example of such caring solidarity between professionals and patients. Jim and his daughter Amy* set out on a fathers and daughters outing one Saturday morning – cycling. On this trip they were involved in an accident – Jim's daughter was killed and Jim had a spinal injury and was in intensive care, unconscious with no clear prognosis as to whether or when he would regain consciousness. Jim's family had to decide whether to continue with the daughter's funeral or postpone it. The family decided to proceed without Jim. When he regained consciousness, he was faced with the painful information that not only did he have a spinal injury, but he had lost his only child, Amy. The family carefully constructed a DVD of Amy's funeral and informed Jim of this.

Jim longed to watch the DVD, but was mindful that it might be too painful and unfair to expect his wife to watch it with him. She was grieving the loss of her daughter and he did not want to inflict more pain and hurt. In the counselling conversations at the spinal unit, he kept telling Susan, the counsellor, how he wanted to watch the DVD but he was afraid of doing this, since he knew grief would overwhelm him. He wanted to watch it but he did not know how he could actually manage to. Witnessing his distress and agony, Susan asked him if he had any ideas, even tentative ones, about what would make it possible for him

to watch it. Together they discussed options – was he thinking of watching it on his own? Would he prefer someone with him, if so, who would that be? Jim wanted to watch the DVD with someone, so Susan started exploring with him who might be a suitable person. During this conversation, he looked at Susan and very quietly asked, almost mumbling: "Would you be willing to watch it with me?" Susan, moved by compassion (tinged with some trepidation) was touched and honoured that he asked her to share something so personal. She responded to him as one human to another, one parent to another and remembers saying:

It would be a privilege to share this experience with you. Could I ask that as we watch it together, I watch with you as a parent and a person who will, I think, be profoundly moved by the experience? I am asking for space to respond in a way that shows what I am experiencing. I will be deeply moved, with you in what I see, and I may cry. Please accept my tears as care.

Careful planning, paying attention to detail, went into the preparations to watch the DVD together, deciding when would be a good time for Jim and how he wanted to prepare himself. Consequently we planned carefully, paying attention to detail such as appropriate timing and preparatory steps Jim wanted to take. Susan also paid careful attention to small details for example: the positioning of the remote control (with his limited hand functioning, he could not reach for it to stop the video if it became too difficult for him to watch), where to discretely place the Kleenex so it would be within his reach if and when he needed it. The reflection on this detail was shaped by Susan's intention to open space for patient agency. Susan also put thought into where to physically position herself, how close or far away to sit in relation to Jim and where she herself would feel comfortable. As the professional, Susan was doing self-care, while also doing care with and for him (Charon, 2001a). Part of this involved being transparent in explaining to Jim that if she watched the DVD with him, it was very likely she would be moved and touched by what she would experience and might cry if she felt moved. This step reminded them both of a humanness that connects them and the invitation to do collaborative care. Such utterances (Bakhtin, 1986), responses and small acts invite a "dialogical responsiveness" (Katz & Shotter, 1996, p. 928) that helps to story a "caring solidarity" (Sevenhuijsen, 1998, p.147). Susan remembers a poignant moment of professional and patient connecting:

As we sat crying, watching the footage of the funeral of Amy, Jim was able to stop the DVD when emotions were just too overwhelming. He could, however, not dry his own tears, as he had limited hand and arm functioning and so, with his permission, I carefully wiped the tears from his eyes.

The above example highlights a number of aspects of relationship-centred care (Beach et al., 2006) where the social role and privileges of the healer are founded upon meaningful relationships in health care, not just technically appropriate transactions within these relationships. It recognises the central importance of affect and emotion in developing, maintaining and terminating relationships. This resonates with the work of Kaethe Weingarten (2003, p 115), who questions the way in which professionals sometimes have to blunt their emotions "in order to stay sane". She talks about the dilemma of how professionals are submerged in a wider culture that believes that the expression of emotion is healthy, whilst continuing to subscribe to professional norms that argue that emotionality on the job undermines performance. Weingarten encourages professionals to witness themselves and to be aware of physical and emotional symptoms of distress. She encourages them to respond to themselves, patients and other colleagues with compassion and care. This compassion and care towards others endorses another

principle of narrative medicine (Charon, 2001a) and relationship-centred care (Beach et al., 2006): all health care relationships occur in the context of reciprocal influence. "Whilst achievement of the patients goals and the maintenance of health are the more obvious focus of any encounter, allowing a patient to have an impact on the clinician is a way to honour that patient and his/her experience" (Beach et al., p.s4).

Relationship-centred care also supports ideas of a weaving and a co-creation of knowledge. It promotes a practice of including "your knowing" and "my knowing" and it strives for an "our knowing" that transcends both – what Paré (2002) calls discursive wisdom. Paré (2002, p. 15) uses the simple analogy (borrowed from Strong, 2001) of "my house", "your house" and "our house". My house includes theoretical concepts and models, and the ideas, beliefs and practices the health practitioner holds. Your house are the ideas, beliefs and practices and unique personal histories the client holds. In relationship-centred care one aims for a construction of "our house", which promotes collaboration and co-construction. This analogy suggests that to privilege one or the other's knowledge (patient and/or medical practitioner) perpetuates relational violence – the aim is a practice that seeks to open conversational spaces which includes both your knowing and my knowing, which then becomes our knowing and transcends both. This conversational space gives opportunity for patients to step into collaborative meaning making with the medical team. Patients then have the opportunity to decide to what extent, if any, they would like to respond to this invitation.

Katz and Shotter (1996) use the idea of a cultural broker – brokering between the medical voice, which is located in the body and is then translated into medical language, and the patient's voice, which relates to cultural and social processes. How might a medical conversation become relational so that the patient feels involved and respected and the conversation is not an alienating event? They pose the following questions:

How might a language be created such that the tacit, the unsaid, the nature of "her world", could be articulated in her terms, instead of being translated into the already accepted, traditional world of medicine? How might this privileging of ordinary language create a more two-way exchange in which she has as much command and import as the other? What possible "topics" or "common places" could we find to create a "common ground" between us, to create a "sensed" or "sensible" space full of "things" about which both she and we could speak? (Katz & Shotter, 1996, p.923)

In Susan's story of her mother's cancer and the multidisciplinary team's limited explanation of the cancer, the important information for the doctors was that the cancer was inoperable. For the family, what was important was how to make sense of the information so that they could be an emotional support to each other and to her mother. What a difference relationship-centred care would have made for the family! Conversations between the multidisciplinary team and the patient team could have worked towards those common places, and collaborative meaning-making could have resulted in an "our knowing" (Paré, 2002, p. 15). This form of collaboration strengthens connection to humanness, respectful listening and compassion for both patient team and the multidisciplinary team.

This section has focused on relationships with the patient. In the next section, the focus is family and support people who are part of the patient team.

The research at the Spinal Unit (Sliedrecht, 2007) identified the importance of including family members. It also highlighted that some of the structures in place to promote family inclusion needed revision. Brief examples are given of how patients' voices shaped goal-setting meetings.

Incorporating Families in Treatment Plans

Participants emphasized the importance of assistance for their families to hear and understand the disruption and adjustment they might have to face after a spinal cord injury. Janet*, a married woman and mother of three children, said:

My first thought went out to my family. I thought I need to get my family in order, my focus was on my family rather than myself... as to understand the whole aspect. They were unsure about what was going to happen and they were worried. It would have been useful if staff shared information to equip them to face the dilemmas and challenges of living with a spinal cord injury. (Sliedrecht, 2007, p. 62)

Studies on caregivers' adjustment to physical disability (Elliot, Shewchuk, & Richards, 1999) and patient education in rehabilitation (May, Day, & Warren, 2006) emphasises the significant contribution many families (caregivers) make to patient well-being. Participants in the research done at the Spinal Unit wanted to work towards meaningful storylines of their families' involvement and contribution to the treatment plans (Sliedrecht, 2007).

One research participant Matthew* said the effect of his injury was more difficult for his family than what it was for him. He felt that they were in some ways "outside of the situation … with all the emotions" and all the focus of care was on him. He felt that lack of knowledge both for himself and his family created stress. He said that his family "were unsure about what was going to happen and they were very worried" (Sliedrecht, 2007 p. 133).

Important forums for family involvement at the spinal unit are the fortnightly goal setting meetings (GSM). Hearing from the participants the importance to them of collaboration and partnership between patient team and multidisciplinary team provided the impetus for staff to reflect on the micro-skills, strategies and steps that shape goal-setting meetings. They reflected on questions such as these: Who sets the agenda for the discussions? How is this done? Who gets first speaking rights – the doctors or the patient and/or family member? Who is part of the patient's team? What information is shared and how is this shared during the meeting?

Through these reflections the purpose of the GSM shifted to a "commitment to mutual knowledge-making" (Paré, 2002, p. 10). This shift provided the space not only to make meaning, but also to acknowledge the "limits of the knowing" and alternating between the positions of knowing and the suspension of knowing which calls forth other voices (Paré, 2002, p.10). This adjusted goal of mutual construction of meaning made possible the unpacking of the taken-for-granted notion that a multidisciplinary team holds the knowledge, and that the family and patients only receive that knowledge. It opened up the possibility of agency and communion, where agency is seen as the possibility of making personal choices in dealing with illness and the healthcare system and as inviting a sense of activism about one's own life in the face of all that is uncertain (McDaniel et al., 2005, p. 6). Agency is an important position for someone with a spinal cord injury to be invited into / offered, especially in dealing with the debilitating effects of disability. Communion refers to emotional bonds that often are frayed by illness, disability and contact with the health care system. The goal-setting meetings assist family members to join together to carefully address the challenges and to "do so within the context of allowing the patient the maximum feasible autonomy and agency" (McDaniel, Hepworth, & Doherty, 1992, p. 10).

The extent to which these GSMs create opportunities for agency for patients and their family depends on the way the meetings are structured and facilitated. The team has worked to put practices of relationship-centred care (Beach et al., 2006;

Williams, Campbell, & Deci, 2000) in place to increase the likelihood of partnership between the multidisciplinary team and the patient team. The team hoped that these practices would allow families agency to seek clarification, ask questions and share information that they regard as important. Detailed below are some of the steps that were taken to promote agency and communion. The preparation for the meeting and the actual meeting itself is discussed.

As part of the preparation for such a meeting, the patient's key worker meets with the patient, and explains the intention, purpose and format of the meetings, and the topics that are likely to be discussed. Patients are encouraged to invite family, friends and support people to this meeting. To ensure that the multidisciplinary team's practice is culturally appropriate, the key worker verifies with the patient whether there are any areas of conversation he or she would not feel comfortable discussing in such a forum, for example, some patients prefer not to discuss bowel and bladder cares in this forum.

In the preparatory meeting (may only take 15 minutes), it is emphasised that the patient team's input is valuable, as the patient and his/her team have expert knowledge about themselves and that this information is very important for reasonable goal-setting. It is the team's hope and intention that patients come "aware and empowered" (Weingarten, 2003, p. 95) to the goal-setting meeting. In this way the power-knowledge relations (Foucault, 1980) between the multidisciplinary team and the patient team are attended to in a small but significant way. Patients select to what extent they take up this invitation.

At the actual meeting, the multidisciplinary team introduces a number of practices to promote information-sharing and mutual meaning-making. Mindful of different cultural practices in New Zealand, the multidisciplinary team offers the family the opportunity to open and close the meeting with a blessing, prayer or a *karakia* (a significant and respectful invitation that honours elders). This gives the family some control of the proceedings.

The multidisciplinary team take care in how members are introduced, making eye contact (if and when doing so is culturally appropriate) and speaking as clearly as possible, so that the patient and family are aware of team members' roles and why team members are attending the meeting. The family members introduce themselves and their relationship to the patient. This introduction is a basic courtesy, as well as a culturally appropriate practice and ensures that people can be identified by their names, re-emphasising the personalised interaction.

The key worker facilitates the meeting – not the medical doctor. The purpose of the meeting is explained again and the patient and family are asked if they have any questions or concerns that they want addressed at this meeting. Time is given for this before any person from the multidisciplinary team gives feedback or discusses the patient's medical situation. Questions, concerns and comments are noted on the agenda and the key worker ensures that these are addressed at some point in the meeting.

Taking the time and respecting the specific wishes of patients and their families attends to the power-knowledge (Foucault, 1980) relation between the medical staff and the patient team. It also positions patients as members of the rehabilitation team and not as patients experiencing multidisciplinary team acting upon them. The example below highlights how beneficial it is to have family and patient involvement in this partnership.

Moana* fell off a ladder whilst pruning a tree. She was admitted to the Spinal Unit for in-patient rehabilitation. During the accident, Moana hit her head, but did not lose consciousness. From a history taken at admission, it was also known that Moana had been diagnosed with severe depression and was taking medication (Citalopram). She also informed the multidisciplinary team that she had learning difficulties.

At the first GSM, Moana and her daughter, Kate*, were asked if they had any particular questions or concerns that they wanted to be paid attention to. They indicated that there was nothing in particular that they wanted to raise.

Radical listening (Weingarten, 1995) or double listening (Denborough, 2005) invites the team to reflect on the available ideas and practices that might shape Moana and Kate's silence, for example, whether or not they believed that the multidisciplinary team holds the knowledge and that the experts should speak first and that Moana and Kate's local knowledges may not be relevant for the discussion. Listening with this in mind, the team kept the following interpretations of their silence available: "no thanks, not yet", or "yes, but we do not yet feel safe" or "we are overwhelmed and cannot think of anything at the moment." The latter position is described by Katz and Shotter (1996) as the "not-yet-known" (p. 923) that can be "experienced by the patient as not making sense" (p. 923) or "as [their knowledge] being heard by the doctor as 'nonsense'" (p. 923). Considering these possible interpretations of their silence facilitates mutual meaning-making between the world of the patient team and the multidisciplinary team. Listening in this way also gives the team an opportunity to be informed by appropriate cultural practices, especially where these may differ from those of the majority of the multidisciplinary team.

The medical consultant showed Moana's x-rays and MRI scan of the spine at the meeting. The implications of the injury and the prognosis were discussed at a pace that seemed, from observation, comfortable for Moana and Kate and they were again invited to raise any concerns, ask questions or make comments, but they declined. It was emphasised that if they wanted any clarification about any aspect, this could be re-visited. They indicated that they understood the information shared with them. They were then asked whether they were ready to hear feedback from the nursing staff and once again they were invited to ask questions, make comments, slow the process down or get clarification. At this point, Kate said: "Actually, there is something that I would like to ask – why is my mother's memory so poor? For example, she can't remember visitors' names."

This information about memory loss had potential significance for the understanding of Moana's behaviour in the ward. Moana was assuring the nursing staff that she was safe to do bed to chair transfers independently, without hands-on or standby assistance. However, she had not been assessed by the physiotherapists as safe to do this independently. The physiotherapists and the nursing staff had noted that at times Moana struggled with the execution of the sequence of the transfer. Staff had also noted that Moana responded impulsively for example she would not wait for assistance with her transfers or mobilising. At times she would become verbally aggressive towards staff. Kate's question about memory loss and the nursing team's observations opened up new meanings of Moana's responses.

The question was then raised whether Moana could not remember that she had not yet been cleared for independent transfers or whether it was a sign of holding onto independence. Alternatively, was her sequencing problem possibly related to learning difficulties and / or brain injury? In addition, were some of her outbursts related to a possible brain injury and had nothing to do with difficulties to accept the effects of the spinal cord injury? Kate's question opened possibilities for mutual meaning-making between the multidisciplinary team and the patient team.

A follow-on of this discussion was exploring how these possibilities might position Moana and Kate, enabling them to story an understanding of the implications for Moana's return home. The narrative was shaped from Kate's local knowledge of her mother when she asked: "Why is my mother's memory so poor?" Kate's question generated important discussions, and relationally, an agentic position was offered. She realised that what she asked and said, made sense and that she held important knowledge. It is in the territory

between the patient team and multidisciplinary team and "in those living moments of talk that we can find the patient, their 'world', and what it is like for them, trying in the face of their illness, to live in it" (Katz & Shotter, 1996, p. 921).

A scientifically competent multidisciplinary team alone cannot help a patient grapple with the loss of health or find meaning in suffering. Along with scientific ability, physicians have to develop the skill to listen to the narratives of the patient, grasp and honour their meanings. Families can help health practitioners to listen, grasp and honour the patients narratives so that practitioners can absorb, interpret, and respond to these stories (Charon, 2001b).

Flexible and Multiple Ways of Speaking Of Grief and Loss

This section of the chapter looks more closely at the spectrum of losses and grief as a result of a spinal cord injury, as well as how patients and families "do hope together" (Weingarten, 2000, p. 399) in the face of these losses. In the research study (Sliedrecht, 2007), participants were very explicit about the significance and variety of losses they experienced. They identified loss as part of the journey of living life with a spinal cord injury. Patients reported that they value more flexible ways of speaking about grief and loss and the importance of holding onto hope.

There are many available discourses about grief and loss. The more readily available medical and psychological accounts of grief centralise a linear or cyclical process – denial, anger, bargaining, depression, with acceptance as a successful result or desired destination (Kübler-Ross, 1970). This then becomes storied as a taken-for-granted "right way to grieve". Even although this is a dated discourse, the traces of this discourse still have significant ripple effects in current day discourse around grief and loss.

Discourses about denial and acceptance, that are the ripple effects of the abovementioned discourse, can position medical professionals to subscribe to ideas that information about a patient's prognosis should be shared as soon as possible (within one or two weeks of a patient being injured) and that it should be factual, clear (sometimes blunt) and to the point. This approach is informed by discourses of "the need to accept reality before you can move on".

Martin* was admitted to the Spinal Unit and informed Susan that one of the hardest things he has had to manage is what he called "the cruel and uncaring way in which the doctor informed me that I would not be able to walk again". Martin was admitted into a tertiary hospital for a planned medical procedure (unrelated to the spine) and had spinal anaesthesias with L3/L4 block. After the surgery, he noticed that there was reduced sensation in his right leg and he was unable to move his left leg. He had an MRI scan to establish the reason for this reduced sensation. Martin's preferences in how he wanted this information shared was not considered. Martin voiced the lack of agency he experienced when he received his prognosis:

The doctor [at the tertiary hospital] walked into my room, and whilst still standing, informed me that he had some bad news for me. He told me he was sorry but there had been a complication with the operation and that I would not be able to walk again. I had no family member present when the news was shared, it was just given straight. It just keeps going around and around in my head. I keep having bad dreams of that doctor walking into my room. At times I am even afraid to close my eyes because I can see his face.

On the question of how patients prefer the diagnosis and prognosis to be shared with them, a participant responded:

Well, I think you do not want to have your situation mirrored for you. I think you know well enough your situation. It is maintaining the delusion but I think that can be important. I think that people can

only come down on their own steam, they realise they can't do these things anymore. (Sliedrecht, 2007, p. 70)

Holding multiple versions as a possibility in the collaborative meaning-making process between the medical and the patient teams can provide practitioners with opportunities to be forthright, respectful and thorough, as well as empathic and humane. This is a territory where it is important to do reasonable hope together (Weingarten, 2009). Reasonable hope accommodates doubt, contradictions, despair and hope of a different outcome and can sit alongside the medical diagnosis and prognosis. For example, in the excerpts below, one research participant talks about medical diagnosis and hope for a different outcome coinciding very comfortably:

There is a part of me that hopes every day that something is going to click or snap in a good way and that I will have 100% back. But I have realistically been told on a number of occasions that pretty much after two years what you have got is what you have got. I am grateful that I am still walking and that I live in a two storey house and that is fantastic etc. etc. But there is a very strong part of me that is upset; not having 100%, I am not able to run and sprint and I do not have that much feeling in my hands.... (Sliedrecht, 2007, p. 67)

When the primary focus and emphasis in rehabilitation was on making sure that patients understood the full implications of the medical prognosis, patients experienced this often as cruel, negative and unhelpful (Sliedrecht, 2007). In an approach where the diagnosis and prognosis are privileged as a singular truth with no or little space for patients' knowledge, dreams and hope, a potential increase of loss can be experienced. Patients can interpret this as pressure to loosen or relinquish their relationships with their preferred hopes and dreams and to strengthen their relationship with the medical team's version of events.

Patients hold many versions of events such as versions of hope – hope that the medical prognosis is wrong and/or hope that medical science will come up with a cure. There is a "faith version"– "I will be healed". There is a "bodily experience version"– what a person notices about his/her own body and how it responds. There is a "medical version"– what the doctors say. There is a "personal belief version" about positive thinking – "as long as I try my hardest, my body will respond." All these different versions may operate together; they may compete at times; there may be a comfortable relationship between them at times; they may jostle for position, depending on what space is opened up for the patient. Holding contradictory and competing possibilities can deconstruct the notion that there is only one version of events and can pave the way to "do hope together" (Weingarten, 2000) or to do "reasonable hope together" (Weingarten, 2009). These possibilities open up when medical practitioners find ways to work alongside patients, respecting the multiplicity of their versions of events and not regarding the dominant medical discourse as the only version of the "truth".

Linked closely to ideas about hope is the discourse of acceptance as an important destination in rehabilitation to be reaching for. On a number of occasions patients have told Susan during counselling that they never really grieved "properly" for the losses brought on by spinal cord injury. Trying to understand this comment, Susan invited them to explain what meaning they make of "grieving properly". Ngaire* said: "Well, I never really got angry and so I do not think that I went through all the stages properly." Another patient said: "Lately, I have been crying a lot so I think I have not really accepted my injury."

Lequecher* suggested that striving for acceptance may not always be important. At the time of her injury, she was a single mother with young children. As a result of her injury she had very limited arm and hand functioning. This meant that she was unable to care physically for her children. She shared how she hates her caregivers, and at the same time, loves them. She hates them because her children run to them for hugs and cuddles, but she loves them because they care for her children. She said:

I know I must accept my injury but I can't accept my injury I was too much of a sporty person....I never had time to sit around and do nothing, that was not me, I was always on the go... going to play sports, taking my children with me, and the loss of my motherhood has had a very traumatic impact on me. (Sliedrecht, 2007, p. 57)

Ideas about acceptance as a desired destination for managing grief positioned Lequecher as reaching for a destination that for her was not possible (or preferable). These challenges about acceptance resonated with the work of the peer counsellors of the Irish Wheelchair Association and the National Council of the Blind of Ireland (Boyle et al., 2003), who mention how the concept of acceptance can be used to disqualify and categorise people with disabilities. They add that, as peer counsellors, they prefer to ask questions such as: What sort of life is it that you want to lead? What does acceptance mean to you? What parts (if any) of this notion of acceptance are useful to you? One of the writers of that article says, "personally accepting my disability is not something I'm interested in doing. Sure I need to adapt to my disability. But welcome it? Accept it? That's not for me" (Boyle et al., 2003, p. 15).

These questions about the place of acceptance open multiple possibilities health practitioners can invite patients to review when storying their (patients) relational preferences to spinal cord injury and/or the destinations they are reaching for.

Multiple and flexible ways of speaking grief and loss do not undermine the importance of patients' clearly understanding their diagnosis and prognosis from a medical perspective, but it can sit alongside other versions of events and for many patients that can include hope for a different outcome.

Sex, Intimacy and Spinal Cord Injury

Everything from here down was affected. [Paul* indicated just below his belly button] My bowels, my bladder, everything, it does not work the way it is supposed to. That is why I have to wear these silly bags, all piped up and everything. But sexually, no help, absolutely nothing, didn't even talk about it, nothing. And to a man that is very, very important. I do not know, I suppose it is to most men, you know. ...All I ever got for that part [sexuality counselling] was a little page about that size [A5 size] on the exercises you can do to keep your bladder working but hey, you are paralysed from there down, the muscles don't work, how are you supposed to do the exercises? ...it affects you a hell of a lot, I do not want to realise it but it does. Yes, well you see in like in our family, dad has been doing our family history and so far he has gone back eight hundred years. And the way I look at it, it has come to a screaming halt because some bastard sat in the middle of the road and caused my accident. [Paul swerved to avoid hitting someone, lost control of the vehicle, the car rolled and Paul sustained his spinal cord injury.] That is the end of our family tree, just because of some dickhead. Those are the little things [Paul's voice fades away, fighting back the tears]. (Sliedrecht, 2007, p. 84)

Paul's frustration ("they did not even talk about it") seems similar to that of some of the twelve participants with spinal cord injury that McAlonan (1996) interviewed to investigate patients' level of satisfaction with the sexual rehabilitation services they received. "Participants reported feelings ranging from frustration and disappointment to embarrassment and intimidation when encountering health care professionals who seemed to be either unwilling or unable to address sexuality.

Often participants perceived an evasive or avoidant quality during discussions with their physicians" (McAlonan, 1996, p. 830).

In a recent workshop for patients at the Spinal Unit, one panellist, who was injured as an adolescent, spoke about how she had longed for workshops or discussions about the physiological and psychological aspects of sex, intimacy and spinal cord injury. She felt it would have helped her to avoid some of the problems she faced. The purpose of rehabilitation is to assist spinal cord injured patients to live a quality life; and an important part of that quality life is being able to express sexuality the way they choose.

Studies on sexuality and spinal cord injury strongly support sexuality counselling as a standard part of rehabilitation, since sexual activity, sexual desires, body image and self-esteem are activities of daily living (Smith & Bodner, 1995, p.83). Sexuality should be treated like any other aspect of health care and not sectioned off and regarded as out of bounds for discussions. Many clinicians would agree that sex and intimacy should be an integral part of rehabilitation, but the question remains: how does one address a topic so complex, sensitive and culturally informed?

The team at the Spinal Unit found the P-LISS-IT model proposed by Annon (1976) useful. This model has four levels/stages that would be required for a comprehensive sexual rehabilitation service to be in place. According to the model, in a rehabilitation unit, every clinician (nurses, doctors, social workers, physiotherapists, peer support, psychologists) should at least be at the Permission Level (P). This 'permission level' involves acknowledging patients' sexuality concerns and a permitting environment where these concerns can be voiced. This requires a level of comfort in discussing sexuality with a patient or the patient's partner if they bring up the topic of sexuality, albeit in a disguised way (for example, in a passing comment or using humour) or directly. It also includes an ability to competently discuss with the patient and/or the patient's partner who in the multidisciplinary team would be able to talk about sex and intimacy and/or to make a referral to that health practitioner. There is no expectation at this permission level that a health practitioner initiates a detailed conversation about sexuality.

The next three levels – Limited Knowledge (Li), Specific Suggestions (SS) and Intensive Therapy (IT) – require more detailed and specialised knowledge. Ongoing application of this model at the Spinal Unit has shown that different disciplines hold specialist knowledge in different areas in relation to sex and intimacy. For example, physiotherapists may have specialist knowledge about positions and how to manage a spasm; peer counsellors may have specialist knowledge about what to do with a catheter bag when being intimate or some of the pitfalls, successes and fears of erectile-enhancing medication; doctors may have specialist knowledge about autonomic dysreflexia and the advisability of erectile-enhancing medications; counsellors or psychologists may have specialist knowledge about relationships and how to enhance sexual intimacy. Having satisfactory enjoyable sexual experiences possibly depends more on the discourses through which people make sense and make meaning of experiences rather than the actual physical abilities of their bodies.

Acknowledging that each person holds different knowledges reduces the pressure on individual clinicians to be positioned as knowledgeable about all aspects of sexuality. The clinical skill becomes carefully listening to what this particular person wants and needs and if it is not within the team member's area of expertise, connecting that person with the right person to help him or her.

In staff training, clinicians, who are expected to operate at the SS level (doctors, nurses and counsellors), are encouraged to find their own language to introduce the topic to patients – taking into account the age, gender and or culture of the patient, but not using these as a reason not to discuss sex and intimacy. For example, in New Zealand, culturally it is generally inappropriate for a female to discuss sexuality with a Pacific

Island male. Knowing this, it is still important that opportunities are given to Pacific Island men to discuss this topic. Finding words that can bring the topic up for consideration and not just ignoring it because it falls into the culturally 'too hard' basket is important. A man from the Pacific Islands was referred for counselling and during the session, Susan realised that no-one had discussed the effect of spinal cord injury on his sexual life and intimacy. Susan introduced the topic as follows:

I am mindful of the fact that culturally the topic of sex and intimacy is not appropriate for me, as a female, to bring up with you. However, I am also aware of the fact that sex and intimacy is a very important topic for many people and I am wondering if we could find a way to ensure that you have the opportunity, if you would like it, to discuss this topic with someone from the team but also in a way that is respectful of your culture.

By acknowledging the cross-cultural difference and possible constraints regarding cross-gender discussion of sexuality, pathways of conversation were opened. Privileging a culturally appropriate practice was positioned alongside an appropriate invitation to decide what support and information he might require. He was given options of team members to discuss this with. Given this kind of agency, he was very comfortable to discuss the topic with Susan and went on to have a very frank discussion with her. This above example demonstrates what was earlier referred to as relationship-centred care (Beach et al., 2006). It supports ideas of a weaving and a co-creation of knowledge. It demonstrates a practice of including "your knowing" and "my knowing" and it strives for an "our knowing" that transcends both.

Acquiring appropriate cultural knowledge and skill to initiate these pathways of conversation is the responsibility of the therapist. As one research participant said, "When they [medical staff] say nothing [about sex and intimacy] you think 'oh my gosh, all is lost'" (Sliedrecht, 2007, p. 82).

Addressing sex and intimacy should be an integral part of service delivery. It has also been highlighted that different disciplines, including people with a spinal cord injury, hold different but important knowledges about sex and intimacy. For example, counsellors may focus on the emotional aspect of sex and intimacy to the exclusion of more medical options such as medication, while medical doctors may address the topic in such a way that sex is medicalised, with the primary focus on medication and erectile functioning. All aspects of sexuality need to be included – physiological, cultural, psychological and ethical. Paul talked about his sadness that his family history of 800 years was coming to a "screaming halt". Accurate information about physiology and the possible changes that may occur because of illness or disability and accurate information about fertility are crucial – in Paul's situation no-one seems to have explained his options to father a child – the message Paul received was that he could not have children.

Finally, discussing sex and intimacy is important for spinal cord patients and their partners, be they of the same sex or not. Avril* said that couple counselling for her and her husband would have been useful because "it is a whole new world". At the time of Avril's injury, she was given a booklet about sexuality, but for her this was not adequate. As an outpatient she has now received more information on spinal injury and sexuality: "The doctor brought it up [sexuality] and I was quite comfortable. I thought oh cool, I was quite pleased that it was mentioned, and I did ask for more information on it."

SOLUTIONS AND RECOMMENDATIONS

Patients' voices about the counselling service they received provided the momentum to carefully reflect on current practices and make changes. They raised a number of aspects that they wanted re-shaped and this included collaborative relationships with all health professionals, a different structure and procedure to include families in the rehabilitation treatment plan, storying grief and loss differently and wanting to have opportunities to talk and learn about sex and intimacy in a way that is inviting discussion and questions.

The team attended to the above by changing the practice between the multidisciplinary team and the patient team to a collaborative partnership which produced the co-production of knowledge or as Paré (2002) mentioned, building "our house". Philosophies, ideas and practices from approaches such as the relationship-centred model, the cultural-broker model, the discursive wisdom model, the narrative medicine and biopsychosocial models resonated with what patients and their families informed the Spinal Unit team would contribute towards nourishing (Charon 2001a) and sustainable medical care. This helped to shape for example, how goal-setting meetings are structured, planned and conducted so that agency for the patient team is centralised. Staff attended workshops and training to pay attention to working more effectively and collaboratively with issues of sex and intimacy with spinal cord injured patients and their partners. The team adopted strategies to shape relationships so that collaborative meaning-making and doing reasonable hope together became possible.

FUTURE RESEARCH DIRECTIONS

Future research projects can include qualitative research with staff of the Spinal Unit to establish how they perceive the collaborative meaning making with the patient team and whether or not the skills and strategies being introduced brought career satisfaction for them as well as reasonable hope in their professional and personal lives.

Follow-up research with patient team can contribute to ongoing review and re-shaping of professional services provided at the unit.

CONCLUSION

In this chapter we have highlighted the importance of a relational practice that invites and allows for reciprocal caring solidarity of interconnection and interdependence. This practice supports the weaving of a knowing and or at times a not knowing between patient team and medical team that produces collaborative and mutual knowledge-making. This co-production of knowledge incorporates technically competent, empathic and respectful medical practice which is filtered by paying attention to the history, beliefs and ways of doing things for this particular and unique patient team.

ACKNOWLEDGMENT

We would like to thank the research participants for their willingness to be involved in this research and sharing their stories. Thank-you to Idette Noome for her help in editing this article and the New Zealand Spinal Trust for the financial contribution towards the editing.

REFERENCES

Annon, J. (1976). The P-LI-SS-IT model: a proposed conceptual scheme for the behavioural treatment of sexual problems. *Journal of Sex Education and Therapy*, *2*, 1–15.

Bakhtin, M. M. (1986). *Speech genres and other late essays* (Emerson, C., & Holquist, M., Trans.). Austin, TX: University of Texas Press. (Original work published 1979)

Beach, M., & Inui, T.Relationship-Centered Care Research Network. (2006). Relationship-centred Care. A constructive reframing. *Journal of General Internal Medicine*, *21*, s3–s8. doi:10.1111/j.1525-1497.2006.00302.x

Boyle, B., Clancy, A., Connolly, A., Daly, E., Hefferman, B., Howley, E., et al. (2003). The same in difference: The work of peer counsellors of the Irish Wheelchair Association and the National Council of the Blind in Ireland. *The International Journal of Narrative Therapy and Community Work* (2), 4-16.

Charon, R. (2001a). Narrative medicine. A model for empathy, reflection, profession and trust. *Journal of the American Medical Association*, *286*(15), 189–1902. doi:10.1001/jama.286.15.1897

Charon, R. (2001b). Narrative medicine: Form function and ethics. *Annals of Internal Medicine*, *134*(1), 83–87.

Charon, R. (2006). *Narrative Medicine: honouring the stories of illness*. New York: Oxford University Press.

Davies, B. (1991). The concept of agency. *Postmodern Critical Theorising*, *30*, 42–53.

Davies, B., Browne, J., Gannon, S., Hopkins, L., McCann, H., & Wihlborg, M. (2006). Constituting the feminist subject in poststructuralist discourse. *Feminism & Psychology*, *15*(1), 87–103. doi:10.1177/0959-353506060825

Denborough, D. (2005). A framework for receiving and documenting testimonies of trauma. *International Journal of Narrative Therapy and Community Work*, *2*(3 & 4), 34–42.

Drewery, W. (2005). Why we should watch what we say: Position calls, everyday speech and the production of relational subjectivity. *Theory & Psychology*, *15*(3), 305–324. doi:10.1177/0959354305053217

Elliot, T. R., Shewchuk, R. M., & Richards, J. S. (1999). Caregiver social problem-solving abilities and family member adjustment to recent onset physical disability. *Rehabilitation Psychology*, *44*(1), 104–123. doi:10.1037/0090-5550.44.1.104

Foucault, M. (1980). *Power/Knowledge: Selected interviews and other writings, 1972-1977.* Brighton: Harvester Press.

Frank, A. W. (1991). *At the will of the body. Reflections on illness.* Boston, MA: Houghton Mifflin.

Frank, A. W. (1995). *The wounded storyteller. Body, illness and ethics.* Chicago: University of Chicago Press.

Frank, A. W. (2001). Can we research suffering? *Qualitative Health Research, 11*(3), 353–362. doi:10.1177/104973201129119154

Frankel, R. M., & Quill, T. (2005). Integrating biopsychosocial and relationship-centered care into mainstream medical practice: A challenge that continues to produce positive results. *Families, Systems & Health, 23*(4), 413–421.. doi:10.1037/1091-7527.23.4.413

Frisch, B. (2006). *Quality of life therapy: Applying a life satisfaction approach to positive psychology and cognitive therapy.* Hoboken, NJ: John Wiley & Sons.

Katz, A., & Shotter, J. (1996). Hearing the patients "voice": Toward a social poetics in diagnostic interviews. *Social Science & Medicine, 43*(6), 919–931. doi:10.1016/0277-9536(95)00442-4

Kübler-Ross, E. (1970). *On death and dying.* New York: Touchstone.

May, L., Day, R., & Warren, S. (2006). Perceptions of patient education in spinal cord injury rehabilitation. *Disability and Rehabilitation, 28*(17), 1041–1049. doi:10.1080/09638280500494744

McAlonan, S. (1996). Improving sexual rehabilitation services: The patients' perspective. *The American Journal of Occupational Therapy., 50*(10), 826–834.

McDaniel, S., Campbell, T., Hepworth, J., & Lorenz, A. (2005). *Family-orientated primary care* (2nd ed.). New York: Springer.

McDaniel, S., Hepworth, J., & Doherty, W. (1992). *Medical family therapy.* New York: Basic Books.

Murray, M. (2009). A narrative approach to health psychology. Background and potential. *Journal of Health Psychology, 2*(1), 9–20. doi:10.1177/135910539700200102

Paré, D. A. (2002). Discursive wisdom: Reflections on ethics and therapeutic knowledge. *International Journal of Critical Psychology, 7*, 30–52.

Sevenhuijsen, S. (1998). *Citizenship and the ethics of care: Feminist consideration on justice, morality and politics.* New York: Routledge.

Sliedrecht, S. (2007). *Counselling patients with a spinal cord injury.* Unpublished master's thesis, University of Waikato, New Zealand.

Smith, E., & Bodner, D. (1993). Sexual dysfunction after spinal cord injury. *The Urologic Clinics of North America, 20*, 535–542.

Weingarten, K. (1995). Radical listening: Challenging cultural belief for and about mothers. In Weingarten, K. (Ed.), *Cultural resistance: Challenging belief about men, women and therapy.* New York: Haworth.

Weingarten, K. (2000). Witnessing, wonder and hope. *Family Process, 39*(4), 389–402. doi:10.1111/j.1545-5300.2000.39401.x

Weingarten, K. (2001). Making sense of illness narratives: Braiding theory, practice and the embodied life. In *Dulwich Centre Publication Working with stories of women's lives.* Adelaide, Australia: Dulwich Centre.

Weingarten, K. (2003). *Common shock, witnessing violence every day: How we are harmed, how we can heal.* New York: Dutton.

Weingarten, K. (2009, September). *Hope: In a time of global despair.* Keynote address presented at the New Zealand Association of Counsellors, Hamilton, New Zealand.

World Health Organisation (WHO). (2001). *International Classification of Functioning, Disability and Health (ICF)*. Geneva: Williams, G. C., Frankel, R. M., Campbell, T. L., & Deci, E. L. (2000). Research on relationship-centered care and healthcare outcomes from the Rochester biopsychosocial program: A self-determination theory integration. *Families, Systems & Health, 18*(1), 79–90.

Youngson, R. (2008). *Disabled doctoring – how can we rehabilitate the medical profession?* Paper presented at the Australian and New Zealand Spinal Cord Society Conference, Christchurch, New Zealand.

ADDITIONAL READING

Cheek, J. (2000). *Postmodern and poststructural approaches to nursing research*. London: Sage.

Compassion in Health. (n.d.). *Compassion in Health*. Retrieved from http://www.compassioninhealthcare.org/

Drewery, W., & Winslade, J. (1997). The theoretical story of narrative therapy. In Monk, G., Winslade, J., Crocket, K., & Epston, D. (Eds.), *Narrative therapy in practice: The archaeology of hope* (pp. 32–52). San Francisco: Jossey Bass.

Katz, J., & Capron, A. (2002). *The silent world of doctor and patient* (2nd ed.). Baltimore, MD: Johns Hopkins University Press.

Kroll, K., & Klein, E. (1995). *Enabling romance: A guide to love, sex and relationships for the disabled*. London: Woodbine House.

McDaniel, S., Hepworth, J., & Doherty, W. (1997). *The shared experience of illness: Stories of patients, families and their therapists*. New York: Basic Books.

Monk, G., & Gehart, D. (2003). Socio-political activist or conversational partner? Distinguishing the position of therapist in narrative and collaborative therapies. *Family Process, 42*(1), 19–29. doi:10.1111/j.1545-5300.2003.00019.x

Weingarten, K. (1999). The politics of illness narratives: Who tells, who listens and who cares in *Narrative Therapy and Community Work: A Conference Collection*. Adelaide: Dulwich Centre Publications, p.13-26.

Witnessing Project. (n.d.). *Witnessing Project*. Retrieved from http://www.witnessingproject.org/

KEY TERMS AND DEFINITIONS

Agency: Within any discourse there are a range of positions one can take up. If a person is able to select and or resist the position calls that are being offered she/he would then be agentically positioned within that discourse. Agency is the ability to, within discourses, make selections about how you want to be / act in the world.

Cultural Broker: Mediation of dialogue, without rank, from the patient's cultural world to the world of medicine and vice versa. This practice ensures that cultural and social practices are not marginalised and sense can be made of what this particular illness means for this particular person.

Discursive Wisdom: Discursive wisdom is knowledge that is generated /produced through the weaving of your knowledge and my knowledge to become our knowledge. This knowledge also includes a not knowing and a not yet known which can create conversational space for new constructions of meaning making.

Goal Setting Meeting: A fortnightly meeting between the multidisciplinary team and the patient team to discuss fortnightly goals, discuss progress and ensure that the whole team are all working in the same direction for a safe discharge.

Key Worker: A person from the multidisciplinary team who is assigned to a patient and is accountable for ensuring that the patient experiences a personalised and co-ordinated approach to their rehabilitation.

Patient Team: A group of people (family members and or friends) brought together for the common purpose of supporting the patient with his/her rehabilitation.

Relationship Centred Care: Relationship is centred as the context and vessel through which healthcare is offered. This brings to the forefront the meaning of health and illness to this person rather than only relating to the disease or illness.

ENDNOTE

[1] Patients' names and that of their family members have been altered throughout to protect their identity. All such changes have been marked with an asterisk upon first use of the pseudonym.

Chapter 27
Social Construction of Chronic Disease:
Narratives on the Experience of Chronic Illness

Chris Peterson
La Trobe University, Australia

Evan Willis
La Trobe University, Australia

ABSTRACT

In this study of narratives in relation to chronic illness, a number of themes relevant to patients were identified from the literature for discussion and analysis. Themes included responsibility and control of chronic illness, stigma and non-legitimation. Discussions and blogs on the Internet were identified and examined representing patient experiences of chronic illness. For some patients taking responsibility for their chronic illness conflicted with some of their important life roles. There were also questions about the degree to which people who already manage busy lives should also be managing their disease. It was found that some patients experience control over their illness and behaviour as a difficulty they faced with a chronic condition. This included being placed on a regimen and reviewed for compliance. Some referred to the experience as policing. Patients who reported some greater difficulties were those with illnesses which struggled to achieve legitimacy through medical means. Their illness experience and outcomes were largely dependent on seeking out sympathetic medical practitioners. Overall the authors conclude that notwithstanding the benefits of self management programs for patients, the uncertainty surrounding chronic illness creates problems for patients and reinforces the importance of having effective and trusting relationships with their health care providers. A typical biomedical perspective on illness tends to focus on disease and its causes without considering the social world within which health and illness occur, and the way in which social forces shape these concepts and experiences. Sociologists and some progressive medical practitioner researchers are concerned with social process and with the effect of factors such as gender relations, social class and the broader political economy on understanding the experience and prevalence of disease. The aim of this chapter is to present some narratives by patients, consumers, medical and health practitioners, and other stakeholders in blogs, discussions and forums

DOI: 10.4018/978-1-60960-097-6.ch027

on the Internet. This chapter looks at a number of aspects of chronic illness that have been identified in a range of studies, from aspects of responsibility of patients and control processes on chronic illness patients through to non-legitimate and resistance themes.

NARRATIVE ANALYSIS

Williams (2006) argues the way that people's beliefs about the causes of illness or disease can best be understood is by a process of narrative reconstruction. A number of authors have reviewed studies of illness and narrative (for example Hyden, 1997, Kleinman, 1988, Foster, 2008). According to Whitehead 'narrativising the chronic illness within the framework of one's own life history makes it possible to give meaning to events that have disrupted and have changed the course of one's life' (2006: 2236). Key factors to affect narrative reconstruction include the nature of diagnosis, any relapse and conflicts with providers of care (note Whitehead, 2006).

Whitehead argues that 'narrative theory is increasingly employed to understand the subjective experience of illness with growing recognition that narratives are the means by which we render our existence as meaningful' (2006:2237).

Previously the narrative approach was seen as an alternative to positivist approaches to understanding. Frank (1998) explored how stories were an opportunity for self expression and led to more power in wider relations. One example of using Frank's work in linking themes and types of narratives is Ezzy's (2000) study of people living with HIV. Most recently Kahan (2009) has used Frank's framework to investigate narratives of public dentistry patients in Australia.

Other studies to use narrative analysis include Fox and Ward's (2006) exploration of health identities originating in the sociopsychological contexts of modernity. They looked at health experts who took on biomedical explanations of health and illness and 'resistant consumers' who explored experiential models of health and the body.

Writers within the tradition of conflict theory such as Coburn (2004) and Navarro (2007) have ar-

gued that neoliberal interpretations of relationships in modern developed societies, underpin competing narrative about health and illness. Societies pursuing neoliberal policies they argue are creating larger divisions between the wealthy and the poor. Those disadvantaged by lack of income and power are more likely to develop counter explanations of phenomena including for their health and illness. We can see that some of these counter narratives are based on differences in power, influence and opportunity that are reflected in people's stories about their illnesses, as Blaxter (2004) found in her classic study of health. Consequently, based on Coburn (2004) and Navarro's (2007) analysis class difference and disadvantage for some is at the root of differing narratives.

At the core of most medical sociological explanation of chronic illness is a social constructivist epistemological base. Social constructivism became particularly prominent during the 1990s. Brown (1995) argues that while social construction is a commonly used term it has not been defined systematically and therefore has many meanings. In medical sociology he argues there are three versions of social constructivism. The first is concerned with social definitions of illness, and focuses on individual and group activities related to illness conditions. An important consideration often not considered strongly enough is that social structures play an important role in health and illness. The second was based on the work of Foucault and postmodernism and sets about to deconstruct language together with symbols to show knowledge creation, and explore the situation's "realities." (Brown, 1995). This includes some of the important work of Bryan Turner on the Sociology of the Body (2008), and its concerns with symbols. The third version focuses on the proposition that facts are based on mutual actions by scientists at work together with their efforts to promote their work. A number of studies have argued the social construction of chronic illness from various viewpoints (e.g. Charmaz, 1990, Anderson, 2006, and Ware, 1992).

The study reported in this chapter follows the first of these versions of social constructivism. It strongly supports that social structure affects illness experience and definition, and that social structure therefore shapes action. However it focuses on the narratives of people with conditions characterised by uncertainty. The study focuses on the way that patients are dependent on medical practitioners for naming their illnesses as well as managing them, in a context of uncertainty where doctors are often unsure of the passage and outcomes of managing these illnesses., Many patient responses to their illnesses are a result of these and other social processes.

METHOD

An unobtrusive research design was utilised involving the analysis of Internet blogs and discussions. These were selected mainly from patient sites such as 'Patient Like Me" and were selected for their appropriateness in adding a voice to the understanding of the experience of illness together with a social dimension. Permission to study and report the blogs and opinion pieces was not sought as they came from open access by the public sites. In looking at the way in which they inform a debate about social construction of chronic illness, they provide a 'lens' or way of looking at health and illness from this perspective

Most patient text came from correspondents on the 'Patient Like Me' blog site. These narratives were struggles by patients with illness, their problems in finding appropriate medical providers and also their stories of success in finding a cure. Most were quite recent and portrayed as stories that could help other patients. Most medical provider blogs came from sites which provided a critical perspective on the provision of health services,

and many of these focussed on the social dimension of health.

There are a number of themes important in analysing these excepts and stories. These include issues of responsibility, control or accountability, motivation, stigma and resistance or challenging non-legitimacy. These themes have been derived from the conceptual literature on chronic illness, patient and practitioner experiences. Focussed on for the analysis are dilemma's of patient responsibility (see Jallinoja et al, 2007), control (or accountability) (Broome and Whittaker, 2004), stigma (Scambler, 2004 and Charmaz, 1990) and resistance, or non-legitimacy (Whitehead, 2006)

Narratives are not only constructions, where the person from their social position has a particular gaze at phenomena. They also arise from a complex interaction between the body, self and society, perhaps best captured through the work of Foucault (1980) and Turner (2008). Power, domination and marginalisation form the basis of understanding counter narratives.

ISSUES DERIVED FROM PATIENT/ PRACTITIONER ACCOUNTS

Responsibility (or the Lack of)

Jallinoja et al. (2007) argue that in terms of patient responsibility, there are a number of drawbacks when dealing with a lifestyle-related condition. Doctors in their study reported that a major drawback was a change of habit on the part of patients.

One health practitioner's blog (see below) puts responsibility into the context of the broader life of patients, for example with Aboriginal diabetes. The relevance of a broader perspective goes beyond what many practitioners would normally assume for their patients.

The social context) broadens our understanding of diabetes in the way we might never aware of before. Surprisingly, this angle is not something totally new, but in fact, it's one of the basic considerations since the human civilization have been established. A human being is not an individually living creature, but rather a socially connected one and has to interact with others as well as with their environment to meet their need.

Many medical practitioners and researchers fail to take into account this basic general knowledge when they examine diabetes related factors. Merely, they used to think about a diabetic patient as an individual suffering from the disease; and all of the causes, prevention or interventions were seen on this individual basis. This medical perspective is not wrong; it's just not enough or considers only half of the picture.

This points to the) failure of the biomedical model and the success of the social perspective understanding of diabetes through the concept of sociological imaginations and the social model of health.

A social perspective looks at social determinants of illness, for example beliefs, gender, culture, and environment that might contribute to the pattern of disease (http://trias.blog.unair.ac.id/2008/06/04/sociological-shape-of-diabetes/)

In the following chaos narrative the patient who has a severe chronic condition expresses that she is going through an "emotional battering". The issue of responsibility in relation to her other roles emerges (a stay at home mother cannot reconcile her mothering and chronic illness role).

Jo the woman in the blog, reported that the health system did not account for conflicts between some of her life roles and her illness. She says

I'm sicker than them and what I do every day running a household and family is far harder and far more significant and I'm so tired of chronic illness and all the pressure it puts on my life and those around me. (http://lunalanding.blogspot.com/2009/12/sigh.html).

In the health care system, more emphasis has been placed on getting patients to take more responsibility for their care, and this has been evidenced through self management programs. Ryan (2009) argues what he calls an Integrated Theory of Health Behaviour Change approaches where change in health behaviour can be fostered by beliefs and knowledge of patients, and increasing skills and abilities in self regulation, such as with self-management. Self-management can affect long-term health outcomes and interventions focussed on the individual can increase self regulation. When self regulation increases there is more opportunity for patients to gain greater control over their disease management and treatment. The notion with chronic illness that there is nothing that the patient can do in relation to their illness is challenged by the self management approach. It is based on the premise that beyond management by a medical practitioner there are a lot of improvements that can be gained through the patient taking some control (Swerissen et al, 2006).

One patient post considered self management as delegation in order to understand its origins.

Who manages you? You may have a boss, who manages some percentage of your tasks at work. But who manages the entirety of your life? No one, if you don't. Are you willing to supervise yourself, to manage yourself? Are you willing to allow yourself to be so managed? (http://solinkable.com/Business/delegation-the-key-to-self-management/)

In terms of responsibility, as chronic illness is largely a management program involving the patient is important for both management and if there is to be recovery. Later in this chapter it is shown how control is important and in fact influences ideas of responsibility.

Control (or Accountability)

Brown (1995) refers to the social construction of medical knowledge, and ways of knowing based on the dominant biomedical paradigm. Here issues of patriarchal attitudes, professional advancement and needs of the labour market are important.

Broom and Whittaker (2004) focus on the extent to which 'control' is used in the management of diabetes. They found with people who have Type 1 diabetes that social relationships and identity have an associated language of surveillance and control, meaning that some are positioned as disobedient children or foolish adults. Given the stigma they experience, some find it undermining given they are dealing with a demanding regimen and a life threatening illness

In the management of diabetes, which is the seventh leading cause of death in Australia (Broom and Whittaker, 2004) there is an emphasis placed on control and responsibility of patients. Broome and Whittaker analysed patient's accounts of diabetes, focussing on discourses used, and of narratives looking at causes of diabetes and its management. 'They argue a number of studies note the importance of language in the management of the disruption of chronic illness and the integration of positive meanings into people's identities' (Broom and Whittaker, 2004: 2371). People use metaphor to integrate exceptional experiences into their identity. Broom and Whittaker maintain that 'diabetes often threatens to spoil or discredit the identity, and that people counter this threat in various ways through what they say and do… We suggest that the language we describe has a moral dimension as a form of "self making" (2004:2372).

Lisa in talking about disease management says

I'm too annoyed to make any intelligent comments.

"Disease management" means sending a nurse to your house to spy on you when you take a sick day. It means people hiding illness because they are terrified to lose their jobs or lose their insurance.

Employers think all they have to do is have a dumb seminar like "10 Foods to Keep You Healthy"

and that's it and if you get sick it's your fault because you didn't eat enough carrots!(http:// brassandivory.blogspot.com/2008/03/chronic-illness-and-patient.html)

Another patient blog, below, examines 'policing' the chronically ill body.

As societies increasingly come to expect their citizens to manage their own health and take responsibility for their own illnesses, the individual is required to 'police their body'. In the sociology of health, a sociology of the body has emerged as a rapidly expanding area following the impact of post-modernist theory.

Unless…sources of power are recognized post-modern ideas threaten to become little more than a gloss on the continuing trend of widening social inequalities (1998).(http://ivythesis.typepad.com/ term_paper_topics/2009/12/models-of-health-disease-and-illness-.html)

Stockl argues that 'the very act of gaining control over disorder (for biomedicine) generates more "epistemological disorder" instead of lessening it' (2007: 1550) meaning further problems for non-legitimated conditions and the people who suffer from them

Another patient reports on the use of narcotics and how it can be used as a form of control, albeit negated as not legitimate, with a condition such as fibromyalgia.

This is why they scoff at our assertions that our experiences are real. This is why our conditions are jokes to a great many people. This is why "fibromyalgia is bullshit" has been the leading search term to my blog.

This is why they seek so desperately to deny that these drugs — any drug — could be having a legitimate effect on us. This is why they treat us like addicts.

Because they can see how we might reasonably be having real pain, and they can see how these drugs might reasonably be legitimately relieving it (http://disabledfeminists.com/2009/10/23/depending-on-narcotics/).

There is an effect beyond control of treatment for some chronic conditions. The treatment itself may cause other conditions that lead to increasing the medical involvement for the patient. Epilepsy is a case in point. (see Smith et al. 1999).

Gunnarsson and Hyden (2009) focus on child allergies and on how illness experiences are constructed by their parents in the everyday moral context. These authors reconstructed parents' narratives, examining what they experienced before they sought professional help for their children. It looked at how they saw themselves as responsible parents. The children's allergic reactions meant there was a diagnosis given quickly, whereas for more diffuse problems and these went through a process before being constructed as illness symptoms. They argue that when parents' actions do not work in the case of their children's health, that parents look for medical aid, but the moral context of their accountability is also an important consideration.

Stigma

Stigma, a social experience can provide important barriers in the experience of some chronic conditions (e.g. epilepsy) that affect its treatment and are formative in patient experiences. Walker and Millen (2003) argue that 'largely, the foundation of stigma in chronic illness lies in its incurability' (2003, 84). Many patients experience rejection and challenge to some of their social roles through the stigma of having certain chronic conditions, and this can hinder the way they live with their disease. Further, Walker and Millen maintains that 'illness influenced by stigma and the metaphors associated with it are embedded in the wider social frameworks and cultural structures' (2003: 84).

Scambler (2004) whose work focuses on stigma and epilepsy proposes a reframing of the concept of stigma to be more appropriate for a changing world. He argues that little has developed since Goffman's (1968) concept of stigma, and that this aspect needs more work. He maintains that symbolic interactionist theories on deviance and on stigma pay little attention to social structure and the use of power. Scambler refers to a "hidden distress" model that relates to epilepsy. By argues that the effect of biographies of people diagnosed with epilepsy that informed it clearly and has gained most attention. People diagnosed with epilepsy developed new ways of interpreting the world which was associated with their new, "unwelcome" self identification. There were two referents, the first being shame at having the condition, and the second 'fear of encountering enacted stigma' (these are episodes of stigma enacted). (Scambler 2004:33).

Werner et al. (2004) investigated the concepts of shame and self in women with chronic pain, and how closely these accounted were related to ideas of gender and disease in cultural discourses. The authors used a feminist perspective to examine the idea of 'plots', that is attempts to deal with both psychological and alternative discussions of pain causing factors. They report the narratives as performance, with their stories as means of dealing with scepticism that their explanations have been met with. Also as arguments, their stories try to be convincing about the reality of the pain experience. In all, the women's experiences appear organised through medical discourses about disease and gender.

Non-Legitimacy (or Resistance)

One of the fundamental aspects of chronicity is that it doesn't fit in with the 'normal' process of having an illness, that is a 'legitimate' illness. In Talcott Parsons' initial work the 'sick role' (1951) is designed for acute condition where patients become well again and assume their normal social roles and function. However, in this context, chronic illnesses represent 'illegitimate' conditions and do not lead to patients assuming normal social roles. In fact it can lead to their stigmatization due to their inability to be 'cured' and assume normal social roles. Many in the medical profession and in the community look for 'legitimacy' in illness and getting well behaviour: that is there are pre-scribed ways that sick people should behave and in many cases those with chronic illnesses do not behave that way.

Whitehead (2006) identifies chronic fatigue syndrome as a condition which is difficult to diagnose illnesses. She maintains that 'by un-covering a means to interpreting the illness, we become better able to re-establish the relationship between the self, the world and our bodies' and following Arthur Frank, 'narrativised reconstruc-tion is concerned with gaining meaning and import to the illness by placing it within the context of one's own life and reconstructing the narrative of the self' (2006: 2236).

Group stories have been a common form of narrative with chronic fatigue syndrome (White-head, 2006), and this was regarded as therapeutic. In the many stories discussed (see Millen and Peterson, 1998), the common theme was CFS as a disease with identifiable symptoms, and coun-tering claims of malingering. Whitehead argues the 'importance of moving beyond a face value analysis of narratives to explore the meanings as constructed by individuals and groups within them which are "more complex and situated discursive productions" that they may be given credit for (2006:2237).

In a case of a patient with chronic fatigue syndrome, the search for an appropriate diagnosis and doctor to treat the condition led one patient to despair. A male patient from the US explains.

At the worst stage of my (CFS) illness, which was about a year ago, I suffered beyond what most humans can comprehend. I was completely bedrid-den and unable to lean up more than a few inches.

I had spent 10 years searching for help from doctors. I would hear, oh it's JUST allergies, it's JUST chronic Epstein Barr, it's JUST depression, oh it's JUST chronic fatigue syndrome and there is nothing we can do...

(Michael Dessin's blog (http://digdeep1.word-press.com/2010/01/09/michael-dessins-cfsac-testimony-about-cfs-me/)

Conditions such as chronic fatigue syndrome and fibromyalgia have a certain ambiguity about their status as a chronic illness. That is, the have been struggling to gain a status of a legitimate illness (see Peterson et al, 1999). Narratives about these illnesses are couched in a language which acknowledges a high wall of scepticism in the medical community and further disempowered patients.

Tucker (2004) examined how knowledge of chronic fatigue syndrome is constructed as rhetoric by four people who suffer the condition. A discursive psychological approach was used to identify how sufferers represent accountability and blame, and their stake in narratives. The themes all were used to identify chronic fatigue syndrome as a legitimate illness with an organic base. As a consequence those suffering the condition saw themselves as legitimately ill, and consequently avoid stigma and threats to the identity when viewed as a psychological condition.

Sim and Madden (2008) discuss fibromy-algia as a condition recognised at first as a set of distinct symptoms in the 1970s. They argue that many people who have been diagnosed with fibromyalgia identify experienced symptoms within a biomedical perspective where its diag-nosis is based on biomedical testing. However, the subjective experience of patients and the felt legitimacy is shown through narratives which are important to the experience of fibromyalgia. They argue that patients are seen through a particular language to struggle to deal with the condition.

This language includes terms such as "adapting" "despair", "struggling" and "giving up".

A 36 year old patient explained what it was like to have had a debilitating condition over a long period of time,

(I) have dealt with chronic pain since I was 16, possibly fibromyalgia that far back, but after a car accident things got much worse. My FMRS is pretty high right now, and I know that it is better at times and worse at times. (http://www. patientslikeme.com/patients/view/35787)

Another patient describes their response to treatment for fibromyalgia.

My pain was significantly under control with the Lyrica/Flexeril/Requip/Klonopin mix that they have me on. And, when I didn't have the Requip or Lyrica it jumped back up to 9 on that scale.

(http://www.patientslikeme.com/fibromyalgia-and-chronic-fatigue-syndrome/community).

One patient responded to a doctor's analysis of CFS as needing to focus on mental health.

Hasn't it occurred to you that many 'militant' ME patients are complaining (albeit in a very different way) about exactly the same thing as you are?

Namely, the issue of CFS being so loosely classified as to become a catch all, dustbin diagnosis containing a hotch botch mix of people with various illnesses; some entirely mental, some entirely physical and some a combination of both.

As others have said, I have good reason to believe the illness is deliberately being defined in a very vague manner due to the influence of certain vested interest groups. (http://nhsblogdoc.blogspot. com/2009/10/myalgic-encephalomyelitis-me-science.html)

Another condition which has been difficult to legitimate in terms of the biomedical model in assessing symptoms is lupis. Stockl (2007) argues that the complex issues surrounding lupis is part of the epistemological changes that biomedicine is undergoing. She argues that lupis is one of a number of complex conditions which biomedicine finds difficult to accept and deal with, and that this has important implications for the lives of people with these conditions. This also has an effect, argues Stockl (2007), on the doctor and patient relationship..

Stockl presents her informants from her study as being even more uncertain about their condition after medical encounters. She identifies that uncertain diagnosis has an important effect on patients. Further that as they wait for a diagnosis, patients resist a psychological explanation of their symptoms. Finally she says 'informants either integrated the medical model into their reasoning about their disorder or they felt frustrated and let down…The complexity of SLE (lupis) which influenced medical practice and the way information was communicated, shaped the relationship between medical authority and patients' (2007: 1551). In this sense there are many models, such as medical, therapeutic and even alternative models which could provide some forms of legitimation.

DIAGNOSIS AND TREATMENT: IMPORTANCE OF THE MEDICAL PRACTITIONERS IN PATIENTS' EXPERIENCES OF NON-LEGITIMATED ILLNESSES

For patients suffering chronic conditions helpful and sympathetic medical practitioners are important in improving the experiences of patients and diagnoses are also key factors in the healing process (see Millen and Peterson, 1998). Key elements in chronic conditions are diagnosis and management, and an 'enlightened' approach needs to be taken by practitioners and patients, in focusing on ways of improving the 'lived' experience for those who have chronic illnesses

The medical community has quite a degree of knowledge about some conditions striving to achieve medical legitimacy. One of the issues which lead to some stigma faced by people with conditions such as chronic fatigue is that there has been a strong push to replace symptoms of the condition with a psychological/psychiatric diagnosis, whereby if the diagnosis is applied their symptoms are largely discounted. Many people with these types of illnesses voice strong concerns and frustrations about this.

A young woman explains difficulties in getting a suitable diagnosis.

Currently I have been diagnosed with Chronic Epstien Barr Virus (Oct 2005) and Chronic Fatigue Syndrome (Feb 2007) and confirmed diagnosis of Fibromyalgia (Sept 2007). Blood work has ruled out Rheumatoid Arthritis and I have a low positive ANA, but they ruled out Lupus. At this point, they have ruled out MS.

In May 2007 I started to shake down the left side of my body. Then in November 2007 I had a seizure. The first and only Grand Mal seizure. Don't want another one. I was then diagnosed with Periodic Limb Movement Disorder.

My motto has always been, I can't fight it if I don't know what it is. It has taken a long time to get these issues diagnosed. (http://www.patientslikeme. com/patients/view/8783?page=9)

Some patients explain how important it was to work with their practitioner until they get a diagnosis. That opens the option for appropriate treatment and the label helps in explaining to friends and others what her illness is.

I didn't know what was going on. Every time I was sick, I went to my doctor and whined about my symptoms. I must have gone through so many

tests, including tests for Hyperthyroid (I was losing weight fast in the beginning, my heart was beating fast, or it felt like it was), liver disease, ulcers, migraine, etc...you name it, I got tested for it.

Fortunately, i had none of those. But my symptoms were so frequent and not knowing what it was frustrated me so much that i had wished I was finally diagnosed with something.

But no. Finally, my doctor suggested that i may have something called "Fibromyalgia." I had never heard of it back then

(http://www.patientslikeme.com/patients/ view/33709)

A young patient reported the introduction of some of the issues in being diagnosed with fibromyalgia.

At some point along the line, can't remember exactly when to be honest but I think it was 2004 or 2005, I got diagnosed with fibromyalgia which made a lot of sense since there had been certain symptoms I'd been experiencing since I was a child.

But I still feel like fibromyalgia is NOT the full story, not for me. I've undergone full psychiatric testing so thankfully at least I never get told "it's all in your head" anymore.

This problem is too complex, it's confused too many doctors, and it's tormented me far too much for me to just "suck it up" and accept being in pain the rest of my life (and for whatever reason my symptoms seem to be progressive, another thing that can't seem to be explained) without having any real reason why. (http://www.patientslikeme. com/patients/view/73929?page=1)

Another patient confirmed how important it was to have a sympathetic practitioner in order to commence a recovery regimen. Without such support it appears that other people start to doubt the patient and recovery can be marred by episodes of stigma.

Jamie (the patient's son) and I went to see one of the world's top specialists in CFS, especially pediatric CFS, in December 2003. During our visit, he officially diagnosed Jamie with CFS and confirmed my diagnosis (I'm lucky enough to have a family doctor who recognizes and understands CFS). (Sue Johnston http://livewithcfs.blogspot.com/2010/02/orthostatic-intolerance-and-cfs.html).

The fact that this woman referred to an "official" diagnosis, to a label being "officially " applied, shows the extent to which some patients and their carers are dependent on medical practitioners for effective outcomes with their illnesses.

A young woman with epilepsy discusses the use of medication and the rest of life.

The disease in itself isn't what really effects my day to day activities; however it's more the side effects from the medication to treat my epilepsy.

Everyday I'm bound with multiple side effects such as, fatigue, headaches, depression, anxiety, aches and pains, nausea, the list could go on. Some days I wake up fine, others not so fine. I have my good days and bad days.

(http://blog.patientslikeme.com)/

A patient with fibromyalgia commented.

I was diagnosed with Fibromyalgia in 2002. Currently, I have a full-time job in the media industry as a finance executive, and I train for triathlons and other endurance sports on the side.

This is a huge contrast to where I was 3-5 years ago, when I was barely making it to work and

when I was not at work I was bed-ridden and depressed most of the time. How did this change come about? Exercise, healthy eating, healthy thinking and sleeping well. http://www.patients-likeme.com/patients/view/33709).

A patient who has HIV commented on the difficulty specifically in relation to medications, life and death.

I was diagnosed HIV poz in 1996, the symptoms, night sweats, swollen glands. low fevers. started a year prior to being diagnosed. I was put on the meds early because It was thought "Hit Hard And Hit Early" would help retain some immunity for the body to fight HIV.

I was off the meds (on a De-tox program) for 7 months. My body is still fighting once again, low fevers, swollen glands. Now doctors think The "Hurry Up and Wait" Theory (wait until you have AIDS) is better, because of early drug resistance. I think it should be up to the individual when they want to start HIV meds

I just wonder now, how many people have lost their lives, that had immune response like me, because their doctors refused them medication until there T-cells fell into the quote (MED-LINE) rendering them into fever like complacations to their death.

Then of course, the public is then addressed, they just died from complications of AIDS. This is why the (hit hard and hit early) should be used when fevers persist in patients, the chances of early mutations are very slim.

(http://www.patientslikeme.com/patients/view/26215?page=3).

This patient reports the effects of being on HIV medications (and the use of 'hit hard and hit early') and how this contributes to the experience of death from the condition.

PERSPECTIVE OF CHRONIC ILLNESS PATIENTS AND KNOWLEDGE OF DISEASES

Chronic illnesses can be experienced as marked suffering, and this characterises many of these conditions. They often are not cured, but are experienced by patients over a period of time, often getting worse. The term management is more often used in relation to the chronic illness, however, the label of chronic can be seen to be arbitrary and can change in definition over time. Some patients, for example have recovered from chronic illnesses and some progress from acute to chronic. Medical practitioners have a role in the time dimension associated with chronic conditions

A greater understanding of the social context of chronic illness may lead to better management of these conditions (see Patterson, 2001, and Ware and Kleinman, 1992). A practitioner reported that,

Proper understanding of health seeking behaviour could reduce delay to diagnosis, improve treatment compliance and improve health promotion strategies in a variety of contexts' (Dr Nihar Ranjan Ray http://christinepepelyan.com/?p=3).

Patterson et al. (2006) reported on a study where chronic disease, interpreted from a social constructivist perspective, viewed Hep C as both a biomedical entity and a social construction. The authors suggest that while Hep C is constructed as a chronic illness, the care is often based on acute models that acknowledge chronicity in terms of a persistent virus. A model of Hep C care is needed that incorporates the stages of chronic illness experience

Lifestyle and lifestyle changes are aspects of a social construction perspective that also need to be incorporated into the discussion. Tuomilehto et al. (2001) found that lifestyle was an important predictor of the onset of diabetes type 2, and that increased sedentary lifestyle (including changes in diet) led to the increase in that condition.

The role of and conception of the body are important considerations with chronic conditions (Turner, 1997 and Williams 2006). A health practitioner blog looked beyond chronicity to disability to emphasis the conception of the body and medical conditions.

"Disability"(is) ... a way of thinking about bodies rather than as something that is wrong with bodies. Within such a critical frame, disability becomes a representational system more than a medical problem, a social construction rather than a personal misfortune or a bodily flaw, and a subject appropriate for wide-ranging intellectual inquiry instead of a specialized field within medicine, rehabilitation, or social work.

Such a critical perspective extends the constructivist analysis that informs gender and race studies.

This approach to disability looks at such issues as changes in the way disability is interpreted over time and within varying cultural contexts; the development of the disabled as a community and a social identity; the political and material circumstances resulting from this system of assigning value to bodies; the history of how disability influences and is influenced by the distribution of resources, power, and status

(S. Kinsiste, 2009 http://www.planet-of-the-blind. com/2009/10/why-no-one-is-normal-anymore. html).

REFLECTIONS ON CHRONIC ILLNESS

There are a number of issues or themes that have emerged from our work with chronic illness. The theme of uncertainty needs to be considered more in reflecting on the lives and experiences of people with chronic conditions. This uncertainty stems from doctors being unsure of the causes of many chronic illnesses and the most effective way of treating them. In many cases, medical knowledge is incomplete and people find themselves being medically "managed" but with an unclear view of the future.

Different doctors try different approaches to preventing and managing chronic diseases. Nonetheless it may not take away the uncertainty of the future. Patients vary in the extent to which they want to be involved in the process of managing their illness. Some are relatively passively compliant with medical regimens, while others engage in self management and "fight" the condition. For some time now patients have been urged to engage in self management of chronic conditions. In many cases patients engage in "doctor shopping" and try different types of practitioners including complimentary medicine practitioners and alternative therapists, often with a view to reduce uncertainty. Many patients try with some chronic conditions to legitimate the illnesses, and find they need a sympathetic or understanding doctor to help them in this process.

CONCLUSION

Chronic illness patients can have a more difficult illness passage than those with acute illness, as there may be little or no expectation of being cured. Consequently the ill person will not act in a socially sanctioned way to recover as quickly as they can. More emphasis is placed on management of the chronic condition and this requires a working relationship with a medical practitioner.

One of the aspects of having a chronic illness, and being involved in its management is dealing with the various forms of control implied. Firstly, medical practitioners will oversee various controls (e.g. good blood sugar levels for diabetes). there are also other forms of control enforced over exercise, diet and other lifestyle factors. One patient refers to 'policing'. In more recent times there has been a shift to reduce the workload from health practitioners and engage patients in self management activities. This is alleviating the patient but still enforcing controls, which will continue as many patients are not expected to be cured. A number of patient and practitioner blogs and forum comments expressed frustration at the forms of control.

Some chronic conditions have struggled for decades to gain legitimacy from the medical profession, that is to have a set of symptoms assigned and diagnosed biomedically. Patients with these types of conditions are more reliant on sympathetic practitioners. In these cases, as reported by some patients, having a medical diagnosis is a key to successfully managing the condition, and in case such as patients with chronic fatigue syndrome and fibromyalgia, of becoming well again. Particularly important to the healing and wellness process is a constructive relationship between patient and practitioners.

Social processes are important in understanding illness and the experience of patients, in this case for those with chronic conditions. Both patient and practitioner narratives emphasised the importance of the social dimension, for the patient in understanding their suffering and illness experience, and for the practitioner in interpreting chronic illness in the context of an array of social factors impinging on the illness process.

REFERENCES

Anderson, J. M. (2006). Immigrant women speak of chronic illness: the social construction of the devalued self. *Journal of Advanced Nursing*, *16*(6), 710–717. doi:10.1111/j.1365-2648.1991.tb01729.x

Blaxter, M. (2004). *Health Cambridge*. London: Polity.

Broom, D., & Whittaker, A. (2004). Controlling diabetes, controlling diabetics: Moral language in the management of diabetes type 2. *Social Science & Medicine, 58,* 2371–2382. doi:10.1016/j.socscimed.2003.09.002

Brown, J. (1995). Naming and framing: The social construction of diagnosis and illness. [CHECK.]. *Journal of Health and Social Behavior,* (Extra Issue), 34–52. doi:10.2307/2626956

Charmaz, K. (1990). Discovering chronic illness: Using grounded theory Social. *Science & Medicine, 30*(11), 1161–1172. doi:10.1016/0277-9536(90)90256-R

Coburn, D. (2004). Beyond the income inequality hypothesis: Class, neoliberalism and health inequalities. *Social Science & Medicine, 58,* 41–56. doi:10.1016/S0277-9536(03)00159-X

Ezzy, D. (2000). Illness narratives. Time hope and HIV. *Social Science & Medicine, 50,* 605–617. doi:10.1016/S0277-9536(99)00306-8

Foster, S. J. (2008). *Crystallising meaning: attitudes of listening to illness narratives* (Ph D Thesis), University of Melbourne, Melbourne, Australia

Foucault, M. (1980) Power/knowledge. In C. Gordon, Trans L. Marshall, J. Merpham and K. (eds), *Soper Selected interviews and other writings 1972-1977.* New York, Pantheon.

Fox, N., & Ward, K. (2006). Health identities: From expert patient to resisting consumer. *Health, 10*(4), 461–479.

Frank, A. (1998). Stories of illness as care of the self: A Foucauldian dialogue. *Health, 2,* 329–348.

Goffman, E. (1968). *Stigma: The Management of Spoiled Identity Harmondsworth.* New York: Penguin.

Gunnarsson, N., & Hyden, L.-C. (2009). Organising allergy and being a "good" parent" Parents' narratives about their children's emerging problems. *Health, 13*(2), 157–174.

Hyden, L. C. (1997). Illness and narrative. *Sociology of Health & Illness, 19*(3), 48–69.

Jallinoja, P., Absetz, P., Kuronen, R., Nissinen, A., Talja, M., Uutela, A., & Patja, K. (2007). The dilemma of patient responsibility for lifestyle change: Perceptions amongst primary care physicians and nurses. *Scandinavian Journal of Primary Health Care, 25*(4), 244–249. doi:10.1080/02813430701691778

Kahan, E. (2009). *Instrumental, detrimental and transcendental: experiences of dental emergency and micro-rationing practices in a Victorian public dental clinic.* (Submitted PhD thesis), La Trobe University, Dec.

Kleinman, A. (1988). *The illness narratives. Suffering, healing and the human condition New York.* Basic Books.

Martin, C., & Peterson, C. (2009). The social construction of chronicity – a key to understanding chronic care transformations. *Journal of Evaluation in Clinical Practice, 15*(3), 578–585. doi:10.1111/j.1365-2753.2008.01025.x

Millen, N., & Peterson, C. (1998). Chronic fatigue syndrome, legitimation and family support. *The International Journal of Sociology and Social Policy, 18*(2), 127–147. doi:10.1108/01443339810788470

Navarro, V. (2007). *Neoliberalism, Globalisation and Inequalities: Consequences for Health and Quality of Life.* Amityville, Baywood.

Parsons, T. (1951). *The Social System.* London: Routledge, Keegan and Paul.

Patterson, B., Butt, L., Mc, G., Guiness, L., & Moffatt, B. (2006). The Construction of Hepatitis C as a Chronic Illness. *Clinical Nursing Research, 15*(3), 209–224. doi:10.1177/1054773806288569

Patterson, B. L. (2001). The shifting perspectives model of chronic illness. *Journal of Nursing Scholarship, 33*(1), 21–26. doi:10.1111/j.1547-5069.2001.00021.x

Peterson, C., Millen, N., & Woodward, R. (1999). Chronic fatigue syndrome: A problem of legitimation. *Australian Journal of Primary Care – Interchange, 5*(2): 65-79.

Ryan, P. (2009). Integrated theory of health behaviour change. *Clinical Nurse Specialist CNS, 23*(3), 161–170. doi:10.1097/NUR.0b013e3181a42373

Scambler, G. (2004). Re-framing stigma: Felt and enacted stigma and challenges to the sociology of chronic and disabling conditions. *Social Theory & Health, 2,* 29–46. doi:10.1057/palgrave.sth.8700012

Sim, J., & Madden, S. (2008). Illness experience in fibromyalgia syndrome: A metasynthesis of qualitative studies. *Social Science & Medicine, 67,* 57–67. doi:10.1016/j.socscimed.2008.03.003

Smith, D., Defalla, B. A., & Chadwick, D. W. (1999). The misdiagnosis of epilepsy and the management of refractory epilepsy in a specialist clinic. *QJMed: An International Journal of Medicine, 92,* 15-23.

Stockl, A. (2007). Complex syndromes, ambivalent diagnosis, and existential uncertainty: The case of Systemic Lupus Erythematosus (SLE). *Social Science & Medicine, 65,* 1549–1550. doi:10.1016/j.socscimed.2007.05.016

Swerrisen, H., Weeks, A., Belfrage, J., Furler, J., Walker, C., & McAvoy, B. (2006). A randomized control trial of a self-management program for people with a chronic illness from Vietnamese, Chinese, Italian and Greek backgrounds. *Patient Education and Counseling, 64*(1-3), 360–368. doi:10.1016/j.pec.2006.04.003

Tucker, I, M. (2004). "Stories" of chronic fatigue syndrome: An exploratory discursive psychological analysis. *Qualitative Research in Psychology, 1,* 153–167. doi:10.1191/1478088704qp008oa

Tuomilehto, J., Lindstrom, J., Eriksson, J. G, & Valle, T, T, Hamalainen, H., Ilanne-Parikka, P., Keinanen-Kiukaanniemi, S., Laakso, M., Louheranta, A., Rastas, M. Salminen, V., Aunola, S., Cepaitis, Z., Moltchanov, V., Hakumaki, M., Mannelin, M., Martikkala, V., Sundvall, J., & Uusitupa, M. (2001). Prevention of type 2 diabetes mellitus by changes in lifestyle among subjects with impaired glucose tolerance. *The New England Journal of Medicine, 344*(18), 1343–1350. doi:10.1056/NEJM200105033441801

Turner, B. S. (1997). Foreword: From governmentality to risk: Some reflections on Foucault's contribution to medical sociology. In Peterson, A., & Bunton, R. (Eds.), *Foucault and Health.* London: Routledge.

Turner, B. S. (2008). *The Body and Society: Explorations in Social Theory* (3rd ed.). UK: Sage.

Walker, C., & Millen, N. (2003). Stigma as social process: The role of stigma in chronic illness in C. Walker, C. Peterson, N. Millen and C. Martin (eds), *Chronic Illness: New Perspectives and New Directions,* Croydon, Tertiary Press, 82-93.

Ware, N. C. (1992). Suffering and the Social Construction of Illness: The Delegitimation of Illness Experience in Chronic Fatigue Syndrome. *Medical Anthropology Quarterly, 6*(4), 347–361. doi:10.1525/maq.1992.6.4.02a00030

Ware, N. C., & Kleinman, A. (1992). Culture and somatic experience: the social course of illness in neurasthenia and chronic fatigue syndrome. *Psychosomatic Medicine, 54*(5), 546–560.

Werner, A., Isaksen, L. W., & Malterud, K. (2004). I am not the kind of woman who complains of everything': Illness stories on self and shame in women with chronic pain. *Social Science & Medicine*, *59*, 1035–1045. doi:10.1016/j.soc-scimed.2003.12.001

Whitehead, L. C. (2006). Quest, status and restitution: Living with chronic fatigue syndrome/ myalgic encephalomyelitis. *Social Science & Medicine*, *62*, 2236–2245. doi:10.1016/j.soc-scimed.2005.09.008

Williams, S. J. (2006). Medical sociology and the biological body: Where are we now and where do we go from here? *Health (London) 10*(5).

KEY TERMS AND DEFINITIONS

Chronic Illness: A medical condition expected to continue, rather than being cured.

Responsibility: Patient's taking actions to manage their chronic conditions

Control: Patients being under pressure to have their chronic condition monitored closely

Stigma: A negative experience representing low self esteem as a result of having some chronic illnesses (e.g. epilepsy).

Legitimate Illness: A condition accepted for diagnosis and treatment by biomedical approaches

Fibromyalgia: A painful condition that causes severe aches and pains.

Chronic Fatigue Syndrome: A debilitating condition that leads to muscle and joint soreness and extreme fatigue

Social Processes: The social context within which an illness is diagnosed, managed and/or treated.

Chapter 28
Dimensions of the Patient Journey:
Charting and Sharing the Patient Journey With Long Term User–Driven Support Systems

Kresten Bjerg
University of Copenhagen, Denmark

ABSTRACT

The ways a person's illnesses and afflictions are socially constructed and culturally conceived amongst relatives and friends as biographically contextualized in the narratives of a known life-journey are contrasted with modern conceptions of "Patient Journey" in the digitizing of medical care in hospitals and in computerized GP Consultations. In this chapter most relevant dimensions of a personal life-journey support system – across health, handicaps and illness - are outlined. The chapter demonstrates a new road to facilitate private logging of phenomena, a coherent and sedimenting self-narrative not only in text, picture and sound, but also through user-network-developed pictographic fonts. Inclusion of biotelemetric data and virtual body imaging as part of such support systems are considered. And questions are raised concerning the future of thus skilled chronic patients' interfacing most trusted helpers, fellow-sufferers and wider shared social platforms of Patient Journey Records.

INTRODUCTION

Public and private expenses for healthcare are surging. As medical advances are made, unhealthy lifestyles are spreading in the industrialized world and people are living longer. We get more and more chronic patients. Public prophylactic measures and health-educational efforts to increase health-awareness and self-care create numerous private

DOI: 10.4018/978-1-60960-097-6.ch028

profitable health-enterprises. With the spread of Internet access, many offers of such services and drugs, programs and technological gadgets are advertised. The transition to digital records, and networking in professional health-related social networks, brings the medical rationalizing and formalization of descriptions to its force, with many advantages.

The only problem is that while tremendous efforts and results are obtained to digitize and train the medical establishment, exemplified in the Hospital and GP settings, the chronic patients are left at their own to learn how to handle a computer, establish e-mail contact, and to hook up to whatever the digitized medical society has to offer - options, threats and promises - concerning their management of their own health.

Therefore the digitizing of citizen health situations has to be re-examined in the light of what is for now the receiving line of citizens, presently having to cope with their own information across all dimensions of their life-space and eventual patient journey, without adequate tools. This involves life-style, economy, employment, family and home life conditions, relative medical compliance, and the "story" and "role" assumed in family, neighborhood and workplace.

To repair this gap, and truly qualify patients to join and contribute to utilizing collaborative social networks and technologies, we must strive to qualify citizens as administrators of their own health, each developing their personal knowledge management skills, to become "life-long e-learners" (Pettenati 2008). It is proposed that personal healthcare and health-related interfaces of the future shall be considered in the full contexts of the citizens' general interfacing themselves through their everyday use of a personal notebook computer from 1st grade in school to final palliative care. We will gain by broadly conceiving of the citizens as genuine individual explorers on their own personal everyday life-trails, along their own life-trajectories. We must favor their empowerment as self documenting "Citizen Scientists" qualified to reflect and deal with own health-data, physiological data, economical data and environmental data. Therefore we must find ways to at least enable and equip the autonomous individual citizens/patients to develop and maintain their own most basic and private sedimenting digital self-narrative of what seems relevant to them: an electronic diary and time-indexed database, as an empowering empirical tool, not least in health-related, body- and domestic habit-related matters.

MEDICAL PATIENTJOURNEY CONCEPTS

Patient Journey is a pragmatic metaphor, an expression which may need some disambiguation, - especially in the context of patient narratives and experiences of illness. It can be used as referring to how patients proceed through an identified care delivery system. Seen from the angle of process mapping this refers to the total number of steps taken, as well as the total number of people involved, the total time taken to perform each process-step and all documents used.

*"When extensive process mapping for a considerable patient volume is done it is now possible to bring the data together and look at the care process from a unit/department perspective........ and perform a flow analysis (widely used in Manufacturing), and develop a current state flow analysis map: •Analyse patient flow across more complex processes •Identify whether the systems are managed and in control •See what adds value and where waste occurs *Understand roles and responsibilities related to managing patient flows." (NHS Scotland (2006) Understanding the Patient Journey – Process Mapping)*

But with the digitizing of health information, and the adoption of electronic patient records, highly professional tools are developed not only for hospitals but also for GP's to organize and administer their patient scheduling, patient records and patient flows in complex and versatile frameworks. This means that recording of consultations, test results, medication, prescriptions and referrals can be integrated as it is approached by e.g. Microsoft Health Common User Interface (http://www.ms-cui.net/). The idea is, to formalize an interface in such ways, that an integrated patient-centric care record can transition seamlessly between care sessions and care settings. The doctor is offered to have a multidimensional "landing place" with appointment list, email-in box, reports received, repeat prescription requests, practice notice board, medical knowledge support links and health news. With a click, each individual patient record is displayed, with expandable panels of:

- Most recent medical activities,
- Previous consultations,- expandable and comparable as detailed for: problem, history, examinations, medication, impression, plan and comments,
- Current and past medications
- Patient charts, graphical and table, making it possible to examine:
  - levels of medication,
  - BMI
  - BP
  - serum e.g.: creatinine cholesterol, LDL, sodium, potassium urea, related to long term time-lines, and visualized both in condensed and in detailed form in graphic curves.
- Risks: allergies and side effects,
- Lifestyle info, smoker/non smoker and calculated risks

Further linking to secondary-care examinations is also attempted, meaning that the GP may go into detail observing (and annotating) the results of patient respiratory pattern, cardiograms, angiograms, EEG etc from hospital or clinic.

Interfacing with the live patients will still be restricted to the briefest possible consultations. GPs can profitably handle more patients, appointments, referrals and prescriptions. In the prevalent concepts of the GP's digitized record keeping network, the cooperation between patient and doctor may be going to include e-mail, SMS, and, in the long run, perhaps occasional video telephone. But the role of the patient is not fundamentally reconsidered and the empowerment of citizens with personal laptops, everyday access to Internet 2.0 and global landscapes of health-related knowledge sources, has not been taken into account.

USER-DRIVEN PATIENT JOURNEY CONCEPT

Considering all the contemporary efforts of ministries of health and education – and of all kinds of professions, media, businesses and enterprises - to inform citizens of health issues and to the marketing of health related facilities, tools and measures to be taken by every citizen including the importance of self monitoring outputs of calories and intakes of vitamins, medicines and drugs, there would be a good logic in combining these with the general educational goals of *empowering citizens digital knowledge management skills* and growth into *personal lifelong learners*.

Not least is the upsurge of the potential and accelerating spread of biometric sensors for health life logging, implanted sensors, wearable strapped on sensors and in-home-sensors. The frontlines of wireless telemedical technology, as fitted in mobile and target-specific gadgets - as well as with patient notebook - are appearing and growing in many directions. "A whole new universe of *quantitative* health is dawning" (Bell & Gemell, 2009)

This must be kept in mind in electronic collaboration toward social health outcomes. Nor should we forget that personal hospital and GP records are in principle "personal health data", which in the long run may be shareable for the patient. What we now must focus is the question whether *a whole new universe of qualitative health* also is dawning.

To the patients, new horizons are opening. Detailed medical knowledge is traceable e.g. Pubmed http://www.ncbi.nlm.nih.gov/pubmed/ and www.wikipedia.com. New options for the patients sharing the journey with others are also emerging. With patient access to Internet, the world of "Health 2.0" also empowers the patient to dive into a wealth of information on health-economy, storing the diagnoses received, the treatments and pharmaceuticals prescribed, the side-effects met by others. Examples include,

Quickenhealth (http://healthcare.intuit.com/), Microsofthttp://www.healthvault.com) and Google (www.google.com/health). And not least, to join networks, relevant for particular diagnoses, to locate other patients with comparable problems, and to exchange subjective narratives of patient journeys through personal bloggings, e.g. www.patientslikeme.com and http://www.pdsa.org/.

This is the new –and global - noosphere, the soil from which user-driven healthcare is going to grow, crossing the divides between the patients, and permitting them to collaborate toward goals of shared interest, including tools to solidify such cooperation.

PATIENT AS LIFE-EXPLORER

It makes a difference to conceive of a patient journey in the sense of the journey of an individual explorer.

My approach is targeting the citizen as a life-explorer whose journey through the everyday - earlier or later - turns into traveling through pains and problems, encounters with medicine men, passage through admissions, tolls to be paid - or not afforded, waiting times to be endured, encampment in more or less friendly healthcare institutions, undergoing pains and sufferings, deprivations and starvations, uncertainties of outcomes, demands of endurance, and potential return to a continuation of previous life voyage, more or less radical change of life-course, or terminal more or less affordable more or less palliative terminal care.

Genuine explorers accumulate data relating to phenomena encountered / obtained (observations, states, courses, trails) to their log-books, from which they can produce maps and reports. Many people use a calendar and write lists and letters, some maintain a handwritten diary for shorter or longer periods of their lives, accumulating/ sedimenting/ accounting/ referring to what for them, at the time, seemed relevant.

With a notebook, we have to re-invent the diary, as a daily follower (Bjerg, 2008). In the present consumer situation we need a tool which can help patients to document, first and foremost to themselves, how they:

"traverse.. their unique disease and illness pathway through life stages and health systems and external social environments...... potentially numerous care relationships, predictable and unpredictable positive and negative influences, and feedback loops through which the patient must navigate.......; often with no definitive cure and demonstrate gradual changes over time with dynamic and evolving phases of being stable, complicated, complex and or chaotic with ultimate decline."(Martin, Carmel M, 2008)

To the extent we can consider citizens (including chronic patients) as equipped not only with a mobile, but also with a personal laptop computer, we must start caring about *self-narrative tools*, which ought to be close to hand, permitting the chronic patient explorer daily to accumulate the most private experiences of all kinds in an " intimate journal". And thus approach the interfacing to user-driven healthcare from a domestic bottom-up perspective.

THE CREATION OF A PERSONAL JOURNEY SUPPORT SYSTEM

In the industrialized world, the last several generations have seen their habitat equipped with ever new technical inventions, each, in their time, adapted, adopted and integrated in a new everyday life, at the very core of personal human existence: tap-water, cold and hot, water-closet, gas and electricity, stove and sewing machine, vacuum cleaner and electric iron, central heating, telephone and radio, camera, record player, refrigerator, TV, freezer, washing machine, dishwasher, coffee-machine, food-processor, microwave-oven, VCR, and CD-player. With the advent of answering machines, DVDs, video cameras, home-computers etc. we first experience these as "more of the same". But with cellular telephones and SMS, lap-tops, memory-sticks, powerful portable multimedia home computers, wireless access, digital cash, digital TV, two-way video telephony, access from homes to two-way traffic in new infrastructures of telecommunication, virtual reality, optical character-recognition, speech-recognition and speech-synthesis and an unexpected range of other technical inventions, previously only conceived in terms of the needs of professionals, we are forced to reconsider the role of the private household and its members, healthy or sick.

The home-consumer-market has stimulated a global competition to exploit an ever-wider range of technological advances for purposes of profitable marketing. And the health market is no exception.

For the "**home-vessels**" of the citizen explorers, being grounded as they are, a navigable media-landscape and a cyberspace are expanding in place of navigable oceans and voyageable continents. But one can say that we lack a valid paradigm for "**the personal domestic bridge**", and fitting tools for orientation and logging on the trails and through the travels of the life journey.

This new world where the personal (portable) computer, mail and the Internet eventually reaches almost everyone, makes new demands for orienting oneself, learning, keeping track of services and programs, passwords and pin codes, addresses and networks. This will easily become a separate province in our lives, with little consistency with our other everyday life other work, other media, other tasks and hobbies, reading and music, socializing, housekeeping, shopping, cleaning and waste, bodily functions and body care.

To competently manage personal knowledge, we are forced to be a new kind of explorer in a new kind of contemporarity - and need some kind of "log", where we - easily - can tell ourselves what we spent time with, whom we met, what

we found, did, thought (and felt?) on each day's journey, or just in each week.

It can be every day (very short, or along the day), or just sometimes. And it can be restricted to specified dimensions: training, weight, horticulture, nutrition, disease, education, press and TV, football or golf, reading, alcohol, cigarettes, knitting, family, job, colleagues, or it can go across all what they consider relevant. Medical data, yes, but also ongoing – evolving – biography, noting all kinds of subjectively relevant observations, interplay with others, stresses and reliefs, and existential issues, as they weave in with the daily and nightly chores of body-maintenance and domestic householdings. Aspects of sleep-diary, pain-diary, compliance-diary, as well as mobile monitoring of physiological data, including future telemedical appliances, may be built into the network interfacing of such a tool, without exposing the private text-diary.

Seen from an existential mental health viewpoint, but also from a health-educational viewpoint, it is important that the clients have means to journal – for themselves, if they wish - all kinds of experiences, thought and emotions, gratitudes, disappointments, angers and resentments, tacit resignations, etc., without necessarily sharing these with family and caretakers, not to speak of further networks. Journaling just health-related data may in itself not be very attractive. But doing this in a room of one's own, a room of private reflection, a room where memories and dreams, recollections and reflections can unfold as consciousness goes on, and the need for making meaning of one's life persists, may motivate in another way. This applies not least to the chronic patient. The popularity of the "life-long learner" paradigm should reach all the way to palliative care.

If we, for example, can promote the chronic patient to the role of expert patient, "Citizen Scientist", chief specialist in his/her own case, and supply an adequate user-adaptable (Schonewille, 2005) toolset for handling her/his own narrative, as an assembling of layered, systematically structured date/time indexed entries, a most personal evidential database, we may be on the road to empower the individual user to decide, and select, which aspects of this may be shared – with closest relatives or caretakers – with physicians – with networks, in blogging, or even in patients-like-me systems, or with a coming Patient Journey Record (PaJR) - Platform for User Driven Healthcare.

I offer a principal solution to how we can equip individuals, not least chronic patients, to exploit the opportunities that come within reach with a personal notebook computer, without losing the consistency and continuity in their personal lives,

BACKGROUND HISTORY

I developed at the University of Copenhagen, Department of Psychology an experimental home (1972-1997) where I explored ways to help inhabitants represent their domestic everyday life and communication processes for themselves. This involved new options for monitoring bodily states, representing domestic space and the time geography of domestic events. Since the introduction of laptops and interactive programming, I focused on the concept of electronic diary, where time indexing of text entries could be automated. I have daily since 1997 – myself – been the main experimental subject, through generations of laptops and software-programs, and I have been entangled in all possible ruses and ignorances, shortcomings and frustrations, while always trying to put myself into the seat of future users - a kind of general empathy-state based on a still updated stock of European senior knowledge. As systems and software tools were optimized I have strived to clarify how the substantial offer of interactivity from the computer can best be brought to use in a tool like the one I had in mind, a tool which in fact is no more than a further development of the traditions of logging in ships, of journaling in work-protocols for the drawers and shelves

of operating rooms, and of personal diaries, in handwritten volumes.

DEVELOPMENT OF A PRELIMINARY PROTOTYPE

Acknowledging the kind of basis which the domestic scene and the personal body must constitute, I present a preliminary non-proprietary prototype, an empowering innovation, which we should wish for prospective citizens to possess, and for the further development of which I invite cross-cultural, cross-platform and cross-disciplinary collaboration. The tools we have developed are tools of "citizen science", enabling users themselves to pursue a sedimenting empirical logging of whatever they find relevant, around the clock, around the week, the month and the year. It is a diary-tool, while also being a log-book-tool.

We are so used to conceive of "the researcher" as an external observer, interviewer, questionnaire-designer and statistician, but the time has come to admit that the only investigator qualified to examine the personal information-flow and the user as strategic and tactic innovator is the user her/himself.

We offer, with this method, a basic instrument with which users, for themselves, can keep track of the personal ongoings and events, not only on the computer, but also throughout the everyday life, in an ongoing diary.

I think it is important that we enable ourselves to hold on to our personal existence, whom we were, whom we are, whom we shall become, and how we are using the shorter or longer lifespan given us, to enable us, as regards matters of personal relevance, to hold onto this, in order to be enabled to reflect upon it. And thereby perhaps get a somewhat better hold of this life, and perhaps develop it in more desirable directions. The new conditions we all are submitted to pose new demands, create new routines and tear us loose from the life anchors in traditions, and the clear-cut roles, previously readymade for the individual. Young or old, rich or poor, ethnic insider or ethnic outsider, educated or uneducated, employed or unemployed, we are all forced day after day to re-orient ourselves in relation to some of the old, and in relation to all the new, ever coming our way.

It is my conviction that it is of paramount importance that the single citizen in the broadband society, in the midst of and across the information bombardments from mass media, and the increasing involvement with the broadband society, gets equipped with a kind of "tool of self documentation", so that we can hold on to at least a bit of what happens to us, what we think about it, and what is practical for us to keep track of: pin codes, passwords, usernames and –numbers, service providers, tariffs, subscriptions, accounts, internet-addresses, e-mail addresses, telephone numbers, birthdays, medical prescriptions, doctor's appointments. And also which dreams we have, in all senses of the word, and the frustrations and disappointments we meet and recollect.

There will be as many ways to keep an electronic diary, as there will be individuals that will do it, and with different advantages. It is evident that nobody could nor should use time to describe everything they do, are exposed to, think and feel along each and every day. This must depend upon richness or shortness of time and subjective relevancies. Some may centre upon cooking, gardening, books, news, the Internet - or worries, symptoms, cures. Or maybe keeping track of the cigarettes, cigars and pipes smoked where and when, how many holes achieved on the golf course, about the arguments one has, meetings, transportation-problems, or lawsuits against telecompanies.

I think, with Tristine Rainer (Rainer, 1979, 2004), that the most important aspect of keeping a diary is the establishment of an area/arena/platform – a breathing-hole of absolute freedom and autonomy, where one can permit oneself to be honest, where one can make room for all of one's ideas, feelings, secret thoughts and fantasies, grieves and worries,

separated from or contextually anchored in the more trivial, but perhaps quite as meaningful, banal occupations and rituals filling one's life. Some keeping track of what others do for you, and keeping track of own reactions to others, may help us deal with more maturely with others. And accounting, narrating to oneself in writing may often help to clear the thinking, clarify the thoughts.

In this way, being equipped with adequate tools, the citizen is empowered for critical action on documented observations from both a consumer and a patient vantage point. If you have habits, which you hope to control-alcohol, tobacco, drugs, medicine, exercise, eating - you can journal the patterns and circumstances of your focused bad habit, in respect to advances, temptations, relapses and replacement for undesirable fix. But not least for persons, as chronic patients, hit by illnesses like cardiovascular disease, sclerosis, diabetes, Alzheimer's, kidney defects and/or submitted to stressful treatments, e.g. for cancer, or fighting physical and psychic handicaps, there should be a support in a purely personal keeping track of the progress of the battle, both at an outer and an inner level.

Writing a diary, journal or logbook by handwriting, has advantages, for which the present model of electronic diary cannot compensate. The expressivity in sizing and varying the handwriting, ornamentation, mixing written and drawn, dried flowers newspaper-cutting glued in, etc, is lost.

But the advantages of the electronic diary compensate, especially as more and more of the information which reaches us, and which we can reach for, arrives to the computer in digital form. A most central aspect is the automatic time-indexing, organizing all inputs relative to the progression of the diurnal, weekly, seasons and years of personal life.

Two special, related functions have been developed: one, enabling the user to "write into" specified temporal addresses, earlier in the day or a previous day, so it gets into the correct slot in the chronology of the day; and another, making it possible to annotate to lines earlier same day, or any of previous days of current diary, keeping track of when annotation was made. The prototype permits the user to create reporting shortcuts around the diary, to whatever programs or services they utilize. And it facilitates the user's name-giving and access to presently forty thematic drawers with accumulating memo-fields for themes of personal relevance. e.g., one for each of one's children and grandchildren, parents, best friends, theatre, movies, acquisitions, subscriptions, books, music, chat-groups, sermons, medications, prayers, treatments etc. Including calendar and address book (linking to e-mail), integrated in the diary, we are providing the user with a workbench and a private scene, relative to which the events and phenomena in their home, their garden, their neighborhood and their workplace can be contextualized, represented and optionally communicated.

I have tried to develop a preliminary set of demands, to the types of information, which should be equally easy to self-document. I think this is important for an understanding of the full scope of the enterprise. We should collaborate to offer a toolbox for citizens of any culture and age, helping them to keep coherent, contextualized track of (alphabetically ordered):

- Addresses, agreements and appointments
- Childcare
- Browsing WWW
- Cleaning and laundry
- Creative ideas, dreams & fantasies
- Demands & waiting times
- Drug, alcohol, coffee & tobacco use and abuse
- Economy, fees and contributions
- Emerging problems & attempted solutions
- Fitness-measures
- Gaming & gambling
- Handicaps and their handling
- Hygiene
- Illnesses
- Meals, diets and cooking

- Memorable reading, viewing and hearing
- Plans, successes and failures
- Rituals, ceremonies & prayers
- Sex
- Shopping
- Sleep
- Sports
- Stresses and endurances
- Studies, school
- Symptoms & prescription compliance
- TV-consumption
- Usability of habitual and emergent tool

THE ICONOSPHERE

Putting words to cognitive phenomena in moments of shared or private life-space seems to be our most distinctive species-specific feature. Talking with others, and talking with ourselves. And logging. The invention and use of numbers, hieroglyphs, and later the alphabets, (separating the languages, self-fulfilling the myth of the ill planned Tower of Babel (with its left hemisphere bias) is what has brought us to the Obama-decennium and the new options for global brotherhood and outreach.

Dynamic virtual social networks (including senior and patient networks, etc.) are now growing up, and citizens with mobiles, SMS and WWW can suddenly play on our "own court," with biographical unique e-identity, and/or many pseudonyms. And writing is now embedded in – and potentially self-documenting - audiovisual time-space fields, with photos, video clips, voice recordings and conversation-records.

I have studied this frontier field from its first rudiments in the 1980s, and have reached to a new category of characters for logging of everyday life's typical acts and events. This is a principal solution that can bridge the gap between text and image universe, both for the individual and in virtual social networks. I introduce a pictorial writing, to ease our PC logging of everyday life phenomena, multimedia dialogues and correspondence for entirely private confidential personal use. But the possibility that we may also use it in our correspondence with others will also appear as soon as basic pictorial fonts are shared, e.g., in a patient network.

Practical agency in the individual life world implies categories of relevance, which can be considered as elements, molecules and strings of habits. The everyday routines in the home – often considered as trivia - are extensively describable in narrative language, there are thousands of typicality's for which the citizen has concept, and most have words in one or more languages. But referring descriptively to them by words in languages is cumbersome.

Already back in the early 80s, working with an experimental apartment, I found that a short cut to overview and understand the processes and events in a family-home was to use small pictures, fitted to represent what took place when and where for the individual inhabitant(s). There are so many typical generally recognizable phenomena in everyday bodily life in our home, in the daily and weekly life, including the well-known bodily functions and household functions. I started then - in collaboration with students of methods of qualitative research - to construct a system of pictograms for this descriptive purpose. And then the technological development suddenly offered a new opportunity.

I found a second shortcut to the pictorial shorthand needed by avoiding the bit-mapped icon-format, and instead using the character-format, i.e. designing glyphs in a font-suite.

Now, as to general use of an electronic-bridge journaling, we have an apparent dilemma: people, who are active, engaged and involved in life and fellow humans, living under information overload, will have all too much to tell their electronic diaries. Involved with other humans and other tasks, there are only small and sparse time-windows for reporting to the diary. Describing everyday life with words is disproportionally time-consuming, and so some kind of shorthand would be convenient.

The everyday stream of thought, of consciousness or of subjective life and agency is to a wide extent language-independent, and not in the form of propositional thought. But there is a division of labor between the two cerebral hemispheres, of which usually the left is handling language in words, whereas the other, so called recessive hemisphere, usually the right, is dealing in images and sensory-motor figures. (Sperry, Gazzaniga, Bogen, 1969) (Levy, 1974).

The development of human civilizations is, as said, intrinsically based on development of spoken language. And the invention of writing, with its origin in images (the hieroglyphs) is a crucial turning point. But writing has, for millennia, developed in force of a minimal number of letters in alphabets, and basically tied to the sounds of spoken language. The original track of the hieroglyphs, writing with images, has been out of bounds to the handwriting-, typewriting- and printing-cultures, simply because general picture-alphabets had to include so many more characters. The international use of traffic signs was the first forceful penetration to the general public of modern hieroglyphs. And since computers entered the scene and reproduction of such pictures were facilitated, the modern world is replete with icons, pictograms, glyphs, used to identify typicality's of brand, origin, qualities, functions, actions and behaviors of goods, men and machines. We see simple non-verbal symbols heavily used, not only in traffic, but in vehicles, hospitals, newspapers and in most mechanical and electronic tools, including their manuals, toolbars and controls, and even on the child's toys, the clothes we wear and the containers of the foods we eat. Their communicative value lies partly in their at-a-glance recognizability, one-letter briefness, colourability and resizeability. But their cross-language understandability is, in force of migration and globalization of the market, a further incentive to extend their use.

Now, in the habits of everyday personal life, typicality's abound. In dealing with the communication-handicapped, programs have been developed which offer a rich variety of icons for symbol and image-based interpersonal communication about everyday life. But they are bit-mapped pictures, and mainly bound to licensed software. However, pictograms can be considered as a species of characters. Symbol fonts are in fact produced and marketed. This implies that a basic diary writing, which can report habitual situations, everyday events and activities with pictograms as single dedicated characters, under-standable even to the illiterate and the child, is a logical possibility. But, the number of keys on keyboards being limited, the entry of icons must take place otherwise than the entry of words. The solution presented here is to let the user choose and distribute pictograms, stored as characters in a font suite, as screen buttons. Users can arrange and rearrange them on a principal screen-window, surrounding a central scroll field, where text is entered, and they can then, with a single mouse-click, be entered in the (time-indexed) text-lines of the diary. Actually, the day card of the diary is a potentially revolving stage-scene to the user's own body map, virtual home, virtual neighbor-hood, etc, where pictogram-buttons also can be placed, contextualized and grouped according to such structured topologies.

The idea of using glyphs to support the verbal journaling and reflection of personal phenomena may sound like an attempt to square the circle. But understanding such glyphs, not as objective classifications, but as private signs of contextual-ized subjective phenomena points to a future of shared/folk-taxonomy alphabets for the more or less global typicality's of phenomenal event in habitats and in bodies.

The glyphs developed amount presently only to approximately 450, and many are lousy and inadequate. A series of them are not available in Windows version etc. But there are presently 12 root-stems, ready for inclusion of many, many more glyphs.

Figure 1. Glyphs distributed in 12 fonts

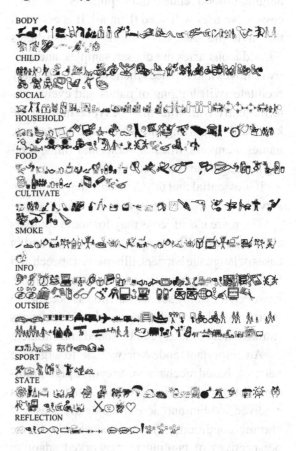

For some, the use of such glyphs in their diary may be uninviting. For others, especially indi-viduals with limited reading writing capacities, lacking language-skills, or anybody in situations where motive for journaling is strong, but time or energy is short, glyphs may provide convenient provisional shorthand.

I am certainly not proud to present this pre-liminary suite of glyphs, with all its weaknesses and shortcomings. In the menus from which they can be chosen, an explanatory label is attached to each, and the ones installed by the user keeps their label as a tool-tip. The glyphs with labels can be closer inspected in www.phenomenalog. dk/glyphs.htm. The user thus has access to an extended library of pictograms, primarily referring to more or less universal all-human – or culture specific - typicality's of bodily, domestic and neighbourhood endeavours, pursuits and processes. No user will need them all. It is essential that it is the user who selects and distributes wanted icons, tries out chosen samples, and easily removes and replaces them with others. They facilitate swift logging of habits and events, intermittently with what may be typed in from the keyboard, reporting in words and sentences, names, numbers, titles of books and films, feelings, thoughts and reflections.

It is essential that the electronic diary thus can serve both cerebral hemispheres in timely ways.[1]

The mere use of icons may for some contexts and purposes suffice, under time-pressure and in cases of language barriers, illiteracy or speech and language-impairment. For adults in literate culture, however, they may sooner function as occasional short hand where qualifying words and sentences (immediately or later) can be added and situated.

An important endeavor will be to organize network-based mechanisms to evolve pictogram-alphabets for subjective symptoms and treatments received, within and across major diseases and chronic conditions. This relates closely to the perspectives of tagging in networked adaptive information systems for chronic care (Biswas, Martin, Sturmberg 2009) (Martin 2009)

THE BODY, THE HOME AND CYBERSPACE IN THE DIARY

From a psychological viewpoint it is crucial, that by ensuring for the members of a household a permanent reference to the solid ground-level of their own particular domestic and bodily time geography, a personal grounded and rooted stem of self-reference can be grown, that can be made to function as a convenient core and anchor point for further personal orientation and reality-testing (Agre& Horswill, 1997). It implies the emergence of a new, coherent potential of demonstrative identifying reference to re-identifiable individual objects, states and event-types in the private life-

world, according to their personal biographical relevance and provide us new means of self-reflection, evaluation and ordination of past and possible future operations, states, informative objects and persons (Bjerg, K, 2008).

In this, one's body constitutes a necessary frame of reference, even for the healthy person. So, before focussing on any specific patient target group, we must cooperate to find general formats for personal body referring over time, in a diary. The day card must include a window to a 2-D or 3-D map of one's body. This constitutes a background scene for distribution of most health relevant glyphs already in the prototype. But it shall also permit a user to bookmark and comment (more permanent and/or on a daily base) spots and areas anywhere in one's body.

General formats are also being created for visualizing in the diary relevant physiologic parameters over time, beginning with the most obvious - accumulating tables of sleep length, number of pills, cigarettes, drinks, and manually entered blood pressure and weight - as basis for occasional reflections. but aiming toward inclusion of illness-specific monitoring, e.g., cholesterol, coagulation, glucose, etc, and zoomable curve-display. Enabling patients to monitor and keep track of bodily states and symptoms will most certainly be the call of the immediate future. The above-mentioned potentials of biotelemetry bring it, so to speak, "under our skin", and highlight the potential intimate, bodily closeness of this "personal level". Some such data might even, if desirable, be accepted for sharing with one or more helpers (Bjerg 2009b). Configuring body-state-representational tools for personal state-reflection is a little-noticed potential, mainly cultivated in circles working with the concept of biofeedback. But seen as one of many keys to a sane health-education, such tools of self-knowledge may reveal a strong prophylactic potential, and thus be worth adding to the domestic tool kit (Baskin, 2004).

The thinking about social processes around the human body includes ranges of social work-

Figure 2.

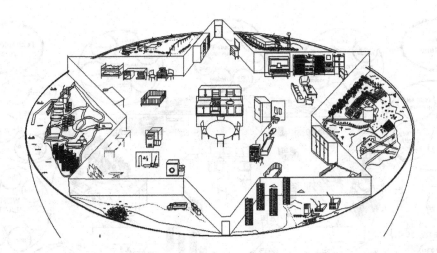

ers, doctors, nurses, secretaries, patient groups, clinics, training facilities etc. And the thinking about technological process, around the human body, includes ranges of diagnostic, maintenance, treatment technologies, prescription and journalizing databases. But the convergence of all these social and technological processes around the human body has an internal double nucleus -the personal body and the personal home, what we term the Somasphere and the Oikosphere.

Whatever measures we take in health and medical care, social and technological, the moment we think of just one citizen we must understand that a convergence of social and technological processes around the body already exists inside the information dynamics of the home and the family. We must build a counterpoint to the systems notion of a patient or client: a view from below, a view from the vantage point of the person-number, a view from the target of the healthcare, the consumer, the citizen's own local and temporal viewpoint, as conscious phenomena in continued personal cognitive and meta-cognitive processes.

As discussed above, one's home also constitutes an essential frame of reference, even for the healthy person. The day card can include a map of the home, being a floor-plan vector graphic representation, or a richer "furnished" "doll-house" top view. This constitutes a background scene for distribution of most household-relevant glyphs already in the prototype. It shall also, in future versions, permit the user on a daily basis to mark, link and comment on spots and areas anywhere in one's home. No doubt such options can have pragmatic value in all kinds of households, not least in cases of brain damage rehabilitation and senile dementias.

As the inclusion of a representation (furnished floor plan) of the user's own home is a complicated endeavour – presently out of reach for most users - a more abstract generalized habitat topology has been designed - the OIKOS –scene.

This constitutes a topology, relative to which glyph-buttons can be distributed, and, not least, demands for coming glyphs arise.

But by the recent inclusion of browser functionality in the diary, the following map may also constitute one of possible backgrounds of the MYCYBERSPACE window, upon which users, here enabled to accumulate and organize Internet bookmarks, can distribute their links, relative to social-ontological contexts.

THE PERSONAL INTERFACE

My method has been to develop an investigative tool, which at a minimum could satisfy the needs

Figure 3.

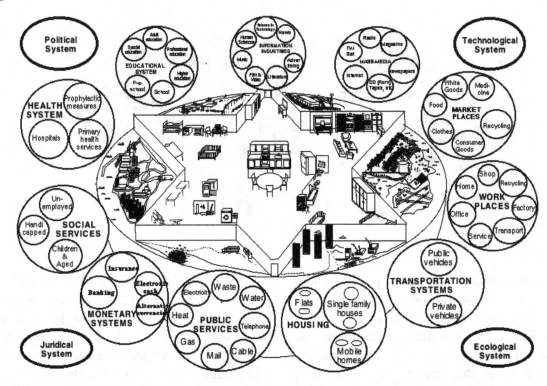

I met in daily use on my personal laptop(s) day in and day out, during all seasons of the year, over a period of 10+ years. The diary opens with a small window on the screen, from which a user can orient.

The moment "Open Diary" is clicked, the full screen is taken over by a window to the last day-card

But the moment the red bottom right button "Hide" is clicked, it vanishes out of sight.

Now, this interface is simplified, and users have direct access to furnish it not only with the glyph buttons they wish, but also with any of the functions shown in the next image.

Shown below is a realistic impression of how a single (male) user has come to personalize his own diary:

ONGOING PROTOTYPING

The latest version of the program, at the time of this writing (v. 18.1.1) has only been in use by a few relatively healthy persons. This version is now going to be tested through an appeal to the 4000+ participants in a Danish senior (age 50+) network (www.ageforce.dk) to join a shared WIKI (www. phenomenalog.wikispaces.com) and involve themselves as beta-testers, with use of the mutual

Figure 4.

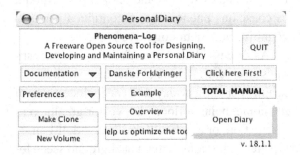

Figure 5. The immediate presentation of an interface to new users, version 18.1.1 (Colours have had to be removed in all illustrations for this publication)

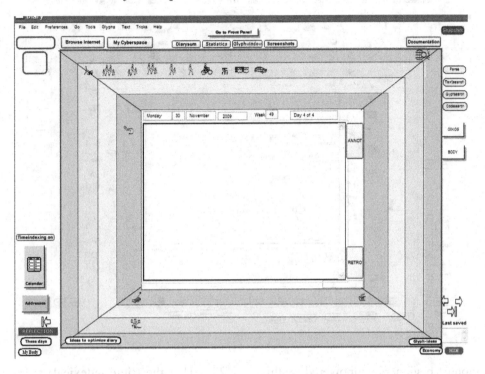

Figure 6. The full range of possible fields and functions

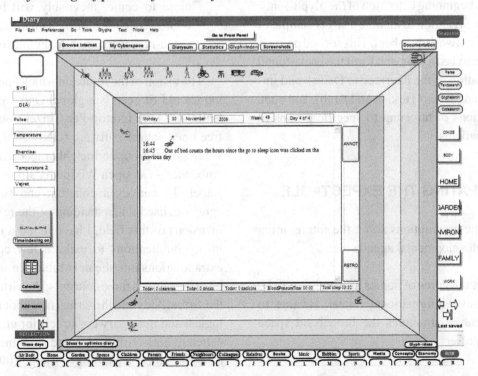

Figure 7. "Inhabited" diary

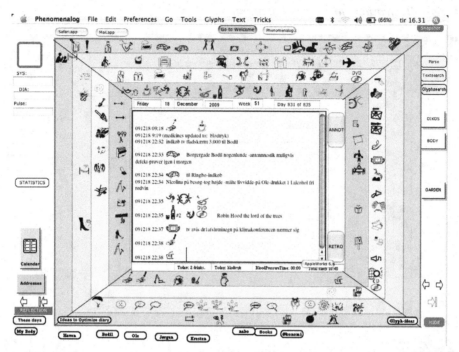

support amongst beginners, empowered by this WIKI. The data from this process shall establish the basis for a thorough revision of the user-interface, beginning extension of the glyph-fonts, and a new invitation to include a larger sample of the senior network members. This second phase is scheduled to last a year, and form the background for translation of the interface to Danish and immigrant languages (Turkish and Arab), and open the questions of targeting to specific groups of chronic patients.

ANTICIPATING THE EXPECTABLE

Among the assumptions about the future going into this developmental agenda are:

1. That the cores of homes and bodies will be massive informational nuclei, relative to whatever structures the broadband space will offer

2. That the (time-indexical) representational options concerning these nuclei with digital text, graphics and audio and video and more to come, inevitably will bloom, as witnessed with mobile technology, digital video-recorders, mobile monitoring, etc.

The vision of the future, in which Phenomenalog should fit best, is a global One-Laptop-Per-Child -> / One-Laptop-Per-Citizen society with free open source software (GNU etc.), and free wireless peer group and neighborhood networking, embedded in an open Wikipedia 3rd millennium Babel. To convey a coherent and sufficiently contextualised understanding of the relevant dimensions of this field, I have found it necessary in my publications to make a few conceptual extrapolations into the near future. In so doing, I have introduced three concepts: the virtual home, the virtual body and the virtual neighbourhood - as logical and necessary constructs for grounding a coherent notion of the demands to future domestic information technology (Bjerg, 2000, Bjerg,

2001). A discussion of these matters should hopefully connect the enterprise at hand with the total recall universe of Gordon Bell and Gemmel (Bell, 2009), and with the "the sixth sense technology "enterprise of Pranav Mistry (Mistry, 2009), and its promises of a wearable gestural interface, e.g. narrating gloves, 3-D pens, and establishment of shortcuts to create virtual objects distributable in virtual spaces, like the virtual home. They are thematically relevant because they can point us to the notion of a fully and coherently contextualized interface, coming to make it possible in timely ways to refer and annotate to any location/area within one's home and any bodily posture and any location/area on or inside one's body.

INTERFACING THE MOST TRUSTED HELPER

Seeing client-helper as a special case of future close multimedia interfacing with trusted others points to important improvements in the long distance person-to person communicative space. Already advanced enterprises setting up frameworks for telehomecare, patients treated at home using telemedicine, are emerging in Denmark, e.g., www.virtuellehospital.dk and www.telekat.dk. To the extent our now-and-here, within-sight and within-reach info-environments (including desktop) now electronically can be made shareable, participants can point in real time to postures, spots and areas both in their own and others' bodies, paraphernalia, instruments, surroundings, practical situations, and sequences of typical events. Interfacing the chronic patient might well empower the patient to display and refer, not only to his body, but also to his room, even showing, in a conversation, by pointing and looking at things (Bjerg, 2009).

Citizens will increasingly depend upon, and anchor themselves through information in and out from their computers. Their acquired orientation, personal inputs and outputs, trails and landmarks across Internet sites and neighbourhoods will increasingly reflect and condition their thinking and problem solving. To the extent the option of showing/sharing what can be seen on one's laptop is an evidently relevant feature in future close communication between laptop users, it enables the sharing of evolving personal patterns of subjective relevance on the Internet in detail and over time - an important aspect of health-education. Citizens´ dealing privately with all this – not to speak of private dealing with IT-tool use – will, also more generally, profit from being shareable in distance-conversations with close friends and trusted helpers.

"Patient literacy" and "patient education" explicitly refer to the knowledge distributed and distributable on websites and WIKI's. If patient education is an aspect of shared health-management, it should support telecoaching within the frames of patients' further orientation on the Internet. Such added features in interfacing the lonely handicapped and chronic patients would at least compensate somewhat for the missing expensive corporeal visits of the helper.

CONCLUSION

In view of the blooming of professional medical technologies, the escalation of healthcare expenses and the spread of health threatening lifestyles in the populations, the importance of increasing health-awareness, self-care and self-monitoring is generally acknowledged, while growing number of chronic patients is escalating. Public health information is intensified. The profitable marketing of drugs, health-related facilities, training, remedies and tools is exploding. But the evolving of patient-driven networks and shared blogging gives unexpected promises of support to the individual patient.

The only problem is, that while tremendous efforts and results are obtained to digitalize and train the medical establishment, the chronic patients are left at their own to learn, how to handle a computer, establish e-mail contact, and to hook up to whatever the digitized medical society has to offer. Therefore the citizen health situation has to be re-examined in the light of the global spread of notebook computers and networks. Personal healthcare and health-related interfacing of the future shall be considered as just one dimension of the citizen's general interfacing him/herself through the everyday use of a personal notebook computer.

We must conceive of citizens as genuine individual explorers on their own personal daily life-trails, along their own life-trajectories. We must favour their empowerment as self documenting "Citizen Scientists" qualified to deal with own health-data, physiological data, economical data and environmental data. We must qualify citizens as administrators of their own health. Therefore we must motivate and equip the autonomous individual citizen/patient to develop and maintain a most basic and private sedimenting digital self-narrative, an electronic diary and time-indexed database, as an empowering empirical tool, not least in health-related, body- and domestic-habit-related matters.

The rationales behind the development of an open source freeware cross-platform tool for this purpose were explained, the dimensions it shall be fit to document were listed, the very preliminary library of pictographic short-hand presented, and the overall design of the interface of the early prototype illustrated. Long term perspectives of the project relate both to the expected spread of bio-telemetric technologies and to interfacing personal health data in the medical systems. Immediate short-term perspectives relate to preliminary testing and user-driven development in a Danish senior citizen network (www.ageforce.dk), and the collective development of a new wiki: www.phenomenalog.wikispaces.com, while developing targeting for broader and more specific chronic patient populations.

ACKNOWLEDGMENT

The development of the concepts and the software described was based on:

- Experimental Home Project, Department of Psychology, University of Copenhagen, Denmark.
- Students involved in Course of Qualitative Research Methods
- Kim Borreby, with whom I co-edited the Proceedings of the IFIP 93 International Cross-disciplinary Conference on "Home-oriented Informatics, Telematics and automation" in Copenhagen, 1994
- A grant from Scandinavian Tobacco Company
- Early programming by Mag.art Bjørn Nake
- Extensive (more than a decade) unpaid voluntary programming help by Steen Kyllesbaek Andersen.
- Extensive unpaid voluntary programming help by Mark Schonewille.
- Economy-X-talk.com - Advice and critique from my wife Beth Bjerg
- And occasional help, over the years, from programmers in the "Revolution" developers community ; Sarah Reichelt and her DateTime.rev collection, Richmond Mathewson for his Paint widgets, Eric Chatonet, Klaus Major, Mark Talluto and others.

REFERENCES

Agre, P., Horswill, I. (1997).Lifeworld analysis. *Journal of Artificial Intelligence Research, 6*(1), 111-145.Baskin, S. M, Kirk, L. P. Lehrer, P. M., Lubar, J. F., & LaVaquue, T. (2004). *Evidence-Based Practice in Biofeedback and Neurofeedback*

Bell, G., & Gemell, J. (2009). *Total Recall*. London: Penguin.

Biswas, R., Martin, C. M., Sturmberg, J., Mukherji, K., Lee, E. W. H., Umakanth, S., & Kasthuri, A. S. (2009) Social Cognitive Ontology and User Driven Healthcare in: Katzipanagos, S & Warburton, S: *Handbook of research on social software and developing community Ontologies*

Bjerg, K. (2000). Citizen Science Implications of Public Access to 3- D Hypermedia Editing and Interactivity in the Home. Consumers as researchers - Homes as laboratories. In Sloane, A., & van Rijn, F. (Eds.), *Home Informatics and Telematics*. Klüwer Academic Publishers.

Bjerg, K. (2001). Towards the virtual home: Construing the multi-media-home to enhance cultural and biographic continuity. In Rasmussen, B., Beardon, C., & Munari, S. (Eds.), *Computers and networks in the age of globalization*. Klüwer Academic Publishers.

Bjerg, K. (2008) "Empowering Citizen Self-Documentation: Re-inventing the diary" Observatorio (OBS*), Vol2, No 2 (2008) www.obs.obercom.pt/index.php/obs/article/view/198 (Paper presented to the COST298 transdiciplinary international conference on "*The user and the future of information and communication technologies*" in Moscow 2007).

Bjerg, K. (2009) Personal Electronic Journaling (Paper presented to the COST298 transdiciplinary international conference on "The *user and the future of information and communication technologies*" in Copenhagen 2009). http://miha2.ef.uni-lj.si/cost298/gbc2009-proceedings/papers/P155.pdf

Bjerg, K. (2009) Self-care, telemonitoring and multidimensionality in person-to-person interfacing: A new angle on self-management in chronic disease (Paper presented to the COST298 transdiciplinary international conference on "*The user and the future of information and communication technologies*" in Copenhagen 2009):http://miha2.ef.uni-lj.si/cost298/gbc2009-proceedings/papers/P154.pdf

Levy, J. (1974). Psychobiological implications of bilateral asymmetry. *In Hemisphere function in the human brain*. Dimond and Beaumont, eds, New York.

Martin, C. M. (2008). *Patient Journey Record (PaJr) Platform for user driven healthcare*. NDRC Translational Research Project Proposal.

Mistry, P. (2009). *The thrilling potential of sixth sense technology*. TED.

Mistry, Pranav m P. Maes (2009) Sixth Sense – a wearable gestural interface. SIGGRAPH Asia 2009

NHSScotland. (2006) Understanding the Patient Journey – Process Mappping http://www.scotland.gov.uk/Resource/Doc/141079/0036023.pdf

Pettenati, M. C., & Cigognini, M. E. Guerin, E. M. C., & Mangione, G. R. (2008). Personal Knowledge Management Skills for Lifelong-learners 2.0 in: Hatzipanagos, S. & Warburton, S. (Eds.), *Handbook of Research on Social Software and Developing Community Ontologies*, Hershey: IGI Global.

Rainer, T. (1979, 2004). *The New Diary. How to Use a Journal for Self-guidance and Expanded Creativity*. Tarcher Publ.

Schonewille, M. (2005). *An adaptive Interface*. (Draft), Nijmegen school of Management

Sperry, R. W., Gazzaniga, M. S., & Bogen, J. E. (1969). Interhemisphere relationship, the neo-cortical commisures, Syndromes of hemisphere disconnection. In *Handbook of Clinical Neurology*. Inken, (ed), Amsterdam.

ADDITIONAL READING

Biswas, R., Maniam, J., Lee, E. W. H., Umakanth, S., et al. (2008). Electronic collaboration toward social health outcomes, in (Eds.) Salmon J, Wilson L, *Handbook of Research on Electronic Collaboration and Organizational Synergy,* Hershey, PA: IGI Global

Biswas, R., Martin, C. M., Sturmberg, J., Shanker, R., Umakanth, S., Shanker, S., & Kasturi, A. S. (2008). User-driven health care - answering multidimensional information needs in individual patients utilizing post-EBM approaches: a conceptual model. *Journal of Evaluation in Clinical Practice, 14*(5).

Bjerg, K. (1996). Home-Oriented Informatics, Telematics & Automation. In *Encyclopaedia of Computer Science and Technology*. Pittsburgh, PA: Marcel Dekker.

Boxer, P. J. (1980). Supporting reflexive learning, - toward a reflexive theory of form. In Bonarius, H., Holland, R., & Rosenberg, S. (Eds.), *Personal Construct Psychology*.

Giddens, A. (1991). *Modernity and Self-Identity*. Oxford: Blackwell.

Hägerstrand. Torsten (1974). Tidsgeografisk Beskrivning- syfte och postulat. *Svensk Geografisk Årbog, 50,* Lund

Hartmann, M. (2008). Everyday life: Domesticating the invisible" in Pierson, Jo (et al) (Eds) '*Innovating for and by users,* Publ. COST – European Co-operation in the field of Scientific and Technical Research.

Kelly, G. A. (1955). *The psychology of personal constructs*. Norton.

Li, I., Day, A., & Forlizzi, J. (2010) A Stage-based model of Personal Informatics Systems, *CHI 2010,* Atlanta, Georgia

Miles, I. (1988). *Home Informatics: Information Technology and the Transformation of Everyday Life*. London: Pinter Publ.

Peña-López, I. (2009). The personal research portal: web 2.0 driven individual commitment with open access. In Hatzipanagos, S., & Warburton, S. (Eds.), *Handbook of Research on Social Software and Developing Community Ontologies*. Hershey: IGI Global.

Proulx, S. (2008). Social innovation among ICT users: Technology as catalyst in promoting social change. In Pierson J.,Mante-Meijer, E, Loos,E and Sapio,B. (Eds), *Innovating for and by Users*. Publ. COST – European Co-operation in the field of Scientific and Technical Research. (de) Saint Laurent-Kogan, A-F. (2008). The evolution of services with ICTs: Remote assistance device for elderly people in (Eds), Pierson J.,Mante-Meijer, E, Loos,E and Sapio,B. *Innovating for and by Users*. Publ. COST – European Co-operation in the field of Scientific and Technical Research

Schutz, A. (1974). *The Structures of the Life-World*. London: Heinemann.

Searles, J. R. (1995). *The Construction of Social Reality*. London: Penguin.

Silverstone, R. (Eds.). (1992). *Consuming Technologies: Media and Information in Domestic Spaces*. London: Routledge. doi:10.4324/9780203401491

Von Hippel, E. (2005). *Democratizing Innovation*. Cambridge, MA: MIT Press.

KEY TERMS AND DEFINITIONS

Biotelemetry: Digital monitoring of various vital signs of ambulatory patients (or healthy persons)

Citizen Science: A term used for projects or ongoing program of <u>scientific work</u> in which individual volunteers or networks of volunteers, many of whom may have no specific scientific training, perform or manage research-related tasks such as observation, measurement or computation.

Cyberspace: The electronic medium of computer-networks in which online communication takes place. The expression "MyCyberspace" designates a mapping of personally most relevant sites on the Internet.

Glyph: Graphic signs of writing. Letters are glyphs, but so are also hieroglyphs, pictograms, ikons, smileys etc. The term is here used to refer to pictograms which – like alphabetic characters- are encoded in fonts

Iconosphere: A sphere of pictorial signs, e.g. glyphs.

Noosphere: (From greek nous (knowledge) The sphere of human thought

Oikosphere: (From greek oikos (home) The sphere of a home and its processes of householding.

Phenomenology: in philosophy and psychology referring to the subjective experience of a person. Experience (or being, or existence itself) is an "in-relation-to" phenomenon, and it is defined by qualities of directedness, embodiment and worldliness which are evoked by the term "Being-in-the-World". This is the background for the term "Phenomenalog".

Propositional Thought: Thoughts in words or sentences, as opposed to non-verbal thoughts in images and gestures.

Somasphere: The sphere of a living human body and its processes

Typicality: referring to a subjective situated category of behaviour or event, which may vary in detail, but function as recognizable token and construct in a persons mental space and metacognition.

Virtual Body: A 3D representation of a body

Virtual Home: A 3D representation of a home

ENDNOTE

[1] The maintenance of time-indexed 24-hours display of inserted icons, as separated from the text written by the user, is an important feature possibility. It means, e.g. in the present prototype, that their distribution around the clock can be inspected in a separate window, where browsing through sequences of days make changes in pattern immediately apparent. And it opens for further developments towards columnar or circular displays permitting their juxtaposition with corresponding curves of vital parameters from body sensors. Physiological curves plotted relative to pictograms referring to behavioural or ideational events may be illuminating not only to researchers and doctors, but also to potential patients. To this end we must approach the logging process from a non-symbolic angle: The more or less automatic inputs of measurements, which a laptop diary can be made to record, along the diurnal cycle

APPENDIX A. IMPLEMENTED FEATURES IN THE DIARY

Features included in the electronic diary (numbered to facilitate further discussion):

1. Freeware (GNU licence)
2. Versions for for Windows (not Vista), Windows 10'inch and Macintosh (unsolved problems with Linux-version).
3. There is a "HIDE" button, removing all traces of the diary from desktop, except link on the taskbar, meaning that its use can switch between all other uses of the computer and the private instantly hidden for casual onlookers.
4. Automation of time indexing, everything is dated, and precise timestamping along the day can be switched on or off.
5. Automatic saving at user defined intervals
6. User defines, how late in the night/how early in the morning new daycards shall be created
7. Automatic backups for last three days complete diary savings
8. As the temporal sequence of inputs to the main diary text field is strictly maintained two "DRAFT" fields are available: one for ordinary textediting, one for simple graphic eding.
9. Option to substitute or supplement text-entries with entries of pictograms (Glyphs) for recurrent typicality's of situations, actions and events in everyday life, as a kind of shorthand,
10. Option for personally selecting which pictograms from an expanding library of glyphs user finds it worth to use screen space for on his/her intra-personal dialogue –scene,- or on one of the 7 one-click-away supplementary side scenes of the daycard (cfr.*21)
11. A retro option to insert text&glyphs to earlier times same day, - to the extent user cares to detail the chronology of the day.
12. An annotation option, enabling time-indexed reflection/commentary/tags to be inserted after any line in the diary.Quoting to the superordinate metacognitive field (cfr. *27) is another tagging-option.
13. Feature of searching and finding each occurrence of chosen word og pictogram in the accumulated diary.
14. Feature of parsing, -producing a file of all time indexed lines (with n lines before n lines after) where a word or a glyph appeared in the accumulated diary
15. Integration with calendar (for fast access to previous days in accumulated day-cards – for swift brief quoting to calendar –and for reminders, to be quoted on opening a specific later day)
16. Integration with address book, (with search function across all fields, including telephone numbers) where also personal notes can be made, from where e.mail to a person can be initiated, and from where www adresses can be opened
17. Options for quoting to and from the diary in relation to files in other programs.
18. There is a large number of separate accumulating thematic fields –Some have default labels, but all can be relabelled by user (E.g symptoms, promises, books read, films seen)
    ◦ They can be opened and added (or deleted) text (they accumulate content over the days)
    ◦ On latest day selected text can be quoted to them, without opening them
    ◦ One is located to permit its continual visibility during diary-use (e.g.as to-do list)
    ◦ One is organized as a (resortable) table for accumulating and refinding personal usernames, customernumbers,, passwords and pin-codes (A virtual digital Key-ring)
19. Option for printing text of any accumulated thematic field

20. Options to print full diary text from single day or span of days
21. Options for user to alter and redesign the interface including showing or hiding the following links and fields:
22. Links to one or more of the supplementary one-click away side scenes of the daycard ("oikosphere", virtual body, home, garden, neighborhood, workplace and family) enabling a more systematic distribution and retrieval of glyph-buttons, and open for users pasting alternative graphic backgrounds and pictures.
23. Fields for
    a. daily counts of use of selected glyphs (e.g. medicine, alcohol, cigarette,) with options for updating along the day
    b. typed physiological data (e.g. blood pressure, weight, temperature)
    c. typed words for symptoms, weather, mood etc
    d. sleep length (as time elapsed between sleep-glyph previous day and "arise" glyph next day.
24. Link to a table, into which the diary for each day accumulates these data on a new line.
25. The option for user to create links (for single days- or permanently) to any application, folder and file on the computer. (Use of such links is automatically timestamped into the diary to make the personal information-handling more transparent in its time-perspectives).
26. A simple browser is included in the program. It is set up to enable user to produce and label Internet bookmarks in a separate editable 2D "MyCyberspace" map. (Use of such links also automatically indicated in the diary)
27. Accumulation of a daily growing, "Diarysum.html" file, containing the full updated content of the diary.
28. A superordinate metacognitive field/file,"REFLECTION" permitting time indexed quotes from any previous daycard and reflective comments
29. An option for any user/caretaker to publish a clone of the program as designed for a chosen client or target-group, e.g. pre-distribution of most relevant glyph-buttons, hiding unnecessary features for that client/group and naming thematic fields for the expected needs of client or group.
30. An option for any user to offer and cooperate on developing a translation of the user-interface to other languages.
31. An option for any user to suggest/co-design new glyphs, found to be missing
32. A forum, www.phenomenalog.wikispaces.com accessible to all users, to discuss their experience, problems met, and ideas for improvement.
33. Installer for Windows
34. Installer for Macintosh
35. Installer for Windows version fitted to 11inch screensize

APPENDIX B: DESIRED FURTHER FEATURES OF THE DIARY

50. Programming the installer download process, so the number of downloads can be counted, and e-mail address of downloader's are obtained

51. Extension of the present logging of use of own (MyCyberspace) browser links to logging of all primary google search terms

52. Installer for Linux, - not least if the built-in browser can be linux-compatible

53. Option to view the accumulated data-table (* 23) as differently colored curves in weekly, monthly and annual perspectives

54. Option to insert repeated recordings the same day for one or more physiological parameters (e.g. bloodpressure, pulse,glycose etc.) and inspect daily sequence as curves

55. Option to display such daily curves in a format permitting curve comparison on a weekly and monthly basis.

56. Expansion and design-improvements of the glyph-library of typicality's from the present app. 450 to at least a couple of thousands. If we could find some designer educations, where such a project could fit in, it would be a nice way to combine teachers professionalism with student work, - and copy free product.

57. Option for user/caretaker to create own small (7-15 characters) text-buttons for typicalities not covered by preliminary glyph supply.

58. Option for user/caretaker to change and modify coloring of the 16 glyph-button background areas surrounding the main diary field

59. Mind mapping options (I am personally using the proprietary program "Inspiration" and looking for a freeware solution to include something like it in the electronic diary)

60. Translation of user-interface to other languages: Arabic, Danish, French, German, Spanish, Japanese, Chinese.

61. Adaptation of the address-book to report and enable Skype calls directly from telephone numbers in address-book

62. Optional time-indexed sound recording of vocal comments (and skype dialogue), retrievable from daycard

63. Prototyping a cigarette lighter, for wireless triggering of time indexed input of numbered cigaretglyphs

64. Option for telemedical input (cfr * 53,* 54 and * 55)

65. Option for synchronizing diary on laptop with input from mobile (SMS, voice or picture) e.g. iPhone.

66. Option for time indexed glyph and text annotation to zoomable virtual home (2D→3D→ QTVR)

67. Option for time indexed glyph and text annotation to zoomable virtual body (2D→3D→ QTVR)

68. Optional time-indexed links to personal photos on later upload automatically retroactively inserted in the diary for the day and time, when photo was taken

69. Future options of making personal GPS data represented in maps of home or neighbourhood on daycard

70. Future options for (even modest) voice-to-text function – not least relating to input from mobile.

Chapter 29
Integrating Medical Education with Medical Practice:
Role of Web 2.0 Tools

Arindam Basu
University of Canterbury, New Zealand

Billy O' Steen
University of Canterbury, New Zealand

Mary Allan
University of Canterbury, New Zealand

ABSTRACT

Education is essentially a social phenomenon. As such, a social constructivist approach to teaching and learning is highly applicable to all disciplines and especially medicine where most graduates are required to deeply engage with society and need to communicate with a diverse array of people as part of their professional responsibilities. While traditional models of medical education are predicated on the establishment of face-to-face interactions, particularly within teaching hospital settings and residencies, there may be some opportunities to utilize current developments in online social networking technologies to enhance students' and instructors' experiences {references}. A review of social networking in the professional preparation of medical students and their subsequent practices would be helpful in determining the viability of such an approach. In this chapter, we provide a review of two key concepts of online social learning (social presence and media richness), explore how they can be implemented in the current wave of web based collaboration tools, and indicate their place in medical education. We provide a few examplars of how educators are incorporating web based or online social tools in student learning in the context of medical education and indicate some ways to extend this approach further.

INTRODUCTION

Learning in an educational setting typically has a strong social activity component. In medical education, a social constructivist approach, where students learn together to inquire and create knowledge on the basis of their experiences, is appropriate. Medical graduates are professionally required to deeply engage with society and need to

DOI: 10.4018/978-1-60960-097-6.ch029

communicate with a diverse array of people as part of their professional responsibilities. While traditional models of medical education are predicated on the establishment of face-to-face interactions, particularly within teaching hospital settings and residency training programmes, there may be some opportunities to utilize current developments in online social networking technologies to enhance students' and instructors' experiences. The purpose and scope of this chapter is to provide a brief review of the current state of and potential directions for online social networking in medical education.

FROM LEARNING THEORIES TO SOCIAL NETWORKING TECHNOLOGIES

In general, we learn from and with others; learning and therefore education is essentially a social activity. In medicine, the social aspects of learning straddle a broad range of experiential learning with teachers, non-teaching academic staff, other students, and colleagues. In addition to learning from and with others, medical education also involves learning from rich media and experiential learning. For example, many medical students' first encounters with real corpses happen when they enter the grim environment of an anatomy dissection room with its display of dissected human remains. This process of learning anatomy is not limited to in the moment experiences with dissected specimens, the accompanying guidance from a teacher', and collaboration with other students but also includes navigating through richly designed anatomical atlases, detailed radiographs, and computerized tomograms and scanned images that were created prior to the in the moment experiences.

Similarly, there are other learning scenarios when students enter hospital wards with expectations of meeting real patients and these encounters involve not only communicating with the patient, learning from other patients, and simultaneously interacting with the teacher and other students but also engagement with sources of information that have been previously created (charts, records, x-rays, etc). Clinical clerkships also offer this kind of integration of information obtained from collaborating with patients, supervisors, colleagues and media. Thus, throughout their professional careers, from medical studentships and clinical clerkships through to advanced professional continuing medical education, physicians learn using a number of different channels of information that include experience, collaboration, and rich media (sight, sound, and senses). Developments in computer science and theoretical advancements in learning have together contributed significantly to the development of a number of rich media applications that provide opportunities to blend collaborative learning and media analysis in diverse fields of study. Given the way that traditional medical education has sought to teach medical students and physicians how to integrate collaboration, experience, and media analysis, it is conceivable that online activities that combine these three elements could play an important role in the professional learning of medical students.

In general, the increasing role that onlne social networking and rich media applications play in education may be attributed to their strong social presence and media richness. Briefly, Social Presence Theory (Short et al., 1976) is based on the premise that the presence of others around a learner, or social presence, has an important influence on the learning process. This implies that technology that allows both interactivity and a sense of others' presence might be interpreted by the learner to exhibit social presence and therefore might positively influence learning. In support of this construct, a review of the role of social presence in fostering social learning in technology-enhanced environments by Tu (2000) found that social presence was essentially subjective and open to interpretation of the learner and was therefore inherently dynamic. This dynamism of social presence was dependent on three key components: social context, online communication, and interactivity. Tu concludes that when, "one examines computer mediated communication as a learning environment ... social presence must be examined" (2000).

This notion of social presence is suggested by education theorists John Biggs and Catherine Tang (2007) in their model for teaching and learning in tertiary education that is based on social constructive alignment. According to their model, teaching should be aligned with learning so that a learner constructs his/her own meaning through lived experiences and in collaboration with others. For this to happen, the teacher and the learner form part of a social relationship where learning is defined by the social transactions that involve a sharing of skills and knowledge among the teacher, the individual learner, and fellow learners (Biggs & Tang, 2007). These ideas thus support a belief that learning is not only a collaborative activity between different stakeholders (learners, teachers, others) but in addition, learning must take into account the learners' lived experiences. In the context of medical education and a physician/surgeon's learning process, this integration of social interaction and lived experiences is already seen as an effective approach. Therefore, new media and emergent online social networking that are used to build on this accepted approach can potentially be seamlessly integrated in medical education.

It may be noted that while the proponents of Social Presence Theory state the importance of a social presence, they do not specify that this strictly means that the physical presence of the teacher and co-learners facilitates learning. Desirable or not, it is not necessarily a requirement. In other words, any form of social transaction or a simulation that facilitates the construction of meaning from lived experiences and allows for collaboration could be enough for constructivist learning, and therefore potentially align with Biggs and Tang's ideas for effective teaching in higher education. Thus, to use Tu's expression, only the "salience

of an interpersonal relationship" is integral to teaching and learning (2000). Hence, those who intend to use technology to create or simulate the social presence and foster communication need to go beyond static presentation of data. At the least, learning content designers must enable interactivity among students and instructors and there is an indication that the content used for interactivity must be media-rich as opposed to the lean nature of text-based media applications (e.g., emails, documents, or static images).

This is related to the second applicable theoretical construct – media richness. Dennis and Kinney (1998) proposed the Media Richness Theory (also referred to as Information Richness Theory), which is a framework that differentiates media as to its ability to facilitate changes in understanding among communicators (Dennis & Valacich, 1999). Within their framework, they suggest that face-to-face (FTF) is the gold standard of communication (Nardi & Whittaker, 2002; Wainfan L. & Davis P.K., 2004) and all other media rank somewhere below it. Prevalent perceptions about FTF interactions suggest that they provide the richest and most effective medium for communication because they contain verbal and non-verbal cues (Billinghurst & Kato, 1999; Daft & Lengel, 1986; Daft & Wiginton, 1979), while at the same time creating a sense of "being there" in each other's presence, or sharing a space (Goffman, 1963; Heeter, 1992; Schroeder, 2006).

The features below highlight these social processes and the non-verbal exchange of information involved in communication between people in FTF communication:

1. Synchronous temporal turn taking interactions that enables the smooth alternation of speaker and listener who are co-present (Bosch, Oostdijk, & Ruiter, 2004),

2. Multidimensional information afforded by Mehrabian's "3 Vs" (Verbal, Vocal and Visual) (1971), and

Figure 1. Media Richness and sense of shared space

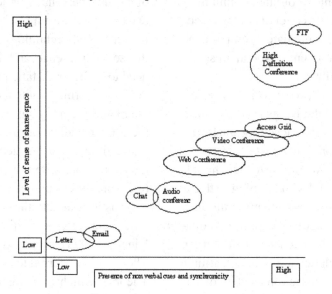

3. A sense of being with another or what Heeter (1992) refers to as presence and co–presence (Goffman, 1963; Schroeder, 2006).

These features are used by Media Richness Theory to rate different media according to the richness of information that they transmit (A.R. Dennis & J.S. Valacich, 1999). In classifying communication media according to their provision of information richness, Daft & Lengel (1986) rank FTF as the richest and then in decreasing richness: telephone, personal documents such as letters or memos, impersonal documents, and numeric documents. The differences in richness measured illustrates a medium's capacity for immediate feedback or synchronicity and the number of social cues and channels transmitted. High levels of richness contribute to an improved sense of shared space, which is the crux of any communication activity.

Building on prior work by Baltes et al. (2002, p.159), and Wainfan and Davis (2004, p.5) that described relationships between degrees of synchronisation and levels of non-verbal cues across various media, Figure 1 shows the relationship between levels of non-verbal cues and synchronisation, and their creation of a sense of shared space.

The correlation between media richness and the levels of shared space can be explained using Social Presence Theory which indicates the degree to which communicants perceive the presence of the other (Biocca, Harms, & Burgoon, 2003; Goffman, 1963; Short, Williams, & B., 1976). It appears that the more social cues that are transmitted and the more synchronicity that is present, then there will be more opportunity for people to perceive each other's presence and experience a feeling of participating in a shared space of communication. Furthermore, the higher the levels of richness and creation of a sense of space, then the closer that mediated communication will resemble FTF (Allan & Thorns, 2009). Social networking technologies, then, have the potential for the facilitation of: social perceptions, socio-emotional communication, a positive socio-emotional climate, and the perceived ability to evaluate others' deception and expertise (Dennis & Valacich, 1999). Further, Dennis and Valacich identified five technology characteristics that can potentially affect communication in those ways. These include: immediacy of feedback, symbol

Figure 2. Quadrants of rich media versus social presence axes

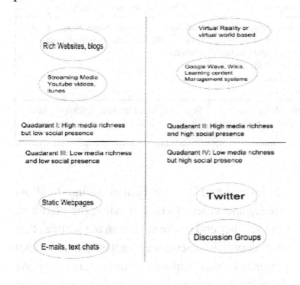

variety, parallelism, rehearsability, and reprocessibility. Of these, immediacy of feedback appears to have the most promise for medical education.

Immediacy of feedback indicates the extent to which the technology allows users to provide feedback and is a measure of the technology's interactivity with the viewer. In the context of social networking in higher education, such immediacy may be achieved by the ability of the student to interact with fellow students and the teacher in real time with a highly rich media tool such as videoconferencing or Twitter and asynchronous interactivity with web-based forums, email, Face-

book, and other formats. This relationship among technology tools and the theories of Social Presence and Media Richness is illustrated in Figure 2.

In higher education, the use of online and Web 2.0 tools are increasing at a rapid pace, as is their adoption in clinical practice. Several features of Social Presence Theory and Media Richness Theory are applicable that may explain the popularity of online social networking and Web 2.0 tools being used. From a social learning and social presence perspective, these include immediacy of feedback, symbol variety, and reprocessibility of the technology. In a technology context, these appear to be key features that would foster social constructivism and would need to be included in implementing Biggs and Tang's (2007) teaching and learning model.

Table 2 illustrates how the two related axes – that of social presence and media richness are related to the education of medical professionals. As can be seen from this table, at various stages, and with various learning contents, different learning styles might utilize different factors that may be more firmly rooted in either media richness and social presence.

If online social collaboration tools and learning in medical topics are plotted along two axes – increasing social presence versus media richness, it is possible to map out tools that fall under one or other quadrant. For instance, tools that

Table 1. Learning theories to support using technology in medical education

Learning Theory Applicable to Using Technology in Medical Education	
Social Presence Theory (SPT)	SPT essentially posits that effectiveness of communication is dependent on the level of social presence. According to this theory, face-to-face interaction has the highest social presence and the further people get away from each other, the effectiveness of the interaction decreases.
Media Richness Theory (MRT)	MRT suggests that task performance will be improved when task needs are matched to a medium's richness. Media capable of sending rich information (such as media that streams simultaneous text, visual, and auditory feeds) are better suited to equivocal tasks or tasks that require multiple interpretations for available information compared to those that do not.

Table 2. The contexts of media richness and social presence in medical education

Axis	Social presence important	Social presence not important
Availability of rich media important or a feature	Learning anatomy dissection, learning surgical techniques, clinical clerkships, internship training, learning from patients and charts by the bedside in collaboration with colleagues and superiors in the field, conference presentations, attending classes	Learning solo, using videos, atlases, picture books, audio files, etc. Essentially personal learning
Availability of rich media not a prominent feature or important	Learning clinical decision making in collaboration with other students, or preceptors, group study	Text book based reading, reflections, note taking by hand

actively use the simultaneous presence of multiple users (e.g., Twitter) to push content to the web are rich in social presence but not in the type of media since most of the work is done over short messages of 140 characters with low resolution and graphics. Recently, newer channels have emerged that combine some aspects of both media richness and strong social presence. For example, Google Buzz does not impose any restriction on the number of characters that can be transmitted and is sophisticated enough to allow images and videos to be posted on the platform. On the other end of the spectrum are sources that offer very rich experiences both in terms of social presence by allowing numerous visitors traversing the same digital "landscape" and sharing conversations with rich media that mimics or simulates the real world closely. Second Life or other virtual world platforms are examples of these sources.

Table 3. How videoconferencing, twitter, facebook, Second life, and now Google Wave weave into the concepts of social presence theory and media richness theory

Concepts	Media Richness	Social Presence
Videoconferencing over internet protocol (Google Chat, Skype, Adobe connect pro, etc)	High media richness, as video/audio can be relayed real time as well as participants can watch movies or multimedia applications while discussing some things together	Strong social presence, where the images and video feed of the inviduals can be transmitted in real time
Twitter	Since twitter is essentially a string of short messages that are sent over cell phones, webpages, media richness is not a feature of twitter	However, collaboration in linking different individuals and users or in the context of education, linking students with each other and students with teachers or fostering team teaching can be highly thematic for using Twitter in a classroom setting
Facebook	Rich media experience that allows posting of text files, audio files, and video files and ability to share with colleagues and students	High social collaboration and enables social presence by allowing several people to simultaneously editing documents.
Youtube	Rich media experience as youtube in the form of streaming media (audio and video media)	Youtube by itself does not provide much opportunities for social presence; however, it is possible to either watch youtube together in a classroom setting or watch youtube videos as part of a chat experience or simultaneously watch youtube videos online. Little social presence and asynchronous, but a social network can be built around youtube.

continued on following page

Table 3. continued

Concepts	Media Richness	Social Presence
Collaborative bookmarking (deli-cious, Connotea, etc)	These are essentially collections of bookmarks or hyperlinks to various resources in the web. By itself these services do not provide any level of media other than textual links. Therefore, they have very poor media richness. However, several educators use them to foster collabora-tion among students and helps the educators to assess some form of internet based research for their students.	Social collaboration is a major theme in col-laborative bookmarking. Therefore, the issue of social presence is comparable as to what hap-pens when several individuals get together to develop or construct or put together resources. Similar to wikis. Like wiki, and commenters on blogs, this medium too, is based on asynchro-nous collaboration.
Blogs	Provides high levels of media richness as blogs can be audio blogs (podcasts), video blogs (vodcasts), inclusion of audio and video feeds in blogs, or incorporation of other types of media	Blogs provide very high levels of social pres-ence for both bloggers as well as users and visitors of these blogs. Moreover, emergent media such as real time collaboration tools such as chats and collaborative diagramming, phone calls), etc can be incorporated in blogs and blogs allow streaming media. Blogs are essentially asynchronous modes of presentation of information and interactivity
Wikis	Possible to embed media during writing (ie read write web). Implementation of rich media	Social presence is a strong feature of wikis as they provide high levels of collaboration among members of the wiki. However, most wikis are asynchronous because most wikis do not allow simultaneous editing
Email based groups	If the group uses html based emails to com-municate among themselves, rich media can be embedded or links to rich media can be embed-ded in emails and transmitted.	It's an asynchronous mode of commuication. For large groups, social presence is featured in the form of active participation of many members
Plain text email	Very little media richness, other than through at-tachments sent in the form of audio files, video files, or other packaged programmes	Minimum sense of social presence, other than textual communication with the recipient, mostly on a one on one basis or reception of one emai from one contact. It's also asynchronous
Websites	Can provide rich media by including audio & video files in the webpage itself and incorpo-rated players that can play the files directly or stream media directly	Issues of social presence (ie one or more individuals) simultaneously browsing a page and providing interaction is not a feature at all. Asynchronous mode of communication between the author of a website and the user who views the site
Html formatted email	Intermediate leve of media richness, because the audio and video files can be played directly from the html formatted email as well as links that can directly link to resources	Ability to learn something in the presence of more than one individual is limited, other than continuously emailing the other learners. Lim-ited sense of social presence
Virtual worlds	Very high sense of media richness because videos can be played in virtual worlds, audio can be played	Individuals through their digital alter egos or avatars can "together" watch or listen to these video/audio feeds, as well as alter them, write on whiteboards, etc. Social presence is a strong feature and virtual worlds can operate in both asynchronous or synchronous modes depending on how they are used.
Social computer games (such as World of Warcraft)	Social, collaborative role playing games (RPGs) provide very high levels of media richness by incorporating sound, images, and video media in them.	Very high as players can play the games together although they may not change anything together.

Just as the sets of online collaboration tools can be considered under the rubric of social presence and media richness, the learning processes in medicine too can be conceptualized along these complementary axes. Thus, framing learning styles, learning content, learning contexts, and tools of learning along a common framework may help an educator select tools that seem most appropriate for specific learning situations. For example, in any setting, correspondence using emails alone may not help attain the desired teaching and learning objectives when multimodality of user experiences determine how 21st century learners are going to approach a specific topic. In other circumstances, where students need to internalize and obtain necessary conceptual background knowledge (e.g., the mechanism of action of pharmaceuticals), highly social networking tools might distract them from grasping the core concepts. Therefore, tools such as information-rich web pages, graphics, and streaming media such as You Tube or podcasting may help to reinforce key concepts but they do not necessarily bring in social presence or social learning. Yet other circumstances may require using tools that have both rich media experiences and social presence, such as videoconferencing over the web with live patients or viewing clinical images and videos for learning clinical medicine, or practicing specific procedures. The optimum combination of providing both rich media as well as devleoping the sense of social presence is ofen created by using tools such as online, virtual world implementations. In the context of medical education, such implementations may be in the form of simulations or interactions in Second Life.

The contextual nature of these various tools are apparent in different learning situations. For example, a group of Polish anatomists (Glinkowsi & Ciszek, 2007) described a curriculum where they created an exhaustive bank of resources on anatomy including atlases, tests (quizzes), and galleries that the students used in addition to their regular dissection, atlas based and lecture

based course implementations. A brief review of their course revealed high student usage and satisfaction with the course. This was an example where rich media alone presented asynchronously provided an opportunity for each student to learn on his or her own time and not necessarily with others. There are yet other instances where the incorporation of social networking technology is essential to teaching core concepts. An example of this might be where an educator is planning to teach clinical decision making using clinical simulations in a multimedia rich environment. In such circumstances, it is necessary for the student to learn in collaboration with the teacher and fellow students on the process of clinical decision making and both the media and the social presence of other learners and the teacher is an essential component of the learning process. Therefore, which tools to use will depend on the teaching and learning context, desired learning outcomes, and available technology.

SOCIAL NETWORKING TECHNOLOGIES IN MEDICAL EDUCATION AND TRAINING

Mcleans et al. (2007) have asserted, "The medical community needs to be aware of these [Web 2.0] technologies and their increasing role in providing health information 'any time, any place'" (p. 174).

Developing a social constructivist paradigm, McLean and his colleagues with the Australian Government Department of Health and Ageing frame the connection of Web 2.0 and education with, "It has been stated that students of all ages learn best when immersed within a culturally and socially rich environment in which learners and peers are committed to achieving the same goals and can regulate each others' performance, and therefore the use of Web 2.0 tools has potential to both liberate and tie learners together in dynamic learning communities" (Ibid, p. 176). In their view, it is incumbent on the medical community to explore the possibilities of using Web 2.0 technologies and state:

Whether these technologies will (r)evolutionise medical education and information distribution will only be known in hindsight. More evaluation of their use in clinical practice and medical education is required, but medical practitioners and educators cannot afford to ignore these developments (Ibid, p. 177).

That medical students are embracing and not ignoring Web 2.0 technologies was made clear in Sandars and Schroter's 2007 study of 3,000 medical students and 3,000 medical practitioners in the UK and their awareness of and interest in using those technologies both personally and academically. They found that both groups had a high awareness of and high interest in Web 2.0 technologies but did not feel that they had the knowledge or skills to use those technologies in either learning or teaching about the medical profession. Like McLean et al., Sandars and Schroter believed that the medical community needs to consider these technologies for education but needs training to do so.

In another study involving medical students, Thompson et al. (2008) collected data from 363 medical students and residents in the US to determine if and how they were using social networking technologies, specifically Facebook, and how that usage might relate to medical professionalism. They found that 44.5% of study participants had Facebook accounts and that activity on those accounts tended to decrease as graduation from their programs approached. Further, because "a significant proportion [of the Facebook sites] had subjectively inappropriate content, Accreditation Council for Graduate Medical Education competencies in professionalism must include instruction on the intersection of personal and professional identities" (Thompson et al., 2008, p. 954). And, it is within this need to educate medical students about professionalism and social networking that the authors see an opportunity for inclusion in medical education:

Since students and residents are participating in online social networks, medical educators need to examine how they can proactively acknowledge and use such sites to teach about professionalism. This could include both discussion and mentoring" (Ibid, p. 956).

Thus, with a consensus from those publications about the need and possibility of using Web 2.0 technologies in medical education, Boulous and Weaver (2007) provide a comprehensive review of the types of technologies that might be most suitable for medicine as well as pointing toward Web 3.0 on the horizon. However, to prevent a rushed adoption of these technologies without due diligence as has happened in other areas of education (Edmundson, 2008; Oppenheimer, 2003), the authors wisely advise consideration with, "Although the tools presented in this review look very promising and potentially fit for purpose in many health care applications and scenarios, careful thinking, testing and evaluation research are still needed in order to establish 'best practice models' for leveraging these emerging technologies to boost our teaching and learning productivity, foster stronger 'communities of practice', and support continuing medical education/professional development (CME/CPD) and patient education" (Boulous and Weaver, 2007, p. 2).

Beyond medical education, these collaborative, and immersive technologies are now being used in the context of the professional traning of physicians, surgeons, and nurses. At the University of Canterbury Health Sciences Centre in New Zealand, tools are being developed to supplement manequin-based simulations and are aimed at teaching clinical decision making skills to first year post graduate residents and nurses. For both groups of health professionals, this simulation teaches students to effectively select the most appropriate treatment option, but also has them respond to changes of the patient, which occur due to the computer programme responding to the students' choices. This provides students with a game-like scenario to rehearse and practice creating channels of communication among themselves.

SUMMARY

Learning to interact, create meaning, apply learning to real world situations, and create new knowledge is essentially a social activity, where students and teachers build knowledge together. This is particularly relevant in the context of medical education where students develop into professionals whose main objective is to interact with patients, other professionals and bring about change in their patients. Therefore, it is essential that medical students learn how to work effectively in a collaborative environment.

In theory, richness of media and social presence highlight the role of social aspects of learning with technology in various contexts. Social presence indicates that as learners study together, they build "presence" around each other. The social presence can not only be a physical nearness to each other but in addition, it may also mean a "nearness" on some other aspects, as fostered in discussion groups, intellectual proximity, or as in case of digital learning, use of digtal spaces where students can form groups and post observations and knowledge bits. However, social presence does not necessarily predicate a physical proximity.

The other aspect of social learning includes richness of media. Media richness is highest with face to face communication, when a number of different ways to convey knowledge and ideas can be adopted; however, media "richness" decreases as one moves from face to face interactions to more text based interactions where textual correspondence is the only mode of learning and teaching. In the context of learning and teaching, these theoretical aspects have been implemented in various ways, particularly in creating and using tool sets for online social learning and to some extent in learning content management systems. In the context of medical education, different

learning and teaching styles fit into a matrix where either social presence dominates or media richness is the key factor, or both, or neither. Learning situations such as learning clinical skills from ward morning rounds, grand rounds in hospitals, learnng operative skills in operation rooms, handling emergencies, anatomical dissections are all learning situations where a high amount of social presence and media richness are necessary. On the other hand, for understaning some key concepts or thought based objects on physiology or biochemical pathways, or understanding the drug dosages, one needs individual understanding. Low levels of media richness is enough to learn form these objects, and richness of social presence may only distract the learner so low levels of social presence is even desirable.

These theoretical constructs are now possible to be used within the context of onlne social learning particularly adaptable to the context of medical education. Specifically, web based online social networking include activities such as maintaining and responding to blogs, identifying web based resources and sharing addresses or hyperlinks to these resources in a shared space (collaborative tagging and sharing of bookmarks), use of wikis where a common shared space is used to write collaboratively, and use of common shared file spaces and videos. The keywords in this new paradigm of learning are "sharing" & "collaboration". The various tools are now widely used in a variety of contexts in medical education and several sterling examples are readily available where the users are deploying these tools for day to day teaching and learning practices in medicine.

The power of online social collaboration and the use of Web 2.0 tools are now well established in medical education. These can be extended now to foster interprofessional communication and as part of a larger scheme of lifelong learning for medical professionals as well. There are ongoing experiments with the use of augemented and virtual reality based scenario development. This work seeks to simulate clinical encounters such as an emergency ward where an emergency physician faces a patient with acute respiratory distress and sets up the next steps of management. Advances in computer based communicaitons and social networking have created opportunities to have students experience the real world of medicine within the safer learning environment of medical education.

REFERENCES

Adams, J. (2006). The part played by instructional media in distance education. *SIMILE: Studies In Media & Information Literacy Education, 6*(2), 1–12. doi:10.3138/sim.6.2.001

Allan, M., & Thorns, D. (2009). Being Face to Face - A state of Mind or Technological Design. In B. Whitworth & A. (de) Moor (Eds.), *Handbook of Research on Socio Technical Designing and Social Networking Systems* (pp. 440-454). Hershey PA: IGI Global Publications.

Baltes, B. B., Dickson, M. W., Sherman, M. P., Bauer, C. C., & LaGanke, J. S. (2002). Computer-Mediated Communication and Group Decision Making: A Meta-Analysis. *Organizational Behavior and Human Decision Processes, 87*(1), 156–179. doi:10.1006/obhd.2001.2961

Beldarrain, Y. (2006). Distance education trends: Integrating new technologies to foster student interaction and collaboration. *Distance Education, 27*(2), 139–153. doi:10.1080/01587910600789498

Bennett, E., & Maniar, N. (2008). *Are videoed lectures an effective teaching tool? Biggs, J., & Tang, C. (2007). Teaching for Quality Learning at University: What the Student does (Society for Research Into Higher Education)*. Mcgraw-Hill Publ.Comp.

Billinghurst, M., & Kato, H. (1999). *Collaborative Mixed Reality- Merging Real and Virtual Worlds*. Paper presented at the First International Symposium on Mixed Reality (ISMR 99), Berlin.

Biocca, F., Harms, C., & Burgoon, J. K. (2003). Towards a More Robust Theory and Measure of Social Presence: Review and Suggested Criteria. *Presence (Cambridge, Mass.), 12*(5), 456–480. doi:10.1162/105474603322761270

Bosch, L. t., Oostdijk, N., & Ruiter, J. P. (2004). *Durational aspects of turn-taking in spontaneous face-to-face and telephone dialogues*. Paper presented at the Text, Speech and Dialogue. Retrieved from http://www.hcrc.ed.ac.uk/comic/documents/

Boulous, M., & Wheeler, S. (2007). The emerging Web 2.0 social software: an enabling suite of sociable technologies in health and health care education. *Health Information and Libraries Journal, 24*, 2–23. doi:10.1111/j.1471-1842.2007.00701.x

Brahler, C., Peterson, N., & Johnson, E. (1999). Developing on-line learning materials for higher education: An overview of current issues. Educational Technology and Society, Vol. 2 (2). Retrieved on 5 October 2009, from http://www.ifets.info/journals/2_2/jayne_brahler.html

Campbell, G. (2005). Podcasting in education. *EDUCAUSE, Nov/Dec, 5.*

Chan, A., Lee, M., & McLoughlin, C. (2006). Everyone's learning with podcasting: A Charles Sturt University experience. *Who's learning? Whose technology? Proceedings ascilite Sydney 2006.*

Chang, C. (2004). Constructing a Streaming Video-Based Learning Forum for Collaborative Learning. *Journal of Educational Multimedia and Hypermedia, 13*(3), 245–264.

Chang, S. (2007). *Academic perceptions of the use of Lectopia: A University of Melbourne example.*

Daft, R. L., & Lengel, R. H. (1986). Organisational Information Requirements, Media Richness and Structural Design. *Management Science, 32*(5), 554–571. doi:10.1287/mnsc.32.5.554

Daft, R. L., & Wiginton, J. (1979). Language and Organisation. *Academy of Management Review, 4*(2), 171–191. doi:10.2307/257772

Dennis, A. R., & Valacich, J. S. (1999). *Rethinking Media Richness: Towards a Theory of Media Synchronicity.* Paper presented at the 32nd Hawaii International Conference on System Sciences, Hawaii.

Dennis, A. R., & Valacich, J. S. (1999). *Rethinking media richness: Towards a theory of media synchronicity.*

Edmundson, M. (2008). Dwelling in possibilities. *Chronicle of Higher Education.* Retrieved on 12 November 2009 from http://chronicle.com/article/Dwelling-in-Possibilities/7083/

Feeney, L., Reynolds, P., Eaton, K., & Harper, J. (2008). *A description of the new technologies used in transforming dental education.*

Goffman, E. (1963). *Behaviour in Public Places: Notes on the Social Organisation of Gatherings.* London: The Free Press of Glenco.

Hartsell, T., & Yuen, S. (2006). Video streaming in online learning. *AACE Journal, 14*(1), 31–43.

Heeter, C., 1(2), pp. (1992). Being There: The subjective experience of presence. *Presence (Cambridge, Mass.), 1*(2), 262–271.

Maag, M. (2006). iPod, uPod? An emerging mobile learning tool in nursing education and students' satisfaction.

McLean, R., Richards, B., & Wardman, J. (2007). The effect of Web 2.0 on the future of medical practice and education: Darwikian evolution or folksonomic revolution? *The Medical Journal of Australia, 187*(3), 174–177.

McLuhan, M. (2003). *Understanding media: The extension of man - critical edition.* Berkeley, CA: Gingko Press.

Mehrabian, A. (1971). *Silent messages.* Belmont, CA: Wadsworth.

Morisse, K., & Ramm, M. (2007). *Teaching via Podcasting: One year of Experience with Work-flows.* Tools and Usage in Higher Education.

Nardi, B. A., & Whittaker, S. (2002). The Place of Face-To- Face Communication in Distributed Work. In Hins, P. J., & Kiesler, S. (Eds.), *Distributed Work* (pp. 83–113). Cambridge, MA: The MIT Press.

Oppenheimer, T. (2003). *The Flickering Mind: The False Promise of Technology in the Classroom and How Learning Can Be Saved.* New York: Random House.

Phillips, R., Gosper, M., McNeill, M., Woo, K., Preston, G., & Green, D. (2007). Staff and student perspectives on web based lecture technologies: Insights into the great divide. Proceedings ascilite Singapore 2007, 854-864.

Sandars, J., & Schroter, S. (2007). Web 2.0 technologies for undergraduate and postgraduate medical education: An online survey. *Postgraduate Medical Journal, 83,* 759–762. doi:10.1136/pgmj.2007.063123

Schroeder, R. (2006). Being There Together and the Future of Connected Presence. *Presence (Cambridge, Mass.), 15*(4), 438–454. doi:10.1162/pres.15.4.438

Shephard, K. (2003). Questioning, promoting and evaluating the use of streaming video to support student learning. *British Journal of Educational Technology, 34*(3), 295–308. doi:10.1111/1467-8535.00328

Short, J., Williams, E., & B., C. (1976). *The Social Psychology of Telecommunications.* New York: John Wiley.

Thompson, L., Dawson, K., Ferdig, R., Black, E., Boyer, J., Coutts, J., & Black, N. P. (2008). The intersection of online social networking with medical professionalism. *Journal of General Internal Medicine, 23*(7), 954–957. doi:10.1007/s11606-008-0538-8

Tu, C.-H. (2000). On-line learning migration: from social learning theory to social presence theory in a CMC environment. *Journal of Network and Computer Applications, 23*(1), 27–37. doi:10.1006/jnca.1999.0099

Wainfan, L., & Davis, P. K. (2004). *Challenges in Virtual Collaboration: Videoconferencing, Audio conferencing, and Computer-Mediated Communications.* Santa Monica: RAND National Defense Research Institute.

Wainfan. L., & K., D. P. (2004). *Challenges in Virtual Collaboration: Videoconferencing, Audio conferencing, and Computer-Mediated Communications.* Santa Monica: RAND National Defense Research Institute.

Chapter 30
Ubiquitous Information Therapy Service through Social Networking Libraries:
An Operational Web 2.0 Service Model

Vahideh Zarea Gavgani
Tabriz University of Medical Sciences, Iran

ABSTRACT

This chapter introduces a model for Information Therapy service through social networks. It discusses how health care providers including physicians, medical specialist and residents can prescribe reliable, evidence based health information to the patients in web 2.0 environment. How evidence based health information incorporated into freely available health information sources? How health information is disseminated to general public through collaboration of health information professional and health care professionals? How health literacy can be improved through social networking health information? And, how user driven health information is disseminated through web 2.0? Recent advances in Information and Communication Technology especially social applications of web 2.0 have given new possibilities and abilities to librarians in rendering better, faster and ubiquitous information services. At the same time, it has created an equivalent right to information for patients/care givers and health providers. Nowadays, the importance of availability and accessibility of health information in healthcare system is realized and emphasized by healthcare providers, policy makers as well as consumers. Provision of reliable, timely, evidence based, right health information to patients/caregivers/consumers in the course of Information Therapy is a necessity for National Health Systems in all countries. This chapter deals with the definition of Information Therapy, importance of information therapy, changes in the preference of information users on how to access right information, Web 2.0, application of Web 2.0 in rendering Information Therapy Service, and a proposal model for Information Therapy service through Web 2.0.

DOI: 10.4018/978-1-60960-097-6.ch030

INTRODUCTION

Recent developments in applications of Web 2.0, social networking and mobile computer technology have created radical change in communication in any sector and field. Web 2.0 tools are used in health and medicine to provide rapid and ubiquitous services for health care consumers and health care providers. Web 2.0 applications have influenced most of today's professions and reshaped their practice, direction and relationships. Medicine 2.0, health 2.0 and library 2.0 are instances of application of web 2.0 tools in practice of medicine, healthcare and library services.

The clear fact is that in none of the new born facets of medicine, healthcare and library built in 2.0 environments, the philosophy and the nature of medicine, healthcare and library are changed. Web 2.0 makes services more social, democratized, connected, available, transparent, interactive and user-centered.

In conventional medicine, physicians always are at the top of pyramid, from which knowledge and practice flow to the patients. They diagnose, they give treatment, information and instruction to patients, and patient should only do whatever is prescribed. In other words, conventional medicine was physician centered and patients were known as passive segments in health care systems rather than active partners.

In the same track, with one way traffic approach, the library's rules and regulations are rigid. Human knowledge and information are organized with controlled vocabularies (pre/post coordination) like MeSh (Medical Subject Headings) that gives some key terms to user to retrieve the information or access the library's material. In other word, in order to access information a user have to think (set his mind) in a way that librarians have already thought and organized the information in that order. In the traditional library and information service, particularly in developing countries, librarians/information pro-

fessionals, play a passive role rather than active in information services.

One of the most substantial achievements of Web 2.0 is that the relationship of the segments in the Web 2.0 based environments is, being two-way/interactive, virtual/remote rather than being in physical contact. Flow of service, knowledge and information is free, transparent, integrated, shared, more democratized, unbiased, participated and more interacted, rather than paternal relationship. It is the right platform for patient centered medicine and user centered library service.

In the course of patient-centered medicine the emerging Information Therapy approach requires a more accessible, rapid, easy, free from commercial bias, transparent, everywhere and every time available, right and timely health information at the moment of care for both patients and physicians to ensure a risk free and shared/right decision making about health problem.

"The challenge is to ensure that everyone in the world can have access to clean, clear knowledge - a basic human right, and a public health need as important as access to clean, clear water, and much more easily achievable." (Pang 2006)

Today, 1.3 billion people lack access to basic health care services. And many more are at risk of receiving poor quality care. A major contributing factor is lack of access to relevant, reliable healthcare information. (HIFA2015, 2008)

To make correct and clear information available for patients and public, librarians prove to have a pivotal and indispensible role to play. Medical/Clinical Librarians, Subject Specialist Librarians in academic, public, medical and health libraries providing information and evidence for physicians and patients through conventional library service(Davidoff and Florance, 2000; William and Zipperer, 2003; Feldman 2003; Weightman 2005), SDI and in some cases through new born Library 2.0 services like library's wiki, Blog,

Face book, etc. However, in today's health care system, patients and physicians need an integral, interactive, easy to use and easy to access platform for information rather than Google amount of information in various format and degree of reliability. Public in general and patients in particular need right information that is easy to understand, evidence based and freely available at the time of care, in order to make a right health decision and manage their health problem(s). But, the question is that is the freely available health information reliable and evidence based? How can a patient access the right information? Do the conventional library services ensure the dissemination of right health information to right health consumer in the right time? How Web 2.0 enhances the dissemination of reliable health information to all through library service?

CURRENT SITUATION OF HEALTH INFORMATION LIBRARY SERVICES AND VISION OF WEB 2.0 BASED HEALTH INFORMATION SERVICES

Librarians as information professional, play a passive role rather than active in information service. They provide health/medical information to their user by a request for information. Usually the information service is rendered based on the availability of information in libraries holdings or consortia.

The library's place and space is limited to physical space of library, a user needs to approach a library to receive health information. Even in Web 1.0, a request for information has to be sent to librarian and the answer will be received from a proper channel such as a printed hand out or by e-mail.

Information dissemination is local rather than global, every library and information center offers information service to its local, regional or national (in case of a national library or informa-

tion center) community. The health and health information services need to be global and without boundaries.

Information is costly and the information sources are not available for everyone, freely. Universities and organizations subscribe to high impact, peer reviewed and accredited journals, based on a limited budget that has been allocated for. They make these resources available to their community by password. The image of chaining the books in middle age's libraries (Churches) is being observed now in the digital age by username and password.

Sources of information are isolated, information is stored in and delivered from separate tools and environments, traditional encyclopedias, journals; books have been incorporated in Web 1.0 with electronic/online format and a user needs to search for information in various places with different strategies. In addition, information is usually offered through different devices like web site, e-mail, mobile-phone, and fax. Therefore, a patient or a physician needs to access information from different files located in different environments.

Health literacy is not a guarantee, in traditional library/information service because in conventional information/library service area, information and knowledge is exclusive rather than being democratized.

In contrast Web 2.0 is a social, user driven, free, ubiquitous environment for dissemination of health information. It ensures democratic flow of information as well as information for all and health literacy. In Web 2.0 librarians and information professionals have the opportunity to play an active role rather than passive. They do not need to sit in the library's physical space and wait for users to come to library and request a piece of information. They can develop user friendly social platforms in Web 2.0 environment and reach out to the people who need information, at any level and category, from general public, patients and care givers to professionals. They can discover health information need of health consumers, patients and public from the news and statistical data published by the WHO, NHS, CMS, IOM, CDC, governmental bodies and organizations or conduct a survey study, then search for the relevant, evidence based, reliable information, restore, reconvert, reform and republish the outcomes to the right contact in Web 2.0 environment. For instance, climate change related diseases are global diseases, and everyone in the world can use such information in the during an epidemic season. An active information provider is aware of the global health problems as well as sources of right information. She/he can provide right information and deliver to the web 2.0 based platform in the benefit of physicians (who may prescribe information following a diagnosis), patients/health consumers (who will receive IP) and general public (who are health literate, interested in gaining information to prevent and control the health problems). Prostate Cancer is another example; the cost of treatment for Prostate Cancer is high, while a right information at the time of care can prevent and help the patients to change the behaviors and make better choices.

A Model for rendering Information Therapy services using Web 2.0 Technology would be an idea for libraries in knowledge sharing era and interactive social networked environment to play their indispensible role in dissemination of right health information for their universal user community.

The pushing Idea behind the proposed model is that the advent of Web 2.0 applications should enable health care professionals and patients to answer their related questions in a more efficient, reliable, connected, and interacted way than have already been possible.

OBJECTIVES OF THE STUDY

The study aims to find out:

1. How Web 2.0 applications like blogs and wikis can be used in Information Therapy Service
2. How health providers and information providers can collaboratively facilitate the flow of right information to right patients through web 2.0.
3. How Web 2.0 provides a proper channel and source for information therapy service.
4. How evidence based health information can be incorporated in freely accessible information on the Web.

Background of the study:

There are many studies on the application of Web 2.0 in library services (Gavgani,Vishwa, 2008; Barsky, 2006) in the relevant literatures, but no study has even addressed service model for information therapy service in Web 2.0 environment. A ubiquitous and social service model for Information Therapy (Ix) or health information to patients proves to be indispensable for right dissemination of right information to right person in healthcare context.

Information Therapy is a recent approach in medicine; therefore a comprehensive definition of Information Therapy will give better clarity to understand its meaning, why patients/caregivers need health Information, how patient's preference in access to the health information changes, and how availability and accessibility of information on the Net especially through Web 2.0 impacts the preference of patients on demanding for health information.

WHAT IS INFORMATION THERAPY?

The concept of Information Therapy in medical science is almost a recent one. Its entrance to medical science is synchronized with the IOM health care quality initiative (IOM, 2001) that emphasizes patients' deprivation of up-to-date health information and role of information in quality of health care. Of course, the practice of information therapy in one of its many forms, formally or informally, has been in vogue since time immemorial.

Information Therapy is utilization of evidence-based, timely, personalized right health information at the moment of care by patients and caregivers to help a right medical decision making and to prevent the likely medical errors. Health information can be prescribed by the concerned physician at the moment of care and during clinical visit or can be searched and accessed by the patient/consumer before consulting physicians. Utilization of health information is not limited to the stage of onset of diseases or after diagnosis, it can be used in the stage of prevention and in daily lifestyle to ensure health for all, healthy community and healthy healthcare system. Information Therapy may take place where the patient needs are limited to appropriate information to solve his/her health care needs (also labeled clinical counseling). There are many common diseases where there is no effective medication or surgical cure (e.g. Irritable Bowel Syndrome) and counseling (particularly making the patients aware of the origin and nature of the disease) is the only therapy.

Information Therapy has been previously defined as follows: "Information therapy is the prescription of evidence-based medical information to a specific patient, caregiver, or consumer at just the right time to help the person make a specific health decision or behavior change." (Kemper-Metler, 2002). However, Information Therapy is an umbrella concept that covers various form of use of information in healthcare. It can be prescribed to a specific patient or a group of patients (Gavgani, 2009).

Information Therapy and dissemination of right health information at the right time can prevent onset of diseases and control the progress of diseases through awareness and behaviors change. It also can reduce the risk of misdiagnosis/medical errors through patients' attitude in/while taking their health history and their partnership in decision making about health problem. In addition, the most important and primary rights of any human being are the right to health and the right to information. Thus, Information Therapy service provides a right track towards both human right to medical information and right to health.

PATIENTS' PREFERENCE IN ACCESSING HEALTH INFORMATION

There are many choices for consumers to access health information. Patients may seek for health information through media such as TV, newspaper, books, family, friends, other co-patients (who had/have the same ill-health), doctors, etc.

Patients have more confidence on their doctors as the reliable sources of health information. However there are many obstacles for physicians in patient education/giving health information to patients. Doctors do not have time to access, appraise, and offer information/evidence to their patients in the limited visiting time. The longstanding mouth-to-ear method of giving health information by doctors to patients also is inefficient because of patients' conditions and anxiety that reduce the concentration; patients' lacks of knowledge of medical terminology that makes most of the orally prescribed information remain unperceived. In addition to above mentioned problems/barrier in the side of patients there are barriers in the side of doctors and information delivery channels too. Doctors' time pressure and information oversupply adds to the limitation of offering health information by doctors to patients.

Therefore, patients/consumers prefer to find information through the internet. In this connection, availability of health information in abundance through the Internet, applications of web 2.0 and potential of social networks for working together from different geographical locations and different background of knowledge has given rise to introduction and demand for online health information. There is increasing demand for online health information for patients, consumers, clinicians and the general public. There are also new opportunities to share evidence globally about the outcomes and effectiveness of health care that can be used for right decision making by patients and clinicians. These opportunities create new environments for health librarians to play their central role in ensuring dissemination of right health information/evidence to meet their right contact. Because in spite of availability of abundant health information on the Internet and patients' preference to find health information online, there should be accessible united and reliable resources to rely on that rather than searching many places for information and comparing the content, evaluating the reliability and accuracy of them to find right information among ocean of mixed information and misinformation on the Internet. The risk of using misinformation is riskier than lack of information. Therefore proliferation of health information does not guarantee optimal care and shared decision making in patient centered medicine. According to Biswas and his colleagues (2008) In spite of the unprecedented expansion in medical information we still do not have the types of information required to allow us to tailor optimal care for a given individual patient. As our current information is chiefly provided in disconnected silos, we need an information system that can seamlessly integrate different types of information to meet diverse user group needs.

Health libraries in collaboration with academic and public libraries, physicians, healthcare experts and health/medical inforamationist can render Information Therapy service in the existed web 2.0 environments.

HOW THE WEB 2.0 APPLICATIONS CAN BE UTILIZED FOR RENDERING INFORMATION THERAPY SERVICE BY THE LIBRARIES/ LIBRARIANS?

Web 2.0 is a term coined by O'Reilly Media in 2004 to describe a second generation of the web. This describes more user participation, social interaction and collaboration with the use of blogs, wikis, social networking and folksonomies (Williams, 2007). Practically, it is application of easy to use, interactive and freely available open software on the Internet. Web 2.0 has created a radical evolution in the information communication, worldwide. It has granted opportunities for people to communicate globally despite the geographical distances and limitations of differences in languages. People, who can access Internet, use Web 2.0 in different ways to express the Ideas, create awareness, and meet the marketplace in more effective, efficient and convenient way. In healthcare delivery also wikis, blogs, podcasts, facebook and other forms of Web 2.0 are used in patient information as well as medicine 2.0 (Gavgani, Vishwa, 2008). The potential of the Web 2.0 as an interactive, rapid, timeline, easy to use and ubiquitous tool has made it a popular culture among internet residents. Organizations use the 2.0 style in developing new software and application to deliver healthcare to patients in an effective mode/style. According to the e-health insider (2008) patient will able to carry out email consultation with GPs [General Physicians] and other clinicians using a Face Book style tool called Communicator. Communicator will be launched as part of ambitious development plans for HealthSpace, the online organizer that gives patients access to their NHS Summary Care Record. (e-health insider, 2008)

The U.S. Department of Health and Human Services (HHS), Food and Drug Administration (FDA), and Centers for Disease Control and Prevention (CDC) are working together to provide consumers and partners with social media tools to access information about the ongoing peanut butter and peanut-containing product recalls (CDC, 2009). They are using various forms of Web 2.0 tools, from Blogs, Online Video, Phone/Email, Podcasts, RSS Feeds, Social Networks, Badges for Social Networks, Twitter, Virtual Worlds, Web Sites, Widgets to keep a right track to patients and their continues easy connection with National Health System.

Medpedia (www.medpedia.com) is another example of collaborative Web 2.0 based information sources for medicine. It has been developed in association with Harvard Medical School, Stanford School of Medicine, UC Berkeley School of Public Health, and University of Michigan Medical School. It is a new online health information resource, a medical encyclopedia that only health professionals will be able to produce and edit the content, the feature that ensures the reliability of information in the field of medicine. Because health information produced by non-health information resources is controversial by itself and there are examples of survey done on Wikipedia about drug information revealing that "Wikipedia are missing out on the vital details of medications like harmful drug interactions and adverse effects" (RedOrbit Staff & Wire Reports,2008).

However, the challenges for medical librarians are that how effectively they can apply Web 2.0 into their services, such as Information Therapy Services, Patient Information, Evidence Based Medicine to provide their users with timely, reliable and right information. What medical librarians can do to create more specific application of Web 2.0 to ensure the dissemination of right information to right person at the right time that help them make a right health decision and improve the quality of healthcare?

In Information Therapy, personalized, evidence-based, timely and specific health information need to be delivered to the right contact. Patients with different level of knowledge, different individual abilities and medical conditions may need different forms of information. Therefore, Web 2.0 with its widespread social tools and software proves to be a right platform for Information Therapy services.

Wiki and Blog, the earlier forms of Web 2.0, are used for various purposes by librarians as well as healthcare professionals. "Wikis are now used for all kind of projects from managing internal library content to revising important references sources such as the International Classification of Diseases (ICD)" (Guistein, 2006). *St. Joseph County Public Library's* uses wiki as a Subject Directory or Subject Guide for information sources. (http://www.libraryforlife.org/subjectguides/index.php/Main_Page). *ListenNJ* is instances of utilizing wiki for joint project managing, according to the ListenNJ, for FY2009 there are 26 library system members representing 105 individual libraries. (http://listennj.pbwiki.com/). *Wiki Thing* or *Library Things* could be another example of wiki for collaborative Library service that is a cumulative Catalog, a subject Guide, a library information resource or according to wiki's page everything about libraries and library things.

Blogs are the other most applicable Web 2.0 tool in the library services, which are used for many purposes such as information sharing, Current awareness services library website, and book reviews. Just to name an example *St. Josef County Public Library* uses blogs as a way to share news about the library, like "Musical Notes," "Movies & More," "Programs, Classes & Events," "To Read or Not to Read."

Ann Arbor District Library (www.aadl.org) has created its website on blog platform and for any type of materials a blog has been created namely: Audio Blog(www.aadl.org/catalog/audio), Books Blog, Video Blog and Media Mentions blog, etc. (OW1SWEB, 2009).

Waterloo Public Library (http://www.wplbookclub.blogspot.com*uses blog as a* book club /) for gathering the Ideas and reviews and Critics of the readers about book /library material.

Among other Web 2.0 tools Really Simple Syndication (RSS) feeds are being used immensely by libraries. Libraries also offer RSS service for its latest news, An example of this is the University of Otago (http://www.library.otago.ac.nz/otagolibrary.rss).

Face book and Twitters also have been newly added to library services. Face book and twitters are used for short and fast messaging purpose among a group of professionals or people with same interests. "Twitter's simplicity of functional design, speed of delivery and ability to connect two or more people around the world provides a powerful means of communication, idea-sharing and collaboration. There's potency in the ability to burst out 140 characters, including a shortened URI." (Baumann,2009) Among 140 characters counted by Phill in his blog, many are applicable in medical libraries Information Therapy service such as: Supportive care for patients and family members, disease management especially chronic diseases like Diabetes management, etc. He refers to doctors and nurses sharing medical information, often as short bursts of data (lab values, conditions, orders, etc.) as an example. Although there is no example of application of Twitter in medical libraries for Ix but there are examples of its application in library service.

East Brunswick Public Library uses Face book page for gathering theternal library content to revising important references sources such as the International Classification of Diseases (ICD)" (Guistein,2006).

These are examples of application of Web 2.0 in library services that create prospects for a free and collaborative global library service without considering geographical boundaries.

However utilization of Web 2.0 for specific purposes like information therapy services has not been developed so far by libraries' services.

POWER OF INFORMATION IN THERAPY THROUGH COLLABORATION /RELATION BETWEEN PHYSICIANS, PATIENTS, LIBRARIANS (INFORMATION PROFESSIONALS)

Information is an auxiliary and complimentary therapy when it is evidence based, relevant, reliable, unbiased, up-to-date, and easy to understand and personalized (Gavgani, 2009). In addition it must be received in right dose and right time. But the very question is that: Who is right source to provide the information in therapy?

Kemper counts three ways for Information prescription namely: "Doctor prescribed information, system prescribed information and consumer prescribed information" (Kemper-Metler, 2002) in which he refers to library and librarians too. It is clear that in Information prescription, physicians are first trusted choice to be refered, because they diagnose the diseases, know the patients health and mental health condition, and they know the necessary information, its dose/scope that the patient nee to receive. But in a limited visit time physicians do not have time to search for information, evaluate, personalize and prescribe it to patient.

Patients are aware of their illness but not aware of diagnoses, prognosis, therapy, side effects, because they do not have medical knowledge. Patient and other consumers are not eligible to prescribe the right information because the danger of wrong information is more risky than lack of information, when it come to making decision on the live or death of a person based on a wrong data.

System prescribed information also needs a standing order, physicians involvement. In addition, it is not ensured if a reliable and evidence based information is prescribed to a person or not, whether the other factors in the health condition of person is also considered by system or no.

Patients (or career who will share in decision making) are right person to give information about their health problem and physical condition, to receive the information on diagnoses, treatments, diseases management, to make and share decisions, and feedback to physician/health provider. Physicians are the right person to diagnose and prescribe treatment and health/medical information controls the health outcomes. Librarians (health information professional) are right person to search, retrieve, evaluate, organize, personalize and deliver the information prescription. In this case the information will be risk free, reliable, cost effectiveness and auxiliary and complementary medicine. Consequently, "Information is medicine, a powerful medicine" (Kemper-Mettler, 2002) when it is prescribed and prepared through relations between physicians, patients and librarians (health information professionals).

The following service model, a Social Networking Library System/Center for rendering Ix, illustrates the collaboration of Health Information Centers and Libraries in a 2.0 environment. It will give an Idea and a vision for librarians to render the longstanding Interlibrary Loan, Library Collaboration, Resource Sharing, SDI service through a social Networking System in general, and Information Therapy Service to patients and healthcare providers through a totally collaborative and connected system of Web 2.0 in particular.

SOCIAL NETWORKING LIBRARY (SNL) SYSTEM FOR INFORMATION THERAPY (IX)

The aims of the Social Networking Library System (SNLS) for Information Therapy (Ix) are to provide easy access to right information for patients and improve the patient safety, health literacy, health and health care practice by dissemination of right information trough Web 2.0 platforms. Today's libraries' mission and manifesto in social networking and 2.0 environment is more about making connection rather than making collection, and being in the track for users, always ready to

change by preference of users and more specifically "Always in Beta" as described well by Laura Cohen (Donna, 2007).

The social Networking Library system is a social Information system in 2.0 environment, it consist of two fundamental group of elements and the Social Networking Library (SNL) for Ix at the center of the System, as follows:

1. Virtual or dynamic elements of SNL System: It forms from various facets of Web 2.0 and social open software such as Wikis, Blogs, BlogCarnivals, Podcasts, Face Books, RSS feeds, Twitter, Delicious, Institutional Repositories, Slide share, Video share, Library2.0, Medicine2.0, etc. wherever they are appropriate to information exchange. In this sense the existing Web 2.0 facets developed by libraries, health professionals and institutions as well as information centers, can be utilized, shared and integrated into the SNL system. Also SNL will develop new subject specific blog Carnivals, wikis and podcast, etc. for its service. It will use institutional repositories to make the library of Information prescriptions.

2. Physical or static elements of SNL System: The National Health System (NHS) of participant countries, National Medical Libraries (NMLs) (Such as National Library of Medicine of America), Clinical/Medical Libraries (C/ML), Public libraries (PL), Data Bases (DBs), Health Information Systems/Centers (HIS/C), and Subject Specialist Librarians (SSLs), Health Informationists, and other related human resources such as health/medical experts. These parties will work together under an agreement, protocol, rules and regulation of the system.

3. Social Networking Library (SNL)'s knowledge base will house at the core and will contain its specific database and information center.

Figure 1. Social Networking Library System for Information Therapy (Ix) Service

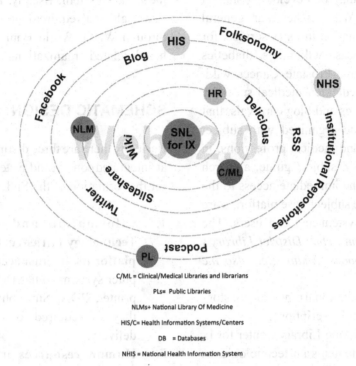

C/ML = Clinical/Medical Libraries and librarians

PLs= Public Libraries

NLMs+ National Library Of Medicine

HIS/C= Health Information Systems/Centers

DB = Databases

NHIS = National Health Information System

Figure 1 illustrates the elements and their relation in the formation of SNL for Ix.

Figure 1 is schematic model that shows the ' Social Networking Library System for Ix ' in the center like a solar system. Any node in the Social Network addresses one of basic physical element/manifestation of Health Information Service Provider such as: NHIS (National Health Information System), NLM (National Library of Medicine), PL (Public Library), Clinical/Medical Libraries and Librarians (C/MLs), Data Bases like Cochrane Reviews, and PubMed Central, that share information and information resources virtually and physically. The human resources clinical medical librarians, who share their expertise to ensure the dissemination of right information at right time for right contact, are implicitly in the SNL Center. They may not be working essentially in the SNL, they can work in any library Research and Development centers any where in the world but share their expertise.

The social networks like Blog(s), Wiki(s), Slideshares, Podcasts, Twitter, BlogCarnivals such as SurgeXperience (http://surgexperiences.wordpress.com/blogroll/), medicine 2.0 blog carnival (http://medicine20.wordpress.com/) in the field of medicine and Medlib's Round (http://blogcarnival.com/bc/cprof_6092.html), in the field of medical librarianship, video and audios, open software, Institutional Repositories are at the background of the system, as applications of Web 2.0 that are used by SNL to provide its accurate, timely, easy to understand, evidence based, free and user driven information service to patients and publics. The other information provision centers like *Center for Diseases Control and Prevention* (CDC), The *Patient Information Centre, MedlinePlus*, Health Information in Multiple Languages, (NLM), *MayoClinic*, and other related websites, blogs, podcasts, etc. can be consulted/ used by SNL as sources of health care information.

SNL incorporate Blogs and Wikis in it information service and it utilizes the existing Blogs and

Wikis as well. SNL may be developing subject oriented Blogs and Wikis rather than general helath/medical infromation in its Ix service. for instance Chronic disease wiki/blogs, diabetics blog, Neoplasm Blogs, Prostate Cancer wiki/blog. Any field of medicine / medical specialty will have specific blogs and blog carnivals, that will be supported and organized with subject specialist librarians and medical professions, in case. Although an A-Z subject guide, a search engine will support the immediate access to the right information, the subject wise platforms are better for both the system and end users. The example could be *Ann Arbor District Library's different Blogs for books, Audio, etc., also the blogCarnivals.*

SNL, also uses institutional repository to store and share Information Prescriptions.

The Social Networking Library Center for Ix includes required equipments and technologies as well as human resources (librarians and research/review groups of such as Cochrane library).

Librarians as indispensable human resources such as patient librarians, clinical/medical librarians, subject specialist health librarians, health informationist, are also implicitly in the SNL system, that will be responsible for organizing the data, assigning the metadata, intelligent codes and standards such as SNOMED, MeSh, UMLS, CPT, etc., personalizing and delivering the information for received prescriptions to the target (patients/career or concerned physician). Other professionals including review groups, translation groups, summarizing group from library professions or maybe other fields, but familiar with heath care subjects and medical languages/terminology and skilled/trained in the required job, also are necessary elements of the system. It neither is essentially physical nor virtual Library. It is about Social Networking Service at 2.0 environments. It will restore collection and also will create connection to other existing information service providers.

The libraries and organization who are contributing in the formation of SNL for Ix can support the library system, fiscally. However, the other financial/fiscal requirements can also be provided through WHO, World Bank, NGO's and other health related organizations and grants.

SCHEMATIC DESIGN

Basically there are three distinguishable layers in an integrated context and system working together for the formation of the SNL system as follows:

1. **Information and communication Technology infrastructures and Web 2.0 platforms**. Internet accessibility and computer systems, other Devices like Scanner, printer, PDA, Smartphone, etc. wherever they are required for information service delivery.
2. **Human resources** including Clinical/Medical Librarians, Health Information specialists, health/medical experts, research and review groups and I T professionals.
3. **Information Center**, that is the Social Networking Library and information centers or knowledgebase.

Figure 2 shows the formation of layers.

Figure 2. Schematic design /Structural layers in Social Networking Library

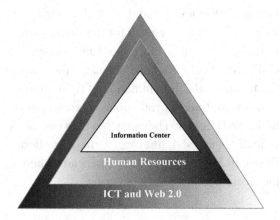

Social networking tools and platforms are freely available on the internet. There are many reliable health information sources like AID WIKI, Ask Dr Wiki, CHIS (Concumer Health Information Service) wiki, clinfowiki, CRI (Clinical Research Informatics) and wiki, WikiSurgery. (Rothman David, 2009).(www.medpedia.com/). In addition, there are free reliable sources like PubMed Central (NLM, 2009), Cochrane Summaries and Systematic Reviews, and other free websites like eMedicineHealth, Patient UK (a comprehensive, free, up-to-date health information as provided by GPs to patients during consultations), Mayo Clinic, Better Health, UK National Health System, and BUPA. These information resources could be used in an integrated environment/platform based on Web 2.0 technology by the 'Information Center'. In addition, SNL will restore the Information Prescriptions in its institutional repository. Information prescriptions can be used by physician to in prescribing information to their patients, or by patients to make an informed decision as well as caregivers to help to patients to control and manage with diseases.

INFORMATION THERAPY SERVICE THROUGH WEB 2.0 SOCIAL NETWORKING LIBRARY SYSTEMS

How Does a Social Networking Model Work?

The Social Networking Library center for Ix evolve a new model for sharing and disseminating knowledge about health, medicine and prescriptions among patients, medical professionals and the general public. It aims to become a repository of up-to-date unbiased and user driven health and medical information environment for all. In the sense of Information Therapy, the information is disseminated by SNL for to two major causes:

1. Health related Current Awareness Services,
2. Information Prescription Services

However, it will deal with any aspects of health information services in the context of library services as well as information prescription.

Its Information Therapy service can be distinguished by two broad stages as follows:

1. Before consulting physicians
2. After consultation or after visit

At the first stage i.e. before visit stage patients try to find health information for many reasons from self diagnosis to healthy living, awareness, and personal interest. But the second stage starts when ill health/diseases are diagnosed and Information Prescription most likely is done by concerned physician. In this concept a patient may consult a Library or Information System with a prescription (that can be a URL, Subject, Metadata, keywords and codes, etc.) addressing a certain piece of information or a certain subject.

According the above categorization and type of information need, the first stage requires general information for awareness purpose, for instance:

- What is lupus?
- What causes Lupus?
- Who is most at risk?
- Signs and symptoms of Lupus
- What can I do to prevent?

The SNL center for Ix play a health information resources role for patients who search for understandable evidence based health information to make a strategic health decision. Therefore integrated system as well as other information systems parties (blogs, wikis, HIS(s) etc.) in the SNL system can be consulted by patient for reliable information. There is increasing number of library blogs and non-library medical, patient education blogs that can be evaluated, and integrated to

SNL for awareness/general information in Ix. In addition there are many best available Institutional repositories in medical/health science. A survey by Oliver Kathleen B. and Swain Robert (2006) reveled that number of 144 institutional repository with medical content (health and medicine) have been developed worldwide. There are still capacities to be filled by Institutions to bridge the gap between best Information and its user in healthcare. Case Reports/studies and pamphlets can be input in institutional repositories as well as wikis to be used in SNL.

However in the post diagnosis/after visit stage the prescribed information will be sought by patient. Therefore in this stage a personalized piece of information will be supplied by SNL. The prescribed information will be retrieved, personalized and delivered by Librarian or health informationist from the resources that are in the different virtual and physical elements but integrated networking system SNL.

1. Naturally in the process of personalization the information trigger is personalized by the name of patient. In addition, according to the patient's preference, level of literacy, physical/individual abilities and situation (maybe audio/video /text format is suitable with patient). Patients can access the health information and evidence that is already provided and are being shared through the Social Networking Library resources like various subject-oriented Blogs and blog carnivals, Wikis and Podcasts, and other platforms. Also they can share their health stories with other co patients, physicians, researchers through the patient's pages (like: blog, wiki and face book, or twitter and comments) that can be used as a self report, self story, user driven information and evidence for more specific research studies.

2. Physician can prescribe information and refer the patient to the Social Networking Library System/Center for Information Prescriptions (IP) by writing the metadata, subject or URL (Uniform Resource Locator) related to the source of information as well as specific information request for special cases. They can also send Information Prescriptions that they have already prepared for their patients, in case it is available, in order to restore in the repository and used by other.

3. When a request for information (Information Prescription) is received by the SNL, for specific case, librarians/system will search and appraise the appropriateness of the information/evidence with the Information Prescription, then personalize and finally send them to the patient/caregivers. In integrated fully networking environment the patient's personal information like name, email/phone/address will be sent along with PI (Prescribed Information) to the SNL. In this way the personalization process will be take place rapidly and the Information will be sent to the required privacy concerns, such as email/phone or home address.

4. If prescribed information is not accessed from the database the moderator will send an urgent or instant message for members of the Social Networking Library Center for Ix, requesting answer for Information Prescription. The responses can be returned to the Social Networking Library Center for Ix to be assessed/approved once more by the experts then it will be personalized and finally targeted to patient or physician.

5. Librarians may access the EMR (Electronic Medical Record) along with the ICD (International Classification of Disease) cod that will be addressing the diseases, in that case the ICD and other codes like CPT (Current Procedural Terminology) (that refers to CT Scan of patient), will be identified /compared by the MeSh, USML, SNOMED cods and the relevant/right Information will be personalized according to the embedded standard cods and will be sent to the target.

6. The review groups in an international collaboration will review, summarize, simplify, and translate the information /evidence and add to the repository /knowledgebase. This will provide a ready, readable (depends on the grade of reading that is usually 6 or 8), understandable, unbiased and free patient education handouts, booklets, leaflets and summaries in any field of medicine.

7. Simultaneously, SNL Center will utilize translation process to include Information in different formats and languages to meet the information needs of the audiences in an information equitable environment such as text, audio, video, podcast, e-file.

This would be the form and nature of the Social Networking Library Center for Ix. The clinical/medical libraries should keep pace with the trends and developments that are taking place in the Information Society or the emerging Knowledge Societies by adapting themselves to the changing technological environment.

CONCLUSION

To keep up with the global move for Open Access to evidence, to ensure health for all by 2020, to ensure availability of clear health information for right person at right time, medical/hospital libraries have an indispensible role to play. Availability of social networking tools and increasing number of health information available in the Internet especially free Web and Web 2.0 is a promising prospect for librarians to keep tune with this global health move. The above presented model is suggested for two considerable evidence 1) the impact and application of social networks in information communication 2) a nonprofit social collaboration is a voluntary service in which any party, library/librarian and health expert/professional cooperates with one another according to their ability, interest, resources and information

at their own time. The paper comes to conclusion with 'How Web 2.0 applications like blogs and wikis can be used in Information Therapy Service.', 'How health providers and information providers can collaboratively facilitate the flow of right information to patients through Web 2.0.' through prescribing information and referring the patients to SNL center for Ix. And it shows 'How Web 2.0 provides a proper channel and source for information therapy service'.

Libraries have accesses to free and fee based resources as well as the library's self processed information and resources like repositories, abstracts, pamphlets and brochures. Librarians have the knowledge of electronic, print and online resources and best evidence in any field and they also have necessary skills of handling them. Librarians have accesses to open source software to make a digital library. Social networks like blogs, wikis, slideshares, podcasts, RSS are freely available. Most of the libraries and librarians all over the world have already developed and created their own social networks/systems. Therefore a 'Social Networking Library Center for Ix' can utilize all the above mentioned facilities or tools in developing its " Social Networking Library Service ".

REFERENCES

Baumann, P. (2009). 140 Health Care Uses for Twitter. *Phill baumann online, health is social*. Retrieved from http://philbaumann. com/2009/01/16/140-health-care-uses-for-twitter/

Biswas, R., Maniam, J., Lee, E. W. H., Das, P. G., Umakanth, S., Dahiya, S., & Ahmed, S. (2008). User driven health care- Answering multidimensional information needs in individual patients utilizing post EBM approaches: An operational model. *Journal of Evaluation in Clinical Practice*, *14*, 750–760. doi:10.1111/j.1365-2753.2008.00997.x

CDC. (Centers for Disease Control and Prevention) (2009). *Social Media Tools for Consumers and Partners.* Retrieved February, 2009, from http://www.cdc.gov/socialmedia

Davidoff, F., & Florance, V. (2000). The informationist: a new health profession? [editorial]. *Annals of Internal Medicine, 132*(12), 996.

E-health insider (2008). *Patients to get facebook style communicator.* Retrieved from www.e-health-insider.com/news/4337/patients_to_get_facebook-style_communicator

Eisenberg, J. M. (2002). Globalise the evidence, localize the decisions: evidence-based medicine and international diversity. *Health Affairs, 21,* 166–168. Retrieved from http://content.healthaffairs.org/cgi/reprint/21/3/166pdf. doi:10.1377/hlthaff.21.3.166

Feldman, S. (2004). *Enterprise search technology: information disasters and the high cost of not finding information.* Portals Mag, 27-28. Retrieved from www.portalsmag.com

Gavgani, V. Z. (2009). *Role of medical librarians in Information Therapy: a study of problems and prospects in India and Iran.* Unpublished PhD thesis submitted to Osmania University, p49-50.

Gavgani, V. Z., & Mohan, V. V. (2008). Application of web 2.0 tools in medical librarianship to support medicine 2.0. *Webology,* 5(1), Article 53. Retrieved from: http://www.webology.ir/2008/v5n1/a53.html

HIFA2015. (2008). *A global Compagine: Health Care Information For All by 2015. HIFA2015 and human rights.* Available at http://www.hifa2015.org/hifa2015-and-human-rights/

IOM (Institute Of Medicine). (1999). *To Err is Human: Building a Safer Health System.* Available at http://www8.nationalacademies.org/onpinews/newsitem.aspx?RecordID=9728

IOM (Institute of Medicine). (2001). *Committee on Quality of Health Care in America.* Crossing the Quality Chasm: a new health system for the 21st cent century. Washington, DC, National Academy Press; 20; 2001. PDF. Retrieved from http://books.nap.edu/html/quality_chasm/reportbrief.pdf

MayoClinic. (2009). *MayoClinic.* Retrieved from http://www.mayoclinic.com/

Medical Malpractice. (2008). *Medical Malpractice.* Retrieved from http://medical-malpractice-flint.com/info.htm

MedPedai. (2009). *MedPedai.* Retreived from www.medpedia.com/

National Library of Medicine. (2009). *MedlinePlus,* Health Information in Multiple Languages. Retrieved from http://www.nlm.nih.gov/medlineplus/languages/languages.html

OW1SWEB (2009). Ow1seb Blog. Retrieved from http://www.owlsweb.info/L4L/blogs.asp#useinlibraries

Oliver, K. B., & Swain, R. (2006). Directories of Institutional Repositories: Research Results & Recommendations. *World Library and Information Congress: 72nd IFLA General Conference and Council,* Seoul, Korea 20-24 August, 2006. Retrieved from http://www.ifla.org/IV/ifla72/papers/151-Oliver_Swain-en.pdf

RedOrbit Staff & Wire Reports. (2008). *Drug Information Often Left Out On Wikipedia.* Retrieved from http://www.redorbit.com/news/health/1602644/drug_information_often_left_out_on_wikipedia/index.html

Rothman, D. (2009). *List of Medical Wikis.* Retrieved from http://davidrothman.net/list-of-medical-wikis/

St. Joseph County Public Library. (2009). *Subject Guide (Wiki).* Retrieved from http://www.library-forlife.org/subjectguides/index.php/Main_Page

Tayson, D. B. (2007). *Library 2.0, Library Service & Web 2.0*. [PPT Slide] Retrieved December, 2009, from www.tbs-sct.gc.ca/im-gi/imday07jourgi/pres/library-biblio/library-biblio-eng.ppt

The Patient Information Centre. (2009). *The patient Information Center, Northumberland, NHS*. Retrieved from http://www.ntw.nhs.uk/pic/?p=about

Tikki, P., Muir, G., & Evans, T. (2006). A 15th grand challenge for global public health. *Lancet, 367*, 284–286. Retrieved from http://www.thelancet.com/journals/lancet/article/PIIS0140673606680501/fulltext. doi:10.1016/S0140-6736(06)68050-1

Transcript of radio broadcast: 28October2008. Retrieved from http://www.voanews.com/specialenglish/2008-10-28-voa2.cfm

University of Otago. (2009). *RSS*. Retrieved from http://www.library.otago.ac.nz/otagolibrary.rss

VOA News. (2008). Almost Half of All Deaths Are in People Under 60

Waterloo Public Library. (2009). *Waterloo Public Library*. Retrieved from http://www.wplbookclub.blogspot.com uses blog as a book club

Weightman, A. L., & Williamson, J. (2005). The value and impact of information provided through library services for patient care: a systematic review. *Health Information and Libraries Journal, 22*(1), 4–25. doi:10.1111/j.1471-1842.2005.00549.x

WHO (World Health Organization). (2009). *World report on child injury prevention*. Retrieved from http://www.who.int/violence_injury_prevention/child/injury/world_report/en/index.html

WHO (World Health Organization). (2003). *Influenza fact sheet*. Retrieved from http://www.who.int/mediacentre/factsheets/2003/fs211/en/

Wiki Thing. (2009). *Wiki Thing or Library Things*. Visited February 2009. Retrieved from http://www.librarything.com/wiki/index.php/WikiThing:About

Williams, D. (2007). *Blog Glossary; Bloging Terms: Popular Products and Services*. Retrieved from http://www.webdesignseo.com/blogging-terms/web-20-terms.php)

Williams, L., & Zipperer, L. (2003). Improving Access to Information: Librarians and Nurses Team Up for Patient Safety. *Nursing Economics, 21*(4), 199–201.

Chapter 31

Bridging Online and Offline Social Networks to Promote Health Innovation:
The CoNEKTR Model

Cameron D. Norman
University of Toronto, Canada

ABSTRACT

Complex problems require strategies that leverage the knowledge of diverse actors working in a coordinated manner in order to address them in a manner that is appropriate to the context. Such strategies require building relationships among groups that enable them to network in ways that have the intensity of face-to-face meetings, but also extend over time. The Complexity, Networks, EHealth, & Knowledge Translation Research (CoNEKTR) model draws upon established methods of face-to-face social engagement and supported with information technology and proscribes an approach to issue exploration, idea generation and collective action that leverages social networks for health innovation. The model combines aspects of communities of practice, online communities, systems and complexity science, and theories of knowledge translation, exchange and integration. The process and steps of implementing the model are described using a case study applied to food systems and health. Implications for health research and knowledge translation are discussed.

"Our Similarities bring us to a common ground; Our Differences allow us to be fascinated by each other."

- Tom Robbins (born 1936); Novelist, Short Story Writer, Essayist

INTRODUCTION

The first decade of the 21st century saw parallel trends that transformed our conceptualization of population health: the shift of burden from acute to chronic disease as the primary driver of healthcare spending; the proliferation of information and communication technologies (ICT) that connect people to ideas and each other on a global scale; and the recognition that social networks impact

DOI: 10.4018/978-1-60960-097-6.ch031

health outcomes and human learning in ways never known before. Each of these trends has meant profound changes in the way that healthcare is experienced both by patients and practitioners, inspiring greater integration between prevention and public health and treatment and palliative care. Disappearing are the silos that create distinct separations between these areas – and the actors within them – and in its place an awareness of the importance of relationships as a conduit for problem solving and innovation. Social networks are the medium by which these factors coalesce.

The term 'social' relates to society and organization with others, while 'network' refers to the linking of these 'others' together. Therefore, the relationship between individuals and groups, how these relationships form, and the patterns that emerge from such engagement represent an opportunity to learn about how knowledge is created, shared, and transformed into value – innovation – and how to achieve the largely unrealized promise of knowledge translation (Graham, Logan, Harrison, & Straus, 2006; Kitson, 2009). Networking knowledge is a means of addressing problems of great social and cognitive complexity, such as those with overlapping causes and possible solutions, ones that are highly dependent on context, and require expertise from multiple actors with different perspectives. Networks consider and articulate a full set of possibilities realized in contextual levels and offers a way to conceive of actionable strategies for enhancing and clarifying communication between them. Because social networks operate differently in different contexts, the ability to create networks that fit the context matters significantly (Pescosolido, 2006).

Networks are social structures that human beings use to build solidarity based on similarities and to bridge differences with multiple actors (Capra, 2002; Gilchrist, 2004; B. A. Israel, 1985). Learning and innovation in healthcare and public health depend both on similarity (e.g., disciplines and specialties) and difference (e.g., inter-professional teams). Building strengths on

similarity, or homophiliy, enables knowledge to be consolidated by leveraging the familiar, tacit practices that come from trust, which forms the foundation for networks to develop (Kliener, 2002; Suitor & Keeton, 1997). Connections based on difference promote new learning by extending an individual or group into a new cognitive space and facilitating the emergence of new pattern formation (Page, 2007; Sawyer, 2006, 2008). This chapter will introduce a model developed that addresses the challenges posed by complex problems and leverages the potential that social networks and information and communication technologies (ICT's) present in building bridges across differences, while reinforcing the strength of similarity with the aim of promoting social innovation in health.

The chapter begins with an exploration of the problems facing knowledge translation and innovation in healthcare and public health, followed by the introduction of a model (CoNETKR) developed to address these issues with reference to work done by others in the facilitation of innovation. The chapter concludes with an example of how the CoNEKTR model has been applied in practice and discussion for future applications.

TRANSFORMING KNOWLEDGE INTO ACTION

The health system faces a paradox where more knowledge is being generated through research and practice than ever before and shared through technologies that enable rapid dissemination to broad audiences, and yet much of what is produced is not being transformed into health value in a manner that keeps pace (Balas & Boren, 2000; Best, Moor, et al., 2003; Davis, et al., 2003; Kiefer, et al., 2005). Under the rubric of knowledge transfer and exchange (Koschatzky, 2002; Norman & Huerta, 2006), knowledge translation (Davis, et al., 2003; Estabrooks, Thompson, Lovely, & Hofmeyer, 2006; Graham, et al., 2006), or knowledge integration (Best, Hiatt, & Norman, 2008; Best, Trochim, Haggerty, Moor, & Norman, 2008; Kerner, 2006), models have been proposed that aim to support putting what is known into practice more quickly. While popular in theory, knowledge-to-action models have not performed well in practice (Best, Hiatt, Cameron, Rimer, & Abrams, 2003; Marincola, 2003) with original research findings still taking a generation before direct benefit to patient care is realized (Balas & Boren, 2000). One of the problems is that different stakeholders– research producers and end users – operate independently from one another throughout the knowledge production, synthesis and integration cycle rather in collaboration. The U.S. Institute of Medicine Clinical Research Roundtable has characterized the field as at a crossroads (Crowley, et al., 2004; Glass & McAtee, 2006), and called for fundamental restructuring of the enterprise that moves research from basic sciences through clinical trials and the development of more effective services to improve the public's health. There are pushes to rethink the organization of knowledge production and translation, including calls to better reflect the multidisciplinary nature of health services and research (Lemieux-Charles & Champagne, 2004), and to conduct more evaluation research on interventions conducted under real-world conditions (Bero, et al., 1998; Kiefer, et al., 2005) to reflect the practical nature of the problems the models seek to address. Yet, few practical strategies have emerged in response to these calls.

These models have also been critiqued for being divorced from the evidence on how people actually generate knowledge, learn and communicate those lessons to others (Bransford, Brown, & Cocking, 2000), nor do they reflect the role of practice-based knowledge in evidence creation (Green, 2006; Green & Glasgow, 2006). The criticisms levied against dominant knowledge-to-action models point to the absence of discussion on experiential learning, tacit knowledge, and

how exchanges between individuals incorporate teaching and learning simultaneously.

All of these challenges and opportunities suggest a need to examine the entire system, not just the components within it in isolation (Best, Trochim, et al., 2008; Kitson, 2009). It also points to the need to consider ways in which interaction between agents in that system lead to the emergence of new patterns or knowledge that cannot be ascribed to planning or linear processes of information sharing. Thus, a systems-oriented strategy that focuses on developing relationships between diverse agents and facilitates interactions that will produce emergent properties (innovations) is likely to provide greater benefit than one that approaches knowledge exchange in a linear manner.

THE CONEKTR MODEL

The Complexity, Networks, EHealth, & Knowledge Translation Research (CoNEKTR) Model represents an attempt to resolve these issues using an approach based on complexity science, social learning theories, and models of knowledge exchange, translation and integration. The CoNEKTR Model incorporates many shared elements germane to existing theories and models as well as processes for social engagement: Unconference/Open Space, electronic social networking platforms, blogging and theories of collective action, design thinking, leadership, and community development. Some of these theories are well established (e.g., social cognitive theory), while other relevant concepts are still emerging in their application to human services work (e.g., Unconferences, design thinking). Akin to systems thinking, the value of the model is not in its attendant sub-components, but rather the manner in which the components form a cohesive learning experience. Consistent with complexity science is the importance of creating flexible boundaries around the system, rather than proscribing the way in which interactions are expected to occur. This flexibility supports diversity in the system and the emergence of new patterns (learning opportunities) that cannot be predicted from the outset. Thus, the theories are combined in a manner that suits the context.

The CoNEKTR model is centred on a five-step process that involves a facilitated face-to-face group interaction between individuals with diverse interests on a single topic followed by an extended knowledge development and exchange process that can take place at a distance using electronic communication tools and further face-to-face meetings. The model draws on a variety of social learning and exchange theories or processes:

1. **Community of Practice (CoP).** A CoP is a self-organized, voluntary, and focused collective of agents (people and organizations) who collaboratively work towards understanding on an issue or problem (Wenger, 1998; Wenger & Snyder, 2000). A CoP is designed in a manner that leverages resources from the user base; shapes a strategy for learning and developing better or best practices, cultivates partnerships; fosters skill development; and promotes dissemination of knowledge (Wenger & Snyder, 2000). The CoP approach encourages self-organization and network formation, where leadership emerges from within the network and is widely distributed, and has been effective as a mechanism for health sciences where there is diverse expertise and many experts are not co-located (Li, et al., 2009; Norman & Huerta, 2006).

2. **Self-organized group learning.** Among the most widely used models of self-organized group learning are Open Space Technology (Owen, 1997) and the World Café approach (J. Brown, 2005). More recently, the concept of the unconference, which has similarities to both models, has gained popularity, particularly within the technology and information

science sectors (Crossett, Kraus, & Lawson, 2009; Greenhill & Wiebrands, 2008). These models are employed to foster interaction between stakeholders and create space for engagement, idea generation, and issue identification and all are designed primarily around face-to-face creative dialogue.

3. **Online Communities.** Electronic tools provide methods of interaction that extend the face-to-face encounter and provide opportunities for dialogue beyond specific one-time events. There exist a wide variety of social network tools that enable collaboration and participation across time and distance. Personal network platforms like Facebook (http://www.facebook.com), professional-oriented networks like LinkedIn (www.linkedin.com) or customizable tools like Ning (http://www.ning.com) provide a means to create communities of practice that extend beyond the face-to-face. Electronic communities of practice (eCoP) can serve as ways to link health professionals who may not have the means due to physical proximity or time to otherwise collaborate and share experiential practice knowledge (Ho, et al., in press).

4. **Social Media.** Social media refers to a constellation of tools that derive their value from the participation of users through direct contribution of original content, editing existing material, providing comments or integrating various media together to create something unique. In 2008, the U.S. presidential campaign of Barack Obama provided one of the most visible examples of ways in which social media can influence mass action and social innovation (Harfoush, 2009). Blogs, wikis, instant messaging software, or collaboration platforms like Google Wave (http://www.wave.google.com) represent various forms of social media.

5. **Collaborative decision-making and emergent action.** Using technologies to

Figure 1. CoNEKTR network of network development

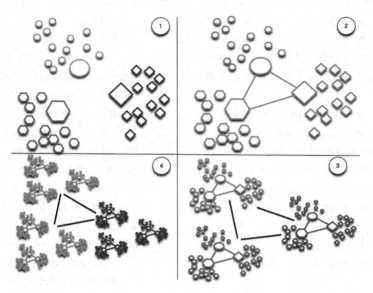

leverage creative ideas has been discussed widely within the popular business literature (Howe, 2008; Surowiecki, 2004; Tapscott & Williams, 2007) under various names such as 'crowdsourcing' or 'collective innovation' and reflects a process of collaborative decision making and social emergence (Sawyer, 2005, 2008). Through exchange of very little information and simple rules, complex patterns can emerge that can produce knowledge or action that was unanticipated and impossible to create if developed by individuals working independently aided by tools that maintain communication (Gloor, 2006).

The CoNEKTR model is designed to leverage the potential for innovation contained within social networks by initiating development of new ties within clusters of agents that are disconnected, but related in their scope of interest and activity. In complexity terms, the model employs the use of a catalytic probe, a conceptual device that focuses attention and initiates the emergence of attractors, which instigates creativity by providing a set of boundary conditions in which cognitive energy can be directed to yield innovations (Sawyer, 2006).

A balance between encouraging the bridging of structural holes in a network, thereby increasing the number of weak ties, through the introduction of new agents to a network is maintained by emphasizing the importance of parallel collaboration within existing, more homophilous agents (groups or individuals) – and extending outward to those agents with more heterogeneous characteristics (Aral & Van Alstyne, 2009). Emphasis is on creating networks of networks, rather than completely reconfiguring existing agent networks in a manner that could have unintended negative consequences (Figure 1).

The network of networks concept emphasizes the scaling effect of interconnectedness that forms when small, local networks of agents are connected to a larger web of similar networks. Figure 1 illustrates this effect by demonstrating how a cluster of activities (quadrant 1) connect together (quadrant 2) and how this larger network cluster is further connected at different levels (quadrants 3 and 4). The colours demonstrate how a network culture forms from distinctive clusters and how, as the network effect is scaled up, new meta-cultures form as connections are made. This ability to scale up through linking one network

Figure 2. CoNEKTR model flow diagram

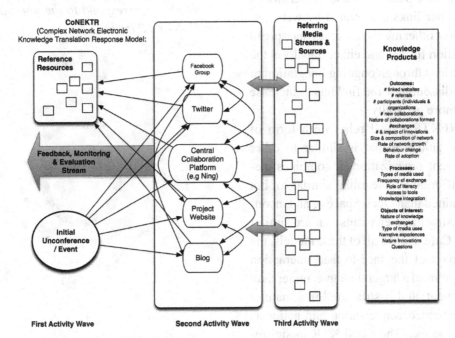

(e.g., a family practice) to another similar network and connecting these to a larger cluster of practice networks such as in the case of local area health networks.

The catalytic probe is a problem or topic of interest to a diverse audience that is still focused enough to that concrete, solution-oriented discussions may be created around it. The probe is one that is able to stimulate intrinsic and extrinsic motivators for action among participants (Deci & Ryan, 2008; Ryan & Deci, 2000). Extrinsic motivators may come from pressures from an industry to adapt to changing market conditions or a health threat to a community. Intrinsic motivation comes from individuals' self interest in the topic and the opportunity to realize certain aspirations through the group process initiated through the CoNEKTR model. Grounding knowledge generation and exchange in a social process also has the benefit of encouraging ideas to be prototyped, consistent with a design thinking strategy for change (T. Brown, 2009), and developed with the benefit of collective feedback allowing ideas most likely

to achieve wider acceptance (and subsequent adoption) to emerge. The model emphasizes not only knowledge exchange, but also the long-term opportunity to integrate that knowledge through practice and skill-building by having groups apply lessons learned to specific projects developed in the course of the interaction. By placing this knowledge within a wider media ecology through online tools and collaboration methods, the CoNEKTR model also holds promise for attracting other unidentified relevant stakeholders to the process.

Figure 2 illustrates the way in which networks of communication tools and social media are created and coordinated throughout the CoNEKTR process. The process unfolds in a series of waves that begin with the initial event, which generates information that is extended outward on to social media platforms to enable that content to be refined, edited and extended. Throughout this foray into the online environment, reference resources are used to support arguments (i.e., provide evidence) and aid in decision-making about actions or activities to take place. As these conversations take place, other links are created by websites, Twitter feeds or other media resources that spread the conversation further and either transform the ideas into actions through ongoing integration of feedback or disseminate the findings to increase knowledge more generally.

The CoNEKTR model relies on a form of participatory guidance that is similar to other models of event organization. It combines elements of self-organized learning similar to, but more constrained than Open Space or an Unconference and structured elements that are similar to the World Café. Unlike all of these models, the model asserts that the face-to-face interaction serves as the start of a larger dialogue, rather than as a single event, and is structured in a manner where the extended conversation and action is essential to success. The CoNEKTR model involves 10 key steps for full implementation and like the other social organization models mentioned, the number of steps and the degree of adoption can be modified to suit the needs of participants, the scope of the problem, and the resources available. Like other models of organizing, the CoNEKTR model may be modified based on the resources available and expressed needs associated with the participants and the problem at hand. The model encompasses five key processes utilized over 10 steps: 1) face-to-face interaction, 2) social modulation, 3) evaluation, 4) feedback and 5) integration. The first two processes are the most intense and interactive, while the latter provide the momentum for action beyond the initial event.

The five processes work in a cyclical manner, building on the work done in successive steps. With each step, the outreach of the processes increases along with the potential for new information to be generated (Figure 3).

As with each process, the reach of the influence becomes wider and more encompassing, reflected in the larger overlapping circles in the figure.

Figure 3. Cycles of activity in CoNEKTR Model
* Numbers correspond to the appropriate steps in CoNEKTR cycle

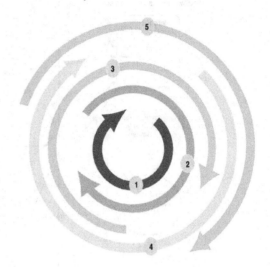

Key Processes:

1. **Face-to-face interaction**. Invited participants are put together in an event that alternates between a modeled and self-organized state that is closely modeled on the Unconference method of social organizing. The Unconference is similar to other participatory organization models such as Open Space Technologies (Owen, 1997) or the World Café (J. Brown, 2005), in that the bulk of the content development for the day and organization of that content is done by the participants. Unconferences have been used successfully in supporting learning in a variety of contexts (Greenhill & Wiebrands, 2008) and create potential for new emergent properties to form from novel information. Unlike the The Unconference, which has a convenor, but relies on self-identified and emergent leadership to take the ideas and plans developed at the event further, conveners employing the CoNEKTR model adopt a more robust leadership role that extends beyond the initial face-to-face event. This

leadership role is one that is guiding rather than prescriptive in nature and intended to provide focus based on the wishes of the group.

The decision to use a convener-led versus a largely self-organized approach as part of the model is grounded in the experience of the author and his research group arising from attending and hosting events using the Unconference, Open Space, and World Café models (among others) and the dissatisfaction with the outcomes they produced relative to the needs and context of healthcare and public health. Specifically, the aforementioned models are effective at provoking new ways of seeing problems, and eliciting feedback and ideas from a diverse collection of actors, however the emphasis on *self-organized* follow-up, whereby individuals are expected to take the ideas and apply them into practice has been found by the author to yield disappointing mid- and long-term results in achieving the vision set out by participants in the initial event. Lack of knowledge of the boundaries and components of the system (e.g., invitation list, participant backgrounds) coupled with the absence of resources to support follow-up activity are possible reasons that impede further actions from taking place. Such models also rest on the assumption that individuals attending these events have the skills and knowledge necessary to transform the knowledge generated into a change strategy and have the resources to lead or support this change process, which has not been observed in practice.

2. **Social modulation**. Facilitators employing the CoNEKTR model actively modulate discussion and interaction among attendees, both in the face-to-face and later online environments. Such active participation is designed to provoke discussion and draw connections between topics of relevance, while also ensuring that a diversity of voices is heard. This last point is of particular im-

portance in mediating the potential effects of social power and perceived authority. Although the model encourages interaction among a diverse range of participants in a non-judgmental, open manner, it is naïve to expect that power imbalances will not be expressed in conversation potentially limiting the willingness of some actors to fully express themselves within the social space created by the face-to-face meeting (Bourdieu, 1995).

Implementation of the model requires acknowledgement of the potential barriers that can emerge when participants feel uncomfortable presenting ideas when they lack the resources to adequately lead or follow-up on ideas or perceive themselves as not having resources viewed as desirable by others. Here, attention to the *nature* of the resources that participants bring to the event is essential. That is, not all resources are equal, as social connectedness, money, influence or social position will have different potential to shape outcomes depending on the issue and the participants attending the initial interaction event. Furthermore, the value of these resources will change as connections are made and the network evolves. The CoNEKTR organizers are to match resource needs with what is available while also balancing the inequality of certain resources. There is no imbalance in the ability to be creative (Sanger, 1994; Sawyer, 2008) so that is where the largest amount of energy is directed by the conveners. The facilitation team (and its useful to have a team) serve as modulators for eliciting or channeling creativity by encouraging participants to self-organize into groups based on an initial process of issue identification, which is done in a free-form manner with facilitators encouraging all participants to voice suggestions.

The modulation role also means serving as an observer and influencer on the process. Unlike a method like Open Space, which encourages creation of as many groups for discussion as there are ideas (with some limitations), the facilitators of the CoNEKTR model aim for preliminary synthesis on areas of loose organization using a content analysis process and seek agreement from the participants on the choice of a limited number of emergent themes rather than leave the options unconstrained. Rather than have participants self-organize the themes of each group, a content analysis is done by the convening organizers and presented back to the group for approval and refinement before moving on to the next step. Qualitative data analysis skills are an asset in order to provide rapid coding and synthesis of the information, which is usually done during a break from the initial introductory session. This ensures that the process can move forward in an orderly and expedient manner, while still providing participants with an option to have the information presented to them in a transparent manner without getting stuck on details. It also introduces a systematic process to organizing the material and limits the amount of detail that participants need to attend to, thus increasing focus.

The day begins with a structured introduction to the topic along with provision of key definitions to ensure that the group is speaking to the same issue and to reduce confusion about terminology. Participants then generate ideas in a scrum facilitated by the convenor followed by a process where individuals are asked to write their topics of interest on sticky notes and place them on a wall or set up space (See Figure 4). These topics are then organized using the process described above. Synthesized topics are used to seed discussions in one or two waves, which are held in 60-minute sessions over the course of a morning and afternoon with snack and lunch breaks in between. No more than two formal discussion sessions are held on a single day in order to reduce participant fatigue. Opportunities for unstructured conversation exist before the introduction session, a coffee break before the first and after the second breakout session, a lunch and a concluding coffee break. Participants are encouraged to bring the content

of these informal discussions to their discussion groups after each break.

The experience of an open, creative process can be exhilarating for some, but also exhausting if extended for long periods of time. The limitation on the length of the discussion ensures that energy is balanced appropriately to fully maintain engagement among individuals and the group (Deci & Ryan, 2008; Loehr & Schwartz, 2003; Ryan & Deci, 2000). If the topic is of such a scope and complexity that more discussion is desired (or necessary), a separate follow-up event is scheduled at a later date. Unconferences and Open Space events can be held over a period of consecutive days, which enables a wider range of discussions, but can also be physically and mentally fatiguing, limiting the ability or willingness of participants to maintain the momentum after the event concludes. The tight focus in the CoNEKTR model is suited to the time constraints of many health professionals and provides a highly focused, guided process.

At the end of the day the lessons are synthesized and a flexible path for action is developed by the group as a whole to maintain focus. These lessons are posted to a central online social networking hub (e.g., Ning or Crowdvine)[1] and used to seed groups or engagement with other common spaces for discussion (Surman & Weshler-Henry, 2001). These social networking hubs are set up in advance or immediately after the event to ensure that they are available once the face-to-face interactions are finished. Catalytic probes are then generated from each theme to invoke further conversation and used to create attractors to stimulate further idea generation and action. As networking takes place online, facilitators scan the network as a whole and help identify connections within the community to spot the emergence of new patterns, to reinforce existing ones that are helpful, and disrupt unhelpful patterns. For examples, a topic like food security and health might invoke discussion of a myriad set of social issues that are likely to create or potentially alleviate the problem, which may set forth discussions on other larger issues. Some of these are more proximally relevant (e.g., income), while others are less so (e.g., design of grocery shopping carts). The modulation process seeks to amplify ideas that are more likely to receive wide purchase (as determined from the discussion in groups and events as well as evidence) through promotion and active participation by leaders, while possibly ignoring or discouraging discussion on areas that are too tangential to the central issue.

3. **Evaluation.** Using a sense-making process that involves a multi-method approach to study, a series of tools are implemented that help collect data throughout the process. Evaluation data collected provides a form of feedback and, consistent with an action research strategy, data is used in an iterative manner to inform decision making, further action and ongoing evaluation (Skinner, Maley, & Norman, 2006). Evaluation methods can vary, however those most likely to capture the effects of social networks, to reflect activity within the system as a whole, and provide clear, utilization-focused feedback, are preferred. Some methods that are well-suited include: 1) qualitative interviews (Patton, 1990, 1996), 2) spidergrams (Lynam, et al., 2003; Rifkin, Muller, & Bichmann, 1988), 3) analysis of narrative fragments (Snowden, 2002), 4) social network analysis (Kane, Robinson-Combre, & Berge, 2010; Mehra, Dixon, Brass, & Robertson, 2005; Norman & Huerta, 2006), and 5) system dynamic models (Fredericks, Deegan, & Carman, 2008; Hirsch, Levine, & Miller, 2007; Stave, 2002). Methods that provide visual assessment of impact are preferred as they provide high levels of information when sharing across distances and contexts through social networks.

4. **Feedback.** The model is to be employed using an approach consistent with community-based research (B. Israel, Schulz, Parker, & Becker, 1998), whereby data is collected,

analyzed and shared in a manner that is transparent to the participants. Feedback also serves as a self-correcting method of dampening attractors that are not productive and supporting those that are. Ongoing waves of data collection with feedback consistent with a developmental evaluation (Patton, 1994, 2008; Westley, Zimmerman, & Patton, 2006) or an action-research approach (Argyris, Putnam, & Smith, 1985; Stringer, 1996; Whyte, 1991) provide ongoing information about the performance of the system. Providing evaluation data to participants in a form that is clear and easy to interpret serves both to validate the knowledge development process and is a form of network guidance/reinforcement in its own right (Norman & Huerta, 2006).

5. **Integration**: Knowledge integration occurs when what has been learned has been integrated into normal practice (Best, Hiatt, et al., 2008; Best, Trochim, et al., 2008; Kerner, 2006). This integration involves taking the innovation and using it to create new ways of working, policies and strategies, and having such innovations sustain themselves over time. Although the steps are akin to the Diffusion of Innovation model (Oldenburg & Parcel, 2002; Rogers, 1995), the process of knowledge integration describes an active, iterative process of putting knowledge into action that goes beyond adoption. Knowledge integration is not just additive; it is synthetic, influencing the entire system that it becomes a part of where learning is transformative.

IMPLEMENTING THE CONEKTR MODEL IN PRACTICE

The CoNEKTR model is implemented in 10 stages to which the five processes are overlaid. The steps involved in the model are:

1. Convene group of diverse, invested agents related to the topic of interest;
2. Introduce topic, including operational definitions of key terms to ensure a common starting point;
3. Engage the participants as a group in collective and independent brainstorming;
4. Collate the ideas and conduct a thematic content analysis of the ideas presented in the brainstorming session;
5. Develop discussion groups based around each major theme;
6. Re-convene and summarize the key points arising within each discussion group;
7. Plan for future actions and activities based on the ideas presented in a manner that encourages participation and leadership from the group and broad-based ownership of the strategy;
8. Collate the ideas and notes and make them available for all participants online and through methods appropriate to them (e.g., Facebook group, email, website);
9. Use participant notes and summaries to seed online discussions and modulate these discussions, identifying key connectors within the community and connections between relevant agents;
10. Identify emergent ideas for action and support from among the interactions and repeat the process as necessary.

The *Food4Health Project*, by the Youth Voices Research Group (http://www.youthvoices.ca) provides an example of the application of the CoNEKTR model in practice. The *Food4Health* project, funded by the Ontario Ministry of Health Promotion, sought to test a systemic intervention strategy aimed at fostering cooperative interconnections across the broad food system – including growing, processing, distributing, marketing, retail and disposal. Participating in the project were representatives of small and large for-profit and non-profit organizations, educators, researchers,

citizen advocates, and food service leaders. The overall goal was to strengthen awareness within the system and overall capacity for collaborative action on issues of food system health including: food security, environmental stewardship, and agri-food innovation. Youth and young adults were among the principal populations of interest.

The project incorporated two phases. The first phase was a 10-week rapid-response, proof-of-concept project that incorporated several layers of innovation guided by the CoNEKTR model. These included:

- Initiating a multi-sectoral, participatory strategy for issue identification, exploration and solution generation through face-to-face and social software platforms;
- Engaging youth in food systems issues using social media (e.g., Facebook, Twitter, TakingITGlobal);
- Fostering collaboration between different sectors that had overlapping agendas (food system, health), but hadn't purposefully worked together before;
- Employing a research methodology grounded in theories of complex adaptive systems (e.g., social network analysis, study of emergent properties within systems) along with deployment of a rapid-response action research approach to data collection and knowledge translation (KT);
- And, an integrated feedback generation system that linked data through a central repository that supported rapid, coordinated KT across programs.

The initial face-to-face event was entitled *Food4You!*, the first four such events that would be held over 6 months. This event represented the first step in the process: convening the group. The initial event was held in Toronto, Canada, one of the world's most multicultural cities with a population of 2.5 million people and surrounded by a protected greenbelt that serves to shield high-quality

Figure 4. Photograph of idea sort on issues of food security from Food4Health Project

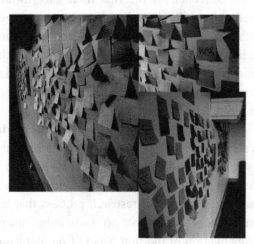

farmland from urban encroachment. Thirty-four youth and 25 adults participated in the event. A strategy aimed at maximum variation was used to identify participants for the event and relied on a snowball approach whereby engaged partners nominated other organizations and individuals who were not involved, but represented a differing perspective. Special attention was paid to those groups least represented in decision making and often most in need of voice such as those from low-income areas of the community, those from visible minorities, immigrants and refugees, and individuals from rural centres. The broad categories of diversity meant that not every group was represented, however the best effort was made for as broad of a sample as possible.

Participants were given a small orientation kit with information on the Food4Health project and its aims at the event where the topic was introduced (step 2 in the process). Once a brief orientation presentation was made regarding the operating definition of food security used to inform the event (step 2), participants participated in a large-group brainstorm session, where ideas were noted on flip-chart paper to ensure transparency. Once an initial set of ideas were discussed as a group, participants independently nominated ideas and

posted them on the wall using sticky notes (step 3). Each participant had multiple sticky notes that they could use to nominate ideas, although participants were not required to use all of the pages. An illustration of this is in Figure 4, which was taken at the initial Food4Health Unconference in Toronto.

The ideas presented on the wall and then sorted using a rapid content analysis by members of the research team (step 4). Together, a set of distinct themes emerged from the initial sort of ideas posted on the wall using the sticky notes. These themes involved: 1) the food industry (production), 2) food availability and selection, 3) taste and appeal, 5) cultural appropriateness, and 5) the ability to access self-sustaining methods for food production (e.g., urban gardening). These themes formed the basis for discussion groups for the afternoon session (step 5).

Participants agreed that the themes were appropriate and did not recommend changes once they were presented by the convenors. The five participant-designed breakout sessions addressed varying topics, several thematic issues and solutions were found across the board from the various discussions (step 6):

1. The idea that food is too expensive and choice is limited in places where youth spend time, particularly schools, including university campuses;
2. Food education is not comprehensive enough (both in terms of physical health, such as nutrition, and mental health, such as eating disorders) and that young people often are mislead or ill-informed about food choices and their consequences for themselves and their communities;
3. *"We are the food industry"* and thus, through action, have control over what foods we eat, how they are produced, and where they come from.

Based on these ideas, a series of actionable steps were proposed for how the group could support moving them into action (step 7). In some cases, leaders (individuals or organizations) stepped forward to take ideas on, while in others there were general recommendations for next steps.

These ideas served as a platform for further discussion on the Youth Voices Research Group Facebook page, TakingITGlobal action page, and for posts to the Twitter feed (steps 8 & 9). At the time of the project, Facebook and TakingITGLobal were both attractive options, while Twitter was still in its emergent phase. Nonetheless, the Twitter feed managed to attract over 225 individuals within its first year. These tools were all considered of interest to participants, however they did not provide the more focused interaction that was initially expected. Thus, a new tool was added for the second phase, described below.

One of the points raised in the face-to-face group and online was a desire to develop a food policy strategy process for the University of Toronto with members of the community (including students). This provided the foundation for the next phase of the project (step 10) and provided punctuation to the first phase of the project and the seeding of a new round of activity.

The success of the first phase of the project in bringing groups together and fostering dialogue, as evidenced from evaluations conducted of the *Food4You!* event and project exit interviews with collaborating organizations and participants, led to the creation of a second phase of the project focused on campus food systems at the University of Toronto. Over four months, three additional face-to-face events were held and supported with the Facebook group, Twitter feed (@food4health), and via a Web-based networking platform (http://studentlife-engagement.ning.com/). The Ning platform was chosen based on its usability and security and was deemed by the research team to be the most appropriate vehicle for online communication and document sharing among the many options available.

The Youth Voices Research Group, served as the convener for the first three face-to-face meetings, while a student-led group emerged as the leader for the final group and continued leading the initiative more than a year after the initial project phase began. The project started in spring 2009 and has remained an ongoing part of the University of Toronto community.

Food4Health demonstrated that social media creates knowledge exchange opportunities and vastly increases the speed of KT across programs, allowing evidence to be mobilized immediately resulting in an action research process that becomes more responsive to knowledge users. An evaluation of the first wave of project using document review, social media use statistics and monitoring, and qualitative interviews with the staff and participants suggested that the project was successful in creating new connections, promoting knowledge translation, and generating useful innovations. Over the extended life of the project a training initiative on food security that was seeded in phase one grew to become a national program, while many new collaborations were formed to produce new funding applications, joint ventures, and strategic partnerships.

CONCLUSION

Scholars looking at the social media sphere have argued that there is a need for some form of political or coordinating overlay to support collaborative decision-making on a broad scale on issues of sensitivity, such as health (Halamka, et al., 2005; Shirky, 2009). The suggestion is not that such interactions should be tightly controlled, but rather that complete self-organization may not be practical or useful to advancing knowledge in a way that is likely to get transmuted into some form of action. The CoNEKTR model aims to balance the benefits of self-organization and self-determined action with a coordinated approach that provides boundaries and stimulates appropriate attractors within the system to provoke change. It was designed to adapt to the needs of busy people who nonetheless face complex problems and seek opportunities to leverage the power of networks to address them.

The CoNEKTR model is employed within flexible constraints and has been used in a variety of different contexts related to health promotion and public health including food security, campus food system health, and global health innovation in business sectors and academic medicine.

Consistent with a public health ethics approach or framework and set of value propositions, the emphasis of the model is on ensuring a diversity of voices are articulated. The problems addressed by the CoNEKTR model are complex ones; those where no single participant in the process has the expertise required to address the problem in its entirety. The model recognizes diverse strengths and knowledge, which provides motivation for a wide range of meaningful participation and effective treatment of complex, perhaps contradictory information by connecting people together. However, these connections and networks also require that attention is paid to the ways in which networks can exacerbate inequalities, rather than reduce them.

Mario Luis Small (2009) has explored this problem and makes seven recommendations on how to reduce potential unintended consequences of social networking and enhance social capital:

1. Create frequent opportunities for interaction;
2. Ensure frequent and regular interactions between agents;
3. Interactions must be long lasting and exist beyond simple, quick exchanges;
4. Interactions are minimally competitive;
5. Interactions are maximally cooperative;
6. Intrinsic motivation consistent with that of the organizations or networks drive interactions and encourage engagement over time;
7. Extrinsic motivators must also be present to support the maintenance of ties over time.

The CoNEKTR model has been designed to realize as many of these elements as possible, which is why the emphasis is on extended, modulated network development using multiple methods (online and offline). It also places explicit emphasis on transparent communication and rapid feedback through evaluation and providing the results to participants quickly after data is collected to inform decision-making. This provides continued evidence of effectiveness to support organizations (or agents affiliated with organizations) to show the return on investment in time and resources for networking.

Like any social process, the CoNEKTR model will evolve over time, refining the processes and steps that produce knowledge and innovation and transform both into social value. Applied in multiple contexts, it has shown itself to be an attractive process for participants looking to develop new knowledge of complex problems and create viable response options. Further evaluation of the model on long-term outcomes is necessary and part of a long-term research strategy by the Youth Voices Research Group and affiliated research projects. In the meantime, the model continues to be used to support the ongoing challenge posed by complex health problems and the opportunity that social networking presents as one means of addressing such issues.

ACKNOWLEDGMENT

The author would like to acknowledge (alphabetically) the following colleagues for providing valuable contributions to the development and implementation of this model over the years: Jill Charnaw-Burger, Monika Goodluck, Charlotte Lombardo, Tamar Meyer, Annie Roy, Samy Saad, Weibke Stoppleman, Richard Streiner and Andrea Yip, who also assisted with the visuals for this chapter.

REFERENCES

Aral, S., & Van Alstyne, M. (2009). *Networks and Novel Information: The Diversity–Bandwidth Tradeoff*. Paper presented at the Workshop on Information in Networks (WIN).

Argyris, C., Putnam, R., & Smith, D. (1985). *Action science: concepts, methods, and skills for research and intervention* (1st ed.). San Francisco, CA: Jossey-Bass.

Balas, E. A., & Boren, S. A. (2000). Managing clinical knowledge for health care improvement. In J. Bemmel & A. T. McCray (Eds.), *Yearbook of Medical Informatics*. Stuttgart, DE: Schattauer Verlagsgesellschaft mbH.

Bero, L., Grilli, R., Grimshaw, J., Harvey, E., Oxman, A., & Thomson, M. (1998). Closing the gap between research and practice: an over view of systematic reviews of inter ventions to promote the implementation of research findings. *British Medical Journal, 317*, 465–469.

Best, A., Hiatt, R., Cameron, R., Rimer, B. K., & Abrams, D. B. (2003). The evolution of cancer control research: An international perspective from Canada and the United States. *Cancer Epidemiology, Biomarkers & Prevention, 12*, 705–712.

Best, A., Hiatt, R. A., & Norman, C. D. (2008). Knowledge integration: conceptualizing communications in cancer control systems. *Patient Education and Counseling, 71*(3), 319–327. doi:10.1016/j.pec.2008.02.013

Best, A., Moor, G., Holmes, B., Clark, P., Bruce, T., & Leischow, S. (2003). Health promotion dissemination and systems thinking: Towards an integrative model. *American Journal of Health Behavior, 27*(Supplement 3), 206–216.

Best, A., Trochim, W. K., Haggerty, J., Moor, G., & Norman, C. D. (2008). Systems thinking for knowledge integration: New models for policy-research collaboration. In McKee, L., Ferlie, E., & Hyde, P. (Eds.), *Organizing and reorganizing: Power and change in health care organizations* (pp. 154–166). Houndsmill, UK: Palgrave Mc-Millan.

Bourdieu, P. (1995). Social space and symbolic power. In McQuarie, D. (Ed.), *Readings in contemporary sociological theory: From modernity to post-modernity* (pp. 323–334). Englewood Cliffs, NJ: Prentice Hall.

Bransford, J. D., Brown, A. L., & Cocking, R. R. (Eds.). (2000). *How people learn: brain, mind, experience, and school*. Washington, DC: National Academy Press.

Brown, J. (2005). *The World Cafe: Shaping our futures through conversations that matter*. San Francisco: Berrett-Koehler.

Brown, T. (2009). *Change by design*. New York: Harper Collins.

Capra, F. (2002). *The hidden connections: integrating the biological, cognitive, and social dimensions of life into a science of sustainability*. New York: Doubleday.

Crossett, L., Kraus, J. R., & Lawson, S. (2009). Collaborative tools used to organize a library camp unconference. *Collaborative Librarianship, 1*(2), 66–69.

Crowley, W. F., Sherwood, L., Salber, P., Scheinberg, D., Slavkin, H., & Tilson, H. (2004). Clinical research in the United States at a crossroads: Proposal for a novel public-private partnership to establish a national clinical research enterprise. *Journal of the American Medical Association, 291*, 1120–1126. doi:10.1001/jama.291.9.1120

Davis, D. A., Evans, M., Jadad, A. R., Perrier, L., Rath, D., & Ryan, D. (2003). The case for knowledge translation: shortening the journey from evidence to effect. *British Medical Journal, 327*(7405), 33–35. doi:10.1136/bmj.327.7405.33

Deci, E. L., & Ryan, R. M. (2008). Self-determination theory: A macrotheory of human motivation, development, and health. *Canadian Psychology/ Psychologie canadienne, 49*(3), 182-185.

Estabrooks, C., Thompson, D., Lovely, J., & Hofmeyer, A. (2006). A guide to knowledge translation theory. *Journal of Continuing Education in the Health Professions*.

Fredericks, K. A., Deegan, M., & Carman, J. G. (2008). Using System Dynamics as an Evaluation Tool: Experience From a Demonstration Program. *The American Journal of Evaluation, 29*(3), 251–267. doi:10.1177/1098214008319446

Gilchrist, A. (2004). *The Well-Connected Community: A Networking Approach To Community Development*. Bristol, UK: Polity Press.

Glass, T., & McAtee, M. (2006). Behavioral science at the crossroads in public health: extending horizons, envisioning the future. *Social Science & Medicine, 62*(7), 1650–1671. doi:10.1016/j.socscimed.2005.08.044

Gloor, P. A. (2006). *Swarm creativity: competitive advantage through collaborative innovation networks*. Oxford, UK: Oxford University Press.

Graham, I. D., Logan, J., Harrison, M. B., & Straus, S. E. (2006). Lost in knowledge translation: Time for a map? *The Journal of Continuing Education in the Health Professions, 26*(1), 13–24. doi:10.1002/chp.47

Green, L. (2006). Public Health asks of systems science: To advance our evidence-based practice, can you help us get more practice-based evidence? *American Journal of Public Health, 96*(3), 406–409. doi:10.2105/AJPH.2005.066035

Green, L., & Glasgow, R. (2006). Evaluating the relevance, generalization, and applicability of research: issues in external validation and translation methodology. *Evaluation & the Health Professions, 29*(1), 126–153. doi:10.1177/0163278705284445

Greenhill, K., & Wiebrands, C. (2008). *The unconference: a new model for better professional communication*. Paper presented at the LIANZA Conference Papers 2008.

Halamka, J., Overhage, J. M., Ricciardi, L., Rishel, W., Shirky, C., & Diamond, C. (2005). Exchanging health information: local distribution, national coordination. *Health Affairs, 24*(5), 1170–1179. doi:10.1377/hlthaff.24.5.1170

Harfoush, R. (2009). *Yes we did: an insider's look at how social media built the Obama brand*. Berkeley, CA: New Riders Press.

Hirsch, G. B., Levine, R., & Miller, R. (2007). Using system dynamics modeling to understand the impact of social change initiatives. *American Journal of Community Psychology, 39*, 239–253. doi:10.1007/s10464-007-9114-3

Ho, K., Jarvis-Selinger, S., Norman, C. D., Li, L., Olatunbosun, T., & Cressmen, C. (in press). Implementing Electronic Community of Practice for Interprofessional Learning and Knowledge Translation: Two Examples. *The Journal of Continuing Education in the Health Professions*.

Howe, J. (2008). *Crowdsourcing: why the future of the crowd is driving the future of business*. New York, NY: Crown Business Publishing.

Israel, B., Schulz, A., Parker, E., & Becker, A. (1998). Review of community-based research: assessing partnership approaches to improve public health. *Annual Review of Public Health, 19*, 173–202. doi:10.1146/annurev.publhealth.19.1.173

Israel, B. A. (1985). Social networks and social support: Implications for natural helper and community level interventions. *Health Education & Behavior*, *12*(1), 65–80. doi:10.1177/109019818501200106

Kane, K., Robinson-Combre, J., & Berge, Z. L. (2010). Tapping into social networking: Collaborating enhances both knowledge management and e-learning. *Vine*, *40*(1), 62–70. doi:10.1108/03055721011024928

Kerner, J. (2006). Knowledge translation versus knowledge integration: A" funders" perspective. *Journal of Continuing Education in the Health Professions.*

Kiefer, L., Frank, J., Di Ruggiero, E., Dobbins, M., Manuel, D., & Gully, P. (2005). Fostering evidence-based decision-making in Canada. *Canadian Journal of Public Health*, *96*(3), 1–18.

Kitson, A. L. (2009). The need for systems change: reflections on knowledge translation and organizational change. *Journal of Advanced Nursing*, *65*(1), 217–228. doi:10.1111/j.1365-2648.2008.04864.x

Kliener, A. (2002). Karen Stephenson: A quantum theory of trust. *Content: The creative mind*, 1-14.

Koschatzky, K. (2002). Networking and Knowledge Transfer Between Research and Industry in Transition Countries: Empirical Evidence from the Slovenian Innovation System. *The Journal of Technology Transfer*, *27*(1), 27. doi:10.1023/A:1013192402977

Lemieux-Charles, L., & Champagne, F. (Eds.). (2004). *The use of knowledge and evidence in health care: multidisciplinary perspectives*. Toronto, ON: University of Toronto Press.

Li, L., Grimshaw, J., Nielsen, C., Judd, M., Coyte, P., & Graham, I. (2009). Evolution of Wenger's concept of community of practice. *Implementation Science; IS*, *4*(1), 11. doi:10.1186/1748-5908-4-11

Loehr, J., & Schwartz, A. (2003). *The Power of Full Engagement: Managing Energy, Not Time, is the Key to High Performance and Personal Renewal*. New York, NY: Free Press.

Lynam, T., Bousquet, F., Le Page, C., d'Aquino, P., Barreteau, O., & Chinembiri, F. (2003). Adaptive science to adaptive managers: Spidergrams, belief models, and multi-agent systems modeling. In Campbell, B. M., & Sayer, J. A. (Eds.), *Integrated Natural Resource Management: Linking Productivity, the Environment and Development* (pp. 157–174). Cambridge, MA: CABI. doi:10.1079/9780851997315.0157

Marincola, F. M. (2003). Translational Medicine: A two-way road. *Journal of Translational Medicine*, *1*(1), 1. doi:10.1186/1479-5876-1-1

Mehra, A., Dixon, A. L., Brass, D. J., & Robertson, B. (2005). (in press). The social networks of leaders: Implications for group performance and leader reputation. *Organization Science.*

Norman, C. D., & Huerta, T. (2006). Knowledge transfer & exchange through social networks: building foundations for a community of practice within tobacco control. *Implementation Science; IS*, *1*(1), 20. doi:10.1186/1748-5908-1-20

Oldenburg, B., & Parcel, G. S. (2002). Diffusion of innovations. In Glanz, K., Rimer, B. K., & Lewis, F. M. (Eds.), *Health behavior and heath education* (3rd ed.). San Francisco, CA: Jossey-Bass.

Owen, H. (1997). *Open space technology: A user's guide*. New York, NY: Berrett-Koehler.

Page, S. E. (2007). *The difference: how the power of diversity creates better groups, firms, schools and societies*. Princeton, NJ: Princeton University Press.

Patton, M. Q. (1990). *Qualitative evaluation and research methods* (2nd ed.). Newbury Park, CA: Sage.

Patton, M. Q. (1994). Developmental Evaluation. *Evaluation Practice, 15*(3), 311–319. doi:10.1016/0886-1633(94)90026-4

Patton, M. Q. (1996). *Utilization-focused evaluation: The new century text* (3rd ed.). Thousand Oaks, CA: Sage.

Patton, M. Q. (2008). *Utilization-focused evaluation* (4th ed.). Los Angeles, CA.

Pescosolido, B. (2006). Of pride and prejudice: the role of sociology and social networks in integrating the health sciences. *Journal of Health and Social Behavior, 47*(3), 189–208. doi:10.1177/002214650604700301

Rifkin, S., Muller, F., & Bichmann, W. (1988). Primary health care: on measuring participation. *Social Science & Medicine, 26*(9), 931–940. doi:10.1016/0277-9536(88)90413-3

Rogers, E. M. (1995). *Diffusion of innovations* (4th ed.). New York: Free Press.

Ryan, R., & Deci, E. (2000). Self-determination theory and the facilitation of intrinsic motivation, social development, and well-being. *The American Psychologist, 55*(1), 68–78. doi:10.1037/0003-066X.55.1.68

Sanger, J. (1994). Seven types of creativity: looking for insights in data analysis. *British Educational Research Journal, 20*(2), 175–185. doi:10.1080/0141192940200203

Sawyer, R. K. (2005). *Social emergence: societies as complex systems*. Cambridge, UK: Cambridge University Press. doi:10.1017/CBO9780511734892

Sawyer, R. K. (2006). *Explaining creativity: The science of human innovation*. Oxford, UK: Oxford University Press.

Sawyer, R. K. (2008). *Group genius: The creative power of collaboration*. New York: Basic Books.

Shirky, C. (2009). *Here comes everybody: the power of organizing without organizations*. New York: Penguin.

Skinner, H. A., Maley, O., & Norman, C. D. (2006). Developing Internet-based eHealth promotion programs: the spiral technology action research (STAR) model. *Health Promotion Practice, 7*(4), 406–417. doi:10.1177/1524839905278889

Small, M. L. (2009). *Unanticipated gains: origins of network inequality in everyday life*. New York: Oxford University Press.

Snowden, D. (2002). Narrative patterns: uses of story in the third age of knowledge management. *Journal of information and knowledge management.*

Stave, K. (2002). Using system dynamics to improve public participation in environmental decisions. *System Dynamics Review.*

Stringer, E. T. (1996). *Action research: A handbook for practitioners*. Thousand Oaks, CA: Sage.

Suitor, J., & Keeton, S. (1997). Once a friend, always a friend? Effects of homophily on women's support networks across a decade. *Social Networks, 19*, 51–62. doi:10.1016/S0378-8733(96)00290-0

Surman, M., & Weshler-Henry, D. (2001). *Common space: beyond virtual community*. Toronto, ON: Pearson - Financial Times.

Surowiecki, J. (2004). *The wisdom of crowds*. New York: Doubleday.

Tapscott, D., & Williams, A. D. (2007). *Wikinomics: how mass collaboration changes everything*. Toronto, ON: Portfolio / Penguin.

Wenger, E. (1998). *Communities of practice: Learning, meaning and identity*. Cambridge, UK: Cambridge University Press.

Wenger, E., & Snyder, W. (2000). Communities of practice: The organizational frontier. *Harvard Business Review, 78*(1), 139–145.

Westley, F., Zimmerman, B., & Patton, M. (2006). *Getting to maybe: How the world is changed.* Toronto, ON: Random House Canada.

Whyte, W. F. (1991). *Participatory action research.* Newbury Park, CA: Sage.

ENDNOTE

[1]   Ning: http://www.ning.com is a tool designed to enable groups to create customized social networks for a monthly fee; Crowdvine (http://www.crowdvine.com) charges a fee up-front as its revenue model. Both enable users to create their own social networks with features like bulletin boards, photo- and document-sharing.

Chapter 32

Emerging Trends in User–Driven Healthcare:
Negotiating Disclosure in Online Health Community Organizations

Handan Vicdan
Eastern Kentucky University, USA

ABSTRACT

The purpose of this chapter is to explore transformations in market roles and relations that reflect collaborative, connective and communal characteristics among healthcare market actors, in light of technological advances and changing consumer-marketer institutional relationships. I exemplify how these transformations influence current market dynamics by providing a deep understanding of Web 2.0 applications in healthcare, specifically organizations that turn social networking into an enterprising virtual community in healthcare. In doing so, I explore how and why such systems develop and function, what makes patients and other actors in healthcare become a part of these systems, and how their interest and participation in these systems are maintained as they share their private health information and contribute to real-time medical research. Consequently, I suggest that current market dynamics in healthcare may be changing as a result of these systems utilizing social networking and engaging in reformation/reconstitution in the healthcare market.

MARKET RELATIONS AT A GLANCE

Past studies of markets and marketing relations have articulated the structure of relationships between consumers and organizations they interact with in the market largely exhibiting dialectical processes (Murray & Ozanne, 1991; Peñaloza & Price, 1993; Slater & Tonkiss, 2001). That is,

scholars generally adopted oppositional and distinct constitution of market actors. For example, some scholars have conceptualized the consumer as (1) a sovereign rational actor (Kotler, 2003, classical economic thought), (2) passive, obedient, and powerless dupe (Horkheimer & Adorno, 1993; Marcuse, 1991), (3) resisting, subversive and confrontational agent (Fiske, 1989; Peñaloza & Price, 1993), and (4) adopting emancipatory/liberatory interests in escaping the market (Kozinets,

DOI: 10.4018/978-1-60960-097-6.ch032

2002a). Some scholars argued that as opposed to the consumer, the marketer is exploiting, powerful, commodifying, and having central role in co-creation (provisioning in a linear and sequential manner) (Terranova, 2004; Zwick et al., 2008). In addition, hegemonic market thrives on these dialectical tensions (Holt, 2002; Kozinets et al., 2004; Thompson, 2004). It has also been suggested that the conventional market order serves as *an* institution (Slater & Tonkiss, 2001), through which market actors are constituted as agents or means to achieve market exchanges rather than ends in themselves (Peñaloza & Venkatesh, 2006).

Recent theories of market relations have adopted a more modest view of consumer-marketer relations, emphasizing co-creation of value, collaboration among market actors (Denegri-Knott, 2004; Holt, 2002; Kozinets et al., 2004; Thompson, 2004; Vargo & Lusch, 2004, Zwick & Dholakia, 2004). Nonetheless, in these theories, the marketer seems to be assigned to institutionalize the 'proper' way of conduct and engage in interactions with consumers in provisioning what they need and want (Firat & Dholakia, 2006), and has central role in co-creation: Provisioning consumer needs/wants (Vargo & Lusch, 2004). In fact, critical scholars have considered co-creation as an exploitation and control tool of corporations (Terranova, 2004; Zwick et al., 2008).

These views of the market and market relations rest mainly on modern conceptions of power including domination, confrontation (Venn, 2007) and unilateral governing of relationships (one way of dictating and imposing), and advocate the use of maximizing, and normalizing discourses by marketers. Such discourses in healthcare include fear of loss of life, normalization of body, prolonging lifespan, and threat of death (Rose, 2007). Medical interventions generally involved this top-down approach: Doctors, researchers, pharmaceuticals and other influentials in the market tell patients what/ what not to do and decide on what patients need to know. Hence, human body in modern society has become an object of one-way scrutiny and surveillance by a superior and rational medical gaze (Foucault, 1975).

Technological advances have remediated the superior-inferior dialectics between the physician and the patient. That is, informed patients have become partners with their receptive physicians (Jadad, 1999; McGregor, 2006). In addition, recent transformation of social networking (Web 2.0) into a business phenomenon (Tapscott & Williams, 2008) has served as a potential to challenge the conventional forms of business, which treat organizations and consumers as distinct entities. In modern market society, organizations were considered as distinct/detached entities from consumers in the market, providing goods/services to satisfy the needs of their target markets (Firat & Dholakia, 2006; Peñaloza & Venkatesh, 2006), which led to explaining consumer-marketer relations in oppositional constitution. Nonetheless, in light of technological transformations, organizations seem to be not separate from their markets, serve as a system of real-time processes (not in sequential or linear ways), where performers of the market together discover and design their needs in actual or virtual collectivities (Firat & Dholakia, 1998; Kozinets, 2002a).

As newer technologies (Web 2.0[1] and social networks) enable the transformation of roles and relations among market actors, they also increase the potential for collaboration among actors in market systems that now function on more complex set of relations. Web 2.0 technologies emphasize innovative, data-oriented, service-centered collaboration, increased levels of user contribution, organization of content through non-hierarchical methods, and increased aspirations of community building, sharing and interaction (Bleicher, 2006). Despite conflicting views (Eysenbach et al., 2004; Jadad et al., 2006), Web 2.0 applications in healthcare present the potentials to transform the long dominating top-down approach in healthcare and change patient-healthcare provider roles and relations: Patients now get involved in clinical research and in determination of their and others' care along with other healthcare market actors, and manage medical knowledge (Jadad, 1999). Such transformations could decentralize the control and use of personal health data, change the mindset of physicians concerning patients as incompetent and solely recipients of information and service (Deshpande & Jadad, 2006), and bring about institutional change in healthcare in a mode of collaboration rather than in a mode of provision.

As scholars discuss potential transformations in market systems, which emphasize learning and co-creating value in networked relations, along with recent transformations in emerging Web 2.0 technologies (Tapscott & Williams, 2008), particular examples as to where and how these transformations are occurring are generally missing. To close this gap, following observations from netnographic (Kozinets, 2002b) inquiry of a specific Health 2.0 community organization, PatientsLikeMe (PLM), which seems to exhibit the potential for such transformations and novel organizations of relations among healthcare market actors, I explore (1) why and how such systems develop and function (2) institutionalizations that develop and maintain these new forms of interactions and relationships, make people become a part of these systems, and share their private health information.

What prompted me to look into this community organization was the cover story of Business 2.0 magazine. Eric Schonfeld and Chris Morrison (2007) talked about a specific healthcare website called PatientsLikeMe (PLM) in Business 2.0 magazine, and argued that PLM is one of the ten organizations that have the potential to rewrite the rules of existing industries and open up entirely new markets. Briefly, PLM is a for-profit (only profit source is the sale of aggregated anonymous patient data to pharmaceuticals) web-based community organization that involves patients, physicians, pharmaceutical companies, healthcare providers and researchers, and the administrators of the website, and uses social networking for clinical trials. Patients manage their and others'

disease through aggregation and organization of personal health data at no monetary cost, and we observe real-time partnership among healthcare actors (data-sharing partnerships with doctors, pharmaceutical and medical device companies, research organizations, and non-profits in pursuit of acceleration of medical research) as well as real-time research (open and non-blinded, patient-driven and patient generated clinical trials). Hence, the site features various types of relationships – both discursive and substantive – with different healthcare players, and engages in clinical research – which was traditionally the remit of academics and clinicians – through experience mining.

Recent trends in the healthcare market, such as the transformation of social networking in health-care (Health 2.0[2]) into a business phenomenon, and the use of social networking for clinical trials are some of the novel establishments these systems offer (Kliff, 2009). Patients now have increased access and potential to become a part of clinical trials, and such patient generated clinical trials attract more funding from pharmaceuticals and future patient recruitment for randomized controlled clinical trials. The collective wisdom that initiates clinical trials through aggregation and analysis of anecdotal personal health information and experience mining is noteworthy, since clinical trials were traditionally the remit of academics and clinicians (physicians determine the eligibility of the patient to become a part of a clinical trial) and were generally considered as a distant hope and not a real world solution for diseases. In fact, many patients are not found eligible to take part in these clinical trials or are not even asked to participate, removing options and control from patients. Yet, observations from recent Web 2.0 applications in healthcare reveal that the real-time research conducted with patients and other actors in online communities gives the vast majority of patients to participate in such trials and have their voices be heard. Patient generated clinical trials in online communities may also serve as a potential and unique source of information (body of medical knowledge generated with many patients with diverse profiles) for traditional clinical trials due to their discovery oriented nature and hypothesis generation orientation (Arnquist, 2009; Arnst, 2008; Johnson, 2008). Such clinical trials may also increase the potential for accelerated trials and faster discovery of diagnosis, prognosis and treatment knowledge, and be more cost effective compared to traditional medical research (Sheridan, 2008).

Consequently, the above observations indicate that the potentials of novel roles and organizations of relations between consumers (patients) and other members of the healthcare market seem to be on the rise. Such relations seem to be qualitatively different from the conventional market relations based on modern marketing principles. That is, there may be different kinds of market models where consumers become involved as partners in decisions that are made together with marketers in a mode of collaboration rather than in a mode of provision. Hence, the exploration of how such systems develop and function, and maintain people's interest will likely attract attention to changing consumer-marketer value systems, roles and relationships in such systems, and the constitution of the consumer and the marketer in dialogue (interacting without necessarily establishing dominancy), collaboration, connectivity and community, rather than in a dominant/dominated dialectic. Ultimately, I aim to discuss overall implications of such consumer-marketer collaboration on the healthcare market.

The contribution of this research is threefold:

1. Shed light on understanding of new systems of marketing roles and relationships
2. Provide insights into developments in healthcare provision and changes in healthcare marketing systems as a result of these systems utilizing social networking and engaging in reformation/reconstitution in healthcare

3. Reconsider previous theories of market and market relations, which have articulated the structure of relationships between consumers and organizations they interact with in the market largely exhibiting dialectical processes:
   a. oppositional constitution of consumer and marketer in dominant/dominated dialectic,
   b. Unidirectional provisioning that gives control and primacy to the marketer, hierarchical relations among actors in market systems,
   c. One way governing of relationships through normalizing and maximizing discourses.

DYNAMICS OF A HEALTH 2.0 FORMATION IN HEALTHCARE

As I engaged in this specific Health 2.0 community organization, PLM, I observed how patients, organization administrators and other healthcare market actors communicate and form and maintain relations with each other, and negotiate the disclosure of private health information in this system. I focused on patient-to-patient, patient-to-organization founders and administrators, and patient-to-physician/caregiver/researcher interactions, and how patient-healthcare provider relations outside of the community are influenced as a result by paying attention to patients' own accounts. In the following section, I aim to unravel the dynamics of this Health 2.0 community organization by laying out the observations, which seem to exhibit potentials for novel constitution of market roles and relations.

Sharing of Private Health Information Redefined

First, such a system brings a structural approach to sharing private health information. Stories, narratives, anecdotal sharing of experiences are turned into systematic, structural sharing for research) for research conducted by a community of patients and other healthcare actors brought together in this platform. This is a sharp distinction from online health information sites such as WebMD or DailyStrength, which serve as providers of online health information sites and platforms for sharing medical information at the anecdotal level. Sharing of private health information among diverse actors and the subsequent experience mining may have the potential to contribute to paradigm change in medicine, where all is considered private. In addition, the alternative to opt-in and opt-out of this system in the form of lurking and temporary detachment for the patient provides feelings of freedom to choose/not choose to share his/her private health information. It allows for observation only, which indicates that a patient does not have to actively participate in discussions, as is the case in support groups. S/he can just observe or lurk or listen, rather than feel the pressure to participate, hence enjoy temporary detachment. S/he does not have to complete profile information to participate in discussions or become a member of the community either. The system is open to everyone (patient's family members and friends, caregivers, researchers, pharmaceuticals and the like), not just limited to doctors or patients. Patients quantify their personal health information and turn it into hard data through a sophisticated system designed by the organization. They keep journals of their own individual experiences. They list symptoms of the disease, treatments received, and different lifestyles led. This individual patient information is then pooled, systematically recorded for analysis, and visualized by the designers of the system. In addition, there are sub-communities formed by patients, who have life-changing diseases (e.g., ALS, MS, Mood, Parkinson Disease, HIV), and other actors such as caregivers, patient family members, researchers, physicians and the like. Patients and other actors in the community interact with each other anecdotally through private

messaging or public messaging in forums and the website's general community blog. They create profiles and share their experiences in forums and community blogs. Although, the organization encourages public profiles and most of the profiles are indeed public, patients have the option to either make their profiles visible only to community members or public. The aggregated information from patient profiles and forums is created in collaboration with the organization, and the system functions well only if patients update their data. Another noticeable fact is that the system forgoes advertising and relies only on word-of-mouth sustainability, which provides feelings of safety for patients in terms of sharing their data, another distinction from other online virtual health communities. Patients also feel safe and get help whenever they need (real-time help). Through a sophisticated search mechanism, patients can have access to personal information of other patients, who have similar or different experiences worldwide. They list their symptoms, treatments that worked or did not work for them, their progression of the disease, alternative lifestyles they lead and engage in mutual sharing and learning.

Value Systems and Forms of Discourse among Healthcare Actors Transform

Second and most importantly, we observe that the value systems and forms of discourse among diverse healthcare actors in this community seem to transform. For example, institutionalizations of relations and conduct between consumers and marketers appear to be performed by a community of diverse actors in search for the 'possible' instead of the 'proper'. Orders in the community are not determined but constantly negotiated in non-confrontational modes. Value systems are established on recognizing and keeping differences despite conflicting positions among healthcare actors. There is also a shift from confrontational and representational discourses to presentational discourses and tolerance for difference (move away from search for resolution for the benefit of one party's self interest). Patients seek for conflict, challenge and acceptance simultaneously. Patients and other healthcare actors engage in presentational modes of sharing of experiences and provide support for each other. They present their experiences with incidents in their lives. They talk about how they've treated their diseases, so others can read and learn from them. Hence, arguing the 'rationale' of what ought to be done is abandoned, 'telling' others what to do is discouraged, 'exhibiting' what can be done through example is preferred (Firat & Dholakia, 1998). Furthermore, the forms of discourse that promote maximization (Jackson, 2000; Sarup, 1993), universal emancipation, and *an* order of organizing lives also seem to be waning. Patients and other healthcare actors engage in both formal and informal sharing. For example, members adopt ironic, critical, and playful engagement with diverse modes of life, and seek for friendly and humorous seriousness in sharing and suffering. They remind each other that they are there to do research and accelerate the discovery of cures, not just have fun, socialize, and seek emotional support by discussing off-topic, non-disease related issues. Yet, at the same time, such ironic engagement seems to help patients cope with their diseases and make the community not only a care-bear community. Members also engage in material and immaterial sharing. They express their desire to exploit their disability for material gain, and turn participatory culture into a business phenomenon, hence leading to material manifestations of their immaterial labor. They seek for both goal achievement (e.g., discover cures for diseases and increase disease awareness) and lifestyle enhancement (e.g., share different lifestyles they lead when coping with their disease).

Meanings of Community Transform: From Belongingness to Connectedness

Third, with these specific Web 2.0 applications in healthcare and in medicine, the meaning of community seems to be transformed. We observe a shift in the meaning of community from a social phenomenon outside of organization (Peñaloza & Venkatesh, 2006) to a business phenomenon (Hummel & Lechner, 2001). Community becomes the enterprise, not outside of the organization, and not temporarily or locally bound. Online communities can be empowering in that they enable access to information and knowledge, and experiencing of the other. In addition, the sense of collectivity is forged with other consumers (Fischer et al., 1996). Nonetheless, the meaning of collective is not about *belongingness* but about *connectedness*. As we keep personal information to ourselves or to the community members, we simultaneously detach ourselves from others. This is due to the fact that secrecy or privacy, while bonding community members (as personal information is only accessible by community members), isolates the individual from others, and removes the heterogeneity of the community and interactions of members and others (Appadurai, 1991). Yet, through Web 2.0 applications in healthcare, we observe a shift in emphasis from belongingness to connectedness in communities and in healthcare. Patients link and tag their existences in various virtual spaces (e.g., myspace, facebook, youtube) and invite other actors to navigate among these virtual platforms. The consumer transforms from someone who *belongs* to a culture, a society, or a lifestyle; to someone who actively *negotiates* one or more communities; a cultural constructor, and a *player* (Bauman, 1996) but always necessarily with(in) and as part of a community. Hence, encounters with other actors in this market system involve immersion in the experience as players and recognizing each other's differences, rather than detaching themselves from these encounters and contesting the other's differences.

As patients connect with other patients from other countries in this community, their learning experience is not only limited to learning in the community. They do not only learn from each other's experiences but also from the multitudes of valuable links they provide on several topics. In addition, collaboration intensifies the connectivity among market actors both within the community and outside of the community. For example, the system contributes to increased disease literacy of the patient and the physician. Patient disease literacy is increased through mediation between patient self-report and interpretation of private health data, which fosters patient-physician relations outside of the community. Patients become more equipped with disease knowledge and engage in proactive relations with their receptive physicians, with the hope that they earn their physicians' respect. Physicians also get more information about diseases by tracking down different patients with specific diseases in this community. Physicians also provide several links of information in their interactions with patients in the community. Therefore, we observe increased aspirations of sharing and increased connectedness between patient-patient, patient-physician, patient-pharmaceutical, patient-government in and/or through this system. Doctor visit sheets and mood charts created in the community help patients track their diseases, compare their conditions with other patients and empathize with them (which also increases their tolerance for each other), and allow for better management of their care through this aggregated private health information. Patients also share these charts and visit sheets with their physicians outside of the community. In addition, a 'share this' button on each patient's profile enables patients to share their knowledge and experiences with others outside of the community. Another recent development also indicates intensified connectedness in healthcare through this community. Patients can directly

report drug side effects to Food and Drug Administration, which may accelerate the years-long traditional clinical research process, and enable effective supervision by FDA on pharmaceuticals. In addition, ongoing clinical research by patients and other healthcare actors in this community scientifically supports off-label drug use. Such information is then delivered to pharmaceuticals and clinicians, once again intensifying collaboration between patients and other healthcare actors. The community engages in the scientific discovery of new uses of existing medications, and new side effects of existing drugs, all of which may serve as a useful check for errors for pharmaceuticals. By bridging the gap between anecdote based medicine and evidence based medicine, the community also has the potential to inform and guide future clinical practice and serve as a useful check for pharmaceuticals, healthcare providers and governmental institutions (FDA).

Constitution of the Consumer and the Marketer Transforms

Fourth, observations from this community seem to exhibit potentials for the constitution of consumer and marketer as collaborative subjects, who opt to act jointly rather than individually or in opposition. For example, the patient adopts diverse roles: S/he serves as an experiential expert, presentational mentor, and confirmer (validation) of one's and others' health status: S/he exhibits her/his experiences of how s/he manages the disease, without preaching or giving advice to others. Preaching is also discouraged by the organization administrators. Community members' actions are results of presentational modes of sharing of experiences, stories, and self-revelations. They do not urge each other to take action or suggest issues that would require them to determine and coordinate actions. Instead, members tend to present their tendencies of thinking and acting, and their experiences with incidents in their lives (talk about what they've done, how they've treated their diseases, so others can read and learn from them), which then find allure among other members of the community. Patients now have increased feelings of license to exert control over their and others' bodies and the doctor's expert power. Nonetheless, many patients are willing to complement the doctor's expert power with their experiential knowledge. Even though they may be inclined to resist, this resistance is to reliance on a single source of information and expert opinion, not the expert opinion itself. Hence, physician comes to be one of the many experts patients rely on. Patients engage in a *presentational* mode of suggesting the potentials and possibilities of including the 'other', the 'unrepresentable' and the unfamiliar (Caputo, 1997), in order to seek and create rich and meaningful life experiences. In effect, arguing the 'rationale' of what ought to be done is abandoned, 'telling' others what to do is discouraged, 'exhibiting' what can be done through example is preferred (Firat & Dholakia, 1998). These burgeoning cultural orientations have also prompted people to readily adopt new communication technologies that enable linking to communities for envisioning new and enticing modes of living and being. They avoid representing reality to others or suggesting unique solutions to their communities. Instead, they present their experiences, ideas about potentials, feelings about events.

The marketer in this constitution serves as a real-time partner, a co-constructor and co-analyst of medical knowledge and experience. Patients no longer consider the doctor as a consultant, who tells them what to do or who is a pure authority figure. Rather, the doctor serves as an analyst, who integrates her/his knowledge and skills with the knowledge and experience of patients, and constructs alternative modes of life with the patients. With the tracking tools in the community, patients constantly monitor their conditions and analyze the progression of their diseases with their physicians outside of the community. Health 2.0 community organizations that gather different market actors in its constitution serve as a co-mediated market platform. They enable organized decentralization of sharing private health data and mobilize market actors as a non-state institution through organized ethos of hope (Rose, 2007).

Community Dynamics of Sharing Private Health Information

Fifth and another important aspect of this community is that different market actors gather and share their 'private' health information. Yet, what are the community (meso level) dynamics that make these actors share their private health information? Sharing of personal health information was impossible to have access and give away due to privacy regulations and proprietary policies. Yet, today, patients engage in mutual sharing of private health data, and seek knowledgeable patients and physicians and learn from them as well as from other actors on a global scale. They add brief autobiographies to their profiles, and describe their conditions in precise detail (e.g., potentially embarrassing information on sexual function, bladder control or constipation). Most patients have pseudonyms, yet many of them use their first names when discussing issues in the forums. Along with sharing of personal health data and how they cope with the disease and lead alternative lifestyles, patients also share their private pictures, poems, videos, links to personal web pages, other social networking sites and the like. Mutual learning also stimulates the desire to share and inform others, make themselves and others suffer well. More sharing also leads to more acceptance of one's status, more mentoring of others, and more humanizing of the disease. Consequently, mutual sharing of personal health information eliminates ignorance and fear about the disease and increases disease literacy of patients and other actors in the system.

More importantly, we observe a move beyond regimes of domination that promotes fear and contestation (Fillion, 2005; Hardt & Negri, 2000) to regimes of collaboration that promotes hope and negotiation. By providing consumers with meaning, substance, continuity, and alternative possibilities for organizing their lives and changing the meaning of diseases a result of mutual discourses among community members, such communities alleviate the likely fear and loss of ownership of private information associated with the definition of privacy as well as mortality salience formerly stimulated by governments and other influentials in the healthcare market (hide it or lose it, panoptic fear). Dialogues and communications in this community encourage the transformation from proprietorship to partnership in disclosure and distribution of health data, which challenges the very definition of privacy: Control over externalization of one's personal information, which *belongs* to the person (Benn, 1971; Culnan, 1993; Gavison, 1980; Goodwin, 1991). Hence, patients now advocate the sharing of private health information as a fundamental human right, as was the case for privacy.

Also, dialogues and interactions among diverse healthcare actors indicate that the boundaries of coercion and consent are blurred through non-dominating discursive regimes (e.g., quality of life) and cultural values (e.g., voluntarism, transparency/openness). The organization collects, analyzes, aggregates, and disseminates collective experience and knowledge of actors with openness philosophy. Patients especially advocate open sharing of private health information as long as it increases accessibility to disease related information and drives treatment research, improves patient-physician relations, enables both social and knowledge support among members, and stimulates patient learning of diseases in diagnosis, prognosis, and treatment stages. Such systems identify themselves as opt-in services, not healthcare providers (changes in healthcare provision), which upends the HIPAA rules for patient privacy (Goetz, 2008). As discussed earlier, prior conceptualizations of privacy suggested that privacy is related to secrecy, which implies the deliberate concealment of one's private in-

formation from others. In addition, this private information is owned by an individual and the individual has sole control over disclosure of his/her private information. With the advent of new technologies, we observe an increase in the number of institutions and people who cross the borders of one's privacy and have a say in the construction of this privacy. With privacy borders becoming more permeable in the digital age and disclosure becoming more of a communicative and relational process, private information is no longer something that is owned by private entity but has become public entity that is co-owned, as patients disclose their private information to others in the community. Patients voluntarily, that is, without deception, coercion, or threat, choose to share or not share their private information. Hence disclosure involves a certain degree of voluntariness, with the system serving as an arbitrator blurring the boundaries of coercion and consent.

In addition, patients and other market actors in this community emphasize more personalization in healthcare and increase in quality of life, and less normalization of bodies, or maximization of life spans. There seems to be an increased focus on the enhancement of lifestyle (as a result of observing diverse patient profiles, different lifestyles they lead, and different forms of medicine they apply) rather than maximization of lifespan formerly stimulated by healthcare providers and the government. Medical interventions seem to transform with the changing consumer culture, since patients as consumers make choices based not only on a medical enforcement of curing the disease and optimizing their health but also on a variety of factors that enhance their and others' vitality and quality of life, their knowledge about diseases, and enable them to live diseases better.

Self and/through Communal Modulation of Sharing Private Information

Dynamics of the community culture also shape the extent and appropriateness of disclosure and the type of the relationship between the discloser and the recipient of this private information. When a patient discloses her/his private health data to others in this community, s/he first quantifies that information in her/his profile, and continues to discuss about her/his experiences in community forums. Then, the designers of the system aggregate and visualize this information. Such information is then disseminated to other patients, who will slice and splice this information based on similarities and differences with others in terms of their diseases. Preceding this process, the organization, following its transparency philosophy, declares the design of the business. PLM declares upfront, how the collection, deployment, analysis and dissemination of patient data will be performed, and who are the partners (e.g., research institutions, pharmaceutical companies) to whom aggregated patient data are sold anonymously.

Patients constantly negotiate their decisions to disclose personal health information in forums, blogs etc, with other actors. Hence, rules that control the level of revealing and concealing private information are negotiated among the actors and are influenced by the community culture in the system. The script of sharing and organizing in the community is constantly negotiated by all members of the community. Patients actively engage in organization of shared health information, forum discussions and create solutions for making sharing easier for members. The system also enables the patient to have a say in the organization of sharing private health data through light-touch moderation. Administrators of the community let members create their own norms of sharing, work out their own disputes, and decide on the extent and form of disclosing their health information. Compared to a lot of other online communities where a moderator might have to approve every post or delete things inexplicably, light moderation in this community emphasizes that patients are the experts about their conditions, and administrators do not delete posts unless they violate user agreement.

Members also recommend each other to focus more on self-censorship in order not to create excessive feud in forums. At times, members feel that administrators serve as a shield for those who are uncomfortable with improper posts, medical advice posts (specifically those that preach about certain medications or treatments), which are not welcomed by the members of the community. Administrators and members continuously emphasize this light moderation and tolerance (allowing others to have different opinions), and administrators are willing to police the community only when members cannot find a solution for disputes and they seek help from the administrators. In addition, patients use private and public messaging and profile options to alleviate tensions when conflicts arise. Patients argue that feuds are considered a part of the community and they should not be the reason to leave the community, since their primary goal is to fight with the disease. Patients can temporarily detach themselves in the form of lurking private messaging as they share their private information. All in all, they perceive this community as the best platform to cope with such problems, and a classroom to accept differences, practice and get ready for the real world and practice a different life in the community. They consider the community as not just a supporter but also a field to grow and look at their illnesses constructively rather than just acknowledge the fact that they are ill.

IMPLICATIONS ON HEALTHCARE MARKET

From government intervention to community intervention in organizing sharing of private health information:

Perception of privacy as a fundamental human right seems somewhat *absolutist* and it may be the case in many cultures; yet in the U.S., privacy is treated as a matter for contractual negotiations (Chan et al., 2005, p. 283), and becomes a tangible entity to organize relationships. Perception of privacy as a fundamental human right indicates that the right to protect privacy –to determine and control the fate of one's own personal information – is led by the individual himself/herself, not the government (Cavoukian & Tapscott, 1995). Nonetheless, governments still intervene in this process. Governmental efforts to protect patient privacy resulted in the establishment of Health Insurance Portability & Accountability Act of 1996 (HIPAA). As Brown (2008) suggests, HIPAA, which strictly sets boundaries on the flow of patient health records to third parties such as insurance companies and employers, controls the private citizens and increases their sensitivity about privacy (e.g., privacy rules concerning disclosure of consumer personal health information thrived on the preceding creation of fear-based societies), has served as a barrier to research and discovery.

Contemporary medicine had long served as a disciplinary entity to maximize our lifespan and normalize our bodies, hence prevent us from death. Governmental institutions utilized 'security' as a discourse of power in this process (Epstein, 2006), particularly as a means to protect patient privacy. For example, they referred to discourses of fear and restitution of normality (healthy body) through threat of death, which had the potential to increase mortality salience among patients. With the increased use of Internet for acquisition, analysis, aggregation, dissemination, deployment and sharing of private health data and information, healthcare industry and governments established policies to protect patient privacy, which rested on the 'hide it or lose it' perspective concerning online privacy (Weitzner et al., 2008). As Weitzner et al. (2008) also suggest, these parties' excessive reliance on secrecy and desire to have control over patient health information caused information privacy rights to be established as a means to provide safety to patients and protect their autonomy against those who are likely to violate or invade their privacy rights. HIPAA – though considered unsatisfactory and insufficient by some privacy advocates and a stumbling block by medical researchers – is now being challenged by Web 2.0 formations in healthcare. Through social networking, individuals 'share' their knowledge and experiences, and engage in clinical research with other healthcare actors, and embrace the 'shared' world that provides new possibilities of organizing lives. One of the patients in the community suggests that current HIPAA regulations, while well intentioned, keep researchers from connecting the dots to understand what causes life changing diseases (e.g., ALS), hence serving as a stumbling block to discovery and research.

As also discussed in the forums and blogs of this community, patients in this community assess the past physician-patient relationship as a top-down relationship, a one-way governing and surveillance by the physician. They argue that physician was considered the sole authority of health and treatment of diseases in the past. Information sharing was minimal not only between patients and physicians but also among physicians themselves. Hence, they concur that openness and privacy are much bigger concerns out in the real world when patients and other healthcare actors interact with each other. Physicians generally withheld information in order not to burden patient with unnecessary info. Some patients in the community also complain about their physicians that they treat them like a number or a piece, not as a whole. Such issues raised by patients may stem from the long dominating paternalistic approach to patient care (physician with white uniform and stethoscope is an authority figure and s/he knows it all), leaving limited room for partnership. Patients in this community argue that physician knowledge was generally limited to literature s/he has read, patients s/he has treated and colleagues s/he has talked to. In addition, clinical trials would include only a small number of patients and the results would be published in medical journals, hence limiting the number of people who benefit from such results. Along these arguments, patients also add that physicians are eventually limited to theoretical knowledge and unable to offer real-time, on-demand health. Consequently, disconnection among these healthcare actors was inevitable. Even pharmaceutical sales reps in this community stressed their disconnection from the patients they assisted.

With the advent of new technologies, physician is no longer considered the sole source of information, sole conduit of specialist knowledge, and sole authority of treatment. Patients are beginning to control their own and others' disease as a means to enhance their lifestyles and improve their quality of life. As discussed by patients and researchers in the community blog, although approached critically by some of the influentials in the market based on the premise that these hyperinformed patients engage in guerilla science and self-medication and increase their risk of death through becoming a part of online health communities (Haig, 2007), social networking technologies enabled consumers to gain more control over their personal health data and in management of their health, and actively engage in conducting clinical trials. For example, some drug side effects discovered in ALS community through a clinical trial was criticized as not scientific enough. In addition, such user-generated trial was approached skeptically by some medical experts and peer-reviewed medical journals. Despite these criticisms, patients in this community also attract attention to the drawbacks of traditional clinical trials. That is, patients have limited access to randomized clinical trials research; clinicians and academics are in full control of who to choose for trials and what information to make accessible, which made information available to limited group of people. In addition, traditional clinical trials are perceived as a distant hope and not a real-world solution for many people. Patients emphasize the importance of fast and real-time clinical trials, particularly for life-changing diseases. They argue that the use of social networking for clinical trials brings the accessibility to various patients to clinical trials with no set rules/criteria, as opposed to traditional

clinical trials, which are under the control of clinicians and academics, and limit patient access. In addition, mutual sharing of health information, learning and doing research help patients better understand their conditions and increase their quality of life through making adjustment to their lifestyles, treatments and the like. Patients also become a part of these communities and actively engage in clinical research with the hope that such engagement improves patient-physicians relations outside of the community as patients become proactive in their care, and accelerates the discovery of cures of life changing diseases.

As mentioned earlier, medical knowledge generated in this community serves as a potential source of hypothesis generation and be validated by traditional clinical research. Patients are actively involved in creation of services (including clinical research). They contribute to the development of new treatments, accelerate medical research and bring better treatments to the market faster than ever before. They become more active in their care, discover their diseases or symptoms, generate data about their symptoms, medications and treatments, and present alternative ways of coping (scientific or alternative forms of healing) with diseases to create a patient experience database. Consequently, they also manage others' care. Empowered and informed patient also has the potential to stimulate more knowledgeable, talented physicians, and enhance physician knowledge and expertise.

Through Web 2.0 applications in healthcare, our corporeal experiences are now (re)constructed by new forms of intervention with other consumers, medical experts, researchers and the like, hence leading to a move away from self-medication to self and/through other medication. As we observe the waning of unidirectional provisioning and overly deterministic actions of marketers – which were prominent in dominant marketing approaches –, and attract attention to the fact that consumers and marketers are in fact both a part of a social system and a market system (Cova,

2005, p.210), governing of relations becomes a multidirectional process rather than a top-down or a bottom-up process with communities formed by organizations and consumers. Actions and (dis)agreements mainly emerge from non-linear, multi-way negotiations when patients share their private health information and continue to be a part of these communities. Increased connectivity among diverse healthcare actors within and outside of this community may also bring about the transformation of new roles and relations in healthcare as well as multi-way communications that are hard to be classified as sovereignty and exploitation. Power disparities may exist among the actors of the system and serve as enablers or delimiters of sharing and disclosing of private health information. But the important issue is how the system can maintain itself despite power disparities and how power becomes a productive force and brings about institutional change in healthcare through this meso level context.

(Re)institutionalizing Surveillance in Healthcare

As previously discussed, the dominance of the top-down approach in healthcare has led to the constitution of patient-physician relations in a one-way surveillance in favor of the rational medical gaze, the physician. Technological and cultural transformations have moved the building blocks of this top-down relation, while empowering the patient to have control over her/his management of health. Nonetheless, the use of social networking in healthcare presents the potentials that patients and other performers of the healthcare market engage in *mutual surveillance* of their diseases. They create a systematic, real-time process that involves collection, analysis, aggregation, and dissemination of shared private health information and the resulting discovery of disease related information through collectivities enabled by Health 2.0 community organizations. Hence, surveillance is institutionalized by a community

of diverse healthcare actors, and discourses among community members influence the decision to share/not share private health information and sustain their interest in the community.

Although recent evidence suggests that consumers are almost never willing to share their medical information online[3] (Lenhart & Madden, 2007), consumer decisions to disclose such private information and the ongoing negotiation concerning disclosure of personal health information among the members of this community is intriguing. This does not mean that they have no privacy concerns. Discourses among the members of this community reveal that the decisions to disclose/not disclose private health information are shaped by both individual and macro concerns: (1) access to identity or revealing of personally identifiable information (e.g., social security numbers, credit card numbers, mailing addresses) is not wanted, (2) employment issues, (fear of losing jobs due to disclosure of private health information), (3) insurance companies could have access to patient private health information, (4) pertinence of information sought for to patient care, (5) government patriot act rendering privacy meaningless at this time in history (belief that we are always being watched), (6) stigmatization associated with revealing information about their diseases, (7) possessive and fear focused characters, and (8) familial reasons (families cannot relate to their diseases, hence they find more people that can relate to them in this community and empathize, which makes disclosure process easier). However, despite these micro and macro concerns about privacy, several factors affecting disclosure decisions are related to the community. For example, some of these meso level factors include the existence of trolls, social status in the community (oldie-newbie member disputes, newbies feel they intrude oldies' private club), cliques occurring within the community (due to the newbie perception that those who contribute the most seem to create cliques, and disease illiteracy of the newbie, which especially discourage new members to share their information). In addition, some members interpret the script of sharing being negotiated constantly in this community as a lack of organization and leadership, which hinders their communication in the community. Moreover, quality of contribution of members, feeling disconnected due to not finding a fit in the community are some of the many factors affecting the disclosure of private health information in this community.

Consequently, despite the individual concerns for privacy, community dynamics may influence privacy saliency and change the meanings and perceptions of privacy. Members also alleviate each other's privacy concerns through recommendations, such as the use of common or unique names in order not to be identified easily by others. They suggest each other alternative ways to protect security on the Internet. The amount of information they provide in their profiles or in the forums encourages others to trust and do more research about each other, which also leads to increased disclosure of private health information. What is secret becomes a strategic tool and a cultural marker that form alliances and deep, intimate relationships and affiliations among community members. During this process of sharing secrets, individuals gain mutual understanding of what is to be shared, how it is shared, kept, used under what circumstances (Dourish and Anderson, 2006), hence leading to interoperability and seamless flow of information and experience among actors in the network. Framing information disclosure as loss of privacy may backfire and increase concerns for privacy. Members of this community, on the other hand, disclose their private health information within a hope based culture. This hope entails the anticipation that, in the future, with the body of knowledge generated through aggregation of private health information of several patients worldwide, medical research process would be fastened and better treatments would be generated for the cure of life-changing diseases. Construction of hope by the members of the community does not just include anticipation

or wishing for future better health outcomes and human lives. Patients also act on their hope for the future (e.g., find a cure for the disease) in the present moment, actively engage in clinical research and the discovery of new medical knowledge. Many patients trade anonymity for getting their voices heard and take advantage of the enabling and empowering role of the Internet, not just as consumers who accept whatever is provided to them but as active negotiators with other actors in online communities, hence negotiating the meanings of privacy.

Different institutional forces other than the government and healthcare providers begin to have a say in the way privacy is constructed, private health information is shared, and clinical research is conducted. These institutions, by using social networking in healthcare and serving as community organizations, bring healthcare actors together in a platform to actively engage in the creation of new medical knowledge, adopt new roles and relations, and increase their connectivity. As we see such transformations emerging and contributing to change in healthcare dynamics, inquiries will be necessary concerning trust and credibility of these institutions and the actors that design them. More importantly, the issue to be explored is how effectively they can gather healthcare actors to collaborate in a seamless manner as a means to contribute to medicine on a global scale and establish an effective flow of information in a real-time process. The interplay of culture and technology and the resulting networked relations among healthcare actors will nevertheless bring about the demise of provision and the rise of collaboration in healthcare, as patients get more involved in the design and creation of health information, not just stay as recipients of health information and care. Despite concerns for privacy, and the accuracy or truthfulness of the medical knowledge generated by diverse healthcare actors in this community, technology enables people to have a voice in the decisions that are made about their and others' health. Recent research indicates the increasing trust of patients in online medical information (Schwartz, 2008), as more people engage in the creation of that information, set avenues to make comparisons in order to contextualize their diseases, observe others' experiences and learn from them, and validate or legitimize their own opinions and behaviors. Better healthcare outcomes are yet to come if more and more healthcare actors engage in creation of these communities without bypassing each other or standing separate from each other, and accelerate medical research through increased mobility of health data as a result of intensified connectivity among multiple healthcare actors.

REFERENCES

Appadurai, A. (1991). Global ethnoscapes: Notes and queries for a transnational anthropology. In Fox, R. G. (Ed.), *Recapturing Anthropology: Working in the Present* (pp. 191–210). Santa Fe, NM: Sch. Am. Res. Press.

Arnquist, S. (2009). Research trove: Patients' online data. *New York Times,* (August 24), available at: http://www.nytimes.com/2009/08/25/health/25web.html

Arnst, C. (2008). Health 2.0: Patients as partners. *BusinessWeek,* (December 4), Retrieved from http://www.businessweek.com/magazine/content/08_50/b4112058194219.htm

Bauman, Z. (1996). From pilgrim to tourist – or a short history of identity. In Hall, S., & du Gay, P. (Eds.), *Questions of Cultural Identity* (pp. 18–36). London: Sage.

Benn, S. I. (1971). Privacy, freedom and respect for persons. In Pennock, R. J., & Chapman, J. W. (Eds.), *Privacy* (pp. 1–26). New York: Atherton Press.

Bleicher, P. (2006). Web 2.0 revolution: Power to the people. *Applied Clinical Trials,* 34-36.

Bonsu, S. K., & Darmody, A. (2008). Putting consumers to work: 'Co-creation' and new marketing govern-mentality. *Journal of Consumer Culture,* 8(2), 163–196. doi:10.1177/1469540508090089

Brown, B. (2008). Research and the privacy rule: The chill is on. *Journal of Health Care Compliance,* 35-36.

Caputo, J. D. (Ed.). (1997). *Deconstruction in a nutshell: A conversation with Jacques Derrida.* New York: Fordham University Press.

Cavoukian, A., & Tapscott, D. (1995). *Who knows: Safeguarding your privacy in a networked world.* Toronto: Random House.

Chan, Y., Culnan, M., Greenaway, K., Laden, G., Levin, T., & Smith, H. J. (2005). Information privacy: Management, marketplace, and legal challenges. *Communications of the Association for Information Systems,* 16, 270–298.

Cova, B. (2005). Thinking of marketing in meridian terms. *Marketing Theory,* 5(2), 205–214. doi:10.1177/1470593105052476

Culnan, M. J. (1993). How did they get my name? An exploratory investigation of consumer attitudes toward secondary information use. *Management Information Systems Quarterly,* 17(3), 341–363. doi:10.2307/249775

Denegri-Knott, J. (2004). Sinking the online music pirates: Foucault, power and deviance on the web. *Journal of Computer-Mediated Communication,* 9(4).

Deshpande, A., & Jadad, A. R. (2006). Web 2.0: Could it help move the health system into the 21st century? *JMHG,* 3(4), 332–336.

Epstein, C. (2006). Guilty bodies, productive bodies, destructive bodies: Crossing the biometric borders. Paper Presented at International Studies Association Conference.

Eysenbach, G., Powell, J., Englesakis, M., Rizo, C., & Stern, A. (2004). Health-related virtual communities and electronic support groups: Systematic review of the effects of online peer-to-peer interactions. *BMJ (Clinical Research Ed.), 328,* 1166–1170. doi:10.1136/bmj.328.7449.1166

Fillion, R. (2005). Moving beyond biopower: Hardt and Negri's post-foucauldian speculative philosophy of history. *History and Theory, 44,* 47–72. doi:10.1111/j.1468-2303.2005.00342.x

Firat, A. F., & Dholakia, N. (1998). *Consuming people: From political economy to theaters of consumption.* London: Routledge. doi:10.4324/9780203449813

Firat, A. F., & Dholakia, N. (2006). Theoretical and philosophical implications of postmodern debates: Some challenges to postmodern marketing. *Marketing Theory, 6*(2), 123–162. doi:10.1177/1470593106063981

Fischer, E., Bristor, J., & Gainer, B. (1996). Creating or escaping community?: An exploratory study of internet consumers' behaviors. *Advances in Consumer Research. Association for Consumer Research (U. S.), 23,* 178–182.

Fiske, J. (1989). *Understanding popular culture.* London: Routledge.

Foucault, M. (1975). *The birth of the clinic: An archeology of medical perception.* New York: Vintage Books.

Gavison, R. (1980). Privacy and the limits of the law. *The Yale Law Journal, 89*(3), 421–471. doi:10.2307/795891

Goezt, T. (2008). Practicing patients. (March 23), *New York Times.*

Goodwin, C. (1991). Privacy: Recognition of a consumer right. *Journal of Public Policy & Marketing, 10*(1), 149–166.

Haig, S. (2007). *When the patient is a googler. Time,* (Nov 8). Retrieved from http://www.time.com/time/health/article/0,8599,1681838,00.html

Hardt, M., & Negri, A. (2000). *Empire.* Cambridge, MA: Harvard University Press.

Holt, D. B. (2002). Why do brands cause trouble? A dialectical theory of consumer culture and branding. *The Journal of Consumer Research, 29*(1), 70–90. doi:10.1086/339922

Horkheimer, M., & Adorno, T. W. (1993). *Dialectic of enlightenment.* New York: Continuum.

Hummel, J., & Lechner, U. (2001). Communities: The role of technology. In *Proceedings of the 9th European Conference on Information Systems.*

Jackson, M. (2000). *Systems approaches to management.* New York: Kluwer Academic/Plenum Publishers.

Jadad, A. R., Enkin, M. W., Glouberman, S., Groff, P., & Stern, A. (1999). Promoting partnerships: Challenges for the internet age. *BMJ (Clinical Research Ed.), 319,* 761–764.

Jadad, A. R., Enkin, M. W., Glouberman, S., Groff, P., & Stern, A. (2006). Are virtual communities good for our health? *BMJ (Clinical Research Ed.), 332,* 925–926. doi:10.1136/bmj.332.7547.925

Johnson, C. Y. (2008). Through website, patients creating own drug studies. *The Boston Globe,* (November 16), available at: http://www.boston.com/news/health/articles/2008/11/16/through_website_patients_creating_own_drug_studies/?page=full

Kahn, J. S. (2008). The wisdom of patients: Health care meets online social media. *California Health-Care Foundation,* 1-24.

Kliff, S. (2009). Pharma's facebook. *Newsweek,* March 10, Available at: http://www.newsweek.com/id/187882

Kotler, P. (2003). *Marketing management.* Upper Saddle River, NJ: Prentice-Hall.

Kozinets, R. V. (2002a). Can consumers escape the market? Emancipatory illuminations from burning man. *The Journal of Consumer Research, 29*(1), 20–38. doi:10.1086/339919

Kozinets, R. V. (2002b). The field behind the screen: Using netnography for marketing research in online communications. *JMR, Journal of Marketing Research, 39*(1), 61–72. doi:10.1509/jmkr.39.1.61.18935

Lenhart, A., & Madden, M. (2007). *Teens, privacy and online social networks: How teens manage their online identities and personal information in the age of MySpace.* Pew Internet and American Life Project. Retrieved from http://www.pewinternet.org/pdfs/PIP_Teens_Privacy_SNS_Report_Final.pdf

Marcuse, H. (1991). *One dimensional man.* London: Abacus.

McGregor, S. (2006). Roles, power, and subjective choice. *Patient Education and Counseling, 60,* 5–9. doi:10.1016/j.pec.2004.11.012

Murray, J. B., & Ozanne, J. L. (1991). The critical imagination: Emancipatory interests in consumer research. *The Journal of Consumer Research, 18*(2), 129–144. doi:10.1086/209247

O'Reilly, T. (2005). *What is web 2.0? Design patterns and business models for the next generation of software.* Retrieved from http://www.oreillynet.com/pub/a/oreilly/tim/news/2005/09/30/what-is-web-20.html

Peñaloza, L., & Price, L. L. (1993). Consumer resistance: A conceptual overview. *Advances in Consumer Research. Association for Consumer Research (U. S.), 20,* 123–128.

Rose, N. (2007). *The politics of life itself: Biomedicine, power, and subjectivity in the twenty-first century.* NJ: Princeton University Press.

Sarup, M. (1993). *An introductory guide to post-structuralism and postmodernism* (2nd ed.). Athens, GA: University of Georgia Press.

Schonfeld, E., & Morrison, C. (2007). The next disruptors: The 10 game changing startups most likely to upend existing industries and spawn new entrepreneurial opportunities. *Business 2.0, 8*(8), 56-64.

Schwartz, J. (2008). Logging on for a second (or third) opinion. (Sep 29), *New York Times.*

Sheridan, B. (2008). Open wide: The open-source movement worked wonders for software. Can it do the same for diabetes and other illnesses?" *NewsWeek.* Retrieved from http://www.newsweek.com/id/164231

Sherry, J. F., Storm, D., Duhachek, A., Nuttavuthisit, K., & Deberry-Spence, B. (2004). Ludic agency and retail spectacle. *The Journal of Consumer Research, 31*(3), 658–672. doi:10.1086/425101

Slater, D., & Tonkiss, F. (2001). *Market society: Markets and modern social theory.* London: Polity Press.

Tapscott, D., & Williams, A. D. (2008). *Wikinomics: How mass collaboration changes everything.* New York: Portfolio Penguin Group.

Terranova, T. (2004). *Network culture: Politics for the information age.* London: Pluto Press.

Thompson, C. J. (2004). Marketplace mythology and discourses of power. *The Journal of Consumer Research, 31*(1), 162–180. doi:10.1086/383432

Vargo, S. L., & Lusch, R. F. (2004). Evolving to a new dominant logic for marketing. *Journal of Marketing, 68*(January), 1–17. doi:10.1509/jmkg.68.1.1.24036

Venkatesh, A. (2006). Further evolving the new dominant logic of marketing: From services to the social construction of markets. *Marketing Theory, 6*(3), 299–316. doi:10.1177/1470593106066789

Venn, C. (2007). Cultural theory, biopolitics, and the question of power. *Theory, Culture & Society*, *24*(3), 111–124. doi:10.1177/0263276407075957

Weitzner, D. J., Abelson, H., Berners-Lee, T., Feigenbaum, J., Hendler, J., & Sussman, G. J. (2008). Information accountability. *Communications of the ACM*, *51*(6), 82–87. doi:10.1145/1349026.1349043

Zwick, D., & Dholakia, N. (2004). Consumer subjectivity in the age of internet: The radical concept of marketing control through customer relationship management. *Information and Organization*, *14*(3), 211–236. doi:10.1016/j.infoandorg.2004.01.002

ENDNOTES

[1] Web 2.0 is considered a technological, social, cultural and even political phenomenon and is coined with terms, such as collective intelligence, architecture of participation, and user-generated content (O'Reilly, 2005).

[2] Health 2.0 is a sub-generation of Web 2.0 social media and is defined as "the use of social software and its ability to promote collaboration between patients, their caregivers, medical professionals, and other stakeholders in health" (Kahn, 2008, p. 2).

[3] Pew Internet Project/Harris Interactive teen focus groups, June 2006

Chapter 33
Global Health Google

Ronald LaPorte
University of Pittsburgh, USA

Faina Linkov
University of Pittsburgh, USA

Eugene Shubnikov
University of Pittsburgh, USA & Institute of Internal Medicine, Russia

Mita Lovalekar
University of Pittsburgh, USA

Ayesha Aziz
University of Pittsburgh, USA

Francois Sauer
University of Pittsburgh, USA

Supercourse Team
University of Pittsburgh, USA

ABSTRACT

We evaluate and illustrate the utility of Google Tools for assessing research communications in Global Health. Page Ranks (PR) appear to be an important tool or utility for ranking the impact pages with the logic that PR determine which pages will be seen in a search. Google Trends provided very intriguing results as with this one can assess the temporal trends in searching. Google analyses appear to be very powerful to evaluate the translation of scientific knowledge.

INTRODUCTION

AIDS, Global Warming, SARS, Avian Flu, Obesity, Drug Addiction: These global conditions reach the front pages of our newspapers and

televisions every day. Global Health impacts us all. Scientists need the latest and most accurate data and information concerning global health. But where can it be found? It cannot be exclusively through journal articles as the information is 1 year old by the time of publication. Citations could be used to find the best quality material (Lundberg,

DOI: 10.4018/978-1-60960-097-6.ch033

G., 2003) however, citations are even more dated than journals, e.g. 2-3 years. Also, citations focus exclusively on journals.

Over the past 15 years, Internet emerged as an alternative way of biomedical information storage. Over the course of the past 10 years we have seen much of our best scientific information exchanged in blogs, emails, chat rooms, etc. We also have been especially interested in Power-Point on the web as a major carrier of research communications (LaPorte, R. E., Linkov, F., Villasenor, T., Sauer, F., Gamboa, C., Lovalekar, M., et al., 2002) and the use of open source model for scientific information sharing (Sa, E., Seki-kawa, A., Linkov, F., Lovalekar, M., & LaPorte, R. E., 2003). Specifically, in our previous stud-ies we evaluated the quality of the Supercourse online lecture library (Linkov, F., LaPorte, R., Lovaleka,r M., & Dodani, S., 2005), (Linkov, F., Lovalekar, M., & LaPorte, R., 2007) leading us to the conclusion that online methodologies for quality control need to be evaluated further. Due to the ever growing nature of the Internet, it is hard to evaluate online materials using citations or traditional peer review mechanisms.

As Internet use grows, health interventions are increasingly being delivered online, with pioneer-ing researchers using the networking potential of the Internet (Griffiths, F., Lindenmeyer, A., Powell, J., Lowe, P., & Thorogood, M., 2006). Similarly, the internet has become a frequently used and powerful tool for patients seeking medi-cal information (Selman, T. J., Prakash, T., Khan, K. S., 2006).

An on-line survey of 164 local health depart-ments' staff in five US Northwestern states in 2006-2007 to assess Internet access and use by staff demonstrated that the most important selection criterion for selecting Web sites was credibility of the sponsoring organization (55%). Accuracy (46%), reputable source (30%), and currency of information (19%) were considered most critical for assessing information quality (Turner, A. M., Petrochilos, D., Nelson, D. E., Allen, E., Liddy, E.

D., 2009). Thus, Internet is becoming an important tool that cannot be ignored in today's research en-vironment. Our previous publications emphasized the importance of information sharing using the Internet (LaPorte, R. E., Linkov, F., Villasenor, T., Sauer, F., Gamboa, C., Lovalekar, M., et al., 2002), LaPorte, R. E., Marler, E., Akazawa, S., Sauer, F., Gamboa, C., Shenton, C., et al., 1995, Laporte, R. E., Omenn, G. S., Serageldin, I., Cerf, V. G., Linkov, F., 2006, & Laporte, R. E., Sekikawa, A., Sa, E., Linkov, F., & Lovalekar, M., 2002), however this is the first publication where our group is emphasizing the importance of Google Trends and Page Rank for measuring the impact of online materials. Google Trends and Page Rank are very new tools and virtually unexplored by scientific community. This chap-ter is emphasizing the need for the use of new technologies in tracking scientific publications and materials online. This article has not been designed as a traditional research articles, it is an exploration of the concept of applicability of Page Ranks to biomedical literature.

PAGE RANKS

A web revolution has taken place with the develop-ment of Google. We are not affiliated with Google, but admire the impact it is having on biomedical science. The use of Google Tools such as Page Rank and Google Trends may be powerful tools for evaluating scientific impact. The concept of Google Page Ranks is straight forward. When one does a Google search on "Global Health," the pages of the search are presented in order. A page that appears as first or second in a search will be seen, one that appears 23,987 will not. The algo-rithm that Google uses to determine Page Ranks is simple. When one searches on Google using a key word or key phrase, the results are displayed in order of the "Google Page Rank."(Wikipedia, 2006) The Google Page Rank system interprets a link from page A to page B as a vote, by page

A, for page B. In addition to the number of links, Google also evaluates number of sites linking into specific pages. Additionally, Google also looks at the relevance of the page in regards to the keywords used to search. It combines Page Rank with text-matching techniques to find pages that are both important and relevant to the search (from Google). One obviously wants to be in the top 20, as you will not otherwise be seen (Wikipedia, 2006). Page Ranks provide an excellent (but not perfect) evaluation of the impact and quality of scientific work which could provide a more accurate evaluation of the impact of journals, institutions, individuals and programs. The idea of page rankings in general is very easy. If you do not see a page on the top of your search, it cannot have impact.

GOOGLE TRENDS

Google recently developed an application called Google Trends. (http://en.wikipedia.org/wiki/Google_Trends). This feature, along with Page ranks allows you to evaluate the temporal trends on searching. For example, immediately after the 2004 Indian Ocean Earthquake (Tsunami) there was a huge spike on the term "tsunami." Jagged trends can be evaluated for Tony Blair, and for SARS with a declining number of searches. With Google it is now very simple to monitor the interest, trends, and specific potential determinants using Google Trends. We, therefore, also examined Google Trends analysis as a means to evaluate scientific impact. When we started to develop this paper we thought that we would examine the web health of e-BMJ, thinking that it would be a great model to show the robustness of the flagship e-journal. Much to our surprise, there appears to be impending web health problems of e-BMJ, which made our Google web results more interesting, but brought concern about e-BMJ.

METHODS

Page Ranks: To illustrate the use of Page Ranks for Impact assessment, we performed a Google search on the term "Global Health" and amazingly close to half a billion sites were identified. Google does not have a simple system to identify specific page ranks, unlike Yahoo or MSN. We therefore did a search within the first 300 entries in order to see the Page Ranks of different sites where Global Health Information could be found.

Three hundred is an arbitrary number. The reality is that in a search few people look at more than 50 pages. However in some cases, such as with Global Health, there are millions of pages. We selected 300 as manageable for hand searches.

Example 1: Global Health Google PR, Impact

To evaluate this we examined selected organizations (e.g. WHO, PAHO, etc.), journals (e.g. BMJ, Lancet, etc.) and new systems, e.g. the global PowerPoint collection of health (the Supercourse) and Wikipedia. In addition, PowerPoint presentations on the web have become a very important means of research communication, we therefore examined Global health and its impact for PowerPoint lectures.

The two tables in Figure 1 present the Page Ranks for global health in the various searches overall and then just for PowerPoint lectures.

The results are very interesting. First, the numbers of sites with the reference to Global Health are enormous. For a site to obtain rankings below 300 means that they are having a very large impact as this represents the upper .00006% of the distribution, well beyond the magical 6 sigma. What is fascinating is that there is broad variability in the leading indices, with surprisingly the highest impact sources being USAID, a collection of PowerPoint lectures in the Supercourse, and the CDC. Journals do not fare well in PRs with JAMA, NEJM and BMJ being the leaders,

501

Figure 1. Page Ranks for "Global Health"

Search on All Files N = 112,000,000			Search on .ppt Files N = 48,500	

Source	PR
WHO	5
Wikipedia	6
USAID	7
Supercourse	11
CDC	24
JAMA	135
NIH	144
NEJM	183
BMJ	273
World Bank	***
PAHO	***
Lancet	***
UN	***

Source	PR
UN	7
Supercourse	10
PAHO	26
WHO	57
CDC	58
BMJ	112
NIH	153
World Bank	190
USAID	***
JAMA	***
NEJM	***
Lancet	***
Wikipedia	***

*** = PR > 300

but well down in the pack. The Lancet did not reach the PR radar screen.

With Google one can also limit the search to educational institutions. As a part of this study, we performed a search for.edu sites, and over a million were found, the first being our Supercourse site, and the second an article by us in the BMJ. Google can examine PR in other languages. Choosing Arabic, for example, there are 121,000 sites found, the first two were from WHO, and the 5th from our Supercourse. Supercourse is an online library of over 3000 lectures on prevention, shared for free, by over 42,000 members of the Global Health Network. (Linkov, F., Ardalan, A., Dodani, S., Lovalekar, M., Sauer, F., Shubnikov, E., et al., 2006)

This information points out the importance of translation to have impact in other countries and languages. A power of the PR is that we can examine impact at a much higher degree of resolution and granularity than we could before. The leaders in all files tended to have similar Page Ranks for lectures in the second table, but not quite. USAID fell down, for example, and PAHO and BMJ jumped forward. The major point of this exercise is to demonstrate that PR can be used to identify the sources that have the greatest

impact on the web for Global Health or, in fact, any other topic.

GLOBAL HEALTH GOOGLE, TEMPORAL TRENDS AND THE DECLINE OF E-BMJ

With Google Trends, we can map the changing patterns of searches on the web. We initially decided to examine the term "Global Health." Then we researched the term "British Medical Journal" because of the long history of the BMJ in the area of e-journals, and its global reach. The results were very surprising.

Global Health Google Trends: As can be seen, during the 2 year period between 2004 and 2006 there has been a major increase to 2005 in the searches and mention of Global Health news. The Google Trends also provides indications as to possible events that might have caused spikes or dips in the searches. Here we can see the patterns in the searches for "global health" during this period of time, with potential precipitators.

We then examined the trends in the searches for the British Medical Journal. Interestingly, there was at least a 30% dip in searches beginning in the second quarter of 2006. It was not clear as to what is the cause. We did a similar temporal analysis for the NEJM, JAMA and Lancet. For these 3 journals, there was no decline in the numbers of searches in 2006. We then did a direct comparison of the British Medical Journal and the Lancet over time. It appeared in 2004, there were about 25% more searches for the BMJ, and in contrast, in 2006 this was reversed with ~ 0-15% in increased searches being for the Lancet. It thus appears to be a true decline in BMJ web searches that is not seen for other major journals.

DISCUSSION: SUMMARY AND IMPORTANCE OF THIS RESEARCH

In summary, this chapter presents interesting data on Page Ranks and Google trends for BMJ and several other journals. The analyses presented are primitive; however, they could not have been done using any approach other than with the Internet and Google. The potential is enormous. This study is different from existing studies in many different ways. This is one of the first studies to use novel Google applications for the investigation of scientific publications online. Secondly, it emphasizes the importance of Internet based approaches in scientific literature quality control, something that most likely needs to be done but is not being done yet. There are many advantages of using Google PR as a measure of impact. These include cross-domain comparisons, e.g. comparing Ron LaPorte with the BMJ and the University of Mexico. Also, there is a simple logic that if it is not ranked high, it is not seen. The database is huge with Google and the web. The information is timely and considerable work has already been done in PR by Google, Yahoo, and MSN. In addition, we can examine impact domain specific and in different countries to evaluate the diffusion of knowledge. Finally, new and better "info-tools" are being established by the major search engines, which can potentially be harnessed for science.

There are, however, disadvantages. This is a new field and there are no "rules". We do not have a good definition of "Impact" or "Web Quality" or "Web Health". Also, it is not clear whether a high page rank for "Nature Jobs" is a measure of "Nature Impact." We need to operationally define these variables before moving forward. Also, the tools for assessment are not yet evolved. We found that we would obtain different results when we searched for "diabetes epidemiology" than when we searched "epidemiology and diabetes." Also, if you do these searches now, the results will differ from our November 2006 analysis as PR fluctuate and the PR methods are constantly being revised. We need to be able to look at trend analyses for PR as was presented for Google Trends for search topics.

The second analysis of search patterns is also very intriguing and surprising. We were able to use the BMJ as an example; we did not expect to see that the searching on the web for the BMJ had a marked decline last year and that the Lancet overtook the BMJ on the web. Much needs to be done to understand this phenomenon. If one uses the search item "lancet" the pattern is quite different than using the term "the lancet." Part of this is due to other companies having the name "lancet" and other items in the search. The power of this approach raises a red flag to the web health of the BMJ, which needs to be examined in more detail in future investigations. The point for us is not the web health of the BMJ, but the power of PR and web statistics. We believe it is real as other major journals demonstrating increases at this time. This analysis can point out problems that need to be looked into.

Search engines only have a 15 year history. During this time they have become very successful in searching through terabytes of information to find that one piece of information you need in milliseconds. Page Ranks are very new on the landscape having been rolled out in only 2001 and trend analysis only in the past year. Remarkable progress has been made in using and understand-

What This Means for Medical Literature Improvement

Important component of our research is the quest for finding applications of automatic Internet based methodologies for improving biomedical literature. Plethora of medical knowledge exists on the Internet, however the quality of this information is in question. On the other hand, there is an abundance of medical textbooks and scientific journals, however not all medical libraries have access to them due to high cost. This problem is especially prevalent in developing countries. Additionally, information published in the textbooks may be outdated, as there is a significant gap between original research and publication of a textbook. Thus, Internet is potentially an important source of medical information, but it can also serve as a tool for assessing the need for biomedical information in certain areas. It also has important implications for quality control. Page ranks can potentially improve biomedical literature in several ways:

- Identify areas of need for medical information. For example, Swine Flu has been identified as one of the most requested information modules in the Supercourse libarary.
- Identify gaps in the biomedical literature;
- Identify geographic areas where certain information is needed;
- Identify areas that do not need to as much attention anymore. This can potentially be used to save valuable resources.
- Lead to improved ways of quality control for biomedical literature on the web. In this instance, it would also be important to develop systems for identifying fraudulent Page Ranks.

What this Means for Users

With more and more health information popping up on the internet, users worldwide are empowered like never before. A user can find just about anything he or she desires just by entering a vague search term and a few clicks of the mouse. Global Health information on the Worldwide Web is especially beneficial to those in areas where experts on the subject, libraries, books, and schools are not readily accessible – those in developing countries or rural, out-of-the way areas. Laypersons who want to know more about something they heard on the news or in a discussion with their doctor can find a plethora of information from all over the world.

As with almost all things, there are positives and negatives to relying on the Internet to provide information. Advantages to locating global health information online include, but are certainly not limited to, a large amount of information, the availability of information in real time, the ability to access expert information from half a world (and further) away, as well as many individual reasons specific to each user. Disadvantages may include out of date information that has been posted and long since forgotten about, information ranging from 'not entirely factual' to downright wrong, as well as literature that has been written in technical language (rendering it inaccessible to the layperson). Ronald E. Rice also adds the classifications "obstacles" and "dangers" when discussing using the Internet for searching for health information which provide broader groupings, while still incorporating most of the aforementioned advantages and disadvantages.(Rice, R. E., 2006) An additional point that Rice includes in his "disadvantage" classification is unequal access to online resources. Access to specific websites, the internet, or even a computer varies greatly between countries.

Worldwide, Internet usage has increased by approximately 360% since the year 2000 with nearly a quarter of all people using, or having used, the Internet at some point.(Internet Usage Statistics) The most marked increase in users over this 9 year span have occurred in the world regions defined as "Africa" (i.e. the countries composing the continent of Africa) and "Middle East" (i.e. Bahrain, Iran, Iraq, Israel, Jordan, Kuwait, Lebanon, Oman, Palestine, Qatar, Saudi Arabia, Syria, U.A.E., and Yemen) with user increases at a little over 1300% in each region. With these dramatic increases in web usage in the African and Middle Eastern regions, a larger audience is able to be reached. This audience has a need for relevant and timely global health information as books, pamphlets, and any information spread by way of mouth could potentially be out of date or inaccurate. While the combined 2009 populations of the "Africa" region and "Middle East" region are 3 and a half times that of the "North America" population, their combined Internet users is a mere 5 million more than the 108 million North American users in 2000.

Until the global digital divide can be conquered, users in developing nations – ones who could benefit most from information "on demand" – will be underrepresented in access to and the viewing of online global health documents. However, the vast percent increase in new users in developing regions can provide hope that information gleaned by these 'pioneers' is being passed on to peers the old fashioned way – by way of mouth.

In conclusion, PR now can do more than any impact assessment. It holds enormous promise to further our understanding of how scientists share and translate knowledge as that this can be improved.

REFERENCES

Griffiths, F., Lindenmeyer, A., Powell, J., Lowe, P., & Thorogood, M. (2006). Why are health care interventions delivered over the internet? A systematic review of the published literature. *Journal of Medical Internet Research, 8*(2), 10. doi:10.2196/jmir.8.2.e10

Internet Usage Statistics. (n.d.). *Internet World Stats*. Retrieved August 27, 2009, from http://www.internetworldstats.com/stats.htm

LaPorte, R. E., Linkov, F., Villasenor, T., Sauer, F., Gamboa, C., & Lovalekar, M. (2002). Papyrus to PowerPoint (P 2 P): metamorphosis of scientific communication. *BMJ (Clinical Research Ed.), 325*(7378), 1478–1481. doi:10.1136/bmj.325.7378.1478

LaPorte, R. E., Marler, E., Akazawa, S., Sauer, F., Gamboa, C., & Shenton, C. (1995). The death of biomedical journals. *BMJ (Clinical Research Ed.), 310*(6991), 1387–1390.

Laporte, R. E., Omenn, G. S., Serageldin, I., Cerf, V. G., & Linkov, F. (2006). A scientific supercourse. *Science, 312*(5773), 526. doi:10.1126/science.312.5773.526c

Laporte, R. E., Sekikawa, A., Sa, E., Linkov, F., & Lovalekar, M. (2002). Whisking research into the classroom. *BMJ (Clinical Research Ed.), 324*(7329), 99. doi:10.1136/bmj.324.7329.99

Linkov, F., Ardalan, A., Dodani, S., Lovalekar, M., Sauer, F., & Shubnikov, E. (2006). Building just-in-time lectures during the prodrome of Hurricanes Katrina and Rita. *Prehospital and Disaster Medicine, 21*(2Suppl 2), 132.

Linkov, F., & LaPorte, R., Lovaleka,r M., & Dodani, S. (2005). Web quality control for lectures: Supercourse and Amazon.com. *Croatian Medical Journal, 46*(6), 875–878.

Linkov, F., Lovalekar, M., & LaPorte, R. (2007). Quality control of epidemiological lectures online: scientific evaluation of peer review. *Croatian Medical Journal, 48*(2), 249–255.

Lundberg, G. (2003). The "omnipotent" Science Citation Index impact factor. *The Medical Journal of Australia, 178*(6), 253–254.

Rice, R. E. (2006). Influences, usage, and outcomes of Internet health information searching: Multivariate results from the Pew surveys. *International Journal of Medical Informatics*, *75*, 8–28. doi:10.1016/j.ijmedinf.2005.07.032

Sa, E., Sekikawa, A., Linkov, F., Lovalekar, M., & LaPorte, R. E. (2003). Open source model for global collaboration in higher education. *International Journal of Medical Informatics*, *71*(2-3), 165. doi:10.1016/S1386-5056(03)00108-4

Selman, T. J., Prakash, T., & Khan, K. S. (2006). Quality of health information for cervical cancer treatment on the internet. *BMC Women's Health*, *6*, 9. doi:10.1186/1472-6874-6-9

Turner, A. M., Petrochilos, D., Nelson, D. E., Allen, E., & Liddy, E. D. (2009). Access and use of the Internet for health information seeking: a survey of local public health professionals in the northwest. *Journal of Public Health Management and Practice*, *15*(1), 67–69.

Wikipedia. (2006). *Page Ranks*. Retrieved from Wikipedia.com

Chapter 34
Testing the Waters:
Participant Focus Testing of Well-Being Indicators forthe Development of an Inuit Health Statistics Directory

Tom Axtell
National Aboriginal Health Organization, Canada

Cassandra Chaulk
Nunatsiavut Health & Social Development, Canada

Dianne Kinnon
National Aboriginal Health Organization, Canada

Carmel M. Martin
Trinity College Dublin, Ireland

Michele Wood
Nunatsiavut Health & Social Development, Canada

ABSTRACT

This chapter describes focus group testing in a small community in the Labrador Inuit Land Claim area of the online information system 'Community Accounts,' developed by the province of Newfoundland and Labrador. Key data users were engaged in a hands-on process to help determine what information and data would be useful in an Inuit Web directory. The purpose was to obtain a better understanding of how Inuit use statistics to better understand the broad determinants of health. Inuit continue to take further steps toward managing Inuit specific data in order to create comprehensive health policies and programs and affect decision-making.

DOI: 10.4018/978-1-60960-097-6.ch034

INTRODUCTION

Inuit Health and Statistics

Naasautit: Inuit Health Statistics is a national project created to enable Inuit regional organizations and communities in Canada to make better use of existing statistics to improve health outcomes. The key deliverable is an Inuit health statistics Web directory. The two-year project is funded through the Aboriginal Health Transition Fund of Health Canada (AHTF) as part of a larger Inuit Pan Canadian AHTF project. The *Naasautit:* Inuit Health Statistics[1] project aims to capture the available statistics on the determinants and health conditions of the 50,485 Inuit in 52 remote Arctic settlements in Canada.

This case study describes the focus group testing, in a small community in the Labrador Inuit Land Claim area, of the <u>Community Accounts</u>[2] online information system, developed by the Province of Newfoundland and Labrador. Key data users were engaged in a hands-on process to help determine what information and data would be useful in an Inuit Web directory. The purpose was to obtain a better understanding of how Inuit can use statistics to better understand the broad determinants of health. Inuit explored their own use of statistics and the meaning and value of indicators of "how people are doing". Inuit continue to take further steps towards managing Inuit specific[3] data in order to create comprehensive health policies and programs and affect decision-making.

THE *NAASAUTIT:* INUIT HEALTH STATISTICS PROJECT – BRINGING THE NUMBERS HOME

Naasautit: Inuit Health Statistics aims to help fill gaps in the understanding of health issues facing Inuit communities, Inuit regions and Pan-Canadian Inuit. The objectives of the project are to:

Figure 1.

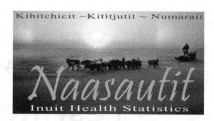

- significantly contribute to the current state of knowledge of Inuit population health indicators;
- facilitate future Inuit population health research by greatly improving access to relevant information; and
- empower[4] Inuit communities through capacity development to conduct their own Inuit perspective health research, thus providing a basis for more fully-informed Inuit knowledge translation and utilisation.

Naasautit: Inuit Health Statistics is a partnership between the Inuit Tuttarvingat, an Inuit research and information sharing centre of the National Aboriginal Health Organization (NAHO), Inuit Tapiriit Kanatami (the national Inuit representative body), and the four land claim organizations: Inuvialuit Regional Corporation, Nunavut Tunngavik Inc., Nunavik Regional Board of Health and Social Services (delegated by Makivik Corporation), and the Nunatsiavut Government in Labrador. Project direction and oversight comes from a Management Group of representatives from the project partners.

THE INUIT POPULATION IN CANADA

Census data show that on average the Inuit population in Canada is much younger than the non-Aboriginal population, and other Aboriginal Peoples. In 2006, the median age of the Inuit population was 22 years, compared with 40 years for non-Aboriginal people, 25 years for First Nations, and 30 years for Métis (Statistics Canada, 2006a). The potential implications of a young, growing Inuit population are numerous. These include an increasing demand for housing and for schooling at all levels. There also will be a greater demand for skills training as young Inuit adults make the transition from school to work in the wage and traditional Inuit economies.

On most indicators where there is health data available for Inuit, Inuit report greater health disparities than not only their non-Aboriginal Canadian counterparts, but First Nations and Métis as well. In 2001, the estimated life expectancy for Inuit was 64 years for men and 70 years for women (INAC, 2004). The average lifespan for Inuit women is 14 years less than that of the average Canadian woman (Statistics Canada, 2004).

The 2006 Canada Census found that 31% of all Inuit live in overcrowded housing compared to three percent in the rest of Canada. While half of Inuit adults have completed high school only four per cent have a university degree compared to 23 per cent for other Canadians (Statistics Canada, 2006a). The unemployment rate among Inuit is more than three times the Canadian average of seven per cent, at 23%. Environmental concerns, such as contaminants and climate change, are having a disproportionately high impact on Inuit

INUIT LANDS: *NUNANGAT*

"Inuit Nunangat" is the Inuktitut expression for "Inuit homeland", an expanse comprising more than one-third of Canada's land mass, extending from northern Labrador to the Northwest Territories. Inuit have inhabited this vast region of Canada, for approximately 5,000 years. In recent times, four Inuit land claims have been signed. While Inuit in each of these regions share a common culture and many traditions, each region is, at the same time, distinct. For example, traditions can sometimes vary and there is much linguistic and geographic diversity from one region to the next.

These four regions are:

- **Nunatsiavut:** This is the most easterly region, encompassing five communities along the northern coast of Labrador. The word "Nunatsiavut" means "our beautiful land" in Inuktitut. This regional government was created through the settlement of the 2005 Labrador Inuit Land Claim Agreement and includes about 120,000 square kilometres of land and the adjacent ocean zone.
- **Nunavik:** This region in northern Quebec was established through the James Bay and Northern Quebec Agreement. This was the first modern land claims agreement in Canada, signed in 1975. Nunavik covers 660,000 square kilometres of land. More recently, the Nunavik Inuit Land Claims Agreement has given Nunavimmiut (Inuit of Nunavik) ownership of many of the islands off the coast of Nunavik.
- **Nunavut:** The 1993 Nunavut Land Claims Agreement led to the creation of the territory of Nunavut in 1999. It was formed out of the eastern part of the Northwest Territories. This agreement is the largest land claim settlement negotiated between a state and Indigenous people in the world. The territory spans 2 million square kilometres. There are three main regions within Nunavut: Qikiqtaaluk, Kivalliq and Kitikmeot.
- **Inuvialuit Settlement Region:** In 1984, the Inuvialuit Final Agreement (IFA) was signed, giving ownership to 90,650 square kilometres of land in the Northwest Territories to the Inuvialuit (Inuit of the western Arctic). The IFA lists six Inuvialuit communities, five within and one outside the Settlement Region. For the purposes of this report, all six Inuvialuit communities have been included.

Figure 2. Source: Inuit Relations Secretariat, Indian and Northern Affaires Canada, Government of Canada

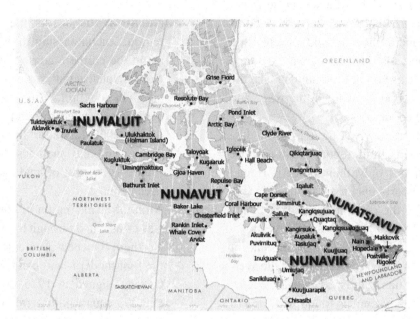

There are 52 Inuit communities across Inuit Nunangat. Because of a lack of road access, these remote communities can, for the most part, be accessed only by air year round and by sea during the summer months. Most communities are small; well over one-third (38%) have a total population under 500 people. About 29% have between 500 and 999 people, while 33% have 1,000 or more. A significant (22%) and growing number of Inuit live outside Inuit Nunangat with 8% in larger Southern urban centres such as Ottawa, Edmonton, Montreal, and Winnipeg (Statistics Canada, 2006a).

Nain (approx. pop. 1,200) is the largest of the five Inuit communities that form the Nunatsiavut region. It was chosen because of the availability of community level data on the Community Accounts Web site. As an administrative centre, Nain is similar to roughly ten other larger Inuit communities across the Arctic where local people are managing a variety of health, education, and municipal services. Nain is home to many administrators and leaders of the regional ethnic government for Labrador Inuit, who saw the training and

focus testing sessions as a way to build capacity and provide participants with the opportunity to further explore how statistics can be used within communities. After the formalization of the Nunatsiavut Government in 2005 through the signing of the Labrador Inuit Land Claim with the provincial and federal governments this regional government has, within the Canadian framework, achieved new rights and responsibilities for lands, resource sharing, and self-government. The way is being paved for the devolution of many provincial and federal responsibilities where statistics will be an important tool.

USING HEALTH STATISTICS IN INUIT REGIONS AND COMMUNITIES

In discussions between the project partners, around the development of how to show health related statistics on the Web site, it was important to understand more about how Inuit administrators and managers in the communities might use statistics and in what form they would like to receive them. With the focus on the social determinants of health, more information was needed about how future users of the Web site directory would respond to statistics describing those determinants. Participatory Web site user testing with residents of Nain, and the graduates of a planned Statistics Canada workshop, would also assess their abilities to use statistics about their own community. This component of Web site user testing was conducted with the approval of the Nunatsiavut Government and with the informed consent of the Nain participants.

The testing provides insight into the suitability of adapting features of the Community Accounts model Web interface, the first information system on the Web to provide social and economic statistics at the community level. Community Accounts is widely used as a credible source of statistics in Newfoundland and Labrador and therefore provided a reasonable "proxy" for how the *Naasautit:* Inuit Health Statistics Web site would be received.

The combination of the Statistics Canada statistics workshop and *Naasautit:* Inuit Health Statistics user testing trip to Nain, Dec 4-6ᵗʰ 2008 was an ideal opportunity to further explore the following questions with participants:

- How would community-level statistics consumers interact with the Community Accounts Web site?
- How would they feel about seeing their community described based on statistics that have both positive and negative meaning for people?
- What kind of questions would they ask?
- What indicators would they choose in comparing communities?
- Was comparing a good thing to do?
- What health statistics did they most want?

Based on participant feedback, along with input from the *Naasautit:* Inuit Health Statistics partners,

the project's national coordinator undertook to design the first round of demonstration Web pages to show the scope of the content and navigation/structure for the future Web application. These demo pages provided a point of reference for making concrete decisions on the Web site for use by each region. The result was a flexible Web site that can expand from a basic data set for each region, to showing community level data if and when communities ask and if the data is available.

"INTRODUCTION TO STATISTICAL TECHNIQUES" COMES TO NAIN

As part of the human resource development plan for the project staff, Statistics Canada, through their *Aboriginal Statistics Training Program*, agreed to provide training in statistics in the Nunatsiavut region. Partners agreed to hold the training session in the small coastal community of Nain, Labrador because similar training had recently been offered in Happy Valley-Goose Bay (a larger hub community). Partners of the project agreed to add at the end of training a short Web site user testing session to elicit valuable information using community-level statistics.

Figure 3. Jim Lyall, President of the Nunatsiavut Government in a speech presented to the participants can be viewed on Isuma TV

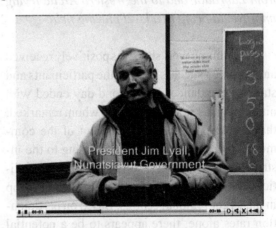

On the first afternoon of the workshop, newly elected Nunatsiavut Government President, Jim Lyall and First Minister Anthony Andersen were present to give short speeches and commence the training. President Lyall thanked the Nunatsiavut Government, the National Aboriginal Health Organization and Statistics Canada for their efforts to bring statistical training to Nain,

"I encourage you to make the most out of the training that you receive as it will enable you to make the better use of statistics. ...I am sure that the end result will be positive for the Nunatsiavut Government in that the training will give us a better understanding of what the numbers mean to Labrador Inuit, as we set priorities for the future, while striving to improve the overall health of our people and our communities".

Minister Andersen encouraged the participants to use statistics for the betterment of communities,

"As Inuit I think we can all agree that we have all been studied quite a lot. It's the conclusions from those studies and stats we've seldomly agreed with. So it's encouraging that Statistics Canada and our national (Inuit) organizations are here to train some of our people so that some of those stats and those studies bring more positive results and results we can begin to agree with will reflect health needs, housing needs that I think we all are, from Labrador and to the Western Arctic trying improve, to bring to a level playing field".

The training workshop was positively received and seen as a success by both the participants and staff in attendance. The second day ended with nine enthusiastic learners, one of whom remarked, that they represented one per cent of the community's entire population. According to the instructors, these learners were equal in their abilities to any drawn to a Statistics Canada workshop in the larger regional centres. Based on participation rates alone, there appears to be a potential

Figure 4. The Nain workshop participants: Fran Winters, Karen Dicker, Gina Dicker, Ernestina Lampe, Pat Foster and Isme Alam (instructors), Sarah Merkuratsuk (seated in front), Jennifer Williams, Edna Winters (seated), and Cassandra Chaulk. Photo Credit: Tom Axtell

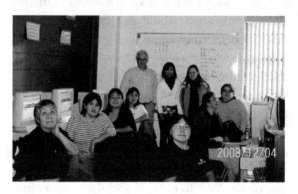

user group for a health statistics Web site in communities the size of Nain. *Naasautit:* Inuit Health Statistics could not have asked for a better prepared focus group.

USER TESTING DESIGN AND RATIONALE

In the past, the work of gathering and analyzing Inuit statistics has been done largely by non-Inuit organizations, with only a few instances of this information reaching Inuit in a usable format. The national Aboriginal People's Survey and Aboriginal Children's Survey data, with over 80% Inuit participation rates, had been used by Inuit Tapiriit Kanatami for advocacy purposes, and some of the data had been used at the regional level, but very little was used by communities themselves. Not only were Inuit health statistics hard to find on the various government Web sites, most people in the communities didn't even know they exist.

The Nunavik Board of Health and Social Services and the Inuvialuit Regional Corporation[5] have used statistics for several years, but their use was not organization-wide and not sustained through core funding. The Nunatsiavut Government through the Department of Health and Social Development works with federal, provincial and regional health authorities towards improving the health and social status of Labrador Inuit through community-based programs and services, advocacy and collaboration. Building the *Naasautit: Inuit Health Statistics Web* directory as a public portal to statistics, it was proposed, can promote use by many more Inuit at the community, regional and national levels.

Comparing populations for the purpose of reducing disparities is the primary use of statistics by large governments. For Inuit, the objective measurement of income and other determinants of health is an attempt to measure and hopefully manage progress toward Inuit identified health goals. But would people in small governments use statistics in a similar way? Having access to accurate data for small, rural/remote populations is new in Canada. How will this new knowledge influence life in rural and remote communities? Will this knowledge contribute (or impact) the development of appropriate programs and services by governments?

WHY WE USED COMMUNITY ACCOUNTS TO TEST INTEREST IN COMMUNITY-LEVEL STATISTICS

Community Accounts is an innovative, user-friendly information system that provides reliable statistics on social, economic and environmental matters. The Government of Newfoundland and Labrador developed Community Accounts and the concept has spread to Nova Scotia and Prince Edward Island (in progress). Community Accounts had been under active consideration as a model for certain features of the *Naasautit: Inuit Health Statistics* Web site user interface since the project took shape in the summer of 2008. Compared to other Web sites providing statistics around the world, Community Accounts presents community-level statistics in a form that is understandable and fairly easy to navigate.

The Community Accounts Web site was first created by Dr. Doug May of Memorial University and the staff of the Newfoundland and Labrador Statistics Agency. Previous to the sites' creation, provincial leaders had few ways to measure socio-economic progress within the province. Memorial University created the benchmarking system for communities enabling leaders to measure change and the impact of programs and services. It is a nine-year experiment in government accountability that the government believes has changed the way communities in Newfoundland and Labrador see themselves. Providing communities with rich data and showing trends over time, is at the heart of the Community Accounts experience. According to one of the co-creators of Community Accounts, Alton Hollet, Assistant Deputy Minister of Economics and Statistics Branch, Government of Newfoundland and Labrador,

People in the communities are no longer arguing about what the numbers are, they are arguing about the issues.[6]

The 400 or more Community Profiles and Well-being Index[7] pages of Community Accounts, were designed for access by people living in Newfoundland and Labrador's many small communities. The communities of Nunatsiavut are included in Community Accounts, and because Inuit comprise 90% of the population in Nain, the profiles and wellness indicator pages presented very relevant statistics for Inuit. Community Accounts provides an in depth demographic profile of each community as well as changes reported over time, in plain language. Of particular interest was Community Accounts' extensive use of graphics and a narrative that provides some context.

The Community Accounts management had offered to assist the *Naasautit:* Inuit Health Statistics project to implement an Inuit version of Community Accounts for the Nunatsiavut region.

Figure 5. Community Accounts Web site, Nain Profile Government of Newfoundland and Labrador

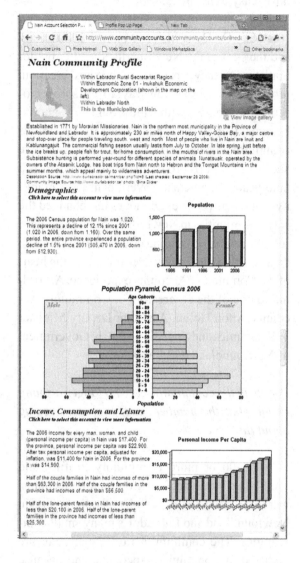

Testing the Community Accounts site with Nunatsiavut residents was a logical way to "cherry pick" features that had undergone years and millions of dollars of information technology development. *Naasautit:* Inuit Health Statistics Web site developers also considered aspects of the navigation, content and forms of statistics presentations used in other important Web resources for Inuit. The other Web-based statistics sites, Nunivaat and Statistics Canada, were assessed at the beginning of the project, but their overwhelming size or the

way numbers were presented did not offer easy access to statistics for analysis by the anticipated user group.

The *Naasautit* Management Group, tasked with building the directory, did not want a database Web site designed solely for government and academic use. Users information needs, and their numeracy and information technology skills will vary considerably. Some officials will have a great deal of familiarity with statistical data while other individuals and groups may have no experience with data retrieval at all. Most sites proved too difficult to navigate. But within most, there were many user-friendly tools that Inuit communities could use. For example, the ability to compare community's side-by-side on the Statistics Canada Community Profile sections was a valuable tool, but with a huge Web site serving all Canadians, this section was nearly impossible for most users to find on the site.

In the earliest discussion about possibly adapting Community Accounts for the *Naasautit* project in July 2008, concerns were raised about the negative impressions and stigma that could result if communities were ranked against each other. The creators of Community Accounts faced the same dilemma. Would this new information reveal previously unknown disparities? From anecdotal accounts by officials within the Government of Newfoundland and Labrador, no, "it has made communities stronger".[8] The Community Accounts Web site testing, undertaken in Nain, allowed the project partners to observe how the ranking system was perceived by the focus testing participants and whether facilitating comparisons between communities or regions would be welcome. While it worked between the nearly 400 communities of Newfoundland and Labrador it was hard to speculate what impact such a health information system would have on the 52 Inuit settlements.

The group was asked to gather data from the Community Accounts Web site, compare communities, generate hypothesis and express their opinions about the process through discussion. This discussion was audio recorded.

The test used only the *Community Profiles* and *Well-being Indicators* pages of the Community Accounts Web site. This was for practical reasons—slow connectivity at the test site meant that six people could not access the site at the same time. Instead, we downloaded and stored all the relevant pages on the computer lab's network server. This enabled participants to flip between the relevant pages (HTML files that opened in their browsers) instantly. Participants did the comparison task in 10 minutes. They spent another 10 minutes reporting interesting facts from the profile pages and reflecting on their experiences.

THE NAIN FOCUS GROUP

The research was conducted with six members of the 11 Nain residents who completed a three-day intensive Introduction to Statistical Techniques workshop, provided by Statistics Canada through the Aboriginal Statistics Training Program. The trainees volunteered to come for the optional Saturday afternoon research activity. This focus group included several prominent community members including Inuit Tuttarvingat's governing committee member, a retired CEO of the regional broadcaster and a former nurse. Two employees of the Nunatsiavut Government, Department of Health and Social Development attended; as well, another participant was a former nursing student. Two others were public administrators with the Nain Community Government.

THE HEALTH STATISTICS WARM-UP EXERCISE

Each participant was asked to select 10 health statistics or indicators from 39 posted on the walls of the computer lab classroom that they felt would be important or useful to them. These

Table 1. Meaningful Statistics Warm Up Exercise Rank Order and Selection: Top 10 Items

Ice retreating – global warming	8
Population increase	6
Overcrowded housing (for children)	5
Family relationships	5
University graduates	4
Physical Inactivity	4
Housing costs	3
Child chronic conditions	3
Traditional medicine	3
Harvesting	3

statistics described various health determinants and conditions, such as disease rates. The selected indicators were transferred to flip chart sheets that were taped to the walls of the computer lab for the entire workshop. Participants were given 10 red stickers and were asked to place the stickers on the indicators that were meaningful to them. These statistics were among over 100 compiled from readily available sources and are illustrated in the following table.

This poll is consistent with how the group rated similar items in the online Nain Health Data Needs Assessment Survey (described later in the chapter). It proved to be an effective way to engage the group in exploring what data and statistical information would be useful and to generate priorities. Notably, this group identified population growth and the importance of relationships (kinship) which was not identified in prior work. The growth of the Inuit population has increased the need for adequate housing, appropriate education spaces and programs, and access to wildlife. The demographic faced by Inuit communities with a growing ratio of more youth to fewer elders, the impact of young families, and other changes as a result of population growth is not being experienced, on average, across Canada as it is in the North. This focus group activity suggests that

Figure 6. Community Accounts Web site, Government of Newfoundland and Labrador

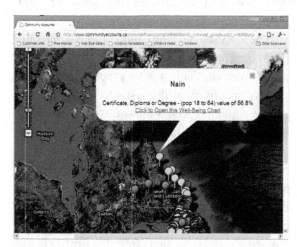

Economic Self-Reliance Ratio – 2006 (left) chart compares Nain and another Nunatsiavut community, two Inuit communities that participants selected for comparison. The Google Map (right) can be used to view the educational attainment levels in another Nunatsiavut community, or any other indicator. Due to limited bandwidth in Nain at the time, participants did not have time to use these tools for their assignments. They compared communities using the Well-Being Index page in Figure 7.

further exploration across the other northern jurisdictions needs to take place to ensure that awareness is raised regarding the determinants of health in various settings, and ensure that indicators important to Inuit are highlighted in the development of health indicators throughout the North.

COMMUNITY ACCOUNTS TESTING

The group took 35 minutes to complete their main research activity in which they were asked to use the Community Accounts Web site to compare their home community of Nain with another randomly assigned Nunatsiavut community; and then to reflect on this experience. This short assignment would determine what statistics Inuit would choose to compare, how they would use the Community Accounts' ranking system to describe the differences between communities, and importantly, was there value in comparing communities. They did their comparative work using the ranking system presented on the Com-

munity Accounts pages of Well-being indicators for each community (Figure 7).

FINDINGS

First Impressions of Community Accounts

Focus group participants all liked navigating within the Community Accounts Web site pages that were made available and found the pages easy to understand and use for the comparison activity. Only one participant had ever visited the Community Accounts Web site before and one other had heard of it. None of the participants in the workshop had ever visited the Statistics Canada Web site before this week.

Group members were surprised to discover how Nain ranked on a number of indicators they choose to look at and compare. One positive comment from a participant was "People make a lot of money!" The Voisey's Bay mining and other socio-economic changes attributed to the

Figure 7. Nain Indicators of Well-being selected for comparison with other Inuit communities: Nain Well-Being Index

Participants that selected indicator		Value	Community Rank	Well-Being Rank
2	Economic Self-Reliance Ratio	80.1%	20th	
3	Income Support Assistance Incidence	33.6%	352th	
1	Personal Income Per Capita	$16,900	392st	
2	Average Couple Family Income	$68,600	26th	
2	Change in Employment	17%	16th	
0	Employment Insurance Incidence	22.2%	13th	
2	Population Change	-12.1%	268th	
0	Migration Rate	.7%	33rd	
3	High School or Above - (18 to 64)	56.7%	270th	
0	Bachelor's Degree or Higher - (25 to 54)	10 %	103rd	
2	Employment Rate - (18 to 64)	80.3.%	74th	
1	Life Expectancy	70	173rd	

Legend: ■ Ranks Low ☐ Ranks Average ▨ Ranks High

This Figure shows the indicators from the Community Accounts Well-being Index page that were chosen by the focus group. They compared Nain with either Hopedale, Postville, Makkovik, Rigolet or Happy Valley- Goose Bay. The legend on the Web site explains how to interpret the colours for the ranking system. Green indicates that Nain is among the top quarter of communities in the province on the Economic Self-Reliance Ratio while they are in the lower quarter in Income Support Assistance. Yellow means that Nain is in the middle 50%. (Community Accounts)

Land Claim have raised Nain to the 20th in rank in the province (out of nearly 400 communities) for the "economic self-reliance ratio". Prior to the focus testing, the group already had a sense that the community was experiencing prosperity, but this was the first time that it was confirmed with statistical information. While no-one knew exactly what was being measured by the indicator of "economic self reliance", they understood that it was showing high self-reliance compared to the rest of the province. There is no doubt that this positive first impression influenced how most of the group thought and felt about the use of statistics and their positive feelings towards the information presented on the Community Accounts Web site.

Comparing Communities

Participants, for the most part, demonstrated great expertise in completing the comparison activity. They accurately copied the numbers into their worksheet in less than five minutes and more importantly found a range of ways to report the differences between communities. Participants did not have the time to explore the indicator charts or the maps (Figure 6) that provided more visual ways to see their communities, due to slow download speeds. While everyone recorded rank in their worksheets, five people also used "%" or "times" to describe differences, which is a technique that demonstrates their statistical literacy. One also described the difference in ranking by stating that the difference between the change of employment between Nain and another community in the region is "a 12.5% difference and a 192 difference in rank." Nain's growth in employment gave it a 16th place rank in positive employment change in the province.

Sensitivity to community realities throughout the *Naasautit:* Inuit Health Statistics development process is first and foremost on the minds of all partners of the project. One person discovered that Nain did not compare so well with another Nunatsiavut community on social assistance and education level indicators. This person did not think that comparing was a good idea and brought this up in the group discussion. Issues of disparities that arise from comparing different communities is unavoidable whenever statistics are published and thus this work will always be contentious for some and deserves close consideration and ongoing discussion as to whether the publishing of this information is beneficial for communities, or better left unsaid.

Participants also generated some research questions from the comparison exercise. However tentative, these are the "golden nuggets" from this activity, indicating that Community Accounts was a useful tool for research exploration and knowledge acquisition. After one person reported the difference in education in high school graduation rates between Nain and a smaller community, a group member wondered if, "the larger the population, the better the education?" Someone else noted the opposite trend between Nain and one of the smaller communities: "Nain, with the higher population, has a lower % of high school graduates!"

There was not enough time to explore the many determinants that influence learning capacity but by exploring the existing statistics the participants were able to ask some relevant and meaningful questions of what might be happening in their communities, and were intuitively looking for associations and explanations. This can also illustrate the potential for statistics to be used by some to rush to false and unproven conclusions, suggesting that clear, bias-free messages need to be developed to accompany the statistics on the *Naasautit* Web site.

HOW WOULD YOU DESCRIBE NAIN AS A PLACE TO LIVE?

Participants answered this question in writing after the main comparison activity, and without any discussion between themselves about the statistics found on the site. They described Nain with what appears to be a mix of prior knowledge and new knowledge acquired from the Community Accounts statistics, primarily the Nain profile page. One declared Nain as a "healthy place to live", adding that the statistics had affirmed what she perceived prior to the activity. Two others (#1 & #4) reported that the reasons Nain was a "have" community was due to new jobs created by the Voisey's Bay nickel mine and the new Inuit government, and the income that followed. Two people (#3 & #6) described Nain as the absence of some of the problems they saw elsewhere Nain is "not a bad place" is compared to conditions elsewhere and compared to the "too busy and hectic" life in the city.

Participants wrote:

Nain is a good community to live in – in terms of economics.

[It's a] healthy place to live

Not a bad place to live because people seem to be living a pretty good life compared to poverty, bad conditions or situations.

Nain has more available resources, jobs, help (i.e. social services).

If I wasn't from Nain, I would choose X (a comparative community from exercise) to live [in] because high school rates are higher and income support is lower and income is about the same.

Community closeness, I love to live here because the city is too busy and hectic. Nain makes it [life] that much [more] stress free, etc.

HOW PARTICIPANTS FOUND NAIN PORTRAYED IN THE COMMUNITY PROFILE

The participants felt that the Community Accounts profile page (Figure 6) for Nain did well to combine contextual information, statistics, basic analysis and trends to provide an overall picture of community wellness. If *Naasautit: Inuit Health Statistics* produced similar profile pages for all 52 settlements, this would be a major analysis activity for the project. Participants demonstrated that new knowledge was acquired from the narrative and analysis presented on the Community Accounts profile page for Nain. Two individuals identified their preference for illustrating the change between two time periods (i.e., a trend) which suggests that this is perhaps a good way to present changes over time, as opposed to presenting columns of numbers (i.e., 2001, 2006) to illustrate the same demographic. In describing how Nain is portrayed, all participants provided further comments, as follows:

Economic self-reliance (80.1%), population change (-12%) and employment rate (pop. 18-64 = 80%.) It shows that Nain's economy is doing well – thought we were much lower in rank.

A bit higher [than expected] at 80.1% self-reliance, and couples had more than $64,800 [in annual income]

Makes Nain look like a pretty decent place to live and we are working toward making Nain a better place to live.

The education, population rate declined. Nice to know for improving areas to look into.

The total number of children 0 to 17 in Nain who were in families on Income Support Assistance was 110. The figure in 1991 was 270. By 2006 it dropped to half. (statement copied verbatim from the Web site). This may show that people are finding jobs instead of relying on the government.

The number of individuals in Nain who collected E.I. (unemployement insurance) at some point in the year 2007 was 140. The 1992 figure was 240.

Showing these facts may have something to do with Voisey's Bay.[9]

SELECTING STATISTICS

One of the purposes of the focus group research was to identify if any of the Community Accounts statistics (Figure 7) was more interesting to participants than others. Focus group members were asked to "pick three statistics that they found interesting". Participants quickly selected indicators relevant to their communities. In presenting the activity, the terms of "well-being" and "indicators" were specifically avoided so participants would interact directly with the numbers and not be too concerned about the importance of their selection. Instead they were asked to look at the more concrete, "statistics" or "measures". The group did not question why so many economic measures (determined by the provincial government) were on the list instead of others that might be equally important to Inuit. As this was not a test of whether this was a good list of well-being indicators for Inuit, the facilitator did not try to solicit this feedback.

Eleven measures out of 12 (Figure 7) were selected once, with two statistics (high school rates and income support) selected by three people. The Bachelor's Degree or higher, for which Nain rated 100th in provincial rank (fairly high) was notably not selected by anyone. The test indicates that most of the Community Accounts statistics that reflect well-being are of some interest and relevance. The findings for this were inconclusive and further testing in other regions may help to further identify what indicators or statistics are of interest across the North.

The Management Group did not have the mandate to develop a Well-being framework or index, therefore the *Naasautit*: Inuit Statistics Web site will not provide ranking across the regions and communities in the first edition.

RELIABILITY AND VALIDITY OF COMMUNITY ACCOUNTS STATISTICS

In asking about the reliability (i.e. accuracy, credibility, trustworthiness) of the statistics on Community Accounts, half of the participants felt that the statistics were accurate and the other half were unsure. In the group discussion it was pointed out that the data sources were not clearly stated. This skepticism may be a result of the workshop that taught participants that mistakes are made and that there is a margin of error in all statistical information. One person believed that income support statistics may not be accurate citing some examples of suspicion around people in communities not using programs for their intended purposes. Skepticism appears to have been set aside for the activity but suggests that building trust and confidence in the numbers on the *Naasautit: Inuit Health Statistics* Web site may take some time and that the indicators developed need to also look at the community context to ensure that the numbers accurately reflect community realities.

REFLECTING ON COMPARING COMMUNITIES

Would the negative numbers contribute to the stigmatization, anger and resignation by members of those communities, or would they lead to something being done about the situation? To understand this more, the focus group was asked if comparing was a good thing to do.

This question elicited strong support for the idea of using statistics for comparison. Five out of six participants agreed that comparing was positive, for the compelling reason offered by one of the leaders in the final group discussion, "It shows us where we are at, so we know where we have to go".

However, one person reported the opposite view about the experience of comparison when the community does not compare as well. In her analysis two indicators were chosen in which Nain did not score as highly as the other community: high school graduates and income support. The participant wrote that she did not want "to feel bad about the community I love". If this test were done in another community which is not as "well off" as Nain, there may be other individuals or groups that feel this way.

Participants wrote:

Yes, it is a good idea; it clearly indicates where each of the communities are.

Yes, for sure.

Depends on what you are comparing?

It's a good idea in a sense that Inuit people know what's going on among themselves.

Gives us an idea.

Not a good idea. I love Nain, my home. Don't want to feel bad about being compared to another community.

Yes, I found it helpful because it shows which communities may be in need of certain things such as employment, schooling etc.

SUMMARY OF FINDINGS FROM THE NAIN FOCUS TESTING

- Community members from Nain, a medium size Arctic community of about 1,200 people, are very interested in learning more about how to use statistics. The 11 people who registered for the statistics training course represented one per cent of the community population. Interest was high enough that six trainees also voluntarily attended for the testing session on a Saturday. Their worksheets on the Community Accounts activity demonstrated both interest and some advanced skills in working with statistics.

- Focus group members found the information easily and quickly in the Community Accounts Web site format. Overall, they enjoyed using the Web site, which was used as a proxy for the future *Naasautit* Web site.
- Participants felt positive about the overall representation of Nain in statistics. That Nain ranks fairly high compared to other Newfoundland and Labrador communities on several economic indicators probably explains this reaction.
- They asked if the education outcomes were related to the community size, showing the potential of statistics to generate questions and the opportunity to conduct research to obtain greater knowledge of an issue.
- In comparing their community with others, they chose to use most of the Community Accounts well-being indicators, which may well demonstrate that Inuit see such universal indicators like income and education as relevant and important. Further testing and feedback from the *Naasautit* Web site will help determine which ones are most important to Inuit. This is a step toward developing Inuit indicators that reflect community realities.
- Most (five of six) of the participants thought that comparing communities using these indicators was a good thing to do for very compelling reasons; simply put, to know where the community has to improve, which is the primary purpose of measuring health indicators. It is notable that one of the six participants was not happy with Nain's lower ranked performance in education and rates of social assistance support use compared to another community in the region. This person's experience shows us that the process of comparing really depends on what is being compared.
- As people will generate their own hypotheses about what is happening, the *Naasautit* Web site needs to provide more than just the numbers. Users need the context and the tools to help them develop their knowledge of the relationships among determinants and outcomes.

In the follow-up to the Nain research one week later, the six participants were asked to take part in the online survey of health statistics needs. Results showed that in the past month, one person looked for data five to nine times, two looked 10-19 times and one other looked over 20 times. Three of these respondents are working in the health field and one is currently a frontline health care provider. This sample of data users was useful for further "testing the waters", confirming they could use all the health indicators that *Naasautit:* Inuit Health Statistics is attempting to collect. They were most interested in the determinants of health, such as food security, access to health services, Inuit language, income, education and water quality. They were interested in health behaviors such as substance use and wanted statistics describing all health conditions.

PLANNING IMPLICATIONS

The *Naasautit:* Inuit Health Statistics project was extremely fortunate to have the opportunity to explore these topics with the very capable learners and public sector workers in Nain. Through their enthusiasm, dedication to learning statistics, and their proven ability, the *Naasautit* project team learned that health statistics are useful and needed in communities such as Nain.

THE "NUMBERS" AND THEIR EFFECT ON COMMUNITY MOBILIZATION

In Canada, disparities in health determinants and health conditions are apparent between north and south, between small and large communities and between geographic regions (PHAC, 2009 and INAC, 2007). Through this examination of statistics, issues relating to Inuit health, of importance to Inuit will be brought to light that illustrate the disparities that communities often face, that governments need to acknowledge, and that individuals have often known over the years but were unable to substantiate until now. Whether the Inuit audience will interpret these numbers as representations of wellness or health deficits and how they integrate this "reality" over time is difficult to predict. Perhaps, in the face of this concern, and to mitigate the *downside* of how statistics can be perceived in a negative light, *Naasautit:* Inuit Health Statistics can promote the use of statistics and the process of comparing them as *tools for change.*

In the weeks before Community Accounts launched, according to the inventors, there were plenty of doubters. Academics and politicians were divided on the merits of publishing community level statistics. In the nine years since, the people of Newfoundland and Labrador have adopted Community Accounts as part of their data systems. In the very first conversation between the national project coordinator and a regional partner on the Community Accounts topic, she said, "You mean Community Accounts isn't Canada-wide, I thought everyone used that?"

In the focus group testing, the positive reaction, by most, to discovering how well Nain was doing within their province was balanced by the one person who identified two important ways that Nain was NOT better off, and who saw the negative impact of the statistics on her view of the community. How people are ultimately affected by this new knowledge is hard to predict, and should

be tested with more audiences, for example, by repeating the exercise with a relatively less prosperous community and asking for more input on how the numbers are presented, as well as testing new indicators of interest to Inuit data users.

For the number of people who gain knowledge that their situation is more positive in some aspect, there will likely be an equal number where people will understand their conditions as less positive. Because using statistics can involve exposing disparities, there will always be challenges for this initiative.

Because of the many unknown impacts of a Community Accounts style ranking system, including simplistic and reductionist conclusions, the project team is opting for a Web site that facilitates the construction of a richer, more multi-dimensional reality. The Web site design facilitates the scan of the many statistics available, so that users can explore different measures and possible associations between numbers, as opposed to only seeing a few numerical descriptors of their communities.

In the design of the *Naasautit:* Inuit Health Statistics Web directory, users will find regional numbers unranked, but side-by-side in bar graph form. And they are not provided with a short list of *key* health indicators, but a larger collection of indicators grouped by health determinant themes and conditions (Figure 6), from which the users select what is important to them. In the Web 2.0[10] world, people expect no less control and interaction with the content

GATHERING THE STATISTICS THAT MATTER TO INUIT

Within the project, there are several processes underway to determine what Inuit health statistics are important for the project partners. The first is the project evaluation using a series of surveys conducted by the project evaluator to establish the baseline of information needs of the organizations;

Figure 8. Naasautit: Inuit Health Statistics Health and Well-being Data Organization Tool

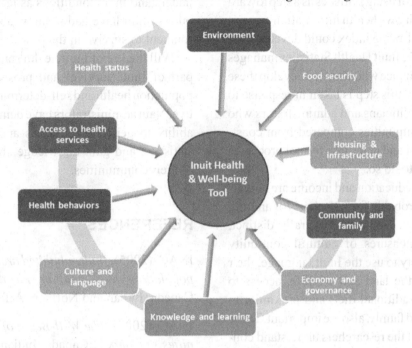

what they now have, and what they would like to concentrate on gathering through the project. In two or more rounds of surveys using the Delphi technique, we have been capturing region-specific priorities and building consensus on what would become common data sets and analysis priorities for the Web site. Given the growing availability of existing data sources and varying levels of use in gathering and disseminating statistics among the partners, time is required to become familiar with the various data sources, and for organizations to establish their role in health monitoring and planning.

The second process was the audience research with the Nain participants that explored how health statistics can be presented and how we might adapt aspects of the Community Accounts system for the Nunatsiavut Government. Other inputs included an on-line health data needs assessment and a determination of priorities from assessing survey questions developed by the staff of the member organizations. Beginning in May 2009, as the Web site is being constructed, there

has been usability testing with the demonstration Web site with the project Management Group and staff at the Inuvialuit Regional Corporation, over 4,000 kilometers to the west of Nain. Finally, a fully functional working model of the *Naasautit:* Inuit Health Statistics Web site with priority indicators provided the Management Group and potential users with a chance to further direct the selection and organization of statistics and refine the presentation. All this interaction with the future Inuit data users *before* committing to the advanced design features, such as intuitive navigation to indicators, user-generated bar graphs and the ability to "stack and scroll" through any number of bar graphs is a process that will hopefully result in a user friendly design that will be popular with Inuit.

CONCLUSION

Inuit have started the process to generate the questions and hypotheses about the meaning, use and potential impact of using statistics as a step toward establishing their own health information system.

An Inuit well-being index could develop over time if *Naasautit:* Inuit Health Statistics manages to engage an audience who wants to develop these concepts. Ideally this step is taken in response to demand from politicians and administrators who want to see communities compared from coast-to-coast-to-coast and enter into formal processes of engagement to do so.

Measures of education and income are universal and would probably form the basis of an Inuit well-being index. However, culturally distinct, Inuit-specific measures of cultural continuity such as the ability to use the Inuit language, their relationship to the land and wildlife, access to country food (traditional diet) and proximity to grandparents and family, also are important. These are numbers that the researchers understand contribute to resilience and community well-being; traits that ensured Inuit survival in past and in modern times. With these measures added to future community well-being and profile pages, we may see a picture of the communities that can explain why most Inuit prefer to stay in the small, close-knit communities where language and traditions are strong, and why, despite over-crowded housing, less access to health care services, food shortages and higher self-reported rates of chronic conditions, half of all Inuit have self-reported that they are in excellent or very good health (Statistics Canada, 2006b).

Promoting the use of Inuit statistics for change at the community and regional level is something newly available to Inuit through statistical databases such as the Aboriginal Peoples Survey and the Aboriginal Children's Survey. Prior to the development of rich data sources such as these, Inuit specific statistics for regional and community use were not available.

For the communities that gain knowledge that their situation is more positive in some aspects, there will be an equal number where people will understand their conditions as less positive than others. Inuit have had to know about their environment to survive in the past.

Will the use of Inuit health statistics becomes part of Inuit survival and prosperity? From a population health and self-determination perspective, Nain administrators have demonstrated their ability to generate questions and answers, use statistics, and gain knowledge about the health of their communities.

REFERENCES

INAC. (2005). *Inuit-inhabited areas from census populations and Canadian Mortality Data Base.* Canada: Indian and Northern Affairs.

INAC. (2006). *The Well-Being of Inuit Communities in Canada.* Canada: Indian and Northern Affairs.

INAC (2007). *Community Well-being: A Comparable Communities Analysis,* Strategic Research and Analysis Directorate: Indian and Northern Affairs Canada, 2007

INAC. (2009). *Measuring Inuit Wellbeing, Inuit Relations Secretariat.* Canada: Indian and Northern Affairs.

PHAC. (2006). *How Healthy Are Rural Canadians? An Assessment of Their Health Status and Health Determinants A Component of the Initiative Canada's Rural Communities: Understanding Rural Health and Its Determinants.* Public Health Agency of Canada.

Statistics Canada. (2006a). *Census of Population.* Statistics Canda.

Statistics Canada. (2006b). *Inuit Health and Social Conditions, Aboriginal Peoples Survey.* Statistics Canda.

The Daily (2004, September 27). Statistics Canada, *The Daily.*

ENDNOTES

1   Naasautit is the Inuit language word for numbers, understood by many people in the Arctic. The project logo includes the regional dialects for this word to express the diversity of the Inuit Nunangat. In Nunavik, they chose to include "to gather" and in this context, "gather meaningful and important numbers".

2   Search for "Community Accounts" or http://www.communityaccounts.ca/

3   Inuit-specific surveillance data are not readily available. Most provincial and territorial governments serving Inuit regions combine Inuit and non-Inuit population health data. For example between 10-20% of the population are non-Inuit, transient "fly-in" guest workers. The Naasautit project is publishing only Inuit-specific data, collected through surveys such as the Aboriginal Peoples Survey (2006). Data on many of the determinants of health are available.

4   While the original project proposal stated that it aimed to "empower Inuit communities", the *Naasautit* Management Group felt that "empower" is an overly ambitious goal, too long-term in nature and difficult to measure in the scope of this project.

5   The Inuvialuit Regional Corporation has gathered existing baseline statistics in order to assess the results of the planned Mackenzie Gas Project on the social, cultural and economic conditions of the Inuvialuit.

6   Alton Hollet, Knowledge in Motion Conference, October 16, 2008, St. John's, Newfoundland & Labrador.

7   It was not known if any Inuit communities had used any form of Well-being index statistics before this testing. The federal department of Indian and Northern Affairs Canada (INAC, 2006) has combined census data to produce "well-being" scores for individual Canadian, First Nations and Inuit populations, including their regions. This is based on the United Nations Human Development Index, which is used by the United Nations Development Program (UNDP) to measure and compare the quality of life in some 170 countries. INAC also created an Inuit Community Well-being Index that combines education, labour force activity, income and housing statistics (INAC, 2009).

8   Ibid.

9   Nain is 50 kilometers from the Voisey's Bay mine, which is the 7th largest nickel deposit in the world, that has led to increased employment opportunities and income rates.

10 Web 2.0 refers to user driven Web applications that are interactive and have user-centered design features and includes social media.

Afterword
User–Driven Health Care:
A Means to Achieve True Health Systems Reform?

Joachim Sturmberg
Monash University and The University of Newcastle, Australia

ABSTRACT

Health, illness and dis-ease are points on the experiential scale of well-being and occur in the presence as well as in the absence of identifiable pathologies. Health, illness and dis-ease in addition are influenced by many contextual factors of a person's life. As such it is not surprising that people require many different inputs into their health care, many of which are non-medical in nature. As yet though, these issues have at best been insufficiently taken into account in the overall planning and provision of care and of health service structures. This chapter will take a conceptual rather than a technical or social perspective towards exploring user-driven health care. It views user-driven health care as an emergent phenomenon in the context of a rapidly evolving web-based communication infrastructure. It highlights that knowledge has many dimensions each of which contributes unique insights to the understanding of health as a personal adaptive experiential state that needs to be distinguished from the health professionals preoccupation with pathologies. Information technologies increase connectivity between people and the sharing of knowledge and experiences narrows the 'gap between the expert in the pathology and the expert in the dis-ease' which finally may give people the power to shift the attractor of the health care system to the health needs of the people, resulting in truly people-centred health care reform.

INTRODUCTION

User-driven healthcare may be defined as 'Improved health care achieved with concerted collaborative learning between multiple users and stakeholders, primarily patients, health professionals and other actors in the care giving collaborative network across a web interface'. (Biswas, et al. 2008) In short user-driven health care promotes the concept of enabling patients and health professionals to meet their individual as well as joint needs – educational as well as emotional and social – whenever they arise. This has become possible by the rapidly developing and expanding IM/IT techniques like mobile phones, internet infrastructure and the Web 2.0 platform (Figure 1) (Biswas, et al. 2009). The increasing awareness, especially of patients, regarding the possibilities and limitations of 'current health care approaches' may enable the user-driven health care movement to become the tipping point to achieve true health care reform, reform that places the person and her health experience at the centre of the health care system.

This chapter will explore the notion of user-driven health care from a conceptual rather than a technical or social perspective. It views user-driven health care as an emergent phenomenon of the rapidly evolving web-based communication infrastructure that allows rapid exchange of information and perspectives between diverse sources with variable degrees of knowledge and/ or authority. To fully appreciate user-driven health care potentials as well as limitations it will explore the notions of knowledge in relation to medicine, and the notion of health, illness and dis-ease in contrast to pathologies. These two concepts are fundamental to understanding the structure and

function of health systems, and together they underpin the proposition of 'patient-centred" health system reform that would result in a truly person-centred health system.

KNOWLEDGE

There have been many philosophical discourses about the nature of knowledge and the following explorations are pragmatic in nature. Knowledge is as much about knowing what – naming facts and relationships – as it is about knowing how – explaining relationships and processes. More importantly though is the fact that knowledge has explicit, i.e. codified and easily communicable, and tacit, i.e. non-codified and therefore difficult to pass on, components. Michael Polanyi (1891–1976) explored the domain of tacit knowledge describing it as the domain of personal knowing.(Polanyi 1958) He contends that tacit knowledge largely shapes the way we perceive the world around us. In relation to medical sciences he stated that:

... personal knowledge in science is not made but discovered, and as such it claims to establish

Figure 1. A framework of user-driven health care (AMIN - xxxx; PHR - Patient Health Record; PSTN - Public Switched Telephone Network ; WAP - Wireless Application Protocol. with permission from Biswas (Biswas, et al. 2009))

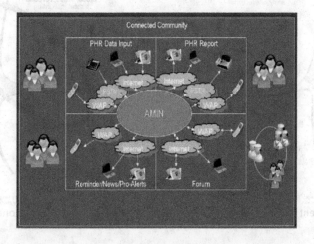

contact with reality beyond the clues on which it relies. It commits us passionately and far beyond our comprehension, to a vision of reality. Of this responsibility we cannot divest ourselves by setting up objective criteria of verifiability – or falsifiability, or testability, or what you will. For we live in it as in the garment of our own skin.

For Polanyi, tacit and explicit are different but inseparable aspects of knowledge. Both can be learnt though the learning modes will be different. Tacit knowledge is largely transferred in an experiential way, it is unfolding as it happens – we see what we know, and we see what we need to know; it identifies our needs in the here and now.

Kurtz and Snowden, through the Cynefin (pronounced kun-ev'in) framework, have taken this further describing knowledge generation and management as both – the state as well as the process – of sense making (Kurtz and Snowden 2003). The Cynefin framework consists of different knowledge domains – the known, the knowable, the complex or emerging, and the chaotic or random – in relation to human thinking and

organisational management. Figure 2 translates 'the business of medicine' into this framework. Looking at the framework makes evident that we always operate in all domains some of the time, or move to and from one domain to another depending on our context or changing circumstances (Sturmberg 2009; Sturmberg and Martin 2008; Sturmberg with a contribution by Martin 2007).

Expanding the static picture into its dynamic underpinnings shows that new knowledge is generated as a continuous flow between the chaotic state of puzzlement to the complex state of relative uncertainty to the state of the known typically associated with expert knowledge. Only occasionally though will some new knowledge become unshakable.

Understanding knowledge as a dynamic phenomenon, and knowledge generation as an iterative process, has important implications for the delivery of health services on the individual level and the way we approach health care reform. At the health care delivery level the lenses of

Figure 2. The Cynefin framework of knowledge and knowledge generation in medicine (with permission Sturmberg with a contribution by Martin 2007)

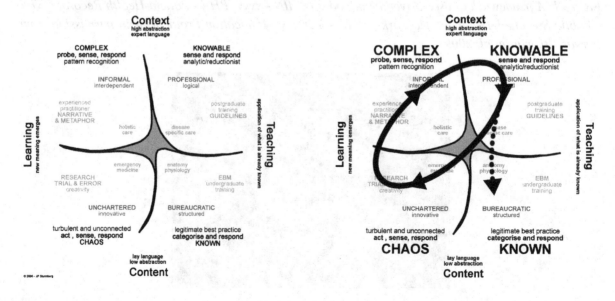

knowledge as a fact and knowledge as a personal event overlap. Sharing the different perspectives allow patient and health care provider to learn, or more precisely, gain new knowledge about each other in the context of the patient's concern. Or put differently new meaning can emerge from the expert knowledge of the health care provider and the lifeworld[ii] knowledge of the patient. (note: the health care provider can be substituted for by any person engaging with a patient, and the sharing itself can be by direct or indirect means).

The dynamic model of knowing is even more important when engaging with the health system and health system reform. No individual will have all the knowledge required to see and understand the interconnections within a huge and diverse health care sector. This is especially true as one also has to take into account the "non-medical" domains impacting on health, such as education, housing, work and working conditions, social and environmental infrastructure and so forth. It should be clear that the prevailing linear hierarchical structures of knowing are incongruent with the dynamic "needs" of knowledge and knowledge generation for a complex adaptive health system.

THE SEMANTICS OF HEALTH, ILLNESS AND DIS-EASE (THE SUBJECTIVE) VERSUS PATHOLOGY (THE OBJECTIVE)

Lakoff alluded to the notion that the way we talk (in metaphors) about things matters as the way we talk reveals how we perceive, how we think, and how we act (Lakoff and Johnsen 2003). Hence the terms health, illness and disease require some a-priori exploration as they are often used interchangeably and have no a-priori relation to the biologically based notion of pathologies. We usually clearly distinguished these from sickness, the social role ascribed to someone who is "not well",

People usually sought and continue to seek medical care when feeling ill or in dis-ease (the literal meaning of the otherwise ambiguous term disease) (Remen 2001). Lewis has argued that health, illness and dis-ease are points on the same subjective scale, and have to be distinguished from the biological changes of pathology (Lewis 2003). On this basis it is no longer tenable to accept equating disease with pathology (Fig 3). It is emphasised here that health, illness and dis-ease can be experienced equally in the presence

Figure 3. The subjective verses the objective nature in health care. The health professional is the translator between the subjective and objective behind the person's experiences about themselves.

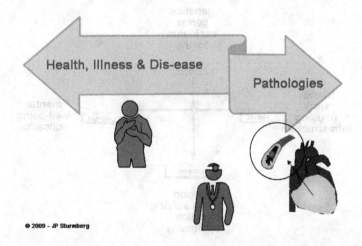

as in the absence of identifiable pathologies, and that the subjective and objective – though often understood as mutually exclusive dualisms – are coexisting experiential realities.[iii]

The notion of pathology, i.e. the biological changes in body structures, as a result of noxious agents is a rather new one. In fact our understanding of most pathologies occurred only since the middle of the 19th century when the newly developing technologies like the microscope allowed us for the first time to see some of the biological changes associated with the phenotypical appearance of some dis-eases. However, as Kerr White and colleagues have shown in a seminal epidemiological study only about 1% of all illness/dis-ease experience has an identifiable underlying pathology (White, et al. 1961).

The most important task of the doctor has been that of the translator between the subjective and objective behind the person's experiences about themselves (Egnew 2005), a point that has been largely lost, but never has it been as important as over the past 150 years, a time in medicine dominated by ever increasing scientific and technological approaches. However the limitations of the scientific and technological approach as the only means to cure humankind are becoming

rapidly evident – for example, the latest belief that the human genome project will be able to clarify once and for all the 'cause' of any health problem is rapidly becoming a myth. The link between the genotypical and phenotypical picture of most pathologies is complex. Latest research has shown that one phenotypical pathology can be 'caused' by a wide variety of genotypes (Beckmann, et al. 2007; Lesnick, et al. 2007; Loscalzo, et al. 2007).

There is an urgent need to refocus on the sense-making work that underpins the healing professions (Egnew 2005; Remen 2001; Sturmberg with a contribution by Martin 2007). Making sense of or coming to terms with one's ailment is essential to achieve health, especially if cure is not possible. Achieving health then becomes a continuous transformative process of adaptation, incorporating the subjective experiences described in the terms health, illness and dis-ease with the objective changes described by pathologies. If health, illness and dis-ease can be experienced as much in the presence as the absence of identifiable pathologies, how can this experience be conceptualised as a coherent whole?

Complex adaptive systems theory offers a framework through which to understand health as a personal experiential construct – health is

Figure 4. The complex adaptive model of health (with permission Sturmberg with a contribution by Martin 2007)

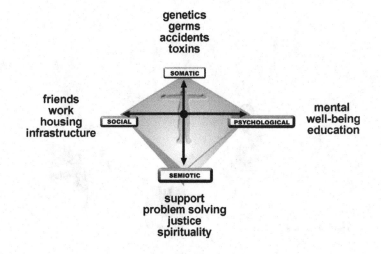

a balanced state between the physical, social, emotional and sense-making dimensions of one's being (Fig 4) (Sturmberg, et al. 2010; Sturmberg with a contribution by Martin 2007). Significant deviation from the balanced state in whatever direction is associated with the experience of illness and dis-ease[iv]. These figures present a particular state of health at a particular time in a particular patient. Reaching a particular point within the 'balance plane' is the result of ongoing dynamic movements within and across all its domains.

HEALTH: A DYNAMICALLY CHANGING STATE

The apparent paradox of health and dis-ease is exemplified in the following two figures. Both patients had a myocardial infarction of varying severity. The first experiences health in the presence of quite severe pathology – ischaemic post-MI cardiomyopathy. Here the patient has done the necessary adaptive work – on his own or through the facilitation of his health care providers – he found new meaning in his altered biological state (Figure 5).

In contrast the other experiences dis-ease in the absence of significant pathology – he sustained a non-transmural myocardial infarction without damage to his heart muscle and its pump function. Here the patient and/or his health care providers failed to do/facilitate the necessary adaptive work to achieve meaning from the experience of a threat to his self (Figure 6).

As these examples illustrate health (and for that matter illness and dis-ease) is a dynamic state. Health is constantly re-interpreted and re-constructed in the context of the myriad of ever changing influences in a person's life. Each new state in the personal health experience generates particular challenges and needs, some of which require simple information, whereas others demand a deep search for knowledge and/or wise counsel.

THE USER-DRIVEN APPROACH REGARDING INFORMATION, KNOWLEDGE AND WISDOM

Getting the right information is only the start towards user-driven health care. E-technologies provide ready access to – often unreliable – in-

Figure 5. Experience of health in the presence of significant pathology (with permission Sturmberg with a contribution by Martin 2007)

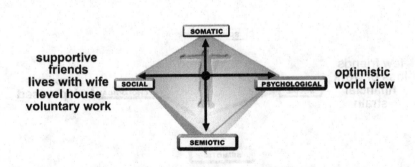

formation, however information alone? does not equate to knowledge. It requires considerable skills to vet the content of websites, and it takes further skill to use reliable information to generate new knowledge.

Blogs and discussion fora allow the sharing of information and experiences between people. This is particularly helpful to people affected by "the same" condition, and much of this sharing enhances their ability to make sense of their symptoms and their illness, both of which strengthen their psycho-immune responses that in turn enhances their self-healing capabilities and enhances their health experience (Kiecolt-Glaser, et al. 2002).

It is the enabling of the person to become an active participant in the consultation – face-to-face or virtual – that contributes to the achievement of good patient care[v]. Good patient care requires an ongoing provider-patient relationship and practical wisdom, also known as phronesis, of the practitioner in helping her patient to adapt to her changing health needs (Egnew 2005; Fugelli 1998).

These are the tenets of this book, and many of the chapters give a deep insight into the wise interactions resulting from a user-driven health care approach, a couple which are highlighted here.

The importance of understanding the patients' context on the structure and function of care delivery is highlighted by Fitzpatrick. Effective and efficient medical care systems must understand the context they operate in and be cognisant about the perceptions, social roles and expectations of the people they cared for (Fitzpatrick - insert reference in relation to book chapter). No two health systems can be structured to operate in the same way, however, health system planner's can aspire health services and their staff to deliver care that meets the needs of their patients.

How important it is to understand context and how easy it is to construe the 'reality' of the people's and community's 'true' context is painfully illustrated by Megan in the context of AIDS in sub-Saharan Africa. A 'single paper' based on speculation has demonised female sex workers as the cause of the AIDS epidemic in sub-Saharan Africa. However poverty is a major factor for women to engage in sex work with its high risk of contracting AIDS, though most see only a small number of clients per week. Their poor health is further compounded by societal stigma, social isolation, and a disinterest of the police and the health care sector for their well-being.

Figure 6. Experience of dis-ease in the absence of significant (with permission Sturmberg with a contribution by Martin 2007)

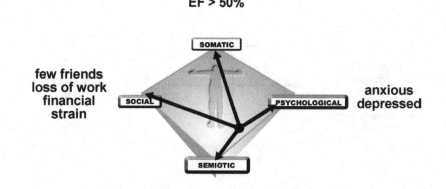

"Because I had a heart attack I now can't do a thing"

The misunderstanding of these interconnected factors perpetuates the poor health of sex workers as it does the spread of AIDS. Interventions that overcome poverty have been shown to get these women away from sex work - a classical example of a small intervention resulting in a major change in a complex adaptive system (Megan - insert reference in relation to book chapter).

Young's personal story illuminates the limitations of the instrumental approach, arising from the belief of certainty inherent in the medical sciences, to health care. Young alludes to the power differential between health professionals and patients, and the perceived inability by many patients to say no to 'well-meaning' treatment suggestions that are incongruent with the patient's beliefs and aspirations. It also highlight an inability of many health professionals to view 'a problem' through the 'patient's lens'. Young's initiative to provide a forum for people affected by her dis-ease provides a new voice as much as it harnesses the 'wisdom of the crowd' to influence clinical decision making and fostering research agendas (Young - insert reference in relation to book chapter).

Sliedrecht and Kotzé's work emphasise the importance for health professionals to 'pro-actively' elicit patient expectations about their care in the context of spinal cord injuries. They also highlight the importance of the 'sense-making' work, as hard as it may be at times, required from patients and their carers to achieve 'healing'. Patient-centred care is clearly more than instrumental care, patient-centred care that aims to heal requires 'to be there in the moment' with the patient, to 'just be human' when it matters most (Sliderich and Kotzé - insert reference in relation to book chapter), a most important skill to be cultivated in all health care providers (Shankar - insert reference in relation to book chapter).

CAN USER-DRIVEN HEALTH CARE BE THE CATALYST FOR TRUE HEALTH SYSTEMS REFORM?

So far the central argument in this chapter has been that knowledge has many dimensions each of which contributes unique insights to the understanding of health as a personal adaptive experiential state. Achieving a good health experience requires the engagement of the person, and the notion of user-driven health care reflects the people's capacity and desire to being an active participant in the healing process.

It naturally follows that health should be the central concern of the health care system. System, or more precisely complex adaptive system, is the imperative term. Complex adaptive systems are characterised by self-organisation, requiring a system to be open and far from equilibrium, with ill-defined boundaries and a large number of non-linear interactions involving short-loop feedback. Most importantly all interactions within the system are focused around its attractor, or core driver.

Capra illustrated the characteristics and functions of complex adaptive systems through the bathtub vortex metaphor (Capra 1996). For the bathtub the attractor is the plug hole – pulling the plug leads to the water forming a vortex, and, as we all recall from our childhood experiences, any disturbance of the vortex in whatever way will always restore the vortex very closely to what it had been before the disturbance, demonstrating the self-organising function around its attractor – the plug hole.

Currently the core drivers of most health systems is either/or or a combination of financial constraint/financial gain and top-down 'pathology' management[vi]. In an ideal health care system the core driver would be the patient's health experience. In operational terms this translates to the needs of the patient being the organising force determining the inter-relationships between all the agents at and between all the levels within the health care vortex.

Figure 7 shows the health care vortex as a representation of the ideal health system driven by patient need. At each level the agents constantly re-organise their relationships and interactions according to this patient's need (Sturmberg, et al. 2009).

A truly responsive health care system would seamlessly integrate the multiple needs of each patient. In such a seamlessly integrated health care system, the medical delivery component is only one part (or sub-system) of the overall system. The medical service delivery sub-system would interact with social, educational, work, transport, housing, environment, and infrastructure and so forth sub-systems, fully cognisant of the role of the interconnected emotional, social and environmental determinants/constraints on the health of this patient. The latter point alludes to the notions of determinants of health at the population level. The terms 'determents' and 'constraints' in the context of complex adaptive systems arises from the interconnected nature of ALL agents and their interactions on the health experience of the patient[vii].

The concept of user-driven health care emerged in the context of improved information technology. Information technologies increase connectivity between people and the sharing of knowledge and experiences narrows the 'gap between the expert in the pathology and the expert in the disease' which finally may give people the power to shift the attractor of the health care system from the top-down, fragmented by specific pathology interests and preoccupied by financial profits, to the health needs of the people. Incidentally this is

Figure 7. The 'Health Care Vortex' as a metaphorical representation of the health care system

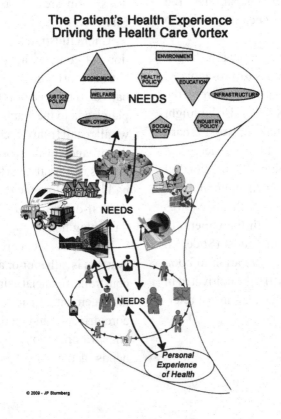

the philosophical and time-proven basis of medical care since time in memoriam across all cultures.

SUMMARY

User-driven health care is more than providing people with access to information through improving technologies. User-driven health care is the expression of people's deep-seated need to be an active participant in the therapeutic relationship with their healer. The user-driven health care technology gives people a voice or the means (or in system terms provides the little nudge or perturbation) that ultimately will shift the system's attractor so that the system will rearrange its structure and interactions to meet their health needs.

ACKNOWLEDGMENT

I am greatly indebted to the critical and insightful comments by Darren Greenop, Joan Young and SD Ross in the preparation of this chapter.

REFERENCES

Beckmann, J. S., Estivill, X., & Antonarakis, S. E. (2007). Copy number variants and genetic traits: closer to the resolution of phenotypic to genotypic variability. Nature Review Genetics, 8(8), 639-646.

Biswas, R., et al. (2008). User-driven health care - answering multidimensional information needs in individual patients utilizing post-EBM approaches: a conceptual model. Journal of Evaluation in Clinical Practice, 14(5), 742-749.

Biswas, R. (2009). Social Cognitive Ontology and User Driven Health Care. In S. Hatzipanagos and S. Warburton, (eds), Handbook of Research on Social Software and Developing Community Ontologies. Hershey, PA: IGI Global.

Capra, F. (1996). The Web of Life. London: HarperCollins Publishers.

Egnew, T. R. (2005). The Meaning Of Healing: Transcending Suffering. Annals of Family Medicine, 3(3), 255-262.

Fugelli, P. (1998). Clinical practice: between Aristotle and Cochrane. Schweizerische Medizinische Wochenschrift. Journal Suisse de Medecine, 128, 184-188.

Kiecolt-Glaser, J. K., et al. (2002). Psychoneuroimmunology: Psychological Influences on Immune Function and Health. Journal of Consulting and Clinical Psychology, 70(3), 537-547.

Kurtz, C. F., & Snowden, D. J. (2003). The new dynamics of strategy: Sense-making in a complex and complicated world. IBM Systems Journal, 42(3), 462-483.

Lakoff, G., & Johnsen, M. (2003). Metaphors we live by. London: The University of Chicago Press.

Lesnick, T. G., et al. (2007). A Genomic Pathway Approach to a Complex Disease: Axon Guidance and Parkinson Disease. PLoS Genetics 3(6), 98.

Lewis, C. (2003). Exploring the Biological Meaning of Disease and Health. Retrieved November 27, 2005, from http://www.chester.ac.uk/~sjlewis/DM/Vienna.htm

Loscalzo, J., Kohane, I., & Barabasi, A.-L. (2007). Human disease classification in the postgenomic era: A complex systems approach to human pathobiology. Molecular Systems Biology, 3(124).

Polanyi, M. (1958). Personal Knowledge. Towards a Post-Critical Philosophy. London: Routledge.

Remen, R. N. (2001). Recapturing the soul of medicine: physicians need to reclaim meaning in their working lives. The Western Journal of Medicin, 174(1), 4.

Sturmberg, J., O'Halloran, D., & Martin, C. (2009). Systems Can Only Do What They Are Designed to Do - Health Care Reform In Australia. In Proceedings of the NAPCRG-Meeting. Montreal.

Sturmberg, J. P. (2009). The personal nature of health. Journal of Evaluation in Clinical Practice, 15(4), 766-769.

Sturmberg, J. P., & Martin, C. M. (2008). Knowing - in Medicine. Journal of Evaluation in Clinical Practice, 14(5), 767-770.

Sturmberg, J. P., Martin, C. M., & Moes, M. (2010). Health at the Centre of Health Systems Reform - How Philosophy Can Inform Policy. Perspectives in Biology and Medicine: In press.

Sturmberg, J. P., & Martin, C. M. (2007). The Foundations of Primary Care. Daring to be Different. San Francisco: Radcliffe Medical Press.

White, K., F. Williams, and B. Greenberg (1961). The Ecology of Medical Care. New England Journal of Medicine 265(18), 885-892.

ENDNOTES

[i] From a medical philosophy point of view I prefer the term 'patient' (meaning the vulnerable) to the term 'user' which has a strong 'instrumental notion' to it, and reflects the sociologicallens of 'the medical encounter'. Pellegrino, ED, and DC Thomasma. 1981. A Philosophical Basis of Medical Practice. Towards a Philosophy and Ethic of the Healing Professions. New York Oxford: Oxford University Press.

[ii] Referring to Husserl's notion of phenomenology

[iii] Lewis refers to Canguilhem as follows: In 1943, the medically trained French philosopher Georges Canguilhem posed an important problem that continues to be relevant to this day. Take a man, he suggested, who complains of no ailments and whose life is suddenly cut short by his being murdered or his dying in a car crash. For various French legal reasons, an autopsy is performed and the dead man is found to have a serious cancerous tumour – in Canguilhem's example, of the kidney. What then do we make of the man – did he have a disease or didn't he? Canguilhem, G. (1989). The Normal and the Pathological. New York: Zone Books. (p92)

[iv] A detailed discussion of these concepts can be found in The Foundations of Primary Care and Health at the Centre of Health Systems Reform – How Philosophy can Inform Policy

[v] The tenet here is that the system is only changing if there is a reason to do so. Enabled patients "demanding" a different approach to their care will "force" doctors and other health care providers to adopt a "different approach" - centred on the patient or people. In this sense the "demand for change" becomes "enabling" for all involved.

[vi] Disease management focuses on the management of patients with discrete pathologies. Disease management programmes place a heavy emphasis on 'correct instrumental management' according to 'best practice guidelines' and vary greatly in terms of addressing patients' needs holistically.

[vii] Traditionally determinism refers to the causality of an unbroken chain of prior occurrences on the event of interest.

Compilation of References

Abbot, J., Dodd, M., Bilton, D., & Webb, A. K. (1994). Treatment Compliance in Adults with Cystic Fibrosis. *Thorax*, *49*(2), 115–120. doi:10.1136/thx.49.2.115

Abbott, J., Dodd, M., Gee, L., & Webb, K. (2001). Ways of coping with cystic fibrosis: implications for treatment adherence. *Disability and Rehabilitation*, *23*(8), 315–324. doi:10.1080/09638280010004171

Acuna, L. E. (2003). Teaching humanities at the national University of La Plata, Argentina. *Academic Medicine*, *78*, 1024–1027. doi:10.1097/00001888-200310000-00017

Adamchak, S. E. (2006). Youth Peer Education in Reproductive Health and HIV and AIDS: Progress, Process and Programming for the Future Youth Issues Paper 7. *Family Health International, Youthnet program*, Arlington, VA.

Adams, J. (2006). The part played by instructional media in distance education. *SIMILE: Studies In Media & Information Literacy Education*, *6*(2), 1–12. doi:10.3138/sim.6.2.001

Agre, P., Horswill, I. (1997). Lifeworld analysis. *Journal of Artificial Intelligence Research*, *6*(1), 111-145. Baskin, S. M, Kirk, L. P. Lehrer, P. M., Lubar, J. F., & LaVaque, T. (2004). *Evidence-Based Practice in Biofeedback and Neurofeedback*

Ahn, Y. S., Horstman, L. L., Jy, W., Jimenez, J. J., & Bowen, B. (2002). Vascular dementia in patients with immune thrombocytopenic purpura. *Thrombosis Research*, *107*(6), 337–344. doi:10.1016/S0049-3848(02)00337-7

Ako, W. Y. (2002). *Factors Affecting the Formulation and Implementation of the 1993 Educational Reforms in Papua New Guinea. Doctoral Thesis*. Bristol: The University of Bristol

Ako, W.Y., & Fitzpatrick, J. (2007, June). Empowering the Initiation of a malaria prevention strategy to combat malaria in Papua New Guinea. *Rural and Remote Health*.

Alarcon, R. D., & Leetz, K. L. (1998). Cultural intersections in the psychotherapy of borderline personality disorder. *American Journal of Psychotherapy*, *52*(2), 176–190.

Allan, M., & Thorns, D. (2009). Being Face to Face - A state of Mind or Technological Design. In B. Whitworth & A. (de) Moor (Eds.), *Handbook of Research on Socio Technical Designing and Social Networking Systems* (pp. 440-454). Hershey PA: IGI Global Publications.

Al-Umran, K. U., Al-Shaikh, B. A., Al-Awary, B. H., Al-Rubaish, A. M., & Al-Muhanna, F. A. (2006). Medical ethics and tomorrow's physicians: an aspect of coverage in the formal curriculum. *Medical Teacher*, *28*, 182–184. doi:10.1080/01421590500271365

American Society of Hematology ITP Practice Guideline Panel. (1997). Diagnosis and Treatment of Idiopathic Thrombocytopenic Purpura. *Recommendations of the American Society of Hematology*, *126*(4), 319–326.

Anand, S. G. (2005). A Content Analysis of E-mail Communication Between Primary Care Providers and Parents. *Pediatrics*, *115*, 1283–1288. doi:10.1542/peds.2004-1297

Andanda, P. (2009). Vulnerability: sex workers in Nairobi's Majengo slum. *Cambridge quarterly of healthcare ethics: CQ: the international journal of healthcare ethics committees, 18*(2), 138-146.

Andersen, R. S. (2008). Learning based on patient case reviews: an interview study. *BMC Medical Education, 8*, 43. doi:10.1186/1472-6920-8-43

Anderson, J. M. (2006). Immigrant women speak of chronic illness: the social construction of the devalued self. *Journal of Advanced Nursing, 16*(6), 710–717. doi:10.1111/j.1365-2648.1991.tb01729.x

Andre, J., Brody, H., Fleck, L., Thomason, C. L., & Tomlinson, T. (2003). Ethics, professionalism and humanities at Michigan state University College of human medicine. *Academic Medicine, 78*, 968–972. doi:10.1097/00001888-200310000-00005

Andrew, J., & Whyte, F. (2004). The experiences of district nurses caring for people receiving palliative chemotherapy. *International Journal of Palliative Nursing, 10*(3), 110–118, discussion 118.

Annon, J. (1976). The P-LI-SS-IT model: a proposed conceptual scheme for the behavioural treatment of sexual problems. *Journal of Sex Education and Therapy, 2*, 1–15.

Anonymous,. (1997). *Confronting AIDS: Public priorities in a global epidemic: World Bank*. Oxford: University Press.

Anonymous. (Participants in the 2001 Conference on Ethical Aspects of Research in Developing Countries). (2002). Ethics. Fair benefits for research in developing countries. *Science, 298*(5601), 2133-2134.

Antman, E. M., Lau, J., Kupelnick, B., Mosteller, F., & Chalmers, T. C. (1992). A comparison of results of meta-analyses of randomized control trials and recommendations of clinical experts. Treatments for myocardial infarction. *Journal of the American Medical Association, 268*, 240–248. doi:10.1001/jama.268.2.240

Appadurai, A. (1991). Global ethnoscapes: Notes and queries for a transnational anthropology. In Fox, R. G. (Ed.), *Recapturing Anthropology: Working in the Present* (pp. 191–210). Santa Fe, NM: Sch. Am. Res. Press.

Aral, S., & Van Alstyne, M. (2009). *Networks and Novel Information: The Diversity–Bandwidth Tradeoff*. Paper presented at the Workshop on Information in Networks (WIN).

Argyris, C., Putnam, R., & Smith, D. (1985). *Action science: concepts, methods, and skills for research and intervention* (1st ed.). San Francisco, CA: Jossey-Bass.

Arias Llorente, R. P., Garcia, C. B., & Diaz Martin, J. J. (2008). Treatment compliance in children and adults with cystic fibrosis. *Journal of Cystic Fibrosis, 7*, 359–367. doi:10.1016/j.jcf.2008.01.003

Armstrong, C. D., Hogg, W. E., Lemelin, J., Dahrouge, S., Martin, C., & Viner, G. S. (2008). Home-based intermediate care program vs hospitalization: Cost comparison study. *Canadian Family Physician Medecin de Famille Canadien, 54*(1), 66–73.

Armstrong, E. C. (2004). *Morning POEMs (Patient Oriented Evidence that Matters): Teaching point-of-care, patient focused evidence-based medicine*. Retrieved August 16, 2007, from http://www.fammed.washington.edu/ebp/media/stfm-9-03-morningpoems.doc.

Arnott, R., Bolton, G., Evans, M., Finlay, I., Macnaughton, J., Meakin, R., & Reid, W. (2001). Proposal for an Academic Association for Medical Humanities. *Medical Humanities, 27*, 104–105. doi:10.1136/mh.27.2.104

Arnquist, S. (2009). Research trove: Patients' online data. *New York Times,* (August 24), available at: http://www.nytimes.com/2009/08/25/health/25web.html

Arnst, C. (2008). Health 2.0: Patients as partners. *BusinessWeek,* (December 4), Retrieved from http://www.businessweek.com/magazine/content/08_50/b4112058194219.htm

Asch, S. M., Kerr, E. A., Keesey, J., Adams, J. L., Setodji, C. M., Malik, S., & McGlynn, E. A. (2006). Who is at greatest risk for receiving poor-quality health care? *The New England Journal of Medicine*, *354*(11), 1147–1156. doi:10.1056/NEJMsa044464

Atherton, J. S. (2009). *Learning and Teaching; Experiential Learning*. Retrieved from http://www.learningandteaching.info/learning/experience.htm

Attwood, T. (1998). *Asperger syndrome: a guide for parents and professionals.* London: Jessica Kingsley Publishers.

AusAID. (2004). *Country Programs: Papua New Guinea.* Retrieved September 22, 2004, from http://www.ausaid.gov.au/country/papua.cfm

Autism Research Centre. (n.d.). *Autism Research Centre.* Retrieved from http://www.autismresearchcentre.com/

Baird, G., Simonoff, E., & Pickles, A. (2006). Prevalence of disorders of the autism spectrum in a population cohort of children in South Thames: the Special Needs and Autism Project (SNAP). *Lancet*, *368*, 210–215. doi:10.1016/S0140-6736(06)69041-7

Baker, A., Jensen, P. J., & Kolb, D. A. (2002). *Conversational learning: an experiential approach to knowledge creation.* Westport, CT: Quorum books.

Bakhtin, M. M. (1986). *Speech genres and other late essays* (Emerson, C., & Holquist, M., Trans.). Austin, TX: University of Texas Press. (Original work published 1979)

Balas, E. A., & Boren, S. A. (2000). Managing clinical knowledge for health care improvement. In J. Bemmel & A. T. McCray (Eds.), *Yearbook of Medical Informatics*. Stuttgart, DE: Schattauer Verlagsgesellschaft mbH.

Ball, M. J., Costin, M. Y., & Lehmann, C. (2008). The personal health record: consumers banking on their health. *Studies in Health Technology and Informatics*, *134*, 35–46.

Ballard, K. (2004). Compliance and concordance. In Gabe, J., Bury, M., & Elston, M. A., *eds.* (2004). *Key Concepts in Medical Sociology* pp.107-112. London: Sage.

Baltes, B. B., Dickson, M. W., Sherman, M. P., Bauer, C. C., & LaGanke, J. S. (2002). Computer-Mediated Communication and Group Decision Making: A Meta-Analysis. *Organizational Behavior and Human Decision Processes*, *87*(1), 156–179. doi:10.1006/obhd.2001.2961

Ban, T. (2001). Pharmacotherapy of mental illness – a historical analysis. *Progress in Neuro-Psychopharmacology & Biological Psychiatry*, *25*, 667–694. doi:10.1016/S0278-5846(01)00160-9

Barnacle, R. (2001). *Phenomenology in education research.* Paper presented at AARE conference, Fremantle

Barnard, A., Hollingum, C., & Hartfiel, B. (2006). Going on a journey: understanding palliative care nursing. *International Journal of Palliative Nursing*, *12*(1), 6–12.

Baron, S. (2009). Evaluating the patient journey approach to ensure health care is centred on patients. *Nursing Times*, *105*(22), 20–23.

Baron-Cohen, S. (2003). *The Essential Difference*. New York: Basic Books.

Baron-Cohen, S., Scott, F., Allison, C., Williams, J., Bolton, P., Matthews, F., & Brayne, C. (n.d.). Prevalence of autism-spectrum conditions: UK school-based population study. *British Journal of Psychiatry*, *194*, 500-509.

Barrett, T. G., & Booth, I. W. (1994). Sartorial eloquence: does it exist in the paediatrician-patient relationship? *BMJ (Clinical Research Ed.)*, *309*, 1710–1712.

Barron-Cohen, S. (2008). *Autism and Asperger Syndrome: the facts*. New York: Oxford University Press.

Basch, E., Artz, D., Dulko, D., Scher, K., Sabbatini, P., & Hensley, M. (2005). Patient Online Self-Reporting of Toxicity Symptoms During Chemotherapy. *Journal of Clinical Oncology*, *23*(15), 3552–3561. doi:10.1200/JCO.2005.04.275

Basic Medical Surveillance Essentials for people with Down's Syndrome (2001). *Basic Medical Surveillance Essentials for people with Down's Syndrome*, Guidelines of the Down's Syndrome Medical Interest Group DSMIG (UK & Ireland) Irish Edition Retrieved from www.dsmig.org.uk

Battling back from childhood sexual abuse and surviving the journey. (1998). *J Psychosoc Nurs Ment Health Serv, 36*(12), 13-17.

Bauman, Z. (1996). From pilgrim to tourist – or a short history of identity. In Hall, S., & du Gay, P. (Eds.), *Questions of Cultural Identity* (pp. 18–36). London: Sage.

Baumann, P. (2009). 140 Health Care Uses for Twitter. *Phill baumann online, health is social.* Retrieved from http://philbaumann.com/2009/01/16/140-health-care-uses-for-twitter/

Bayliss, E. A., Ellis, J. L., & Steiner, J. F. (2009). Seniors' self-reported multimorbidity captured biopsychosocial factors not incorporated into two other data-based morbidity measures. *J Clin Epidemiol, 62*(5), 550-557 e551.

Baynes, K. (1994). Communicative ethics, the public sphere, and communication media. *Critical Studies in Mass Communication, 11*, 315–326. doi:10.1080/15295039409366908

Bazaz, R., & Brown, C. (2007). War on white coats. *Lancet, 370*, 2097. doi:10.1016/S0140-6736(07)61891-1

Beach, M., & Inui, T. Relationship-Centered Care Research Network. (2006). Relationship-centred Care. A constructive reframing. *Journal of General Internal Medicine, 21*, s3–s8. doi:10.1111/j.1525-1497.2006.00302.x

Beldarrain, Y. (2006). Distance education trends: Integrating new technologies to foster student interaction and collaboration. *Distance Education, 27*(2), 139–153. doi:10.1080/01587910600789498

Bell, G., & Gemell, J. (2009). *Total Recall*. London: Penguin.

Bendixen, R. M., Levy, C. E., Olive, E. S., Kobb, R. F., & Mann, W. C. (2009). Cost effectiveness of a telerehabilitation program to support chronically ill and disabled elders in their homes. *Telemedicine Journal and e-Health, 15*(1), 31–38. doi:10.1089/tmj.2008.0046

Benn, S. I. (1971). Privacy, freedom and respect for persons. In Pennock, R. J., & Chapman, J. W. (Eds.), *Privacy* (pp. 1–26). New York: Atherton Press.

Bennett, N. L. (2005). Family physicians' information seeking behaviors: A survey comparison with other specialties. *BMC Medical Informatics and Decision Making, 5*, 9. Retrieved from http://www.biomedcentral.com/content/pdf/1472-6947-5-9.pdf. doi:10.1186/1472-6947-5-9

Bennett, E., & Maniar, N. (2008). *Are videoed lectures an effective teaching tool? Biggs, J., & Tang, C. (2007). Teaching for Quality Learning at University: What the Student does (Society for Research Into Higher Education)*. Mcgraw-Hill Publ.Comp.

Ber, R., & Bar-et, Y. (2003). Faculty of medicine of the Technion-Israel Institute of Technology, humanities in medicine. *Academic Medicine, 78*, 1071–1072. doi:10.1097/00001888-200310000-00044

Berelson, B. (1952). *Content analysis in communication research*. NY: Hafner.

Bero, L., Grilli, R., Grimshaw, J., Harvey, E., Oxman, A., & Thomson, M. (1998). Closing the gap between research and practice: an over view of systematic reviews of inter ventions to promote the implementation of research findings. *British Medical Journal, 317*, 465–469.

Besa, C. E., & Woermann, U. (2009, February 6). *Chronic Myelogenous Leukemia. E Medicine (Medscape)*. Retrieved June 16, 2009 from http://emedicine.medscape.com/article/199425-overview

Best, A., Hiatt, R., Cameron, R., Rimer, B. K., & Abrams, D. B. (2003). The evolution of cancer control research: An international perspective from Canada and the United States. *Cancer Epidemiology, Biomarkers & Prevention, 12*, 705–712.

Best, A., Hiatt, R. A., & Norman, C. D. (2008). Knowledge integration: conceptualizing communications in cancer control systems. *Patient Education and Counseling, 71*(3), 319–327. doi:10.1016/j.pec.2008.02.013

Best, A., Moor, G., Holmes, B., Clark, P., Bruce, T., & Leischow, S. (2003). Health promotion dissemination and systems thinking: Towards an integrative model. *American Journal of Health Behavior, 27*(Supplement 3), 206–216.

Best, A., Trochim, W. K., Haggerty, J., Moor, G., & Norman, C. D. (2008). Systems thinking for knowledge integration: New models for policy-research collaboration. In McKee, L., Ferlie, E., & Hyde, P. (Eds.), *Organizing and reorganizing: Power and change in health care organizations* (pp. 154–166). Houndsmill, UK: Palgrave McMillan.

Bhandari, M., Montori, V., Devereaux, P. J., Dosanjh, S., Sprague, S., & Guyatt, G. H. (2003). Challenges to the practice of evidence-based medicine during residents' surgical training: a qualitative study using grounded theory. *Academic Medicine*, *78*(11), 1183–1190. doi:10.1097/00001888-200311000-00022

Bielli, E., Carminati, F., La Capra, S., Lina, M., Brunelli, C., & Tamburini, M. (2004). A Wireless Health Outcomes Monitoring System (WHOMS): development and field testing with cancer patients using mobile phones. *BMC Medical Informatics and Decision Making*, *4*(1), 7. doi:10.1186/1472-6947-4-7

Biklen, D. (2005). *Autism and the Myth of the Person Alone*. New York: NYU Press.

Billinghurst, M., & Kato, H. (1999). *Collaborative Mixed Reality-Merging Real and Virtual Worlds*. Paper presented at the First International Symposium on Mixed Reality (ISMR 99), Berlin.

Binkley, L. (1999). Caring for renal patients during loss and bereavement. *EDTNA/ERCA Journal (English Ed.)*, *25*(2), 45–48.

Biocca, F., Harms, C., & Burgoon, J. K. (2003). Towards a More Robust Theory and Measure of Social Presence: Review and Suggested Criteria. *Presence (Cambridge, Mass.)*, *12*(5), 456–480. doi:10.1162/105474603322761270

Biswas, R., Martin, C., Sturmberg, J., Shankar, R., & Umakanth, S., Shanker, & Kasthuri A. S. (2008). User driven health care - Answering multidimensional information needs in individual patients utilizing post EBM approaches: A conceptual model. *Journal of Evaluation in Clinical Practice*, *14*, 742–749. doi:10.1111/j.1365-2753.2008.00998.x

Biswas, R. (2009). *The Conscious Notebook*. New York: Nova Science Publishers.

Biswas, R., & Dalal, M. (2003, May). A yoga teacher with persistent cheilitis. *Intl Jl Clin Pract (UK)*, *57*(4), 340–342.

Biswas, R., Paul, A., & Shetty, K. J. (2002, November). A yoga teacher with persistent reflux symptoms. *Intl Jl Clin Pract (UK)*, *56*, 9.

Biswas, R., Maniam, J., Lee, E. W., Gopal, P., Umakanth, S., & Dahiya, S. (2008). User-driven health care: answering multidimensional information needs in individual patients utilizing post-EBM approaches: an operational model. *Journal of Evaluation in Clinical Practice*, *14*(5), 750–760. doi:10.1111/j.1365-2753.2008.00997.x

Biswas, R. (2002). Developing Holistic health care in the third world: A working study proposal. *Eubios Jl Asian Intl Bioethics (Tokyo)*, *12*(4), 143–147.

Biswas, R., & Dhakal, B. (2003). Medical student narratives for understanding Disease and social order in the third world. *Eubios Jl Asian Intl Bioethics(Tokyo)*, *13*(4), 139–142.

Biswas, R. (2003). Patient networks and their level of complexity as an outcome measure in clinical intervention. *BMJ rapid response to Edwards N, Clinical networks. BMJ (Clinical Research Ed.)*, *324*, 63.

Biswas, R., Umakanth, S., Strumberg, J., Martin, C. M., Hande, M., & Nagra, J. S. (2007b). The process of evidence-based medicine and the search for meaning. *Journal of Evaluation in Clinical Practice*, *13*, 529–532. doi:10.1111/j.1365-2753.2007.00837.x

Biswas, R., Umakanth, S., Shetty, M., Hande, M., & Nagra, J. S. (2009). Problem based self-directed life long participatory learning in medical educators and their audience: Reflective lessons learnt from a lecture series. In Geinare, P. F. (Ed.), *Trends in continuing education*. New York: Nova Science Publishers.

Biswas, R. (2009). Open Information Management in User-Driven Healthcare. In Niiranen, S. (Eds.), *Open Information Management: Applications of Interconnectivity and Collaboration*. Hershey, PA: Information Science Reference.

Biswas, R., (2001, January). Irritable Bowel syndrome in the tropics: a possible culprit. *Journal of Indian academy of clinical medicine (letter), 2*(1-2).

Biswas, R., Martin, C. M., Sturmberg, J., Mukherji, K., Lee, E. W. H., Umakanth, S., & Kasthuri, A. S. (2009) Social Cognitive Ontology and User Driven Healthcare in: Katzipanagos, S & Warburton, S: *Handbook of research on social software and developing community Ontologies*

Bjerg, K. (2001). Towards the virtual home: Construing the multi-media-home to enhance cultural and biographic continuity. In Rasmussen, B., Beardon, C., & Munari, S. (Eds.), *Computers and networks in the age of globalization*. Klüwer Academic Publishers.

Bjerg, K. (2000). Citizen Science Implications of Public Access to 3-D Hypermedia Editing and Interactivity in the Home. Consumers as researchers - Homes as laboratories. In Sloane, A., & van Rijn, F. (Eds.), *Home Informatics and Telematics*. Klüwer Academic Publishers.

Bjerg, K. (2008) "Empowering Citizen Self-Documentation: Re-inventing the diary" Observatorio (OBS*), Vol2, No 2 (2008) www.obs.obercom.pt/index.php/obs/article/view/198 (Paper presented to the COST298 transdiciplinary international conference on "*The user and the future of information and communication technologies*" in Moscow 2007).

Bjerg, K. (2009) Personal Electronic Journaling (Paper presented to the COST298 transdiciplinary international conference on "The *user and the future of information and communication technologies*" in Copenhagen 2009). http://miha2.ef.uni-lj.si/cost298/gbc2009-proceedings/papers/P155.pdf

Bjerg, K. (2009) Self-care, telemonitoring and multidimensionality in person-to-person interfacing: A new angle on self-management in chronic disease (Paper presented to the COST298 transdiciplinary international conference on "*The user and the future of information and communication technologies*" in Copenhagen 2009):http://miha2.ef.uni-lj.si/cost298/gbc2009-proceedings/papers/P154.pdf

Blasco, P. G., Moreto, G., & Levites, M. R. (2005). Teaching humanities through opera: leading medical students to reflective attitudes. *Family Medicine, 37*, 18–20.

Blaxter, M. (2004). Life narratives, health and identity. In Kelleher, D., & Leavey, G. *eds.* (2004). *Identity and Health* pp.170-199. London: Routledge.

Bleicher, P. (2006). Web 2.0 revolution: Power to the people. *Applied Clinical Trials*, 34-36.

Blondal, K., & Halldorsdottir, S. (2009). The challenge of caring for patients in pain: from the nurse's perspective. *Journal of Clinical Nursing, 18*(20), 2897–2906. doi:10.1111/j.1365-2702.2009.02794.x

Bluhm, R. (2009). Evidence-Based Medicine and Patient Autonomy. *International Journal of Feminist Approaches to Bioethics, 2*(2), 134–151. doi:10.2979/FAB.2009.2.2.134

BMA Central Consultants and Specialists Committee. *Uniform and dress code for doctors: guidance from the central consultants and specialists committee, 2007*. Retrieved from http://www.bma.org.uk/ap.nsf/Content/CCSCdresscode051207?OpenDocument&Highlight=2, ccsc,bare,below,elbows

Bodenheimer, T., & Grumbach, K. (2003). Electronic technology: a spark to revitalize primary care? *Journal of the American Medical Association, 290*(2), 259–264. doi:10.1001/jama.290.2.259

Bond, A., Jones, A., Haynes, R., Tam, M., Denton, E., & Ballantyne, M. (2009). Tackling climate change close to home: mobile breast screening as a model. *Journal of Health Services Research & Policy, 14*(3), 165–167. doi:10.1258/jhsrp.2009.008154

Bonsu, S. K., & Darmody, A. (2008). Putting consumers to work: 'Co-creation' and new marketing governmentality. *Journal of Consumer Culture*, 8(2), 163–196. doi:10.1177/1469540508090089

Bosch, L. t., Oostdijk, N., & Ruiter, J. P. (2004). *Durational aspects of turn-taking in spontaneous face-to-face and telephone dialogues*. Paper presented at the Text, Speech and Dialogue. Retrieved from http://www.hcrc.ed.ac.uk/comic/documents/

Bottazzi, D., Corradi, A., & Montanari, R. (2006). Context-aware middleware solutions for anytime and anywhere emergency assistance to elderly people. *IEEE Communications Magazine*, 44(4), 82–90. doi:10.1109/MCOM.2006.1632653

Bottiger, B. W., Hans-Richard, A., Chamberlain, D. A., Blukhmki, E., Belmans, A., & Sanays, T. (2008). Thrombolysis during Resuscitation for Out-of-Hospital Cardiac Arrest. *The New England Journal of Medicine*, 359, 2651–2662. doi:10.1056/NEJMoa070570

Boulos, M. G. K., Maramba, I., & Wheeler, S. (2006). Wikis, blogs and podcasts: a new generation of Web-based tools for virtual collaborative clinical practice and education, *BMC Medical Education*, 6, 41. Retrieved from [REMOVED HYPERLINK FIELD]http://www.biomedcentral.com/content/pdf/1472-6920-6-41.pdf

Boulous, M., & Wheeler, S. (2007). The emerging Web 2.0 social software: an enabling suite of sociable technologies in health and health care education. *Health Information and Libraries Journal*, 24, 2–23. doi:10.1111/j.1471-1842.2007.00701.x

Boultier, M., Mason, R., & Rootman, I. (1997). Community action and reflective practice in health promotion research. *Health Promotion International*, 12(1), 60–78.

Bourdieu, P. (1995). Social space and symbolic power. In McQuarie, D. (Ed.), *Readings in contemporary sociological theory: From modernity to post-modernity* (pp. 323–334). Englewood Cliffs, NJ: Prentice Hall.

Bourgeois, F. C., Taylor, P. L., Emans, S. J., Nigrin, D. J., & Mandl, K. D. (2008). Whose Personal Control? Creating Private, Personally Controlled Health Records for Pediatric and Adolescent Patients. *Journal of the American Medical Informatics Association*, 15(6), 737–743. doi:10.1197/jamia.M2865

Bouton-Lewis, G., & Lewis, D. (2002). Conceptions of Health held by Aboriginal, Torres Strait Islander and Papua New Guinean Health Science Students. *Close Up 2 H Higher Education Conference*. University of Lancaster.

Boyle, B., Clancy, A., Connolly, A., Daly, E., Hefferman, B., Howley, E., et al. (2003). The same in difference: The work of peer counsellors of the Irish Wheelchair Association and the National Council of the Blind in Ireland. *The International Journal of Narrative Therapy and Community Work* (2), 4-16.

Brahler, C., Peterson, N., & Johnson, E. (1999). Developing on-line learning materials for higher education: An overview of current issues. Educational Technology and Society, Vol. 2 (2). Retrieved on 5 October 2009, from http://www.ifets.info/journals/2_2/jayne_brahler.html

Bransford, J. D., Brown, A. L., & Cocking, R. R. (Eds.). (2000). *How people learn: brain, mind, experience, and school*. Washington, DC: National Academy Press.

Brase, G. L., & Richmond, J. (2006). The White–Coat effect: physician attire and perceived authority, friendliness, and attractiveness. *Journal of Applied Social Psychology*, 34, 2469–2481. doi:10.1111/j.1559-1816.2004.tb01987.x

Bronagh, W., Helen, R., & Jane, H. (2007). Emergency hospital admissions for ill-defined conditions amongst older people: a review of the literature. *International Journal of Older People Nursing*, 2(4), 270–277. doi:10.1111/j.1748-3743.2007.00093.x

Brook, R. H. (2009). Assessing the appropriateness of Care, its time has come. *Journal of the American Medical Association*, 302(9), 997–998. doi:10.1001/jama.2009.1279

Broom, D., & Whittaker, A. (2004). Controlling diabetes, controlling diabetics: moral language in the management of diabetes type 2. *Social Science & Medicine*, *58*(11), 2371–2382. doi:10.1016/j.socscimed.2003.09.002

Broome, B., & Chen, M. (1992). Guidelines for computer-assisted group problem solving: Meeting the challenges of complex issues. *Small Group Research*, *23*(2), 216–236. doi:10.1177/1046496492232005

Brothers, R. (2000). The computer-mediated public sphere and the cosmopolitan ideal. *Ethics and Information Technology*, *2*, 91–98. doi:10.1023/A:1010073319706

Brown, L., Cai, T., & DasGupta, A. (2001). Interval estimation for a binomial proportion. *Statistical Science*, *16*(2), 101–117. doi:10.1214/ss/1009213286

Brown, J. (1995). Naming and framing: The social construction of diagnosis and illness. [CHECK.]. *Journal of Health and Social Behavior*, (Extra Issue), 34–52. doi:10.2307/2626956

Brown, J. (2005). *The World Cafe: Shaping our futures through conversations that matter*. San Francisco: Berrett-Koehler.

Brown, B. (2008). Research and the privacy rule: The chill is on. *Journal of Health Care Compliance*, 35-36.

Brownstein, C. A., Brownstein, J. S., Williams, D. S., Wicks, P., & Heywood, J. A. (2009). The power of social networking in medicine. *Nature Biotechnology*, *27*(10), 888–890. doi:10.1038/nbt1009-888

Bryan, C. S., & Babelay, A. M. (2009). Building character: a model for reflective practice. *Academic Medicine*, *84*, 1283–1288. doi:10.1097/ACM.0b013e3181b6a79c

Bryar, R. M., Closs, S. J., Baum, G., Cooke, J., Griffiths, J., & Hostick, T. (2003). Yorkshire BARRIERS project. *International Journal of Nursing Studies*, *40*(1), 73–84. doi:10.1016/S0020-7489(02)00039-1

Bud, R. (2007). *Penicillin – Triumph and Tragedy*. Oxford, UK: Oxford University Press.

Burge, P., Devlin, N., Appleby, J., Gallo, F., Nason, E., & Ling, T. (2006). *Understanding Patients' Choices at the Point of Referral*. Santa Monica: RAND Corporation.

Burton, J. L. (1993). The Lips. In: Rook, Wilkinson, Ebling (eds), *Textbook of dermatology*. Oxford, UK: Blackwell Scientific publications.

Bury, M., & Taylor, D. (2008). Towards a theory of care transition: from medical dominance to managed consumerism. *Social Theory & Health*, *6*, 201–219. doi:10.1057/sth.2008.9

Cabana, M. D., Rand, C. S., Powe, N. R., Wu, A. W., Wilson, M. H., Abboud, P. A. C., & Rubin, H. R. (1999). Why don't physicians follow clinical practice guidelines? A framework for improvement. *Journal of the American Medical Association*, *282*(15), 1458–1465. doi:10.1001/jama.282.15.1458

Cai, J., Johnson, S., & Hripcsak, G. (2000). Generic data modeling for home telemonitoring of chronically ill patients. *Proc AMIA Symp*, 116–120.

Campbell, G. (2005). Podcasting in education. *EDUCAUSE, Nov/Dec, 5*.

Capra, F. (2002). *The hidden connections: integrating the biological, cognitive, and social dimensions of life into a science of sustainability*. New York: Doubleday.

Caputo, J. D. (Ed.). (1997). *Deconstruction in a nutshell: A conversation with Jacques Derrida*. New York: Fordham University Press.

Carrasquilla, G. (2001) Cad. Suide Publica, Rio de Jeniro 17. *Suplemento*, 171-179.

Carson, C. F. (2001, August). Riley TV. Safety, efficacy and provenance of tea tree (Melaleuca alternifolia) oil. *Contact Dermatitis*, *45*(2), 65–67. doi:10.1034/j.1600-0536.2001.045002065.x

Carter, R. F. (1991). Comparative analysis, theory, and cross-cultural communication. *Communication Theory*, *1*(2), 151–158. doi:10.1111/j.1468-2885.1991.tb00011.x

Carter, R. (2003). Communication: a harder science. Dervin, B., Chaffee, S., and Foreman-Wernet, L. (Eds). *Communication, a different kind of horse race: Essays honoring Richard F. Carter* (pp. 369-376). Cresskill, NJ: Hampton.

Carter, R. F. (1988). On paradigmatic productivity. In B. Dervin, L. Grossberg, B. O'Keefe, & E. Wartella (eds.), *Paradigm strategies in communication: Vol 1 Issues* (pp. 144-147). Beverly Hills, CA: Sage, 144-147.

Castells, M. (1996). *The Rise of the Network Society.* Oxford: Blackwell.

Cavoukian, A., & Tapscott, D. (1995). *Who knows: Safeguarding your privacy in a networked world.* Toronto: Random House.

CDC. (Centers for Disease Control and Prevention) (2009). *Social Media Tools for Consumers and Partners.* Retrieved February, 2009, from http://www.cdc.gov/socialmedia

Celler, B. G., Lovell, N. H., & Basilakis, J. (2003). Using information technology to improve the management of chronic disease. *The Medical Journal of Australia, 179*(5), 242–246.

Centers, L. C. (2001). Beyond denial and despair: ALS and our heroic potential for hope. *Journal of Palliative Care, 17*(4), 259–264.

CF Trust (2000) *Growing Older with CF: A Handbook for Adults.* Published jointly by the Cystic Fibrosis Trust and Solvay Healthcare Limited.

Cha, A., Hecht, B., Nelson, K., & Hopkins, M. (2004). Resident physician attire: does it make a difference to our patients? *American Journal of Obstetrics and Gynecology, 190,* 1484–1488. doi:10.1016/j.ajog.2004.02.022

Chan, M., Campo, E., & Esteve, D. (2002). Assessment of elderly mobility using a remote multisensor monitoring system. *Studies in Health Technology and Informatics, 90,* 72–77.

Chan, Y., Culnan, M., Greenaway, K., Laden, G., Levin, T., & Smith, H. J. (2005). Information privacy: Management, marketplace, and legal challenges. *Communications of the Association for Information Systems, 16,* 270–298.

Chan, A., Lee, M., & McLoughlin, C. (2006). Everyone's learning with podcasting: A Charles Sturt University experience. *Who's learning? Whose technology? Proceedings ascilite Sydney 2006.*

Chang, C. (2004). Constructing a Streaming Video-Based Learning Forum for Collaborative Learning. *Journal of Educational Multimedia and Hypermedia, 13*(3), 245–264.

Chang, S. (2007). *Academic perceptions of the use of Lectopia: A University of Melbourne example.*

Chapple, A., Ziebland, S., & McPherson, A. (2004). Stigma, shame, and blame experienced by patients with lung cancer: qualitative study. *BMJ (Clinical Research Ed.), 328*(7454), 1470. doi:10.1136/bmj.38111.639734.7C

Charles, C., Gafni, A., & Whelan, T. (1997). Shared Decision-making in the Medical Encounter: What does it Mean? (Or it Takes at Least Two to Tango*). Social Science & Medicine, 47,* 681–692. doi:10.1016/S0277-9536(96)00221-3

Charmaz, K. (1983). Loss of self: a fundamental form of suffering in the chronically ill. *Sociology of Health & Illness, 5*(2), 168–195. doi:10.1111/1467-9566.ep10491512

Charmaz, K. (1990). Discovering chronic illness: Using grounded theory Social. *Science & Medicine, 30*(11), 1161–1172. doi:10.1016/0277-9536(90)90256-R

Charon, R. (2006). *Narrative Medicine: Honoring the stories of Illness.* New York: Oxford University Press.

Charon, R., & Wyer, P.NEBM Working Group. (2008). Perspectives, Narrative evidence based medicine. *Lancet, 371*(9609), 296–297. doi:10.1016/S0140-6736(08)60156-7

Charon, R. (2001a). Narrative medicine. A model for empathy, reflection, profession and trust. *Journal of the American Medical Association, 286*(15), 189–1902. doi:10.1001/jama.286.15.1897

Charon, R. (2001b). Narrative medicine: Form function and ethics. *Annals of Internal Medicine, 134*(1), 83–87.

Chidambaram, L., Bostrom, R., & Wynne, B. (1990). A longitudinal study of the impact of group decision support systems on group development. *Journal of Management Information Systems*, 7(3), 7–25.

Choi, J., Jenkins, M. L., Cimino, J. J., White, T. M., & Bakken, S. (2005). Toward Semantic Interoperability in Home Health Care: Formally Representing OASIS Items for Integration into a Concept-oriented Terminology. *Journal of the American Medical Informatics Association*, 12(4), 410–417. doi:10.1197/jamia.M1786

Christakis, N. A. (2004, Jul 24). Social networks and collateral health effects. *BMJ (Clinical Research Ed.)*, 329(7459), 184–185. doi:10.1136/bmj.329.7459.184

Cines, D. B. (2007). Pumping out platelets. *Blood*, 113(11), 4591–4592. doi:10.1182/blood-2007-03-079483

Cines, D. B., Bussel, J. B., & Liebman, H. A. (2009). The ITP syndrome: pathogenic and clinical diversity. *Blood*, 113, 6511–6521. doi:10.1182/blood-2009-01-129155

Clare, C., & Bullock, I. (2003). Door to needle times bulls' eye or just bull? The effect of reducing door to needle times on the appropriate administration of thrombolysis: implications and recommendations. *European Journal of Cardiovascular Nursing*, 2(1), 39–45. doi:10.1016/S1474-5151(03)00005-7

Clark, C. J. (1998). *Let your online learning community grow: 3 design principles for growing successful Email Listervs and online forums in educational settings*. San Diego State University. Retrieved September 14, from http://www.noendpress.com/caleb/olc/3Principles_Online_Comm.pdf

Classroom organization. (n.d.). *Classroom organization: the physical environment*. Retrieved December 12, 2009, from http://www2.scholastic.com/browse/article.jsp?id=4134

Coburn, D. (2004). Beyond the income inequality hypothesis: Class, neoliberalism and health inequalities. *Social Science & Medicine*, 58, 41–56. doi:10.1016/S0277-9536(03)00159-X

Cohen, L. (1988). *Ain't no cure for love*, I'm Your Man, CBS Records 1988

Coiera, E. (1997). *Guide to Medical Informatics, the Internet and Telemedicine*. London: Chapman & Hall.

Conrad, M. E. (2006, October). *Iron Deficiency Anemia: Treatment & Medication. E Medicine (Medscape)*. Retrieved June 16 2009 from http://emedicine.medscape.com/article/202333-treatment

Conroy, R. M. (2002). Choosing an appropriate real-life measure of effect-size: the case of a continuous predictor and a binary outcome. *The Stata Journal*, 2(3), 290–295.

Conway, S. P., Pond, M. N., Hamnet, T., & Watson, A. (1996). Compliance with Treatment in Adult Patients with Cystic Fibrosis. *Thorax*, 51, 29–33. doi:10.1136/thx.51.1.29

Coulehan, J., Belling, C., Williams, P. C., McCrary, S. V., & Vetrano, M. (2003). Human contexts: Medicine in society at Stony Brook University School of Medicine. *Academic Medicine*, 78, 987–992. doi:10.1097/00001888-200310000-00009

Cova, B. (2005). Thinking of marketing in meridian terms. *Marketing Theory*, 5(2), 205–214. doi:10.1177/1470593105052476

Crespo, R. (2007). Virtual community health promotion. *Preventing Chronic Disease*, 4, A75.

Creswell, J. W. (2003). *Research design. Qualitative, quantitative and mixed methods approaches*. Thousand Oaks, CA: Sage publications.

Crossett, L., Kraus, J. R., & Lawson, S. (2009). Collaborative tools used to organize a library camp unconference. *Collaborative Librarianship*, 1(2), 66–69.

Crossley, M., & Holmes, K. (2001). Challenges for educational research. interantional partnerships and capacity building in small states. *Oxford Review of Education*, 27(3), 395–409. doi:10.1080/03054980120067429

Crossley, M. L. (1999). Making sense of HIV infection: discourse and adaptation to life with a long term HIV positive diagnosis. *Health*, 3(1), 96–119.

Crossley, M. L. (2000). *Introducing Narrative Psychology: Self, Trauma and the Cronstruction of Meaning.* Buckingham: Open University Press.

Crowley, W. F., Sherwood, L., Salber, P., Scheinberg, D., Slavkin, H., & Tilson, H. (2004). Clinical research in the United States at a crossroads: Proposal for a novel public-private partnership to establish a national clinical research enterprise. *Journal of the American Medical Association, 291,* 1120–1126. doi:10.1001/jama.291.9.1120

Culnan, M. J. (1993). How did they get my name? An exploratory investigation of consumer attitudes toward secondary information use. *Management Information Systems Quarterly, 17*(3), 341–363. doi:10.2307/249775

Curry, L. C., & Stone, J. G. (1991). The grief process: a preparation for death. *Clinical Nurse Specialist CNS, 5*(1), 17–22. doi:10.1097/00002800-199100510-00007

Czarniawska, B. (2004). *Narratives in Social Science Research.* London: Sage.

D'Angelo, S. L., & Lask, B. (2001). Approaches to Problems of Adherence. In Bluebond-Langner, A., Lask, B., & Angst, D. B. eds. (2001). *Psychosocial Aspects of Cystic Fibrosis* pp.361-79. London: Arnold.

Daft, R. L., & Lengel, R. H. (1986). Organisational Information Requirements, Media Richness and Structural Design. *Management Science, 32*(5), 554–571. doi:10.1287/mnsc.32.5.554

Daft, R. L., & Wiginton, J. (1979). Language and Organisation. *Academy of Management Review, 4*(2), 171–191. doi:10.2307/257772

Darkins, A., Ryan, P., Kobb, R., Foster, L., Edmonson, E., & Wakefield, B. (2008). Care Coordination/Home Telehealth: the systematic implementation of health informatics, home telehealth, and disease management to support the care of veteran patients with chronic conditions. *Telemedicine Journal and e-Health, 14*(10), 1118–1126. doi:10.1089/tmj.2008.0021

Dartmouth Atlas Project. (2007). *Effective care. A Dartmouth Atlas Project Topic Brief.* Retrieved from http://www.dartmouthatlas.org/topics/effective_care.pdf

DasGupta, S. (2007). Between stillness and story: lessons of children's illness narratives. *Pediatrics, 119,* e1384–e1391. doi:10.1542/peds.2006-2619

DasGupta, S., & Charon, R. (2004). Personal illness narratives: using reflective writing to teach empathy. *Academic Medicine, 79,* 351–356. doi:10.1097/00001888-200404000-00013

Davidoff, F., & Florance, V. (2000). The informationist: a new health profession? [editorial]. *Annals of Internal Medicine, 132*(12), 996.

Davies, M. L. (1997). Shattered assumptions: Time and the experience of long-term HIV positivity. *Social Science & Medicine, 44*(5), 561–571. doi:10.1016/S0277-9536(96)00177-3

Davies, B. (1991). The concept of agency. *Postmodern Critical Theorising, 30,* 42–53.

Davies, B., Browne, J., Gannon, S., Hopkins, L., McCann, H., & Wihlborg, M. (2006). Constituting the feminist subject in poststructuralist discourse. *Feminism & Psychology, 15*(1), 87–103. doi:10.1177/0959-353506060825

Davis, D. A., Evans, M., Jadad, A. R., Perrier, L., Rath, D., & Ryan, D. (2003). The case for knowledge translation: shortening the journey from evidence to effect. *British Medical Journal, 327*(7405), 33–35. doi:10.1136/bmj.327.7405.33

Dawes, M., Summerskill, W., Glasziou, P., Cartabellotta, A., Martin, J., & Hopayian, K. (2005). Sicily statement on evidence-based practice. *BMC Medical Education, 5,* 1. doi:10.1186/1472-6920-5-1

Deci, E. L., & Ryan, R. M. (2008). Self-determination theory: A macrotheory of human motivation, development, and health. *Canadian Psychology/Psychologie canadienne, 49*(3), 182-185.

del Pozo, P. R., & Fins, J. J. (2005). The globalization of education in medical ethics and humanities: evolving pedagogy at Weill Cornell medical college in Qatar. *Academic Medicine, 80,* 135–140. doi:10.1097/00001888-200502000-00005

DeLisa, J. A., Jain, S. S., Kirshblum, S., & Christodoulou, C. (1999). Evidence-based medicine in physiatry: the experience of one department's faculty and trainees. *American Journal of Physical Medicine & Rehabilitation, 78*(3), 228–232. doi:10.1097/00002060-199905000-00008

Demiris, G. (2006). The diffusion of virtual communities in health care: Concepts and challenges. *Patient Education and Counseling, 62*, 178–188. doi:10.1016/j.pec.2005.10.003

Denborough, D. (2005). A framework for receiving and documenting testimonies of trauma. *International Journal of Narrative Therapy and Community Work, 2*(3 & 4), 34–42.

Denegri-Knott, J. (2004). Sinking the online music pirates: Foucault, power and deviance on the web. *Journal of Computer-Mediated Communication, 9*(4).

Dennis, A. R., & Valacich, J. S. (1999). *Rethinking Media Richness: Towards a Theory of Media Synchronicity.* Paper presented at the 32nd Hawaii International Conference on System Sciences, Hawaii.

Denny, C. C., & Grady, C. (2007). Clinical research with economically disadvantaged populations. *Journal of Medical Ethics, 33*(7), 382–385. doi:10.1136/jme.2006.017681

Department of Fusion Technologies and Nuclear Presidium. (2009). *Meta-Knowledge Engineering & Management (MKEM).* Research Server for High-Intelligent Socio-Cognitive Systems.

Department of Health. (2001). *The Expert Patient: A New Approach to Disease Management for the 21st Century.* London: HMSO.

Department of Health. (2006). Supporting people with long term conditions to self care – A guide to developing local strategies and good practice. Available at: http://www.dh.gov.uk/prod_consum_dh/groups/dh_digitalassets/@dh/@en/documents/digitalasset/dh_4130868.pdf.

Dervin, B., Forman-Wernet, L., & Lauterbach, E. (Eds.). (2003). *Sense-Making methodology reader.* Cresskill, NJ: Hampton.

Dervin, B. (2003a). Chaos, order, and Sense-Making: a proposed theory for information design. In Dervin, B., & Forman-Wernet, L. (Eds.), *Sense-Making methodology reader* (pp. 325–340). Cresskill, NJ: Hampton. (Original work published 1999)

Dervin, B. (2003b). Information← → Democracy. In Dervin, B., & Forman-Wernet, L. (Eds.), *Sense-Making methodology reader* (pp. 73–100). Cresskill, NJ: Hampton. (Original work published 1999)

Dervin, B. (2003c). A theoretic perspective and research approach for generating research helpful to communication practice. In Dervin, B., & Forman-Wernet, L. (Eds.), *Sense-Making methodology reader* (pp. 251–268). Cresskill, NJ: Hampton. (Original work published 2001)

Dervin, B., & Clark, K. (2003). Communication and Democracy: Mandate for procedural invention. In Dervin, B., & Forman-Wernet, L. (Eds.), *Sense-Making methodology reader* (pp. 165–193). Cresskill, NJ: Hampton. (Original work published 1993)

Dervin, B., & Schaefer, D. (2003). Peopling the public sphere. In Dervin, B., & Forman-Wernet, L. (Eds.), *Sense-Making methodology reader* (pp. 341–347). Cresskill, NJ: Hampton. (Original work published 1999)

Dervin, B. (1983). *An overview of sense-making research: Concepts, methods, and results to date.* Presented at International Communication Association annual meeting, Dallas, May, 1983.

Deshpande, A., & Jadad, A. R. (2006). Web 2.0: Could it help move the health system into the 21st century? *JMHG, 3*(4), 332–336.

Detmer, D. E., Bloomrosen, M., Raymond, B., & Tang, P. (2008). Integrated personal health records: Transformative tools for consumer-centric care. *BMC Medical Informatics and Decision Making, 8*(1), 45. doi:10.1186/1472-6947-8-45

Dewey, J. (1966). *Democracy and education.* New York: Free Press. (Original work published 1916)

Diaz, J. A. (2005). Brief Report: What Types of Internet Guidance Do Patients Want from Their Physicians? *Journal of General Internal Medicine, 20,* 683–685. doi:10.1111/j.1525-1497.2005.0115.x

Diez Roux, A. V. (2007). Integrating social and biologic factors in health research: a systems view. *Annals of Epidemiology, 17*(7), 569–574. doi:10.1016/j.annepidem.2007.03.001

Doll, R., & Hill, A. B. (1950). Smoking and carcinoma of the lung. *British Medical Journal, 221*(2), 739–748. doi:10.1136/bmj.2.4682.739

Donaghy, B. (2004). Supplementary prescribing in cystic fibrosis: responding to an acute exacerbation. *Nurse Prescribing, 2*(2), 84–88.

Dong, B. R., Hao, Q., Yue, J., Wu, T., & Liu, G. J. (2009). Thrombolytic Therapy for Pulmonary Embolus. *Cochrane Database of Systematic Reviews,* 3.

Dorr, D., Bonner, L. M., Cohen, A. N., Shoai, R. S., Perrin, R., & Chaney, E. (2007). Informatics Systems to Promote Improved Care for Chronic Illness: A Literature Review. *Journal of the American Medical Informatics Association, 14*(2), 156–163. doi:10.1197/jamia.M2255

Douse, J., Derrett-Smith, E., Dheda, K., & Dilworth, J. P. (2004). Should doctors wear white coats? *Postgraduate Medical Journal, 80,* 284–286. doi:10.1136/pgmj.2003.017483

Downie, R. S. (1991). Literature and Medicine. *Journal of Medical Ethics, 17,* 93–96, 98. doi:10.1136/jme.17.2.93

Doyle, C. J., Post, H., Burney, R. E., Maino, J., Keefe, M., & Rhee, K. J. (1987). Family Participating During Resuscitation: an Option. *Annals of Emergency Medicine, 16*(6), 673–675. doi:10.1016/S0196-0644(87)80069-0

Drewery, W. (2005). Why we should watch what we say: Position calls, everyday speech and the production of relational subjectivity. *Theory & Psychology, 15*(3), 305–324. doi:10.1177/0959354305053217

Dunn, J. J., Lee, T. H., & Percelay, J. M. (1987). Patient and house officer attitudes on physician attire and etiquette. *Journal of the American Medical Association, 257,* 65–68. doi:10.1001/jama.257.1.65

Edmundson, M. (2008). Dwelling in possibilities. *Chronicle of Higher Education.* Retrieved on 12 November 2009 from http://chronicle.com/article/Dwelling-in-Possibilities/7083/

E-health insider (2008). *Patients to get facebook style communicator.* Retrieved from www.e-health-insider.com/news/4337/patients_to_get_facebook-style_communicator

Eichhorn, D. J., Myers, T. A., Guzzetta, C. E., Clark, A. P., Klein, J. D., Taliaferro, E., & Calvin, A. O. (2001). Family Presence during Invasive Procedures and Resuscitation: Hearing the Voice of the Patient. *The American Journal of Nursing, 101,* 48–55.

Eisenberg, J. M. (2002). Globalise the evidence, localize the decisions: evidence-based medicine and international diversity. *Health Affairs, 21,* 166–168. Retrieved from http://content.healthaffairs.org/cgi/reprint/21/3/166pdf. doi:10.1377/hlthaff.21.3.166

Elcin, M., Odabasi, O., Ward, K., Turan, S., Akyiz, C., & Sayek, I. The first medical humanities programme in Turkey. *Medical Education, 40,* 278–282. doi:10.1111/j.1365-2929.2006.02390.x

Eliot, T. S. (1967). *Little Gidding.* Four Quartets, New York: Faber and Faber.

Elliot, T. R., Shewchuk, R. M., & Richards, J. S. (1999). Caregiver social problem-solving abilities and family member adjustment to recent onset physical disability. *Rehabilitation Psychology, 44*(1), 104–123. doi:10.1037/0090-5550.44.1.104

Elmore-Meegan, M., Conroy, R. M., & Agala, C. B. (2004). Sex workers in Kenya, numbers of clients and associated risks: an exploratory survey. *Reproductive Health Matters, 12*(23), 50–57. doi:10.1016/S0968-8080(04)23125-1

Ely, J. W., & Osheroff, J. A. (2002). Obstacles to answering doctors' questions about patient care with evidence: qualitative study. *BMJ (Clinical Research Ed.)*, *324*, 710. doi:10.1136/bmj.324.7339.710

Emanuel, R., & Hegde, B. M. (1975). Association of Secundum Atrial Septal Defect with Abnormalities of AV Conduction of Left Axis Deviation. *British Heart Journal*, *30*, 1085–1092. doi:10.1136/hrt.37.10.1085

Emanuel, E. J., Wendler, D., & Grady, C. (2000). What makes clinical research ethical? *Journal of the American Medical Association*, *283*(20), 2701–2711. doi:10.1001/jama.283.20.2701

Emanuel, E. J., Wendler, D., Killen, J., & Grady, C. (2004). What makes clinical research in developing countries ethical? The benchmarks of ethical research. *The Journal of Infectious Diseases*, *189*(5), 930–937. doi:10.1086/381709

Enders, W. (2003). *Applied Econometric Time Series* (2nd ed.). John Wiley & Sons.

Engel, G. L. (1977). The Need for a new Medical Model: a Challenge for Biomedicine. *Science*, *196*, 129–136. doi:10.1126/science.847460

Englund, T. (2000). Rethinking democracy and education: Towards an education of deliberative citizens. *Journal of Curriculum Studies*, *32*(2), 305–313. doi:10.1080/002202700182772

Epstein, C. (2006). Guilty bodies, productive bodies, destructive bodies: Crossing the biometric borders. Paper Presented at International Studies Association Conference.

Ess, C. (2000). Wag the dog? Online conferencing and teaching. *Computers and the Humanities*, *34*, 297–309. doi:10.1023/A:1002075505432

Ess, C. (2002). Computer-mediated colonization, the renaissance, and educational imperatives for an intercultural global village. *Ethics and Information Technology*, *4*, 11–22. doi:10.1023/A:1015227723904

Ess, C. (1996). The political computer: Democracy, CMC, and Habermas. In Ess, C. (Ed.), *Philosophical perspectives on computer-mediated communication*. Albany, NY: SUNY Press.

Ess, C., & Cavalier, R. (1996). Does the Internet democratize? Philosophical dialogue on-line as a microcosm/case study. (Unpublished paper). Retrieved from http://www.lcl.cmu.edu/CAAE/Home/Forum/report.html

Estabrooks, C., Thompson, D., Lovely, J., & Hofmeyer, A. (2006). A guide to knowledge translation theory. *Journal of Continuing Education in the Health Professions*.

Esterman, A. J., & Ben-Tovim, D. I. (2002). The Australian coordinated care trials: success or failure? The second round of trials may provide more answers. *The Medical Journal of Australia*, *177*(9), 469–470.

Evans, D. (2001). Imagination and medical education. *Medical Humanities*, *27*, 30–34. doi:10.1136/mh.27.1.30

Evans, H. M., & Macnaughton, J. (2004). Should medical humanities be a multidisciplinary or an interdisciplinary study? *Medical Humanities*, *30*, 1–4. doi:10.1136/jmh.2004.000143

Evans, M. (2002). Reflection on the humanities in medical education. *Medical Education*, *36*, 508–513. doi:10.1046/j.1365-2923.2002.01225.x

Everding, G. (2002). *Reading Module*. Retrieved December 12, 2009, from http://www.edu-cyberpg.com/culdesac/ReadingModule/EmotionTiesToCognitive.html

Executive Board of the United Nations Development Programme and the United Nations Populations Fund. (2002). *Country Co-operations Frameworks and Related Matters: Country Programme Outline for Papua New Guinea (2003-2007)* New York: UN

Eysenbach, G. (2008). Medicine 2.0: Social Networking, Collaboration, Participation, Apomediation, and Openness. *Journal of Medical Internet Research*, *10*(3), 22. doi:10.2196/jmir.1030

Eysenbach, G., Power, J., & Englesakis, M. (2004). Health related virtual communities and electronic support groups: systematic review of the effects of online peer to peer interactions. *British Medical Journal, 328*, 1166–1171. doi:10.1136/bmj.328.7449.1166

Ezzy, D. (2000). Illness narratives. Time hope and HIV. *Social Science & Medicine, 50*, 605–617. doi:10.1016/S0277-9536(99)00306-8

Fabrega, H. (1997). Historical and cultural foundations of health behaviour. In Gochman, D. S. (Ed.), *Handbook for Health Behaviour Research1 Personal and Social Determinants*. New York: Plenum Press.

Fabris, F., Tassan, T., Ramon, R., Carraro, G., Randi, M. L., & Luzzatto, G. (2001). Age as the major predictive factor of long-term response to splenectomy in immune thrombocytopenic purpura. *British Journal of Haematology, 112*, 637–640. doi:10.1046/j.1365-2141.2001.02615.x

Falik, M., Needleman, J., Wells, B. L., & Korb, J. (2001). Ambulatory care sensitive hospitalizations and emergency visits: experiences of Medicaid patients using federally qualified health centers. *Medical Care, 39*, 551–561. doi:10.1097/00005650-200106000-00004

Family Medicine Net Guide (2004, February). Empowered! Taking Control of Your Health with the Web: advice from a survivor: a talk with Laura Landro. *Family Medicine Net Guide, 2*(1).

Farmer, A., Gibson, O., Hayton, P., Bryden, K., Dudley, C., & Neil, A. (2005). A real-time, mobile phone-based telemedicine system to support young adults with type 1 diabetes. *Informatics in Primary Care, 13*(3), 171–177.

Farquhar, M. C., Barclay, S. I., Earl, H., Grande, G. E., Emery, J., & Crawford, R. A. (2005). Barriers to effective communication across the primary/secondary interface: examples from the ovarian cancer patient journey (a qualitative study). *European Journal of Cancer Care, 14*(4), 359–366. doi:10.1111/j.1365-2354.2005.00596.x

Farraj, R., & Baron, J. H. (1991). Why do hospital doctors wear white coats? *Journal of the Royal Society of Medicine, 84*, 43.

Feeney, L., Reynolds, P., Eaton, K., & Harper, J. (2008). *A description of the new technologies used in transforming dental education.*

Feldman, S. (2004). *Enterprise search technology: information disasters and the high cost of not finding information.* Portals Mag, 27-28. Retrieved from www.portalsmag.com

Felger, I., Tavul, L., Kabintik, S., Marshall, V., Genton, B., Alpers, M., & Beck, H. P. (1994). Plasmodium falciparum: extensive polymorphism in merozoite surface antigen 2 alleles in an area with endemic malaria in Papua New Guinea. *Experimental Parasitology, 79*(2), 106–116. doi:10.1006/expr.1994.1070

Félix-Bortolotti, M. (2009). Part 1 - Unravelling primary health care conceptual predicaments through the lenses of complexity: A position paper for progressive transformation. *Journal of Evaluation in Clinical Practice, 15*(5). doi:10.1111/j.1365-2753.2009.01274.x

Ferguson, A. G., & Morris, C. N. (2007). Mapping transactional sex on the Northern Corridor highway in Kenya. *Health & Place, 13*(2), 504–519. doi:10.1016/j.healthplace.2006.05.009

Ferguson, T. (2007). *ePatients white paper*. Retrieved July 24, 2009 from http://www.e-patients.net/e-Patients_White_Paper.pdf

Fibrinolytic Therapists Trialists' (FTT) Collaborative Group. (1994). Indications for Fibrinolytic Therapy in Suspected Acute Myocardial Infarction: Collaborative Overview of early Mortality and Morbidity results from all Randomized Trials of more than 1000 patients. *Lancet, 343*, 311–322.

Field, D., & Kelly, M. P. (2003). Chronic Illness and Physical Disability. In Taylor, S. & Field, D. Eds. (2003 3rd edn) *Sociology of Health & Health Care* pp. 117-136. Oxford: Blackwell.

Fillion, R. (2005). Moving beyond biopower: Hardt and Negri's post-foucauldian speculative philosophy of history. *History and Theory, 44*, 47–72. doi:10.1111/j.1468-2303.2005.00342.x

Firat, A. F., & Dholakia, N. (1998). *Consuming people: From political economy to theaters of consumption.* London: Routledge. doi:10.4324/9780203449813

Firat, A. F., & Dholakia, N. (2006). Theoretical and philosophical implications of postmodern debates: Some challenges to postmodern marketing. *Marketing Theory, 6*(2), 123–162. doi:10.1177/1470593106063981

Fischer, E., Bristor, J., & Gainer, B. (1996). Creating or escaping community?: An exploratory study of internet consumers' behaviors. *Advances in Consumer Research. Association for Consumer Research (U. S.), 23,* 178–182.

Fisher, B. (1978). *Perspectives on human communication.* New York: Macmillan.

Fisher, E. S., Bynum, J. P., & Skinner, J. S. (2009). Slowing the growth of health care costs – Lessons from regional variation. *The New England Journal of Medicine, 360*(9), 849–852. doi:10.1056/NEJMp0809794

Fisher, E. S., Wennberg, D. E., Stukel, T. A., Gottlieb, D. J., Lucas, F. L., & Pinder, E. L. (2003a). The implications of regional variations in Medicare spending. Part 1: the content, quality, and accessibility of care. *Annals of Internal Medicine, 138*(4), 273–287.

Fitzpatrick (2007). Malaria: promoting awareness and prevention of a critical crisis in a remote area of Papua New Guinea through community involvement. 2006 Volume 5 Number Global connections *CONNECT The World of Critical Care Nursing* 2006 5 1 22

Flflowergirl. Ferritin less than 1? Forum post (2009, January). *Anemia message board, In HealthBoards Message Boards.* Retrieved June 15, 2009, from http://www.healthboards.com/boards/showthread.php?t=666920&highlight=lotsawalls&page=5

Fombonne, E. (2003). Epidemiological Surveys of Autism and Other Pervasive Developmental Disorders: An Update. *Journal of Autism and Developmental Disorders, 33*(4). doi:10.1023/A:1025054610557

Fontana, V., Jy, W., Ahn, E. R., Dudkiewicz, P., Horstman, L. L., Duncan, R., & Ahn, Y. S. (2008). Increased procoagulant cell-derived microparticles (C-MP) in splenectomized patients with ITP. *Thrombosis Research, 122*(5), 599–603. doi:10.1016/j.thromres.2007.12.022

Forman-Wernet, L. (2003). Rethinking communication: Introducing the Sense-Making methodology. In Dervin, B., & Forman-Wernet, L. (Eds.), *Sense-Making methodology reader* (pp. 3–16). Cresskill, NJ: Hampton.

Foster, L. (2009). *Expression of coping with cancer: A content analysis of 'Blog for a Cure.'* Paper presented at the International Communication Association annual meeting, Chicago, IL, May 2009.

Foster, S. J. (2008). *Crystallising meaning: attitudes of listening to illness narratives* (Ph D Thesis), University of Melbourne, Melbourne, Australia

Foucault, M. (1975). *The birth of the clinic: An archeology of medical perception.* New York: Vintage Books.

Foucault, M. (1980) Power/knowledge. In C. Gordon, Trans L. Marshall, J. Merpham and K. (eds), *SoperSelected interviews and other writings 1972-1977.* New York, Pantheon.

Fox, N., & Ward, K. (2006). Health identities: from expert patient to resisting consumer. *Health, 10*(4), 461–479.

Fox, N. J., & Ward, K. J. (2008). What are health identities and how may we study them? *Sociology of Health & Illness, 30*(7), 1007–1021. doi:10.1111/j.1467-9566.2008.01093.x

Foy, J. M., & Earls, M. F. (2005). A Process for Developing Community Consensus Regarding the Diagnosis and Management of Attention-Deficit/Hyperactivity Disorder. *Pediatrics, 115,* e97–e104.

Frank, A. W. (1991). *At the will of the body. Reflections on illness.* Boston, MA: Houghton Mifflin.

Frank, A. W. (1995). *The wounded storyteller. Body, illness and ethics.* Chicago: University of Chicago Press.

Frank, A. W. (2001). Can we research suffering? *Qualitative Health Research, 11*(3), 353–362. doi:10.1177/104973201129119154

Frank, A. (1998). Stories of illness as care of the self: A Foucauldian dialogue. *Health, 2*, 329–348.

Frankel, R. M., & Quill, T. (2005). Integrating biopsychosocial and relationship-centered care into mainstream medical practice: A challenge that continues to produce positive results. *Families, Systems & Health, 23*(4), 413–421..doi:10.1037/1091-7527.23.4.413

Fredericks, K. A., Deegan, M., & Carman, J. G. (2008). Using System Dynamics as an Evaluation Tool: Experience From a Demonstration Program. *The American Journal of Evaluation, 29*(3), 251–267. doi:10.1177/1098214008319446

Frich, J. C., & Fugelli, P. (2003). Medicine and the arts in the undergraduate medical curriculum at the University of Oslo Faculty of Medicine, Oslo, Norway. *Academic Medicine, 78*, 1036–1038. doi:10.1097/00001888-200310000-00020

Friedman, L. D. (2002). The precarious position of the medical humanities in the medical school curriculum. *Academic Medicine, 77*, 320–322. doi:10.1097/00001888-200204000-00011

Friere, P. (1970). *Pedagogy of the oppressed.* New York: Seabury Press.

Frisch, B. (2006). *Quality of life therapy: Applying a life satisfaction approach to positive psychology and cognitive therapy.* Hoboken, NJ: John Wiley & Sons.

Fritz, T. M., Burg, G., & Krasovec, M. (2001). Allergic contact dermatitis to cosmetics containing Melaleuca alternifolia (tea tree oil)]. *Annales de Dermatologie et de Venereologie, 128*(2), 123–126.

Frost, J. H., Massagli, M. P., Wicks, P., & Heywood, J. (2008). How the social web supports patient experimentation with a new therapy: The demand for patient-controlled and patient-centered informatics. *AMIA... Annual Symposium Proceedings / AMIA Symposium. AMIA Symposium, 6*, 217–221.

Frostholm, L., Ornbol, E., Hansen, H. S., Olesen, F., Weinman, J., & Fink, P. (2010). Which is more important for outcome: the physician's or the patient's understanding of a health problem? A 2-year follow-up study in primary care. *General Hospital Psychiatry, 32*(1), 1–8. doi:10.1016/j.genhosppsych.2009.08.004

Fursse, J., Clarke, M., Jones, R., Khemka, S., & Findlay, G. (2008). Early experience in using telemonitoring for the management of chronic disease in primary care. *Journal of Telemedicine and Telecare, 14*(3), 122–124. doi:10.1258/jtt.2008.003005

Gallupe, R., & McKeen, J. (1990). Enhancing computer-mediated communication: An experimental investigation into the use of a group decision support system for face-to-face versus remote meetings. *Information & Management, 18*, 1–13. doi:10.1016/0378-7206(90)90059-Q

Gardner, H. E. (1983). *Frames of Mind: The theory of Multiple Intelligences.* New York: Basic Books.

Gathiqi, H. W., Bwayo, J., Karuga, P. M., Kihara, A. N., Omari, M. A., & Plummer, F. A. *The socio-economic status of prostitutes at a truck drivers' stop and their interaction with male clients.* Paper presented at the Int Conf AIDS. 1993 Jun 6-11;9(2):830 (abstract no. PO-D09-3672).

Gavgani, V. Z. (2009). *Role of medical librarians in Information Therapy: a study of problems and prospects in India and Iran.* Unpublished PhD thesis submitted to Osmania University, p49-50.

Gavgani, V. Z., & Mohan, V. V. (2008). Application of web 2.0 tools in medical librarianship to support medicine 2.0. *Webology, 5*(1), Article 53. Retrieved from: http://www.webology.ir/2008/v5n1/a53.html

Gavison, R. (1980). Privacy and the limits of the law. *The Yale Law Journal, 89*(3), 421–471. doi:10.2307/795891

Gensini, G. F., Conti, A., Lippi, D., & Conti, A. A. (2005). Full integration of teaching 'medical humanities' in the medical curriculum: the challenge of the Florence medical school. *Medical Principles and Practice, 14*, 64–65. doi:10.1159/000081928

Gigerenzer, G. (2008). *Gut feelings: short cuts to better decision making*. London: Penguin.

Gilchrist, A. (2004). *The Well-Connected Community: A Networking Approach To Community Development*. Bristol, UK: Polity Press.

Gillberg, I., & Gillberg, C. (1989). Asperger Syndrome: Some Epidemiological Considerations. A Research Note. *Journal of Child Psychology and Psychiatry, and Allied Disciplines, 30*(4), 631–638. doi:10.1111/j.1469-7610.1989.tb00275.x

Gillick, M. R., Serrell, N. A., & Gillick, L. S. (1982). Adverse consequences of hospitalization in the elderly. [doi: DOI: 10.1016/0277-9536(82)90175-7]. *Social Science & Medicine, 16*(10), 1033-1038.

Giustini, D. (2006). How Web 2.0 is changing medicine [Editorial]. *British Medical Journal, 333*, 1283–1284. doi:10.1136/bmj.39062.555405.80

Gjengedal, E., Rustoen, T., Wahl, A. K., & Hanesta, B. R. (2003). Growing up and living with cystic fibrosis: everyday life and encounters with the health care and social services--a qualitative study. *ANS. Advances in Nursing Science, 26*(2), 149–159.

Glass, T., & McAtee, M. (2006). Behavioral science at the crossroads in public health: extending horizons, envisioning the future. *Social Science & Medicine, 62*(7), 1650–1671. doi:10.1016/j.socscimed.2005.08.044

Glasziou, P. (2006). Why is evidence-based medicine important? *Evidence-Based Medicine, 11*, 133–135. doi:10.1136/ebm.11.5.133

Glasziou, P., & Haynes, B. (2005). The paths from research to improved health outcomes. *ACP Journal Club, 142*, A8–A10.

Glennon, T. (2001). The stress of the university experience for students with Asperger syndrome. Work: Journal of Prevention. *Assessment & Rehabilitation, 17*(3), 183–190.

Gloor, P. A. (2006). *Swarm creativity: competitive advantage through collaborative innovation networks*. Oxford, UK: Oxford University Press.

Goddard, A. F., McIntyre, A. S., & Scott, B. B. (2000, December). Guidelines for the management of iron deficiency anaemia. *British Society of Gastroenterology, 47*(6), 872. Retrieved June 15, 2009 from http://www.pubmedcentral.nih.gov/articlerender.fcgi?artid=1766761

Goffman, E. (1990). *The Presentation of Self in everyday Life*. New York: Penguin Books.

Goffman, E. (1968). *Stigma: The Management of Spoiled Identity Harmondsworth*. New York: Penguin.

Goffman, E. (1963). *Behaviour in Public Places: Notes on the Social Organisation of Gatherings*. London: The Free Press of Glenco.

Goh, J. M. (2008). *Taking Charge of Your Health: The Drivers of Enrollment and Continued Participation? in Online Health Intervention Programs*. Paper presented at the Proceedings of the 41st Annual Hawaii International Conference on System Sciences (HICSS 2008), Hawaii.

Goldberg, M. (1997). Ten rules for the doctor-detective. *Postgraduate Medicine, 101*(2), 23–26.

Goldberger, A. L., Amaral, L. A. N., Hausdorff, J. M., Ivanov, P. C., Peng, C. K., & Stanley, H. E. (2002). Fractal dynamics in physiology: Alterations with disease and aging. *Proceedings of the National Academy of Sciences of the United States of America, 99*(Suppl 1), 2466–2472. doi:10.1073/pnas.012579499

Gonzalez Del Rey, J. A., Paul, R. I. (1995). Preferences of parents for pediatric emergency physicians' attire. *Pediatr Emerg Care, 11*, 361-364.

Gonzalez-Gonzalez, A. I. (2007). Information Needs and Information-Seeking Behavior of Primary Care Physicians. *Annals of Family Medicine, 5*, 345–352. doi:10.1370/afm.681

Gooden, B. R., Smith, M. J., Tattersall, S. J., & Stockler, M. R. (2001). Hospitalised patients' views on doctors and white coats. *The Medical Journal of Australia, 175*, 219–222.

Goodwin, C. (1991). Privacy: Recognition of a consumer right. *Journal of Public Policy & Marketing, 10*(1), 149–166.

Gordon, J., & Finkelstein, J. (2003). University of Sydney medical humanities program. *Academic Medicine, 78,* 1069–1070. doi:10.1097/00001888-200310000-00042

Gorgulu, R. S., & Dinc, L. (2007). Ethics in Turkish nursing education programs. *Nursing Ethics, 14,* 741–752. doi:10.1177/0969733007082114

Gotz, I., & Gotz, M. (2000). Cystic Fibrosis: psychological issues. *Paediatric Respiratory Reviews, 1*(2), 121–127. doi:10.1053/prrv.2000.0033

Goyal, R. K., Charon, R., Lekas, H. M., Fullilove, M. T., Devlin, M. J., Falzon, L., & Wyer, P. C. (2008). A Local Habitation and a name: How Narrative Evidence-based Medicine Transforms the Translational Research Paradigm. *Journal of Evaluation in Clinical Practice, 14*(5), 732–741. doi:10.1111/j.1365-2753.2008.01077.x

Graham, I. D., & Tetroe, J. (2007). CIHR Research: How to Translate Health Research Knowledge into Effective Healthcare Action. *Healthcare Quarterly (Toronto, Ont.), 10*(3), 20–22.

Graham, I. D., Logan, J., Harrison, M. B., & Straus, S. E. (2006). Lost in knowledge translation: Time for a map? *The Journal of Continuing Education in the Health Professions, 26*(1), 13–24. doi:10.1002/chp.47

Grant, V. J. (2003). University of Auckland faculty of medical and health sciences, medical humanities courses. *Academic Medicine, 78,* 1072–1073. doi:10.1097/00001888-200310000-00045

Gratwohl, A., Hermans, J., & Niederwieser, D. (1993). Bone marrow transplantation for chronic myeloid leukemia: Long term results. Chronic Leukemia Working Party of the European Group for Bone Marrow Transplantation. *Bone Marrow Transplantation, 12*(5), 509–516.

Gravelle, H., Dusheiko, M., Sheaff, R., Sargent, P., Boaden, R., & Pickar, S. (2007). Impact of case management (Evercare) on frail elderly patients: controlled before and after analysis of quantitative outcome data. *BMJ (Clinical Research Ed.), 334,* 31–34. doi:10.1136/bmj.39020.413310.55

Graves, D. L., Shue, C. K., & Arnold, L. (2002). The role of spirituality in patient care: incorporating spirituality training into medical school curriculum. *Academic Medicine, 77*(11), 1167. doi:10.1097/00001888-200211000-00035

Grazi, G. L. (2006). Web Relationships Between Physicians and Individuals Seeking Information on Hepatopancreatobiliary Diseases. *Archives of Surgery, 141,* 1176–1182. doi:10.1001/archsurg.141.12.1176

Greaves, D., & Evans, M. (2000). Medical Humanities. *Medical Humanities, 26,* 1–2. doi:10.1136/mh.26.1.1

Green, H., McGinnity, A., Meltzer, H., Ford, T., & Goodman, R. (2005). *Mental health of children and young people in Great Britain, A survey carried out by the Office for National Statistics on behalf of the Department of Health and the Scottish Executive.* London: Palgrave Macmillan.

Green, C. J., Fortin, P., Maclure, M., Macgregor, A., & Robinson, S. (2006). Information system support as a critical success factor for chronic disease management: Necessary but not sufficient. *International Journal of Medical Informatics, 75*(12), 818–828. doi:10.1016/j.ijmedinf.2006.05.042

Green, L. W., & Kreuter, M. W. (1999). *Health promotion planning: An educational and ecological approach* (3rd ed.). Mountain View, CA: Mayfield.

Green, M. L., & Ruff, T. R. (2005). Why do residents fail to answer their clinical questions? A qualitative study of barriers to practicing evidence-based medicine. *Academic Medicine, 80*(2), 176–182. doi:10.1097/00001888-200502000-00016

Green, L. (2006). Public Health asks of systems science: To advance our evidence-based practice, can you help us get more practice-based evidence? *American Journal of Public Health, 96*(3), 406–409. doi:10.2105/AJPH.2005.066035

Green, L., & Glasgow, R. (2006). Evaluating the relevance, generalization, and applicability of research: issues in external validation and translation methodology. *Evaluation & the Health Professions, 29*(1), 126–153. doi:10.1177/0163278705284445

Greenhalgh, T. (2002). Intuition and evidence--uneasy bedfellows? *The British Journal of General Practice, 52*(478), 395–400.

Greenhalgh, T., Robert, G., Macfarlane, F., Bate, P., Kyriakidou, O., & Peacock, R. (2004). Diffusion of innovations in service organizations: systematic review and recommendations. Storylines of research in diffusion of innovation: a meta-narrative approach to systematic review. *The Milbank Quarterly, 82*(4), 581–629. doi:10.1111/j.0887-378X.2004.00325.x

Greenhalgh, T., & B, H. (1998). *Why Study Narrative? Narrative Based Medicine: dialogue and discourse in medical practice.*: BMJ Books.

Greenhill, K., & Wiebrands, C. (2008). *The unconference: a new model for better professional communication.* Paper presented at the LIANZA Conference Papers 2008.

Greenlaugh, T andd Russel J2009 Evidence-BasedPolicymaking *a critique Perspectives in Biology and Medicine, 52*(2), 304–18 Baltimore, MD:The Johns Hopkins University Press

Griffin, I. S., & Fentiman, M. (2002). 17. Psychosocial problems following a diagnosis of breast cancer. *International Journal of Clinical Practice, 56*(9), 672–675.

Griffiths, F., Lindenmeyer, A., Powell, J., Lowe, P., & Thorogood, M. (2006). Why are health care interventions delivered over the internet? A systematic review of the published literature. *Journal of Medical Internet Research, 8*(2), 10. doi:10.2196/jmir.8.2.e10

Griffitsh, K. M., & Christensen, H. (2000). Quality of web based information on treatment of depression: cross sectional survey. *British Medical Journal, 32*, 1511–1515. doi:10.1136/bmj.321.7275.1511

Grol, R. (1997). Personal paper. Beliefs and evidence in changing clinical practice. *British Medical Journal, 315*(7150), 418–421.

Grol, R. (2001). Successes and failures in the implementation of evidence based guidelines for clinical practice. *Medical Care, 39*(8Suppl 2), 1146–1154. doi:10.1097/00005650-200108002-00003

Grol, R., & Grimshaw, J. (2003). From best evidence to best practice: effective implementation of change in patients' care. *Lancet, 362*(9391), 1225–1230. doi:10.1016/S0140-6736(03)14546-1

Gruber, T. R. (1993) What is an Ontology? Toward principles for the design of ontologies used for knowledge sharing. Presented at the Padua workshop on Formal Ontology, March 1993, later published in *International Journal of Human-Computer Studies, 43*(4-5), 907-928.

Guastello, S. J. (2005). Nonlinear methods for the social sciences. In Wheelan, S. (Ed.), *The handbook of group research and practice* (pp. 251–268). Thousand Oaks, CA: Sage.

Guidelines for the management of iron deficiency anaemia (2005). *British Society of Gastroenterology.* Retrieved June 15, 2009, from http://www.bsg.org.uk/pdf_word_docs/iron_def.pdf

Gulpinar, M. A., Akman, M., & User, I. (2009). A course, 'The Human in Medicine', as an example of a preclinical medical humanities program: A summary of 7 years. *Medical Teacher, 21*, 1–8. doi:10.1080/01421590802638014

Gunnarsson, N., & Hyden, L.-C. (2009). Organising allergy and being a "good" parent" Parents' narratives about their children's emerging problems. *Health, 13*(2), 157–174.

Gurak, L., & Antonijevic, S. (2008). The psychology of blogging: You, me, and everyone in between. *The American Behavioral Scientist, 52*(1), 60–68. doi:10.1177/0002764208321341

Guyatt, G., & Rennie, D. (Eds.). (2002). *Users' guides to the medical literature. A manual for evidence-based clinical practice.* Chicago, IL: AMA Press.

Gwee, K. A., Leong, Y. L., Graham, C., McKendrick, M. W., Collins, S. M., & Walters, S. J.The role of psychological and biological factors in postinfective gut dysfunction. *Gut, 44*(3), 400–406. doi:10.1136/gut.44.3.400

Habermas, J. (1984). The theory of communicative action: *Vol. 1. Reason and the rationalization of society.* Boston: Beacon.

Haddon, M. (2005). *The Curious Incident of the Dog in the Night-Time*. New York: Doubleday.

Haig, S. (2007). *When the patient is a googler. Time,* (Nov 8). Retrieved from http://www.time.com/time/health/article/0,8599,1681838,00.html

Halamka, J., Overhage, J. M., Ricciardi, L., Rishel, W., Shirky, C., & Diamond, C. (2005). Exchanging health information: local distribution, national coordination. *Health Affairs, 24*(5), 1170–1179. doi:10.1377/hlthaff.24.5.1170

Hall, B. (2005). Wound care for burn patients in acute rehabilitation settings. *Rehabilitation Nursing, 30*(3), 114–119.

Hanney, S. R., Gonzalez-Block, M. A., Buxton, M. J., & Kogan, M. (2003). The utilisation of health research in policy-making: concepts, examples and methods of assessment. *Health Research Policy and Systems,* 2003.

Hardt, M., & Negri, A. (2000). *Empire*. Cambridge, MA: Harvard University Press.

Harfoush, R. (2009). *Yes we did: an insider's look at how social media built the Obama brand*. Berkeley, CA: New Riders Press.

Harmel, M. H. (1986). Monitoring, past, present, future. A personal journey. *International Journal of Clinical Monitoring and Computing, 3*(2), 147–153. doi:10.1007/BF01880768

Hartsell, T., & Yuen, S. (2006). Video streaming in online learning. *AACE Journal, 14*(1), 31–43.

Hawken, M. P., Melis, R. D., Ngombo, D. T., Mandaliya, K., Ng'ang'a, L. W., & Price, J. (2002). Part time female sex workers in a suburban community in Kenya: a vulnerable hidden population. *Sexually Transmitted Infections, 78*(4), 271–273. doi:10.1136/sti.78.4.271

Hay, M. C. (2008). Prepared Patients: Internet Information Seeking by New Rheumatology Patients *Arthritis & Rheumatism (. Arthritis Care and Research, 59*, 575–582. doi:10.1002/art.23533

Haynes, R. B., Sackett, D. L., Gray, J. R., Cook, D. C., & Guyatt, G. H. (1996). Transferring evidence from research into practice: 1. The role of clinical care research evidence in clinical decisions [Editorial]. *American College of Physicians Journal Club, 125*, A14–A16.

Haynes, R. B., Devereaux, P. J., & Guyatt, G. H. (2002). Physicians' and patients' choices in evidence based practice. Evidence does not make decisions, people do. *British Medical Journal, 321*(7350), 1350. doi:10.1136/bmj.324.7350.1350

Health Economics Research Group, Office of Health Economics, RAND Europe. (2008). *Medical Research: What's it worth? Estimating the economic benefits from medical research in the UK*. London: UK Evaluation Forum.

Heeter, C., 1(2), pp. (1992). Being There: The subjective experience of presence. *Presence (Cambridge, Mass.), 1*(2), 262–271.

Hegde, B. M. (1985). How to detect early splenic enlargement? *The Practitioner, London, 229*, 857.

Hegde, B. M. (1994). *24, 228*. Miscellanea Medical. In Proc Roy Coll Phys Edin.

Hegde, B. M. (1994). Auscultation for MVP. *Lancet, 344*, 1446–1447. doi:10.1016/S0140-6736(94)90619-X

Hegde, B. M. (1995). *Unconventional Wisdom in Medicine* (p. 292). Glasgow: Bull.Roy.Coll.Phys.Surg.

Hegde, B. M. (1995). Mitralklappen - Prolaps? *Medical Tribune(German), 17*, 36.

Hegde, B. M. (1996). Hypertension Â– Past, Present and Future. *Kuwait Med. J.,* (suppl.), 194–198.

Hegde, B. M. (1997). Medical Humanism. *Proceedings of the Royal College of Physicians of Edinburgh, 27*, 65–67.

Hegde, B. M. (1997). Reductio Ad Absurdum. *Briti. Roy. Coll.Physi. Surg. Glasgow, 26*, 10–12.

Hegde, B. M. (1997). Heart of the Matter. *Bull. Roy. Coll. Physi. Surg. Glasgow., 26*, 14–15.

Hegde, B. M. (1998). Cardiological Examinations [letter]. *Jr.Roy.Coll.Physi. Lon.*, *32*, 83–84.

Hegde, B. M. (1999). Exercise Â– Sense Versus Non-Sense - Bull. *Roy. Coll. Physi. Surg. Glasgow*, *28*, 13–14.

Hegde, B. M. (1999). Hypertension Â– the other side of the coin. *Jap.Soc. of Hyper. Int*, *13-14*, 99–100.

Hegde, B. M. (2002, March). Health Care Delivery in India Today. *JAPI*, *50*, 425–427.

Hegde, B. M. (2002). To do or Not to Do-Doctors Dilemma, Plea for Proper Audit. *JIACM*, *3*(3), 236–239.

Hegde, B. M. (2002). Septmeber). Needless Interventions in Medicine. *JIMA*, *5*(3), 153–15.

Hegde, B. M. (2002). Where is the Reality? *Kuwait Medical Journal*, *34*(4), 263–265.

Hegde, B. M., & Chakrapani, M. (1991). Early Renal Involvement in Mild moderate hypertension. *Chinese Medical Sciences Journal*, *6*(3), 46.

Hegde, B. M., & Rao, R. A. C. (1987). Long term Thiazide Therapy and Fat Profile. *Cardiovascular Drugs and Therapy*, *1*, 310.

Hegde, B. M. (1988). *Blood Pressure and Meals*. The practitioner, London, 232, 224-225.

Hegde, B. M. (1992). Materia Paramedica. *Journal of the Royal College of Physicians & Surgeons of Glasgow*, 18.

Hegde, B. M. (1993). Need for change in Medical Paradigm. In *Proc Roy Coll Phy Edin.*, *23*, 9-12.

Hegde, B. M. (1993). The state of Internal Medicine. In *Proc Roy Coll Phy Edi.*, *23*, 511-18.

Hegde, B. M. (1995). Coronary Artery Disease, Time for Reappraisal. In *Proc. R.C.P. Edin.*, *26*, 421-24.

Heilferty, C. (2009). Toward a theory of online communication in illness: Concept analysis of illness blogs. *Journal of Advanced Nursing*, *65*(7), 1539–1547. doi:10.1111/j.1365-2648.2009.04996.x

Henderson, J. V. (1998). Comprehensive, Technology-Based Clinical Education: The Virtual Practicum. *International Journal of Psychiatry in Medicine*, *28*(1), 41–79. doi:10.2190/NQEN-KRT8-19GA-R0BV

Henry, S. G., Zaner, R. M., & Dittus, R. S. (2007). Moving Beyond Evidence-Based Medicine. *Academic Medicine*, *82*, 292–297. doi:10.1097/ACM.0b013e3180307f6d

Herman, S. E., & Onaga, E., Pernice-Duca Fet al. (2005). Sense of community in clubhouse programs: member and staff concepts. *American Journal of Community Psychology*, *36*, 343–356. doi:10.1007/s10464-005-8630-2

Herring, S. (1993). Gender and democracy in computer-mediated communication, *Electronic Journal of Communication, 3* (2).

HIFA2015. (2008). *A global Compagine: Health Care Information For All by 2015. HIFA2015 and human rights.* Available at http://www.hifa2015.org/hifa2015-and-human-rights/

Hiltz, S., & Turoff, M. (1993). *The network nation.* Cambridge, MA: MIT. (Original work published 1977)

Hirsch, G. B., Levine, R., & Miller, R. (2007). Using system dynamics modeling to understand the impact of social change initiatives. *American Journal of Community Psychology*, *39*, 239–253. doi:10.1007/s10464-007-9114-3

Ho, K., Jarvis-Selinger, S., Norman, C. D., Li, L., Olatunbosun, T., & Cressmen, C. (in press). Implementing Electronic Community of Practice for Interprofessional Learning and Knowledge Translation: Two Examples. *The Journal of Continuing Education in the Health Professions.*

Hodgkin, P., Munro, J. (2007). The long tale: public services and Web 2.0. *Consumer policy review, 17*(2): 84-88

Hoge, C. W., Shlim, D. R., & Rajah, R. (1993). Epidemiology of diarrhoel illness associated with coccidian like organism among travellers and foreign residents in Nepal. *Lancet*, *341*, 1175. doi:10.1016/0140-6736(93)91002-4

Hollingshead, A., McGrath, J., & O'Connor, K. (1993). Group task performance and communication technology: A longitudinal study of computer-mediated versus face-to-face work groups. *Small Group Research, 24*(3), 307–333. doi:10.1177/1046496493243003

Holt, D. B. (2002). Why do brands cause trouble? A dialectical theory of consumer culture and branding. *The Journal of Consumer Research, 29*(1), 70–90. doi:10.1086/339922

Holter, I. M., & Scwartz-Barcott, D. (1993). Action research: What is it? How has it been used and how can it be used in nursing? *Journal of Advanced Nursing, 18,* 208–304. doi:10.1046/j.1365-2648.1993.18020298.x

Holter, I. M., & Scwartz-Barcott, D. (1993). Action research: What is it? How has it been used and how can it be used in nursing? *Journal of Advanced Nursing, 18,* 208–304. doi:10.1046/j.1365-2648.1993.18020298.x

Hooker, C. (2008). The medical humanities a brief introduction. *Australian Family Physician, 37,* 369–370.

Horkheimer, M., & Adorno, T. W. (1993). *Dialectic of enlightenment.* New York: Continuum.

Howe, J. (2008). *Crowdsourcing: why the future of the crowd is driving the future of business.* New York, NY: Crown Business Publishing.

Htwe, T. H., Mushtaq, A., Robinson, S. B., Rosher, R. B., & Khardori, N. (2007). Infection in the Elderly. [doi: DOI: 10.1016/j.idc.2007.07.006]. *Infectious Disease Clinics of North America, 21*(3), 711-743.

Hubbard, R. A., Inoue, L. Y., & Diehr, P. (2009). Joint modeling of self-rated health and changes in physical functioning. *Journal of the American Statistical Association, 104*(487), 912. doi:10.1198/jasa.2009.ap08423

Hughes, P. (2008). *Reflections: Me and Planet Weirdo.* London: Chipmunkapublishing.

Hughes, B., Joshi, I., & Wareham, J. (2008). Health 2.0 and Medicine 2.0: Tensions and Controversies in the Field. *Journal of Medical Internet Research, 10,* e23. Retrieved from http://www.jmir.org/2008/3/e23/. doi:10.2196/jmir.1056

Human iron metabolism (2009). *Wikipedia, the free encyclopedia.* Retrieved June 15, 2009, from http://en.wikipedia.org/wiki/Human_iron_metabolism

Hummel, J., & Lechner, U. (2001). Communities: The role of technology. In *Proceedings of the 9th European Conference on Information Systems.*

Humphreys, T. (1993). *A Different kind of Teacher.* Dublin, Ireland: Newleaf, an imprint of Gill and Macmillan limited.

Hurlbutt, K., & Chalmers, L. (2002). Adults with Autism Speak Out: Perceptions of Their Life Experiences. *Focus on Autism and Other Developmental Disabilities, 17*(2), 103–111. doi:10.1177/10883576020170020501

Hyden, L. C. (1997). Illness and narrative. *Sociology of Health & Illness, 19*(3), 48–69.

Idler, E. L., & Benyamini, Y. (1997). Self-rated health and mortality: a review of twenty-seven community studies. *Journal of Health and Social Behavior, 38*(1), 21–37. doi:10.2307/2955359

Idler, E. L., Russell, L. B., & Davis, D. (2000). Survival, functional limitations, and self-rated health in the NHANES I Epidemiologic Follow-up Study, 1992. First National Health and Nutrition Examination Survey. *American Journal of Epidemiology, 152*(9), 874–883. doi:10.1093/aje/152.9.874

INAC (2007). *Community Well-being: A Comparable Communities Analysis,* Strategic Research and Analysis Directorate: Indian and Northern Affairs Canada, 2007

INAC. (2005). *Inuit-inhabited areas from census populations and Canadian Mortality Data Base.* Canada: Indian and Northern Affairs.

INAC. (2006). *The Well-Being of Inuit Communities in Canada.* Canada: Indian and Northern Affairs.

INAC. (2009). *Measuring Inuit Wellbeing, Inuit Relations Secretariat.* Canada: Indian and Northern Affairs.

Infoplease (2005) *Infoplease.* Retrieved April 21, 2005, from http://www.infoplease.com/ipa/A0107875.html

Institute of Medicine. (2008). *Improving the Quality of Health Care for Mental and Substance-Use Conditions*. Washington, DC: National Academies Press.

Institute of Medicine. (2001). *Crossing the Quality Chasm: A New Health System for the Twenty-first Century*. Washington: National Academy Press.

Internet Usage Statistics. (n.d.). *Internet World Stats*. Retrieved August 27, 2009, from http://www.internetworldstats.com/stats.htm

IOM (Institute of Medicine). (2001). *Committee on Quality of Health Care in America*. Crossing the Quality Chasm: a new health system for the 21st cent century. Washington, DC, National Academy Press; 20; 2001. PDF. Retrieved from http://books.nap.edu/html/quality_chasm/reportbrief.pdf

IOM (Institute Of Medicine). (1999). *To Err is Human: Building a Safer Health System*. Available at http://www8.nationalacademies.org/onpinews/newsitem.aspx?RecordID=9728

Ipser, J. C., Dewing, S., & Stein, D. F. (2007). A systematic review of the quality of information on the treatment of anxiety disorders on the Internet. *Current Psychiatry Reports*, *9*, 303–309. doi:10.1007/s11920-007-0037-3

Israel, B., Schulz, A., Parker, E., & Becker, A. (1998). Review of community-based research: assessing partnership approaches to improve public health. *Annual Review of Public Health*, *19*, 173–202. doi:10.1146/annurev.publhealth.19.1.173

Israel, B. A. (1985). Social networks and social support: Implications for natural helper and community level interventions. *Health Education & Behavior*, *12*(1), 65–80. doi:10.1177/109019818501200106

Iverson, S. A., Howard, K. B., & Penney, B. K. (2008). Impact of Internet Use on Health-Related Behaviors and the Patient-Physician Relationship: A Survey-Based Study and Review. *The Journal of the American Osteopathic Association*, *108*, 699–711.

Jackson, M. (2000). *Systems approaches to management*. New York: Kluwer Academic/Plenum Publishers.

Jadad, A. R., Enkin, M. W., Glouberman, S., Groff, P., & Stern, A. (1999). Promoting partnerships: Challenges for the internet age. *BMJ (Clinical Research Ed.)*, *319*, 761–764.

Jadad, A. R., Enkin, M. W., Glouberman, S., Groff, P., & Stern, A. (2006). Are virtual communities good for our health? *BMJ (Clinical Research Ed.)*, *332*, 925–926. doi:10.1136/bmj.332.7547.925

Jallinoja, P., Absetz, P., Kuronen, R., Nissinen, A., Talja, M., Uutela, A., & Patja, K. (2007). The dilemma of patient responsibility for lifestyle change: Perceptions amongst primary care physicians and nurses. *Scandinavian Journal of Primary Health Care*, *25*(4), 244–249. doi:10.1080/02813430701691778

James, D., Hess, S., Kretzing, J. E. Jr, & Stabile, M. E. (2007). Showing "what right looks like"--how to improve performance through a paradigm shift around implementation thinking. *Journal of Healthcare Information Management*, *21*(1), 54–61.

Jayaraman, C., Kennedy, P., Dutu, G., & Lawrenson, R. (2008). Use of mobile phone cameras for after-hours triage in primary care. *Journal of Telemedicine and Telecare*, *14*(5), 271–274. doi:10.1258/jtt.2008.080303

Jenkins, J. (2006). Survivorship: finding a new balance. *Seminars in Oncology Nursing*, *22*(2), 117–125. doi:10.1016/j.soncn.2006.01.007

Johnson, C. Y. (2008). Through website, patients creating own drug studies. *The Boston Globe,* (November 16), available at: http://www.boston.com/news/health/articles/2008/11/16/through_website_patients_creating_own_drug_studies/?page=full

Jones, A. E., Brown, M. D., Trzeciak, S., Shapiro, N. I., Garrett, J. S., Heffner, A. C., & Kline, J. A. (2008). The effect of a quantitative resuscitation strategy on mortality in patients with sepsis: a meta-analysis. *Critical Care Medicine*, *36*(10), 2734–2739. doi:10.1097/CCM.0b013e318186f839

Jones, J., Snyder, C., & Wu, A. (2007). Issues in the design of Internet-based systems for collecting patient-reported outcomes. *Quality of Life Research*, 16(8), 1407–1417. doi:10.1007/s11136-007-9235-z

Jones, T., & Verghese, A. (2003). On becoming a humanities curriculum: the center for medical humanities and ethics at the University of Texas health science center at San Antonio. *Academic Medicine*, 78, 1010–1014. doi:10.1097/00001888-200310000-00014

Jones (1995). *A Short History of Rigour in Mathematics*. Retrieved December 12, 2009, from http://www.rbjones.com/rbjpub/maths/math003.htm

Jordan, D. A., McKeown, K. R., Concepcion, K. J., Feiner, S. K., & Hatzivassiloglou, V. (2001). Generation and Evaluation of Intraoperative Inferences for Automated Health Care Briefings on Patient Status After Bypass Surgery. *Journal of the American Medical Informatics Association*, 8(3), 267–280.

Jordon, M., Lanham, H. J., Anderson, R. A., & Jr, R. R. M. (2010). Implications of complex adaptive systems theory for interpreting research about health care organizations. *Forum on Systems and Complexity in Health Care in Journal of Evaluation in Clinical Practice*, 16(1), 228–231.

Jui-Chih, C. (2009). *Multi-user Narrative Sharing System for Children with Chronic Illness*.

Kahan, E. (2009). *Instrumental, detrimental and transcendental: experiences of dental emergency and micro-rationing practices in a Victorian public dental clinic*. (Submitted PhD thesis), La Trobe University, Dec.

Kahn, J. S. (2008). The wisdom of patients: Health care meets online social media. *California HealthCare Foundation*, 1-24.

Kahneman, D. (2002). *Maps of Bounded Rationality: a perspective on intuitive judgment and choice*. Stockholm: Noble Prize Lecture.

Kane, K., Robinson-Combre, J., & Berge, Z. L. (2010). Tapping into social networking: Collaborating enhances both knowledge management and e-learning. *Vine*, 40(1), 62–70. doi:10.1108/03055721011024928

Kaplan, W. (2006). Can the ubiquitous power of mobile phones be used to improve health outcomes in developing countries? *Globalization and Health*, 2(1), 9. doi:10.1186/1744-8603-2-9

Katerndahl, D. A. (2009). Power laws in covariability of anxiety and depression among newly diagnosed patients with major depressive episode, panic disorder and controls. *Journal of Evaluation in Clinical Practice*, 15(3), 565–570. doi:10.1111/j.1365-2753.2009.01166.x

Katz, A., & Shotter, J. (1996). Hearing the patients "voice": Toward a social poetics in diagnostic interviews. *Social Science & Medicine*, 43(6), 919–931. doi:10.1016/0277-9536(95)00442-4

Kay, S., & Purves, I. (1998). The Electronic Medical Record and the "Story Stuff": a narrativistic model. In Greenhalgh, T., & Hurwitz, B. (Eds.), *Narrative Based Medicine: dialogue and discourse in medical practice* (pp. 185–201). London: BMJ Books.

Kelly, M. J., Lloyd, T. D., Marshall, D., Garcea, G., Sutton, C. D., & Beach, M. (2003). A snapshot of MDT working and patient mapping in the UK colorectal cancer centres in 2002. *Colorectal Disease*, 5(6), 577–581. doi:10.1046/j.1463-1318.2003.00531.x

Kendal, S. L., & Creen, M. (2007). *An introduction to knowledge engineering*. London: Springer.

Kerfoot, K. (1998). Management is taught, leadership is learned. *Nursing Economics*, 16(3), 144–145.

Kerlinger, F. (1986). *Foundations of behavioral research*. New York: Holt, Rinehart, and Winston.

Kerner, J. (2006). Knowledge translation versus knowledge integration: A" funders" perspective. *Journal of Continuing Education in the Health Professions*.

Kidd, M. G., & Connor, J. T. H. (2008). Striving to do good things: teaching humanities in Canadian medical schools. *The Journal of Medical Humanities*, 29, 45–54. doi:10.1007/s10912-007-9049-6

Kiefer, L., Frank, J., Di Ruggiero, E., Dobbins, M., Manuel, D., & Gully, P. (2005). Fostering evidence-based decision-making in Canada. *Canadian Journal of Public Health*, *96*(3), 1–18.

Kim, H. S., & Oh, J. A. (2003). Adherence to diabetes control recommendations: impact of nurse telephone calls. *Journal of Advanced Nursing*, *44*(3), 256–261. doi:10.1046/j.1365-2648.2003.02800.x

Kim, J., Lee, S., & Guild, J. (2009). *Healthy communication: Mere communication effect on managing chronic health problems*. Paper presented at the International Communication Association annual meeting, Chicago, IL, May 2009.

Kirklin, D. (2003). The Centre for Medical Humanities, Royal Free and University College Medical School, London, England. *Academic Medicine*, *78*, 1048–1053. doi:10.1097/00001888-200310000-00023

Kiteley, C., & Vaitekunas, D. (2006). Leaving our imprints: an exploration into the nurse-patient relationship. *Canadian Oncology Nursing Journal*, *16*(3), 180–190.

Kitson, A. L. (2009). The need for systems change: reflections on knowledge translation and organizational change. *Journal of Advanced Nursing*, *65*(1), 217–228. doi:10.1111/j.1365-2648.2008.04864.x

Kittenwithawhip. My anemia story.... Forum post (2005, August). *Anemia message board, In HealthBoards Message Boards*. Retrieved June 15, 2009, from http://www.healthboards.com/boards/showthread.php?t=310085&highlight=kittenwithawhip

Klein, G., Moon, B., & Hoffman, R. R. (2006). Making Sense of Sensemaking 1: Alternative Perspectives. *IEEE Intelligent Systems*, *21*(2), 70–73. doi:10.1109/MIS.2006.75

Kleinman, A. (1988). *The illness narratives. Suffering, healing and the human condition New York*. Basic Books.

Klerman, G. (1977). Better but not well: social and ethical issues in the deinstitutionalization of the mentally ill. *Schizophrenia Bulletin*, *3*, 617–631.

Kliener, A. (2002). Karen Stephenson: A quantum theory of trust. *Content: The creative mind*, 1–14.

Kliff, S. (2009). Pharma's facebook. *Newsweek*, March 10, Available at: http://www.newsweek.com/id/187882

Klinken, W. A., & Black, D. (2007). Integrating Public Health and Medicine: First Steps in a New Curriculum. *Education for Health* 7 (online), 122. Retrieved from http://www.educationforhealth.net/articles/subviewnew.asp?ArticleID=122

Klosterhalfen, B., Offner, F., Vogel, P., & Kirckpatrick, C. J. (1991). Anatomic nature and surgical significance of anal sinus and anal intramuscular glands. Retreieved from http://www.springerlink.com/content/t4rv02umj00h6q77

Kmietowicz, Z. (2007). MPs "dismayed" at confusion about electronic patient records. *BMJ (Clinical Research Ed.)*, *335*(7620), 581. doi:10.1136/bmj.39339.414306.DB

Kobayashi, J. S. (1997). The evolution of adjustment issues in HIV/AIDS. *Bulletin of the Menninger Clinic*, *61*(2), 146–188.

Kojouri, K., Vesely, S. K., Terrell, D. R., & George, J. N. (2004). Splenectomy for adult patients with idiopathic thrombocytopenic purpura: a systematic review to assess long-term platelet count responses, prediction of response, and surgical complications. *Blood*, *104*(9), 2623–2634. doi:10.1182/blood-2004-03-1168

Kolb, D. A., Boyatzis, R., & Mainemelis, C. (2000), Experiential learning theory: previous research and new directions. Prepared for R. J. Sternberg and and L. F. Zhang (Eds.), *Perspectives on cognitive learning, and thinking styles*. NJ: Lawrence Erlbaum, 2000.

Kopelman, L. M. (1998). Bioethics and humanities: what makes us one field? *The Journal of Medicine and Philosophy*, *23*, 356–368. doi:10.1076/jmep.23.4.356.2576

Koschatzky, K. (2002). Networking and Knowledge Transfer Between Research and Industry in Transition Countries: Empirical Evidence from the Slovenian Innovation System. *The Journal of Technology Transfer*, *27*(1), 27. doi:10.1023/A:1013192402977

Kotler, P. (2003). *Marketing management*. Upper Saddle River, NJ: Prentice-Hall.

Kozinets, R. V. (2002a). Can consumers escape the market? Emancipatory illuminations from burning man. *The Journal of Consumer Research, 29*(1), 20–38. doi:10.1086/339919

Kozinets, R. V. (2002b). The field behind the screen: Using netnography for marketing research in online communications. *JMR, Journal of Marketing Research, 39*(1), 61–72. doi:10.1509/jmkr.39.1.61.18935

Kreiss, J. K., Koech, D., Plummer, F. A., Holmes, K. K., Lightfoote, M., & Piot, P. (1986). AIDS virus infection in Nairobi prostitutes. Spread of the epidemic to East Africa. *The New England Journal of Medicine, 314*(7), 414–418. doi:10.1056/NEJM198602133140704

Krumholz, H. M., Currie, P. M., Riegel, B., Phillips, C. O., Peterson, E. D., & Smith, R. (2006). A Taxonomy for Disease Management: A Scientific Statement From the American Heart Association Disease Management Taxonomy Writing Group. *Circulation, 114*(13), 1432–1445. doi:10.1161/CIRCULATIONAHA.106.177322

Kumagai, A. K. (2008). A conceptual framework for the use of illness narratives in medical education. *Academic Medicine, 83*, 653–658. doi:10.1097/ACM.0b013e3181782e17

Kumar, N. K. (2006). Bioethics activities in India. *Eastern Mediterranean Health Journal, 12*(Supplement 1), S56–S65.

Kyriacou, C. (1997). *Effective Teaching in Schools*. London: Nelson Thornes.

Laditka, J. N., Laditka, S. B., & Mastanduno, M. P. (2003). Hospital utilization for ambulatory care sensitive conditions: Health outcome disparities associated with race and ethnicity. *Social Science & Medicine, 57*, 1429–1441. doi:10.1016/S0277-9536(02)00539-7

Lakeland, P. (1993). Preserving the lifeworld, restoring the public sphere, renewing higher education. *Cross Currents, 43*(4), 488–502.

Lancaster, T., Hart, R., & Gardner, S. (2002). Literature and medicine: evaluating a special study module using the nominal group technique. *Medical Education, 36*, 1071–1076. doi:10.1046/j.1365-2923.2002.01325.x

Landro, L. A. (1996, October). Survivor's Tale: How a Wall Street Journal reporter confronted a potentially fatal cancer head-on. *The Wall Street Journal, Health & Medicine (A Special Report): Essay*. Retrieved June 7, 2009, from http://leukemia.acor.org/storydir/landro.html

Lane, J., & Flagg, J. (2010). Translating three states of knowledge - discovery, invention & innovation. *Implementation Science; IS, 5*(1), 9. doi:10.1186/1748-5908-5-9

Laporte, R. E., Omenn, G. S., Serageldin, I., Cerf, V. G., & Linkov, F. (2006). A scientific supercourse. *Science, 312*(5773), 526. doi:10.1126/science.312.5773.526c

Laporte, R. E., Sekikawa, A., Sa, E., Linkov, F., & Lovalekar, M. (2002). Whisking research into the classroom. *BMJ (Clinical Research Ed.), 324*(7329), 99. doi:10.1136/bmj.324.7329.99

LaPorte, R. E., Linkov, F., Villasenor, T., Sauer, F., Gamboa, C., & Lovalekar, M. (2002). Papyrus to PowerPoint (P 2 P): metamorphosis of scientific communication. *BMJ (Clinical Research Ed.), 325*(7378), 1478–1481. doi:10.1136/bmj.325.7378.1478

LaPorte, R. E., Marler, E., Akazawa, S., Sauer, F., Gamboa, C., & Shenton, C. (1995). The death of biomedical journals. *BMJ (Clinical Research Ed.), 310*(6991), 1387–1390.

Lapsley, P., & Groves, T. (2004). The patient's journey: travelling through life with a chronic illness. *BMJ (Clinical Research Ed.), 329*(7466), 582–583. doi:10.1136/bmj.329.7466.582

Larijani, B., Zahedi, F., & Malek-Afzali, H. (2005). Medical ethics in the Islamic republic of Iran. *Eastern Mediterranean Health Journal, 11*, 1061–1072.

Lasser, J., & Corley, K. (2008). Constructing normalcy: a qualitative study of parenting children with Asperger's Disorder. *Educational Psychology in Practice, 24*(4), 335–346. doi:10.1080/02667360802488773

Lau, J., Antman, E. M., Jimenez-Silva, J., Kupelnick, B., Mosteller, F., & Chalmers, T. C. (1992). Cumulative meta-analysis of therapeutic trials for myocardial infarction. *The New England Journal of Medicine, 327,* 248–254. doi:10.1056/NEJM199207233270406

Layder, D. (1994). *New Strategies in Social Research.* Cambridge, UK: Cambridge Polity Press.

Leavitt, F. J. (2002). What is Bioethics? Commentary on Harris & Sass on The Eubios Declaration, Biswas on Holistic Health Care, Yu Kam Por on Futile Medical Treatment. *Eubios Journal of Asian and International Bioethics; EJAIB, 12,* 162–164.

Legall, I. (2009). *Anal Fistulas and Fissures E medicine.* Retrieved Oct 25, 2009, from http://emedicine.medscape.com/article/776150-overview

Lehmann, L. S., Kasoff, W. S., Koch, P., & Federman, D. D. (2004). A survey of medical ethics education at U.S. and Canadian medical schools. *Academic Medicine, 79,* 682–589. doi:10.1097/00001888-200407000-00015

Lehmann-Rommel, R. (2000). The renewal of Dewey - Trends in the nineties. *Studies in Philosophy and Education, 19,* 187–218. doi:10.1007/BF02764159

Lemieux-Charles, L., & Champagne, F. (Eds.). (2004). *The use of knowledge and evidence in health care: multidisciplinary perspectives.* Toronto, ON: University of Toronto Press.

Lenhart, A., & Madden, M. (2007). *Teens, privacy and online social networks: How teens manage their online identities and personal information in the age of MySpace.* Pew Internet and American Life Project. Retrieved from http://www.pewinternet.org/pdfs/PIP_Teens_Privacy_SNS_Report_Final.pdf

Lett, H. S., Blumenthal, J. A., Babyak, M. A., Strauman, T. J., Robins, C., & Sherwood, A. (2005). Social support and coronary heart disease: epidemiologic evidence and implications for treatment. *Psychosomatic Medicine, 67*(6), 869–878. doi:10.1097/01.psy.0000188393.73571.0a

Levine, R. B., Kern, D. E., & Wright, S. M. (2008). The impact of prompted narrative writing during internship on reflective practice: a qualitative study. *Advances in Health Sciences Education : Theory and Practice, 13,* 723–733. doi:10.1007/s10459-007-9079-x

Levy, J. (1974). Psychobiological implications of bilateral asymmetry. *In Hemisphere function in the human brain.* Dimond and Beaumont, eds, New York.

Leykum, L., Pugh, J., Lawrence, V., Parchman, M., Noel, P., & Cornell, J. (2007). Organizational interventions employing principles of complexity science have improved outcomes for patients with Type II diabetes. *Implementation Science; IS, 2*(1), 28. doi:10.1186/1748-5908-2-28

Li, L., Grimshaw, J., Nielsen, C., Judd, M., Coyte, P., & Graham, I. (2009). Evolution of Wenger's concept of community of practice. *Implementation Science; IS, 4*(1), 11. doi:10.1186/1748-5908-4-11

Lim, R. (2003) *Outside the classroom: Oral and visual research methods applied in vernacular settlements.* Conference Proceedings, International Conference on Integrating Teaching with Research and Practice in the Built Environment. Wadham College Oxford.

Linkov, F., Ardalan, A., Dodani, S., Lovalekar, M., Sauer, F., & Shubnikov, E. (2006). Building just-in-time lectures during the prodrome of Hurricanes Katrina and Rita. *Prehospital and Disaster Medicine, 21*(2Suppl 2), 132.

Linkov, F., & LaPorte, R., Lovaleka,r M., & Dodani, S. (2005). Web quality control for lectures: Supercourse and Amazon.com. *Croatian Medical Journal, 46*(6), 875–878.

Linkov, F., Lovalekar, M., & LaPorte, R. (2007). Quality control of epidemiological lectures online: scientific evaluation of peer review. *Croatian Medical Journal, 48*(2), 249–255.

Lipsitz, L. A., & Goldberger, A. L. (1992). Loss of 'complexity' and aging. Potential applications of fractals and chaos theory to senescence. *Journal of the American Medical Association, 267,* 1806–1809. doi:10.1001/jama.267.13.1806

Liu, J. (2008). Bypass of Local Primary Care in Rural Counties: Effect of Patient and Community Characteristics. *Annals of Family Medicine*, *6*, 124–130. doi:10.1370/afm.794

Loehr, J., & Schwartz, A. (2003). *The Power of Full Engagement: Managing Energy, Not Time, is the Key to High Performance and Personal Renewal*. New York, NY: Free Press.

Lotsawalls. Ferritin less than 1? Forum post (2009, Jan). Anemia message board, In *HealthBoards Message Boards*. Retrieved June 15, 2009, from http://www.healthboards.com/boards/showthread.php?t=666920&highlight=lotsawalls&page=5

Louk, W. (2009). Peters, H., Gerjo Kok, Geert T. M., Ten Dam, Goof J Buijs, & Theo G. W. M. Paulussen(2009) Effective elements of school health promotion across behavioral domains: a systematic review of reviews. *BMC Public Health*, *9*, 182. Published online 2009 June 12. doi:.doi:10.1186/1471-2458-9-182

Lowton, K., & Gabe, J. (2003). Life on a Slippery Slope: Perceptions of Health in Adults with Cystic Fibrosis. *Sociology of Health & Illness*, *25*(4), 289–319. doi:10.1111/1467-9566.00348

Lundberg, G. (2003). The "omnipotent" Science Citation Index impact factor. *The Medical Journal of Australia*, *178*(6), 253–254.

Lutfey, K. (2005). On practices of 'good doctoring': reconsidering the relationship between provider roles and patient adherence. *Sociology of Health & Illness*, *27*(4), 421–447. doi:10.1111/j.1467-9566.2005.00450.x

Lynam, T., Bousquet, F., Le Page, C., d'Aquino, P., Barreteau, O., & Chinembiri, F. (2003). Adaptive science to adaptive managers: Spidergrams, belief models, and multi-agent systems modeling. In Campbell, B. M., & Sayer, J. A. (Eds.), *Integrated Natural Resource Management: Linking Productivity, the Environment and Development* (pp. 157–174). Cambridge, MA: CABI. doi:10.1079/9780851997315.0157

Lynn, B., & Bluman, B. (2009). It Takes More than Medical Knowledge and Skills. Retrieved July 24, 2009, from http://www.university-cme.ca/canada/editorial.php?show_id=5&lang=en

Lysaker, P. H., & Buck, K. D. (2007). Neurocognitive deficits as a barrier to psychosocial function in schizophrenia: effects on learning, coping, & self-concept. *Journal of Psychosocial Nursing and Mental Health Services*, *45*, 24–30.

Lyytinen, K., & Ngwenyama, O. (1999). Sharrock and Button... and much ado about nothing. *Computer Supported Cooperative Work*, *8*, 285–293. doi:10.1023/A:1008720609782

Maag, M. (2006). iPod, uPod? An emerging mobile learning tool in nursing education and students' satisfaction.

Mabrito, M. (1992). Real-time computer network collaboration: Case studies of business writing students. *Journal of Business and Technical Communication*, *6*(3), 316–336. doi:10.1177/1050651992006003003

Macnaughton, J. (2000). The humanities in medical education: context, outcomes and structures. *Medical Humanities*, *26*, 23–30. doi:10.1136/mh.26.1.23

Makundi, E. A., Malebo, H. M., Mhame, P., Kitua, A. y., & Warsame, M. (2006). Role of Traditional Healers in the management of severe malaria among children below five years of age: The case of Kilosa and Handeni Districs in Tanzania. *Malaria Journal*, *5*, 58. http://www.malariajournal.com/contents/5/1/58. doi:10.1186/1475-2875-5-58

Battersby, M., Harvey, P., Mills, P. D., Kalucy, E., Pols, R. G., Frith, P. A., et al. (2007). SA HealthPlus: A Controlled Trial of a Statewide Application of a Generic Model of Chronic Illness Care. *The Milbank Quarterly*, *85*(1), 37–67. doi:10.1111/j.1468-0009.2007.00476.x.

Mangione-Smith, R., DeCristofaro, A. H., Setodji, C. M., Keesey, J., Klein, D. J., Adams, M. A., & McGlynn, E. A. (2007). The quality of ambulatory care delivered to children in the United States. *The New England Journal of Medicine*, *357*(15), 1515–1523. doi:10.1056/NEJMsa064637

Marik, P. E. (2001). *Handbook of Evidence Based Critical Care*. New York: Springer.

Marincola, F. M. (2003). Translational Medicine: A two-way road. *Journal of Translational Medicine*, *1*(1), 1. doi:10.1186/1479-5876-1-1

Marín-García, J., Goldenthal, M. J., & Moe, G. W. (2008). Transcriptional, Proteomic, SNPs, Gene Mapping and Epigenetics Analysis. In *Aging and the Heart* (pp. 417–440). Profiling the Aging Cardiovascular System. doi:10.1007/978-0-387-74072-0_13

Marshall, S., Haywood, K., & Fitzpatrick, R. (2006). Impact of patient-reported outcome measures on routine practice: a structured review. *Journal of Evaluation in Clinical Practice*, *12*(5), 559–568. doi:10.1111/j.1365-2753.2006.00650.x

Martin, C. M. (2007). Chronic disease and illness care: Adding principles of family medicine to address ongoing health system redesign. *Canadian Family Physician Medecin de Famille Canadien*, *53*(12), 2086–2091.

Martin, C. M., & Kaufman, T. (2008). (in press). Do physicians have the responsibility to address health inequalities? Going beyond Primary Care to deliver Primary Health Care in our own communities. *Canadian Family Physician Medecin de Famille Canadien*.

Martin, C. M., & Peterson, C. (2008). (in press). The social construction of chronicity:- A key to understanding chronic care transformations. *Journal of Evaluation in Clinical Practice*.

Martin, C. M., & Sturmberg, J. P. (2009). Perturbing ongoing conversations about systems and complexity in health services and systems. *Journal of Evaluation in Clinical Practice*, *15*(3), 549–552. doi:10.1111/j.1365-2753.2009.01164.x

Martin, M., Hin, P., & O'Neill, D. (2004). Acute medical take or subacute-on-chronic medical take? *Irish Medical Journal*, *97*(7), 212–214.

Martin, C. M., Peterson, C., Robinson, R., & Sturmberg, J. P. (2009). Care for chronic illness in Australian general practice - focus groups of chronic disease self-help groups over 10 years: implications for chronic care systems reforms. *Asia Pacific Family Medicine*, *8*(1), 1. doi:10.1186/1447-056X-8-1

Martin, M., Hin, P., & O'Neill, D. (2004). Acute medical take or subacute-on-chronic medical take? *Irish Medical Journal*, *97*(7), 212–214.

Martin, C., & Sturmberg, J. (2009). Complex adaptive chronic care. *Journal of Evaluation in Clinical Practice*, *15*(3), 571–577. doi:10.1111/j.1365-2753.2008.01022.x

Martin, C., & Peterson, C. (2009). The social construction of chronicity – a key to understanding chronic care transformations. *Journal of Evaluation in Clinical Practice*, *15*(3), 578–585. doi:10.1111/j.1365-2753.2008.01025.x

Martin, C. M. (2008). *Patient Journey Record (PaJr) Platform for user driven healthcare*. NDRC Translational Research Project Proposal.

Martin, C. M., Biswas, R., Joshi, A., & Sturmberg, J. (2010). Patient Journey Record Systems (PaJR): The development of a conceptual framework for a patient journey system. Part 1. In Biswas, R., & Martin, C. (Eds.), *User-Driven Healthcare and Narrative Medicine: Utilizing Collaborative Social Networks and Technologies* (Vol. 1). Hershey, PA, USA: IGI Global.

Martin CM, & Sturmberg JP. (2008). Complex Adaptive Chronic Care: a framework for health, health care, health systems and policy. *Journal of Evaluation in Clinical Practice*.

Martin, C. M., Biswas, R., Topps, D., Joshi, A., & Sturmberg, J. (2010). *Patient Journey Systems (PaJS): Narratives and evidence for a paradigm shift. Part 1* (Martin, R. B. C., Ed.).

Martin, C. (1998). *The care of chronic illness in general practice*. (PhD Thesis) Unpublished Epidemiology and Population Health, Australian National University http://normed.academia.edu/CarmelMartin/Papers/74540/The-Care-of-Chronic-Illness-in-General-Practice, Canberra.

Martin, C. (2007). Chronic Disease and Illness Care: Additional Principles of Family Medicine are needed to address ongoing health system redesign. *Canadian Family Physician, Dec;53(12):2086-91.*

Martin, C. M. (1998). *The Care of Chronic Illness in General Practice. PhD Thesis.* Australian National University, Canberra.

Martin, C. M., & Kaufman, T. (2007b). *Glossary of Terms in New Orientations, a Shared Framework: A way forward to adaptive Primary Health Care Systems across Canada: A Discussion Monograph.* Commissioned by the Canadian Association of Community Health Centre Associations, and the Association of Ontario Health Centres (www.cachca.ca)).

Martin, C. M., & Sturmberg, J. P. (2006). Rethinking general practice – Part 2: Strategies for the future: Patient-centred responsive primary health care and the leadership challenges. *Asia Pacific Journal of Family Medicine, 5*(3).

Masefield, J. (1988). *Pompey the Great.* Oxford, UK: Oxford Library of English Poetry.

Maskrey, N., Hutchinson, A., & Underhill, J. (2009). Getting a better grip on research: the comfort of opinion. *InnovAiT, 2*(11), 679–686. doi:10.1093/innovait/inp085

Matsui, D., Cho, M., & Rieder, M. J. (1998). Physicians' attire as perceived by young children and their parents: the myth of the white coat syndrome. *Pediatric Emergency Care, 14,* 198–201. doi:10.1097/00006565-199806000-00006

Matthews, D. A., Suchman, A. L., & Branch, W. T. (1993). Making "connexions": enhancing the therapeutic potential of patient-clinician relationships. *Annals of Internal Medicine, 118,* 973–977.

Maughan, T. S., Finlay, I. G., & Webster, D. J. (2001). Portfolio learning with cancer patients: an integrated module in undergraduate medical education. *Clinical Oncology (Royal College of Radiologists (Great Britain)), 13*(1), 44–49.

May, L., Day, R., & Warren, S. (2006). Perceptions of patient education in spinal cord injury rehabilitation. *Disability and Rehabilitation, 28*(17), 1041–1049. doi:10.1080/09638280500494744

May, C., & Mead, N. (1999). Patient-centeredness: A History. In Dowrick, C., & Frith, L. (Eds.), *General Practice and Ethics: Uncertainty and Responsibility* (pp. 76–90). London: Routledge.

MayoClinic. (2009). *MayoClinic.* Retrieved from http://www.mayoclinic.com/

Mayor, V. (2006). Long-term conditions. 3: Being an expert patient. *British Journal of Community Nursing, 11*(2), 59–63.

McAlister, F. A., Graham, I., Karr, G. W., & Laupacis, A. (1999). Evidence-based medicine and the practicing clinician. *Journal of General Internal Medicine, 14*(4), 236–242. doi:10.1046/j.1525-1497.1999.00323.x

McAlonan, S. (1996). Improving sexual rehabilitation services: The patients' perspective. *The American Journal of Occupational Therapy., 50*(10), 826–834.

McClenathan, B. M., Torrington, K. G., & Uyehara, F. T. (2002). Cardiopulmonary Resuscitation: A Survey of US and International Critical Care Professionals. *Chest, 122,* 2204–2211. doi:10.1378/chest.122.6.2204

McDaniel, S., Campbell, T., Hepworth, J., & Lorenz, A. (2005). *Family-orientated primary care* (2nd ed.). New York: Springer.

McDaniel, S., Hepworth, J., & Doherty, W. (1992). *Medical family therapy.* New York: Basic Books.

McDermott, L. M., & Ebmeier, K. P. (2009). A meta-analysis of depression severity and cognitive function. *Journal of Affective Disorders, 119,* 1–8. doi:10.1016/j.jad.2009.04.022

McGlynn, E. A., Asch, S. M., Adams, J., Keesey, J., Hicks, J., DeCristofaro, A., & Kerr, E. A. (2003). The quality of care delivered to adults in the United States. *The New England Journal of Medicine, 348*(26), 2635–2645. doi:10.1056/NEJMsa022615

McGrath, K. M., Bennett, D. M., Ben-Tovim, D. I., Boyages, S. C., Lyons, N. J., & O'Connell, T. J. (2008). Implementing and sustaining transformational change in health care: lessons learnt about clinical process redesign. *The Medical Journal of Australia, 188*(6Suppl), S32–S35.

McGrath, B. P. (2006). Lack of integration of medical education in Australia: the need for change. *The Medical Journal of Australia, 184*, 346–348. Retrieved from http://www.mja.com.au/public/issues/184_07_030406/mcg10993_fm.pdf.

McGregor, S. (2006). Roles, power, and subjective choice. *Patient Education and Counseling, 60*, 5–9. doi:10.1016/j.pec.2004.11.012

McLean, R., Richards, B., & Wardman, J. (2007). The effect of Web 2.0 on the future of medical practice and education: Darwikian evolution or folksonomic revolution? *The Medical Journal of Australia, 187*(3), 174–177.

McLeod, M. E. (2003). The caring physician: a journey in self-exploration and self-care. *The American Journal of Gastroenterology, 98*(10), 2135–2138. doi:10.1111/j.1572-0241.2003.07719.x

McLuhan, M. (2003). *Understanding media: The extension of man - critical edition.* Berkeley, CA: Gingko Press.

McNeill, B. J. (2001). Shattuck Lecture -- Hidden barriers to improvement in the quality of care. *The New England Journal of Medicine, 345*(22), 1612–1620. doi:10.1056/NEJMsa011810

McNicholl, M. P., Dunne, K., Garvey, A., Sharkey, R., & Bradley, A. (2006). Using the Liverpool Care Pathway for a dying patient. *Nursing Standard, 20*(38), 46–50.

Meadows, L. M., Lackner, S., & Belic, M. (1997). Irritable bowel syndrome. An exploration of the patient perspective. *Clinical Nursing Research, 6*(2), 156–170. doi:10.1177/105477389700600205

Medical Malpractice. (2008). *Medical Malpractice.* Retrieved from http://medical-malpractice-flint.com/info.htm

Medsphere and Webreach. (n.d.). *Medsphere and Webreach.* Retrieved from http://www.medsphere.com/press/20080701

Mehra, A., Dixon, A. L., Brass, D. J., & Robertson, B. (2005). (in press). The social networks of leaders: Implications for group performance and leader reputation. *Organization Science.*

Melnyk, B. M. (2002). Strategies for overcoming barriers in implementing evidence based practice. *Paediatric Nursing, 28*(2), 159–161.

Mikhail Prokopenko, F. B. A. J. R. (2008). An information-theoretic primer on complexity, self-organization, and emergence. *Complexity, 9*(9), NA.

Miles, A., Loughlin, M., & Polychronis, A. (2007). Medicine and evidence: knowledge and action in clinical practice. *Journal of Evaluation in Clinical Practice, 13*(4), 481–503. doi:10.1111/j.1365-2753.2007.00923.x

Miles, M., & Huberman, A. (1994). *Qualitative data analysis.* Thousand Oaks, CA: SAGE.

Millen, N., & Peterson, C. (1998). Chronic fatigue syndrome, legitimation and family support. *The International Journal of Sociology and Social Policy, 18*(2), 127–147. doi:10.1108/01443339810788470

Milligan, E., & Woodley, E. (2009). Creative expressive encounters in health ethics education: teaching ethics as relational engagement. *Teaching and Learning in Medicine, 21*, 131–139. doi:10.1080/10401330902791248

Mirth (n.d.). *Mirth.* Retrieved from http://www.mirthcorp.com/community/overview; http://www.mirthcorp.com/archives/2085

Mistry, Pranav m P. Maes (2009) Sixth Sense – a wearable gestural interface. SIGGRAPH Asia 2009

Miyasaka, M., Akabayashi, A., Kai, I., & Ohi, G. (1999). An international survey of medical ethics curricula in Asia. *Journal of Medical Ethics, 25*, 514–521. doi:10.1136/jme.25.6.514

Mizutani, H., Engelman, R. W., Kurata, Y., Ikehara, S., & Good, R. A. (1994). Energy restriction prevents and reverses immune thrombocytopenic purpura (ITP) and increases life span of ITP-prone (NZW x BXSB) F1 mice. *The Journal of Nutrition, 124*(10), 2016–2023.

Moisseeva, M. (2007). *Online learning communities and collaborative learning. Institute of International Education, New York*. Retrieved July 21, 2009, from http://www.iienetwork.org/?p=41543.

Molinari, G., Valbusa, A., Terrizzano, M., Bazzano, M., Torelli, L., & Girardi, N. (2004). Nine years' experience of telecardiology in primary care. *Journal of Telemedicine and Telecare, 10*(5), 249–253. doi:10.1258/1357633042026297

Morel, V., Chatton, A., & Cochand, S. (2008). Quality of web-based information on bipolar disorder. *Journal of Affective Disorders, 110*, 265–269. doi:10.1016/j.jad.2008.01.007

Morisse, K., & Ramm, M. (2007). *Teaching via Podcasting: One year of Experience with Workflows*. Tools and Usage in Higher Education.

Morris, M. E. (2005). Social networks as health feedback displays. *IEEE Internet Computing, 9*(5), 29–37. doi:10.1109/MIC.2005.109

Moser, R. H. (1973). Mission Possible. *Journal of the American Medical Association, 226*, 350. doi:10.1001/jama.226.3.350b

Mueller, I. (2005). Namuigi, P., Kundi, J., Ivivi, R. Tandrapah, T., and Bjorge, S. Epidemic Malaria in the Highlands of Paua New Guinea. *American Journal of Tropical Medicine, 72*, 554–560.

Muir, F. (2007). Placing the patient at the core of teaching. *Medical Teacher, 29*(2-3), 258–260. doi:10.1080/01421590701291477

Muir Gray, J. (2001). Evidence-based medicine for professionals. In Edwards, A., & Elwyn, G. (Eds.), *Evidence-based patient choice; inevitable or impossible?* Oxford: Oxford University Press.

Murray, J. (2003). Development of a medical humanities program at Dalhousie University faculty of Medicine, Nova Scotia, Canada, 1992-2003. *Academic Medicine, 78*, 1020–1023. doi:10.1097/00001888-200310000-00016

Murray, M. (2009). A narrative approach to health psychology. Background and potential. *Journal of Health Psychology, 2*(1), 9–20. doi:10.1177/135910539700200102

Murray, J. B., & Ozanne, J. L. (1991). The critical imagination: Emancipatory interests in consumer research. *The Journal of Consumer Research, 18*(2), 129–144. doi:10.1086/209247

Nair, B. R., Attia, J. R., Mears, S. R., & Hitchcock, K. I. (2002). Evidence-based physicians' dressing: a crossover trial. *The Medical Journal of Australia, 16*, 681–682.

Nardi, B. A., & Whittaker, S. (2002). The Place of Face-To- Face Communication in Distributed Work. In Hins, P. J., & Kiesler, S. (Eds.), *Distributed Work* (pp. 83–113). Cambridge, MA: The MIT Press.

National Autistic Society. (n.d.). *National Autistic Society*. Retrieved from http://www.nas.org.uk/

National Digital Research Centre. (2010). *Heartphone*. Retreived from http://www.ndrc.ie/projects/heartphone/

National Library of Medicine. (2009). *MedlinePlus, Health Information in Multiple Languages*. Retrieved from http://www.nlm.nih.gov/medlineplus/languages/languages.html

Navarro, V. (2007). *Neoliberalism, Globalisation and Inequalities: Consequences for Health and Quality of Life*. Amityville, Baywood.

Neas, J. F. (2003). Digestive System Development in Embryology Atlas. Upper Saddle River, NJ: Pearson Education Inc Nhieu, J. T., Nin, F., Fleury-Feith, J., Chaumette, M. T., Schaeffer, A., & Bretagne, S. Identification of intracellular stages of Cyclospora species by light microscopy of thick sections using hematoxylin. *Human Pathology*, (10): 1107–1109.

Neito, T., Mendez, F., & Carrasquilla, G. (1999). Knowledge Beliefs and practices relevant for malaria control in an endemic urban area of the Columbian Pacific. *Social Science & Medicine, 49*, 601–609. doi:10.1016/S0277-9536(99)00134-3

Newman, M., Papadopoulos, I., & Sigsworth, J. (1998). Barriers to evidence-based practice. *Intensive & Critical Care Nursing, 14*(5), 231–238. doi:10.1016/S0964-3397(98)80634-4

Ngwenyama, O., & Lyytinen, K. (1997). Groupware environments as action constitutive resources: a social action framework for analyzing groupware technologies. *Computer Supported Cooperative Work, 6*, 71–93. doi:10.1023/A:1008600220584

NHSScotland. (2006) Understanding the Patient Journey – Process Mappping http://www.scotland.gov.uk/Resource/Doc/141079/0036023.pdf

Nicholas, B., & Gillett, G. (1997). Doctors' stories, patients' stories: a narrative approach to teaching medical ethics. *Journal of Medical Ethics, 23*(5), 295–299. doi:10.1136/jme.23.5.295

Norman, C. D., & Huerta, T. (2006). Knowledge transfer & exchange through social networks: building foundations for a community of practice within tobacco control. *Implementation Science; IS, 1*(1), 20. doi:10.1186/1748-5908-1-20

NRC. (1996). *NRC.* Retrieved from http://education-northwest.org/webfm_send/203

O' Rourke, M. F. (1999). William Osler: a model for the 21st century? *The Medical Journal of Australia, 171*, 577–579.

O'Reilly, T. (2005). *What is web 2.0? Design patterns and business models for the next generation of software.* Retrieved from http://www.oreillynet.com/pub/a/oreilly/tim/news/2005/09/30/what-is-web-20.html

Ogur, B., & Hirsh, D. (2009). Learning through longitudinal patient care-narratives from the Harvard Medical School-Cambridge Integrated Clerkship. *Academic Medicine, 84*, 844–850. doi:10.1097/ACM.0b013e3181a85793

Olaniran, B. (1994). Group performance in computer-mediated and face-to-face communication media. *Management Communication Quarterly, 7*(3), 256–281. doi:10.1177/0893318994007003002

Oldenburg, B., & Parcel, G. S. (2002). Diffusion of innovations. In Glanz, K., Rimer, B. K., & Lewis, F. M. (Eds.), *Health behavior and heath education* (3rd ed.). San Francisco, CA: Jossey-Bass.

Oliver, K. B., & Swain, R. (2006). Directories of Institutional Repositories: Research Results & Recommendations. *World Library and Information Congress: 72nd IFLA General Conference and Council*, Seoul, Korea 20-24 August, 2006. Retrieved from http://www.ifla.org/IV/ifla72/papers/151-Oliver_Swain-en.pdf

Oppenheimer, T. (2003). *The Flickering Mind: The False Promise of Technology in the Classroom and How Learning Can Be Saved.* New York: Random House.

Orem, D. E. (2001). *Nursing: Concepts of practice* (6th ed.). St. Louis, MO: Mosby.

Osler, W. (1904). *Aequanimitas with Other Addresses to Medical Students, Nurses and Practitioners of Medicine.* Philadelphia: The Blakiston Company.

Osler, W. (1928). *The Student Life and Other Essays.* London: Constable.

OW1SWEB (2009). Ow1seb Blog. Retrieved from http://www.owlsweb.info/L4L/blogs.asp#useinlibraries

Owen, H. (1997). *Open space technology: A user's guide.* New York, NY: Berrett-Koehler.

Page, S. E. (2007). *The difference: how the power of diversity creates better groups, firms, schools and societies.* Princeton, NJ: Princeton University Press.

Papacharissi, Z. (2002). The virtual sphere: The internet as a public sphere. *New Media & Society, 4*(1), 9–27. doi:10.1177/14614440222226244

Papacharissi, Z. (2004). Democracy online: Civility, politeness, and the democratic potential of online political discussion groups. *New Media & Society, 6*(2), 259–283. doi:10.1177/1461444804041444

Paré, D. A. (2002). Discursive wisdom: Reflections on ethics and therapeutic knowledge. *International Journal of Critical Psychology, 7*, 30–52.

Parkman, H. P., & Cohen, S. (1995). Heartburn, regurgitation, odynophagia, chest pain and dysphagia. In Haubrich, W. S., Schaffner, F., & Berk, J. E. (Eds.), *Bockus Gastroenterology* (5th ed., pp. 30–40). Philadelphia: WB Saunders company.

Parsons, T. (1951). *The Social System*. Glencove, New York: The Free Press.

Pask, G. (1975). Minds and media in education and entertainment: some theoretical comments illustrated by the design and operation of a system for exteriorizing and manipulating individual theses. In Trappl, R., & Pask, G. (Eds.), *Progress in Cybernetics and Systems Research, 4* (pp. 38–50). Washington, London: Hemisphere Publishing Corporation.

Patterson, B., Butt, L., Mc, G., Guiness, L., & Moffatt, B. (2006). The Construction of Hepatitis C as a Chronic Illness. *Clinical Nursing Research, 15*(3), 209–224. doi:10.1177/1054773806288569

Patterson, B. L. (2001). The shifting perspectives model of chronic illness. *Journal of Nursing Scholarship, 33*(1), 21–26. doi:10.1111/j.1547-5069.2001.00021.x

Patton, M. Q. (1990). *Qualitative evaluation and research methods* (2nd ed.). Newbury Park, CA: Sage.

Patton, M. Q. (1994). Developmental Evaluation. *Evaluation Practice, 15*(3), 311–319. doi:10.1016/0886-1633(94)90026-4

Patton, M. Q. (2008). *Utilization-focused evaluation* (4th ed.). Los Angeles, CA.

Pearson, A. S., McTigue, M. P., & Tarpley, J. L. (2008). Narrative medicine in surgical education. *Journal of Surgical Education, 65*, 99–100. doi:10.1016/j.jsurg.2007.11.008

Peersman, G., Flores, S., Zee, A., & Eke, A. (2001) Interventions for preventing HIV in young people in Low Income countries, *The Cochrane Database of Systematic Reviews*, The Cochrane Library. http://www.cochrane.org/colloquia/abstracts/capetown/capetownPD11.html

Peñaloza, L., & Price, L. L. (1993). Consumer resistance: A conceptual overview. *Advances in Consumer Research. Association for Consumer Research (U. S.), 20*, 123–128.

Pena-Purcell, N. (2008). Hispanics' use of Internet health information: an exploratory study. *Journal of the Medical Library Association: JMLA, 96*, 101–107. doi:10.3163/1536-5050.96.2.101

Pescosolido, B. (2006). Of pride and prejudice: the role of sociology and social networks in integrating the health sciences. *Journal of Health and Social Behavior, 47*(3), 189–208. doi:10.1177/002214650604700301

Peterkin, A. (2008). Medical humanities for what ails us. *Canadian Medical Association Journal, 178*, 648. doi:10.1503/cmaj.071851

Peterson, H. E. (2006). From punched cards to computerized patient records: a personal journey. *Yearbook of Medical Informatics*, 180–186.

Peterson, C., Millen, N., & Woodward, R. (1999). Chronic fatigue syndrome: A problem of legitimation. *Australian Journal of Primary Care – Interchange, 5*(2): 65-79.

Pettenati, M. C., & Cigognini, M. E. Guerin, E. M. C., & Mangione, G. R. (2008). Personal Knowledge Management Skills for Lifelong-learners 2.0 in: Hatzipanagos, S. & Warburton, S. (Eds.), *Handbook of Research on Social Software and Developing Community Ontologies*, Hershey: IGI Global.

Pfeffer, P. E., Pfeffer, J. M., & Hodson, M. E. (2003). The Psychosocial and Psychiatric Side of Cystic Fibrosis in Adolescents and Adults. *Journal of Cystic Fibrosis, 2*, 61–68. doi:10.1016/S1569-1993(03)00020-1

PHAC. (2006). *How Healthy Are Rural Canadians? An Assessment of Their Health Status and Health Determinants A Component of the Initiative Canada's Rural Communities: Understanding Rural Health and Its Determinants*. Public Health Agency of Canada.

Phillips, R., Gosper, M., McNeill, M., Woo, K., Preston, G., & Green, D. (2007). Staff and student perspectives on web based lecture technologies: Insights into the great divide. Proceedings ascilite Singapore 2007, 854-864.

Pickering, H., Okongo, M., Nnalusiba, B., Bwanika, K., & Whitworth, J.Sexual networks in Uganda: casual and commercial sex in a trading town. *AIDS Care*, *9*(2), 199–207. doi:10.1080/09540129750125217

Pickering, H., Quigley, M., Hayes, R. J., Todd, J., & Wilkins, A.Determinants of condom use in 24,000 prostitute/client contacts in The Gambia. *AIDS (London, England)*, *7*(8), 1093–1098. doi:10.1097/00002030-199308000-00011

Pitman, B. (2003). Leading for Value. *Harvard Business Review*, (Apr): 41–46.

PNG DoH. (2001). *National Health Plan 2001-2010*. Port Moresby: Department of Health, Government of Papua New Guinea.

Podrazik, P. M., & Whelan, C. T. (2008). Acute Hospital Care for the Elderly Patient: Its Impact on Clinical and Hospital Systems of Care. [doi: DOI: 10.1016/j.mcna.2007.11.004]. *Medical Clinics of North America*, *92*(2), 387-406.

Polat, G., Tamer, L., Tanriverdi, K., Gürkan, E., Baslamisli, F., & Atik, U. (n.d.). Levels of Malondialdehyde, Glutathione and Ascorbic Acid in Idiopathic Thromboctytopoenic Purpura. *East African Medical Journal*, *79*(8), 446-449.

Poole, M., Holmes, M., Watson, R., & DeSanctis, G. (1993). Group decision support systems and group communication. *Communication Research*, *20*(2), 176–213. doi:10.1177/009365093020002002

Pope, C., Ziebland, S., & Mays, N. 1999, E. B. B. (1999). Analysing Qualitative Data In Pope C & Mays N (Eds.), *Qualitative Research in Healthcare* (Second ed.). London: BMJ Books.

Powell-Tuck, J. (2009). Teams, strategies and networks: developments in nutritional support; a personal perspective. *The Proceedings of the Nutrition Society*, *68*(3), 289–295. doi:10.1017/S0029665109001311

Provan, D., Stasi, R., & Newland, A. C. (2010). International consensus report on the investigation and management of primary immune thrombocytopenia. *Blood*, *115*, 168–186. doi:10.1182/blood-2009-06-225565

Pullman, D., Bethune, C., & Duke, P. (2005). Narrative means to humanistic ends. *Teaching and Learning in Medicine*, *17*, 279–284. doi:10.1207/s15328015tlm1703_14

Purcell, G. P. (2005). What makes a good clinical decision support system. *British Medical Journal*, *330*, 740–741. doi:10.1136/bmj.330.7494.740

Qian, H., & Scott, C. (2007). Anonymity and self-disclosure on weblogs. *Journal of Computer-Mediated Communication*, *12*(4), 1428–1451. doi:10.1111/j.1083-6101.2007.00380.x

Radley, A. (1994). *Making Sense of Illness: The Social Psychology of Health & Illness*. London: Sage.

Rainer, T. (1979, 2004). *The New Diary. How to Use a Journal for Self-guidance and Expanded Creativity*. Tarcher Publ.

Rajendra, A., Hegde, B. M., Subbabba, B. P., Ashok, R., & Niranjan, C. U. (2002, September). Wavelet Analysis of Heart Rate Variability: New Method of Studying the Heart's Functions. *Kuwait Medical Journal*, *34*(3), 195–200.

Ralston, J. D., Carrell, D., Reid, R., Anderson, M., Moran, M., & Hereford, J. (2007). Patient Web Services Integrated with a Shared Medical Record: Patient Use and Satisfaction. *Journal of the American Medical Informatics Association*, *14*(6), 798–806. doi:10.1197/jamia.M2302

Rananand, P. (2003). Internet and democracy in Thailand. In Banerjee, I. (Ed.), *Rhetoric and reality: The Internet challenge for democracy in Asia*. Singapore: Times Media.

Red blood cell distribution width (2009). *Wikipedia, the free encyclopedia*. Retrieved June 15, 2009 from http://en.wikipedia.org/wiki/Red_blood_cell_distribution_width

Redley, B., Botti, M., & Duke, M. (2006). Family Member Presence during Resuscitation in the Emergency Department: an Australian Perspective. *Emergency Medicine Australasia*, *16*, 295–308.

RedOrbit Staff & Wire Reports. (2008). *Drug Information Often Left Out On Wikipedia*. Retrieved from http://www.redorbit.com/news/health/1602644/drug_information_often_left_out_on_wikipedia/index.html

Rehman, S. U., Nietert, P. J., Cope, D. W., & Kilpatrick, A. (2005). What to wear today? Effect of doctor's attire on the trust and confidence of patients. *The American Journal of Medicine, 118*, 1279–1286. doi:10.1016/j.amjmed.2005.04.026

Retsas, A. S. (2000). Barriers to using research evidence in nursing practice. *Journal of Advanced Nursing, 31*(3), 599–606. doi:10.1046/j.1365-2648.2000.01315.x

Revere, D., & Dunbar, P. J. (2001). Review of Computer-generated Outpatient Health Behavior Interventions: Clinical Encounters "in Absentia". *Journal of the American Medical Informatics Association, 8*(1), 62–79.

Rice, R. E. (2006). Influences, usage, and outcomes of Internet health information searching: Multivariate results from the Pew surveys. *International Journal of Medical Informatics, 75*, 8–28. doi:10.1016/j.ijmedinf.2005.07.032

Richardson, S., Casey, M., & Hider, P. (2007). Following the patient journey: Older persons' experiences of emergency departments and discharge. *Accident and Emergency Nursing, 15*(3), 134–140. doi:10.1016/j.aaen.2007.05.004

Rier, D. A. (2001). The Missing Voice of the Critically Ill: a Medical Sociologist's First-Person Account. *Sociology of Health & Illness, 22*(1), 68–93. doi:10.1111/1467-9566.00192

Rifkin, S., Muller, F., & Bichmann, W. (1988). Primary health care: on measuring participation. *Social Science & Medicine, 26*(9), 931–940. doi:10.1016/0277-9536(88)90413-3

Rigaux, N. (2005). [Journey to dementia]. *Psychologie & Neuropsychiatrie du Vieillissement, 3*(2), 107–114.

Robinson, S. M., Mackenzie-Ross, S., Campbell-Hewson, G. L., Egleston, C. V., & Prevost, A. T. (1998). Psychological Effect of Witnessed Resuscitation on Bereaved Relatives. *Lancet, 352*, 614–617. doi:10.1016/S0140-6736(97)12179-1

Robinson, I. (1990). Personal narratives, social careers and medical courses: Analysing life trajectories in autobiographies of people with multiple sclerosis. *Social Science & Medicine, 30*(11), 1173–1186. doi:10.1016/0277-9536(90)90257-S

Rockwood, K., Wallack, M., & Tallis, R. (2003). The treatment of Alzheimer's disease: success short of cure. *The Lancet Neurology, 2*(10), 630–633. doi:10.1016/S1474-4422(03)00533-7

Rodeghiero, F., Stasi, R., & Gernsheimer, T. (2009). Standardization of terminology, definitions and outcome criteria in immune thrombocytopenic purpura of adults and children: report from an international working group. *Blood, 113*, 2386–2393. doi:10.1182/blood-2008-07-162503

Rogers, J. A., Vergare, M. J., Baron, R. C., & Salzer, M. S. (2007). Barriers to recovery and recommendations for change: the Pennsylvania consensus conference on psychiatry's role. *Psychiatric Services (Washington, D.C.), 58*, 1119–1123. doi:10.1176/appi.ps.58.8.1119

Rogers, E. M. (1995). *Diffusion of innovations* (4th ed.). New York: Free Press.

Rose, N. (2007). *The politics of life itself: Biomedicine, power, and subjectivity in the twenty-first century*. NJ: Princeton University Press.

Ross, S. (2009). *Travels with Shubh: A Memoir of the MetaWorks Journey*. Bloomington, IN: iUniverse.

Rothman, D. (2009). *List of Medical Wikis*. Retrieved from http://davidrothman.net/list-of-medical-wikis/

Royal Pharmaceutical Society of Great Britain. (1997). *From Compliance to Concordance: Achieving Shared Goals in Medicine Taking*. Published Jointly by RPSGB and Merck Sharp & Dome.

Royston, P., & Altman, D. (1995). Using fractional polynomials to model curved regression relationships. *Stata Technical Bulletin, 4*(21).

Ryan, D., Cobern, W., Wheeler, J., Price, D., & Tarassenko, L. (2005). Mobile phone technology in the management of asthma. *Journal of Telemedicine and Telecare, 11*(Suppl 1), 43–46. doi:10.1258/1357633054461714

Ryan, P. (2009). Integrated theory of health behaviour change. *Clinical Nurse Specialist CNS, 23*(3), 161–170. doi:10.1097/NUR.0b013e3181a42373

Ryan, R., & Deci, E. (2000). Self-determination theory and the facilitation of intrinsic motivation, social development, and well-being. *The American Psychologist, 55*(1), 68–78. doi:10.1037/0003-066X.55.1.68

Sa, E., Sekikawa, A., Linkov, F., Lovalekar, M., & LaPorte, R. E. (2003). Open source model for global collaboration in higher education. *International Journal of Medical Informatics, 71*(2-3), 165. doi:10.1016/S1386-5056(03)00108-4

Sackett, D. L., Rosenberg, W. M., Gray, J. A., Haynes, R. B., & Richardson, W. S. (1996). Evidence based medicine: what it is and what it isn't. *British Medical Journal, 312*(7023), 71–72.

Sackett, D.L. Strauss, S.E. Richardson, W. S. Rosenberg, W.and Haynes, R.B. *Evidence Based Medicine How to Practice and Teach EBM*, 2nd Edition Edinburgh Churchill Livingstone

Salvador, C. H., Pascual Carrasco, M., Gonzalez de Mingo, M. A., Munoz Carrero, A., Marquez Montes, J., & Sosa Martin, L. (2005). Airmed-cardio: a GSM and Internet services-based system for out-of-hospital follow-up of cardiac patients. *IEEE Transactions on Information Technology in Biomedicine, 9*(1), 73–85. doi:10.1109/TITB.2004.840067

Sammet, K. (2003). University hospital Hamburg-Eppendorf, University of Hamburg, Institute for the history and ethics of medicine. *Academic Medicine, 78*, 1070–1071. doi:10.1097/00001888-200310000-00043

Sandars, J., & Haythornthwaite, C. (2007). New horizons for e-learning in medical education: ecological and Web 2.0 perspectives. *Medical Teacher, 29*, 307–310. doi:10.1080/01421590601176406

Sandars, J., & Schroter, S. (2007). Web 2.0 technologies for undergraduate and postgraduate medical education: An online survey. *Postgraduate Medical Journal, 83*, 759–762. doi:10.1136/pgmj.2007.063123

Sanger, J. (1994). Seven types of creativity: looking for insights in data analysis. *British Educational Research Journal, 20*(2), 175–185. doi:10.1080/0141192940200203

Sarbadhikari, S. N. (2005). The State of Medical Informatics in India: A Roadmap for optimal organization. *Journal of Medical Systems, 29*, 125–141. doi:10.1007/s10916-005-3001-y

Sarbadhikari, S. N. (2008). How to design an effective e-learning course for medical education. *Indian Journal of Medical Informatics, 3*(1). Retrieved from http://ijmi.org/index.php/ijmi/article/view/y08i1a3/15.

Sarup, M. (1993). *An introductory guide to post-structuralism and postmodernism* (2nd ed.). Athens, GA: University of Georgia Press.

Save the Children. (2003). Papua New Guinea: Training volunteers to improve community health. Retrieved from http://www.savethechildren.net/new_zealand/what_we_do/our_projects/papua_new_guinea.html

Sawyer, R. K. (2005). *Social emergence: societies as complex systems.* Cambridge, UK: Cambridge University Press. doi:10.1017/CBO9780511734892

Sawyer, R. K. (2006). *Explaining creativity: The science of human innovation.* Oxford, UK: Oxford University Press.

Sawyer, R. K. (2008). *Group genius: The creative power of collaboration.* New York: Basic Books.

Scambler, G. (2004). Re-framing stigma: Felt and enacted stigma and challenges to the sociology of chronic and disabling conditions. *Social Theory & Health, 2*, 29–46. doi:10.1057/palgrave.sth.8700012

Schaefer, D., & Dervin, B. (2009). From the dialogic to the contemplative: A conceptual and empirical rethinking of online communication outcomes as verbing micropractices. *Ethics and Information Technology, 11*(4), 265–278. doi:10.1007/s10676-009-9206-x

Schaefer, D. (1999a). From community to community-ing. *Electronic Journal of Communication, 9* (2, 3, 4).

Schaefer, D. (1999b). *Sense-making design for web sites: Cyber-possibilities for an electronic public sphere.* Paper presented at the session "Methodology between the cracks: Sense-Making as exemplar," International Communication Association 49th Annual Conference, San Francisco, CA, May 27, 1999.

Schaefer, D. (2000). *Rethinking Electronic Public Spheres: Beyond Consensus/Dissensus.* Paper presented at the conference "Social Justice, Peace, and International Conflict Resolution: Civic Discourse beyond the Millennium," Rochester Institute of Technology, Rochester, NY, July 20-22, 2000.

Schaefer, D. (2001). *Dynamics of electronic public spheres: Verbing online participation.* (Doctoral Dissertation, The Ohio State University, Columbus, OH, U.S.A.).

Schaefer, D., & Dervin, B. (2001). *Dialoguing in electronic public spheres: Reconceptualizing participation as verbing micro-practices.* Paper presented at the sixth annual Rochester Intercultural Conference "The Intercultural World and the Digital Connection," Rochester Institute of Technology, Rochester, NY, July 19-21, 2001.

Schaefer, D., & Dervin, B. (2003). *The constitution and distortion of electronic public spheres: A conceptual and empirical rethinking of online communication outcomes as verbing micropractices.* Paper presented at the International Communication Association annual meeting, San Diego, CA, May 23- 27, 2003.

Scherr, D., Zweiker, R., Kollmann, A., Kastner, P., Schreier, G., & Fruhwald, F. M. (2006). Mobile phone-based surveillance of cardiac patients at home. *Journal of Telemedicine and Telecare, 12*(5), 255–261. doi:10.1258/135763306777889046

Schneider, S. (1997). *Expanding the public sphere through computer-mediated communications: Political discussion about abortion in a Usenet news group.* (Doctoral Dissertation, Massachusetts Institute of Technology, 1997).

Schoen, C., Osborn, R., Doty, M. M., Squires, D., Peugh, J., & Applebaum, S. (2009). A Survey Of Primary Care Physicians In Eleven Countries, 2009: Perspectives On Care, Costs, And Experiences. *Health Affairs, 28*(6), w1171–w1183. doi:10.1377/hlthaff.28.6.w1171

Schonewille, M. (2005). *An adaptive Interface.* (Draft), Nijmegen school of Management

Schonfeld, E., & Morrison, C. (2007). The next disruptors: The 10 game changing startups most likely to upend existing industries and spawn new entrepreneurial opportunities. *Business 2.0, 8*(8), 56-64.

Schroeder, R. (2006). Being There Together and the Future of Connected Presence. *Presence (Cambridge, Mass.), 15*(4), 438–454. doi:10.1162/pres.15.4.438

Schroeder, D., & Gefenas, E. (2009). Vulnerability: too vague and too broad? *Cambridge quarterly of healthcare ethics: CQ: the international journal of healthcare ethics committees, 18*(2), 113-121.

Schuster, M. A., McGlynn, E. A., & Brook, R. H. (1998). How good is the quality of health care in the United States? *The Milbank Quarterly, 76*(4), 517–563. doi:10.1111/1468-0009.00105

Schwartz, J. (2008). Logging on for a second (or third) opinion. (Sep 29), *New York Times.*

Scott, P. A. (2000). The relationship between the arts and medicine. *Medical Humanities, 26,* 3–8. doi:10.1136/mh.26.1.3

Selman, T. J., Prakash, T., & Khan, K. S. (2006). Quality of health information for cervical cancer treatment on the internet. *BMC Women's Health, 6,* 9. doi:10.1186/1472-6874-6-9

Sevenhuijsen, S. (1998). *Citizenship and the ethics of care: Feminist consideration on justice, morality and politics.* New York: Routledge.

Shankar, P. R. (2007). Conducting a voluntary module: personal experiences. *Journal of Medical Sciences Research, 2,* 55–58.

Shankar, P. R. (2008). A voluntary medical humanities module at the Manipal College of medical sciences, Pokhara, Nepal. *Family Medicine, 40*, 468–470.

Shankar, P. R. (2008a). Medical students and medical teachers learn together: preliminary experiences from Western Nepal. *South East Asian Journal of Medical Education, 2*, 79–82.

Shankar, P. R. (2009). A Voluntary Medical Humanities Module in a Medical College in Western Nepal: Participant feedback. *Teaching and Learning in Medicine, 21*, 248–253. doi:10.1080/10401330903020605

Shankar, P. R. (2009c). Design the shoe according to the foot! *The Clinical Teacher, 6*, 67–68. doi:10.1111/j.1743-498X.2009.00269.x

Shankar, P. R. (2010). Sir Robert Hutchison's petition and the medical humanities. *International Journal of Medical Education, 1*, 2–4. doi:10.5116/ijme.4b8a.fba9

Shankar, P. R., & Piryani, R. M. (2009). Using paintings to explore the Medical Humanities in a Nepalese medical school. *Medical Humanities, 35*, 121–122. doi:10.1136/jmh.2009.002568

Shankar, P. R. (2008b). Using case scenarios and role plays to explore issues of human sexuality. *Education for Health (Abingdon), 20*.

Shankar, P. R. (2008c). Can medical humanities take root in Asia? *Journal of Clinical and Diagnostic Research*, JCDR (published online first 24 Feb 2008).

Shankar, P. R. (2008d). *Medical humanities: sowing the seeds in the Himalayan country of Nepal. Literature, arts and medicine blog*. Posted April 14th, 2008. Retrieved December 8, 2009, from http://medhum.med.nyu.edu/blog/?p=113

Shankar, P. R. (2009b). Creating and maintaining participant interest in the Medical Humanities. *Literature, art and medicine Blog Posted October 28th, 2009*. Retrieved December 8, 2009, from http://medhum.med.nyu.edu/blog/?p=215

Shankar, P. R., & Piryani, R. M. (2009a). English as the language of Medical Humanities learning in Nepal: Our experiences. *The literature, art and medicine blog Posted on 22nd April 2009*. Retrieved December 8, 2009 from http://medhum.med.nyu.edu/blog/?p=175

Shankar, R. (2008e). *Arts and humanities: a neglected aspect of education in South Asia. BMJ Medical Humanities Blog posted on 17th July 2008*. Retrieved December 8, 2009, from http://blogs.bmj.com/medical-humanities/2008/07/17/arts-and-humanities-a-neglected-aspect-of-education-in-south-asia/

Shankar, R. (2009a). Establishing a medical humanities in Nepal with the help of a FAIMER fellowship. *BMJ Medical Humanities blog* posted 7th December 2009. Retrieved December 9, 2009, from http://blogs.bmj.com/medical-humanities/2009/12/07/establishing-a-medical-humanities-in-nepal-with-the-help-of-a-faimer-fellowship-by-ravi-shankar/

Shapiro, J., Coulehan, J., Wear, D., & Montello, M. (2009). Medical Humanities and Their Discontents: Definitions, Critiques, and Implications. *Academic Medicine, 84*, 192–198. doi:10.1097/ACM.0b013e3181938bca

Shapiro, J., Morrison, E. H., & Boker, J. R. (2004). Teaching empathy to first year medical students: Evaluation of an elective literature and medicine course. *Education for Health (Abingdon), 17*, 73–84. doi:10.1080/135762 80310001656196

Shapiro, J., & Rucker, L. (2003). Can poetry make better doctors? Teaching the humanities and arts to medical students and residents at the University of California, Irvine, College of Medicine. *Academic Medicine, 78*, 953–957. doi:10.1097/00001888-200310000-00002

Sharples, M. (2002). Disruptive Devices: Mobile Technology for Conversational Learning. *International Journal of Continuing Engineering Education and Lifelong Learning, 12*(5/6), 504–520. doi:10.1504/IJCEELL.2002.002148

Sharrock, W., & Button, G. (1997). On the relevance of Habermas' theory of communicative action for CSCW. *Computer Supported Cooperative Work, 6*, 369–389. doi:10.1023/A:1008644224566

Shaughnessy, A. F., Slawson, D. C., & Becker, L. (1998). Clinical jazz: harmonizing clinical experience and evidence-based medicine. *The Journal of Family Practice*, *47*, 425–428.

Shephard, K. (2003). Questioning, promoting and evaluating the use of streaming video to support student learning. *British Journal of Educational Technology*, *34*(3), 295–308. doi:10.1111/1467-8535.00328

Shepperd, S., Doll, H., Angus, R. M., Clarke, M. J., Iliffe, S., & Kalra, L. (2009). Avoiding hospital admission through provision of hospital care at home: a systematic review and meta-analysis of individual patient data. *Canadian Medical Association Journal*, *180*(2), 175–182. doi:10.1503/cmaj.081491

Sheridan, B. (2008). Open wide: The open-source movement worked wonders for software. Can it do the same for diabetes and other illnesses?" *NewsWeek*. Retrieved from http://www.newsweek.com/id/164231

Sherry, J. F., Storm, D., Duhachek, A., Nuttavuthisit, K., & Deberry-Spence, B. (2004).Ludic agency and retail spectacle. *The Journal of Consumer Research*, *31*(3), 658–672. doi:10.1086/425101

Shirky, C. (2009). *Here comes everybody: the power of organizing without organizations*. New York: Penguin.

Shivas, T. (2004). Contextualizing the vulnerability standard. *Am. J. Bioeth*, *4*(3), 84-86; discussion W32.

Short, J., Williams, E., & B., C. (1976). *The Social Psychology of Telecommunications*. New York: John Wiley.

Shreeve, S., Holt, M., & O'Grady, L. (2007). *Health 2.0 Definition*. Retrieved December 2007, from http://health20.org/wiki/Health_2.0_Definition

Sikes, P. (2007). *Auto/biographical and narrative approaches*. Retrieved from http://www.bera.ac.uk/autobiographical-and-narrative-approaches/

Silva, S. A., & Wyer, P. C. (2009). Where Is The Wisdom? II. Evidence-Based Medicine and The Epistemological Crisis in Clinical Medicine. Exposition and Commentary on Djulbegovic, B., Guyatt, G.H. & Ashcroft, R.E. (2009) *Cancer* Control, 16, 158-168. *Journal of Evaluation in Clinical Practice*, *15*, 899–906. doi:10.1111/j.1365-2753.2009.01324.x

Sim, I., Gorman, P., Greenes, R. A., Haynes, R. B., Kaplan, B., & Lehmann, H. (2001). Clinical decision support systems for the practice of evidence-based medicine. *Journal of the American Medical Informatics Association*, *8*, 527–534.

Sim, J., & Madden, S. (2008). Illness experience in fibromyalgia syndrome: A metasynthesis of qualitative studies. *Social Science & Medicine*, *67*, 57–67. doi:10.1016/j.socscimed.2008.03.003

Simms, P. A. (2002) Papua New Guinea needs law and order above all. *British Medical Journal*. 2002 325:914-915 (26 October)

Simon, H. A. (1947). *Administrative behaviour: a study of decision-making processes in administrative organisations*. New York: The Free press.

Simon, H. A. (1982). *Models of bounded rationality*. Vols 1 and 2. Cambridge and London, respectively: MIT press.

Sirovich, B., Gallagher, P. M., Wennberg, D. E., & Fisher, E. S. (2008). Discretionary decision making by primary care physicians and the cost of U.S. health care. *Health Affairs*, *27*(3), 813–823..doi:10.1377/hlthaff.27.3.813

Skelton, J. R. (2000). Teaching literature and medicine to medical students, part I: The beginning. *Lancet*, *356*, 1920–1922. doi:10.1016/S0140-6736(00)03270-0

Skinner, H. A., Maley, O., & Norman, C. D. (2006). Developing Internet-based eHealth promotion programs: the spiral technology action research (STAR) model. *Health Promotion Practice*, *7*(4), 406–417. doi:10.1177/1524839905278889

Slater, D., & Tonkiss, F. (2001). *Market society: Markets and modern social theory*. London: Polity Press.

Sliedrecht, S. (2007). *Counselling patients with a spinal cord injury*. Unpublished master's thesis, University of Waikato, New Zealand.

Smaling, A. (2000). What kind of dialogue should paradigm-dialogues be? *Quality & Quantity, 34*, 51–63. doi:10.1023/A:1004747524463

Small, M. L. (2009). *Unanticipated gains: origins of network inequality in everyday life*. New York: Oxford University Press.

Smith, R. (1996). What clinical information do doctors' need? *BMJ (Clinical Research Ed.), 313*, 1062–1068.

Smith, E., & Bodner, D. (1993). Sexual dysfunction after spinal cord injury. *The Urologic Clinics of North America, 20*, 535–542.

Smith, C., McLaughlin, M., & Osborne, K. (1998). From terminal ineptitude to virtual sociopathy: how conduct is regulated on Usenet. In Sudweeks, F., McLaughlin, M., & Rafaeli, S. (Eds.), *Network and Netplay*. Menlo Park, CA: AAAI/MIT Press.

Smith, D., Defalla, B. A., & Chadwick, D. W. (1999). The misdiagnosis of epilepsy and the management of refractory epilepsy in a specialist clinic. *QJMed: An International Journal of Medicine, 92*, 15-23.

Snowden, D. (2002). Narrative patterns: uses of story in the third age of knowledge management. *Journal of information and knowledge management*.

Sochalski, J., Jaarsma, T., Krumholz, H. M., Laramee, A., McMurray, J. J. V., & Naylor, M. D. (2009). What Works In Chronic Care Management: The Case Of Heart Failure. *Health Affairs, 28*(1), 179–189. doi:10.1377/hlthaff.28.1.179

Sparkes, A. C., & Smith, B. M. (2006). When narratives matter: men, sport, and spinal cord injury. In Rapport, F., & Wainwright, P. *eds*. (2006). *The Self in Health and Illness* pp.53-67. Abingdon: Radcliffe Publishing Ltd.

Sperry, R. W., Gazzaniga, M. S., & Bogen, J. E. (1969). Interhemisphere relationship, the neocortical commisures, Syndromes of hemisphere disconnection. In *Handbook of Clinical Neurology*. Inken, (ed), Amsterdam.

Spike, J. P. (2003). Developing a medical humanities concentration in the medical curriculum at the University of Rochester School of medicine and dentistry, Rochester, New York. *Academic Medicine, 78*, 983–986. doi:10.1097/00001888-200310000-00008

Spiller, R. C., Jenkins, D., Thornley, J. P., Hebden, J. M., Wright, T., & Skinner, M. (2000). Increased rectal mucosal enteroendocrine cells, T lymphocytes, and increased gut permeability following acute Campylobacter enteritis and in post-dysenteric irritable bowel syndrome. *Gut, 47*(6), 804–811. doi:10.1136/gut.47.6.804

Sproull, L., & Kiesler, S. (1991). *Connections: New ways of working in the networked organization*. Cambridge, MA: MIT.

St. Joseph County Public Library. (2009). *Subject Guide (Wiki)*. Retrieved from http://www.libraryforlife.org/subjectguides/index.php/Main_Page

Stark, L. J., Jelalian, E., McGrath, A. N., & Mackner, L. (2001). Behavioural Approaches to Cystic Fibrosis: Applications to Feeding and Eating. In *Bluebond-Langner, A., Lask, B., & Angst, D. B. (2001). Psychosocial Aspects of Cystic Fibrosis* (pp. 348–360). London: Arnold.

Stasi, R., Sarpatwari, A., & Sega, J. B. (2009). Effects of eradication of Helicobacter pylori infection in patients with immune thrombocytopenic purpura: a systematic review. *Blood, 113*, 1231–1240. doi:10.1182/blood-2008-07-167155

Statistics Canada. (2006b). *Inuit Health and Social Conditions, Aboriginal Peoples Survey*. Statistics Canda.

Stave, K. (2002). Using system dynamics to improve public participation in environmental decisions. *System Dynamics Review*.

Stewart, W. F., Shah, N. R., & Selna, M. J. (2007, March/April). Bridging The Inferential Gap: The Electronic Health Record and Clinical Evidence. *Health Affairs*, *26*(2), 181–191. doi:10.1377/hlthaff.26.2.w181

Stockl, A. (2007). Complex syndromes, ambivalent diagnosis, and existential uncertainty: The case of Systemic Lupus Erythematosus (SLE). *Social Science & Medicine*, *65*, 1549–1550. doi:10.1016/j.socscimed.2007.05.016

Storli, S. L., Lindseth, A., & Asplund, K. (2008). A journey in quest of meaning: a hermeneutic-phenomenological study on living with memories from intensive care. *Nursing in Critical Care*, *13*(2), 86–96. doi:10.1111/j.1478-5153.2007.00235.x

Straus, S. (1996). Getting a clue: The effects of communication media and information distribution on participation and performance in computer-mediated and face-to-face groups. *Small Group Research*, *27*(1), 115–142. doi:10.1177/1046496496271006

Straus, S. E., & McAlister, F. A. (2000). Evidence-based medicine: a commentary on common criticisms. *Canadian Medical Association Journal*, *163*(7), 837–841.

Straus, S. E., Richardson, W. S., Glasziou, P., & Haynes, R. B. (2005). *Evidence-based medicine: how to practice and teach EBM*. Edinburgh: Churchill Livingstone.

Stringer, E. T. (1996). *Action research: A handbook for practitioners*. Thousand Oaks, CA: Sage.

Strohman, R. C. (1995). Linear genetics, non-linear epigenetics: complementary approaches to understanding complex diseases. *Integrative Physiological and Behavioral Science*, *30*, 273. doi:10.1007/BF02691601

Sturmberg, J. P., & Martin, C. M. (2006). Rethinking General Practice - Part 1: Far from Equilibrium. Disease-Centred and Econometric-Oriented Health Care and General Practice/Family Medicine. *Asia Pacific Family Medicine*, *5*(2).

Sturmberg, J. P., Reid, A., & Khadra, M. H. (2001). Community Based Medical Education in a Rural Area: A New Direction in Undergraduate Training. *The Australian Journal of Rural Health*, *9*(Suppl 1), 14–18. doi:10.1046/j.1440-1584.9.s1.6.x

Sturmberg, J. P., Reid, S., & Khadra, M. H. (2002). A Longitudinal, Patient-Centred, Integrated Curriculum: Facilitating Community-Based Education in a Rural Clinical School. *Education for Health*, *15*(3), 294–304. doi:10.1080/1357628021000012787

Sturmberg, J., Martin, C., & Moes, M. (2010). (in press). Health at the Centre of Health Systems Reform – How Philosophy Can Inform Policy. *Perspectives in Biology and Medicine*.

Sturmberg, J. P., & Martin, C. M. (2008). Knowing - in Medicine. *Journal of Evaluation in Clinical Practice*, *14*(5), 767–770. doi:10.1111/j.1365-2753.2008.01011.x

Sturmberg, J. P. (2007). *The Foundations of Primary Care*. Oxford, UK: Radcliffe Publishing.

Sturt, J. (1999). Placing empowerment research within an action research typology. *Journal of Advanced Nursing*, *30*(5), 1057–1063. doi:10.1046/j.1365-2648.1999.01202.x

Suitor, J., & Keeton, S. (1997). Once a friend, always a friend? Effects of homophily on women's support networks across a decade. *Social Networks*, *19*, 51–62. doi:10.1016/S0378-8733(96)00290-0

Sumathipala, A. (2006). Bioethics in Sri Lanka. *Eastern Mediterranean Health Journal*, *12*(1), S73–S79.

Surman, M., & Weshler-Henry, D. (2001). *Common space: beyond virtual community*. Toronto, ON: Pearson - Financial Times.

Surowiecki, J. P. (2004). *Wisdom of the crowds*. New York: Random house.

Survey of Non-traditional Treatments of ITP. (2001). *Survey of Non-traditional Treatments of ITP*. Retrieved from http://www.pdsa.org/about-itp/surveys/item/113.html

Sutra (n.d.). *Spiritual-Theosophy Dictionary on Sutra*. Retrieved from http://www.experiencefestival.com/a/Sutra/id/195147

Swami, S. S. (1981). Hathayoga (Kunjal kriya). In Swami, S. S. (Ed.), *A systematic course in the ancient tantric techniques of Yoga and Kriya, Bihar school of Yoga* (pp. 205–214).

Swennen, M. H. J., van der Heijden, G. J. M. G., Blijham, G. H., & Kalkman, C. J. (in press). Career stage and work setting create different barriers for Evidence-based Medicine. *Journal of Evaluation in Clinical Practice*.

Swerrisen, H., Weeks, A., Belfrage, J., Furler, J., Walker, C., & McAvoy, B. (2006). A randomized control trial of a self-management program for people with a chronic illness from Vietnamese, Chinese, Italian and Greek backgrounds. *Patient Education and Counseling, 64*(1-3), 360–368. doi:10.1016/j.pec.2006.04.003

Szumilas, M., & Kutcher, S. (2009). Teen suicidal information on the Internet: a systematic analysis of quality. *Canadian Journal of Psychiatry, 54*, 596–604.

Tan, J. (2005). *E-health care information systems*. New York: Wiley Imprint.

Tan, H., & Ng, J. H. K. (2006). Googling for a diagnosis—use of Google as a diagnostic aid: Internet based study. *British Medical Journal, 333*, 1143–1145. doi:10.1136/bmj.39003.640567.AE

Tang, P. C., Ash, J. S., Bates, D. W., Overhage, J. M., & Sands, D. Z. (2006). Personal Health Records: Definitions, Benefits, and Strategies for Overcoming Barriers to Adoption. *Journal of the American Medical Informatics Association, 13*(2), 121–126. doi:10.1197/jamia.M2025

Tang, W.-Y., & Ho, S.-M. (2007). Epigenetic reprogramming and imprinting in origins of disease. *Reviews in Endocrine & Metabolic Disorders, 8*(2), 173–182. doi:10.1007/s11154-007-9042-4

Tapscott, D., & Williams, A. D. (2008). *Wikinomics: How mass collaboration changes everything*. New York: Portfolio Penguin Group.

Taubes, T. (1998). Healthy avenues of the mind": psychological theory building and the influence of religion during the era of moral treatment. *The American Journal of Psychiatry, 155*, 1001–1008.

Tayson, D. B. (2007). *Library 2.0, Library Service & Web 2.0*. [PPT Slide] Retrieved December, 2009, from www.tbs-sct.gc.ca/im-gi/imday07jourgi/pres/library-biblio/library-biblio-eng.ppt

Teatree Oil. (n.d.). *Teatree Oil Information*. Retrieved April 2002, from http://www.teatree.co.uk/cuttings.html.

Tech, M. M., Radhakrishnan, S., & Subbaraj, P. (2009). Elderly patient monitoring system using a wireless sensor network. *Telemedicine Journal and e-Health, 15*, 73. doi:10.1089/tmj.2008.0056

Terranova, T. (2004). *Network culture: Politics for the information age*. London: Pluto Press.

The Economist. (2007). *Health 2.0: Technology and society: Is the outbreak of cancer videos, bulimia blogs and other forms of "user generated" medical information a healthy trend?* The Economist, September 6: 73-74

The National Institute of Neurological Disorders and Stroke rt-PA Stroke study group. (1995). Tissue Plaminogen Activator for Acute Ischemic Stroke. *New England Journal of Medicine, 333*(24), 1581-1588.

The National Working Group on Evidence-Based Health Care. (2008). Advancing the Evidence of Experience: Practical Issues for Patient/Consumer Inclusion http://www.evidencebasedhealthcare.org/index.cfm?objectid=80363086-1372-4D20-C8275AD-1BBB7C263

The New York Times (March 6, 2007). The Difficult Patient, a Problem Old as History (or Older) by Abigail Zuger.

The Patient Information Centre. (2009). *The patient Information Center, Northumberland, NHS*. Retrieved from http://www.ntw.nhs.uk/pic/?p=about

Thiagarajan P. (2006). *Platelet disorders, E-medicine from web MD*. Retrieved August 16, 2007, from webmd.com

Thiagarajan, P. (2009). *Platelet disorders, E-medicine (Medscape)*. Retrieved June 16 2009 from http://emedicine.medscape.com/article/201722-treatment

Thompson, L., Dawson, K., Ferdig, R., Black, E., Boyer, J., Coutts, J., & Black, N. P. (2008). The intersection of online social networking with medical professionalism. *Journal of General Internal Medicine, 23*(7), 954–957. doi:10.1007/s11606-008-0538-8

Thompson, C. J. (2004). Marketplace mythology and discourses of power. *The Journal of Consumer Research, 31*(1), 162–180. doi:10.1086/383432

Thorne, S., Armstrong, E. A., Harris, S. R., Hislop, T. G., Kim-Sing, C., & Oglov, V. (2009). Patient real-time and 12-month retrospective perceptions of difficult communications in the cancer diagnostic period. *Qualitative Health Research, 19*(10), 1383–1394. doi:10.1177/1049732309348382

Tikki, P., Muir, G., & Evans, T. (2006). A 15th grand challenge for global public health. *Lancet, 367*, 284–286. Retrieved from http://www.thelancet.com/journals/lancet/article/PIIS0140673606680501/fulltext. doi:10.1016/S0140-6736(06)68050-1

Tilburt, J. C. (2008). Evidence bsed medicine beyond the bedside: keeping an eye on the context. *Journal of Evaluation in Clinical Practice, 14*, 721–725. doi:10.1111/j.1365-2753.2008.00948.x

Timmer, J. (2000). *Living Within Intricate Futures: Order and Confusion in Imjan Worlds*. Holland: Centre for Pacific and Asian Studies.

Tokuda, Y., Hinohara, S., & Fukui, T. (2008). Introducing a new medical school system into Japan. *Annals of the Academy of Medicine, Singapore, 37*, 800–802.

Tonelli, M. (2006). Integrating evidence into clinical practice: an alternative to evidence-based approaches. *Journal of Evaluation in Clinical Practice, 12*, 248–256. doi:10.1111/j.1365-2753.2004.00551.x

Transcript of radio broadcast: 28 October 2008. Retrieved from http://www.voanews.com/specialenglish/2008-10-28-voa2.cfm

Trust, C. F. (May 2006). *The Facts: An Introduction to Cystic Fibrosis*. Available at: http://www.cftrust.org.uk/aboutcf/publications/booklets/The_Facts_0506.pdf

Tsai, D. J. (2008). Community-oriented curriculum design for medical humanities. *The Kaohsiung Journal of Medical Sciences, 24*, 373–379. doi:10.1016/S1607-551X(08)70135-9

Tu, C.-H. (2000). On-line learning migration: from social learning theory to social presence theory in a CMC environment. *Journal of Network and Computer Applications, 23*(1), 27–37. doi:10.1006/jnca.1999.0099

Tucker, I, M. (2004). "Stories" of chronic fatigue syndrome: An exploratory discursive psychological analysis. *Qualitative Research in Psychology, 1*, 153–167. doi:10.1191/1478088704qp008oa

Tuomilehto, J., Lindstrom, J., Eriksson, J. G, & Valle, T, T, Hamalainen, H., Ilanne-Parikka, P., Keinanen-Kiukaanniemi, S., Laakso, M., Louheranta, A., Rastas, M. Salminen, V., Aunola, S., Cepaitis, Z., Moltchanov, V., Hakumaki, M., Mannelin, M., Martikkala, V., Sundvall, J., & Uusitupa, M. (2001). Prevention of type 2 diabetes mellitus by changes in lifestyle among subjects with impaired glucose tolerance. *The New England Journal of Medicine, 344*(18), 1343–1350. doi:10.1056/NEJM200105033441801

Turnbull, J. (2007). *9 Habits of Highly Effective Teachers*. New York: Continuum International Publishing group

Turner, B. S. (2008). *The Body and Society: Explorations in Social Theory* (3rd ed.). UK: Sage.

Turner, A. M., Petrochilos, D., Nelson, D. E., Allen, E., & Liddy, E. D. (2009). Access and use of the Internet for health information seeking: a survey of local public health professionals in the northwest. *Journal of Public Health Management and Practice, 15*(1), 67–69.

Turner, B. S. (1997). Foreword: From governmentality to risk: Some reflections on Foucault's contribution to medical sociology. In Peterson, A., & Bunton, R. (Eds.), *Foucault and Health*. London: Routledge.

U.S. Agency for Healthcare Research and Quality. (2007, March 12). AHRQ Quality Indicators—Guide to Prevention Quality Indicators: Hospital Admissions for Ambulatory Care Sensitive Conditions. Retrieved from http://www.qualityindicators.ahrq.gov/downloads/pqi/pqi_guide_v31.pdf

University of Otago. (2009). *RSS.* Retrieved from http://www.library.otago.ac.nz/otagolibrary.rss

User driven healthcare innovation (n.d.). *User driven healthcare innovation.* Retrieved from http://www.pervasivehealthcare.dk/projects/index.php#13

User driven test beds at Lombardi, Italy (n.d.). *User driven test beds at Lombardi, Italy.* Retrieved from http://www.remine-project.eu/index.php?option=com_content&task=view&id=12&Itemid=36

Valacich, J., Dennis, A., & Nunamaker, J. (1992). Group size and anonymity effects on computer-mediated idea generation. *Small Group Research, 23*(1), 49–73. doi:10.1177/1046496492231004

Valacich, J., George, J., Nunamaker, J., & Vogel, D. (1994). Physical proximity effects on computer-media group idea generation. *Small Group Research, 25*(1), 83–104. doi:10.1177/1046496494251006

Van de Ven, A. H., & Schomaker, M. S. (2002). Commentary: The Rhetoric of Evidence-Based Medicine. *Health Care Management Review, 27*, 90.

Van Der Weyden, M. B. (2007). Expanding primary care-based medical education: a renaissance of general practice? *The Medical Journal of Australia, 187*, 66–67. Retrieved from http://www.mja.com.au/public/issues/187_02_160707/van10686_fm.html.

van Manen, M. (1990). *Researching Lived Experience: Human Science for an Action Sensitive Pedagogy.* New York: State University of New York Press.

Vargo, S. L., & Lusch, R. F. (2004). Evolving to a new dominant logic for marketing. *Journal of Marketing, 68*(January), 1–17. doi:10.1509/jmkg.68.1.1.24036

Various authors. (2003). Special theme brief articles: United States. *Academic Medicine, 78*, 1059-68.

Vegni, E., Mauri, E., & Moja, E. A. (2005). Stories from doctors of patients with pain. A qualitative research on the physicians' perspective. *Supportive Care in Cancer, 13*(1), 18–25. doi:10.1007/s00520-004-0714-2

Venkatesh, V., Morris, M. G., Davis, G. B., & Davis, F. D. (2004). User acceptance of information technology: Toward a unified view. *Management Information Systems Quarterly, 27*(3), 425–478.

Venkatesh, A. (2006). Further evolving the new dominant logic of marketing: From services to the social construction of markets. *Marketing Theory, 6*(3), 299–316. doi:10.1177/1470593106066789

Venn, C. (2007). Cultural theory, biopolitics, and the question of power. *Theory, Culture & Society, 24*(3), 111–124. doi:10.1177/0263276407075957

Ventegodt, S., Andersen, N. J., & Merrick, J. (2003). The life mission theory II. The structure of the life purpose and the ego. *TheScientificWorldJournal, 3*, 1277–1285. doi:10.1100/tsw.2003.114

Venter, J. A., & Hannan, S. J. (2009). A complex case management system provides optimal care for all patients. *Journal of Refractive Surgery (Thorofare, N.J.), 25*(7Suppl), S655–S660.

VSO. (1999). *Country Profile PNG.* Retrieved April 5, 2005, from http://vsocanada.ca/attachments/papua_new_guinea.pdf

Wachtler, C., Lundin, S., & Troein, M. (2006). Humanities for medical students? A qualitative study of a medical humanities curriculum in a medical school program. *BMC Medical Education, 6*, 16. doi:10.1186/1472-6920-6-16

Wainfan, L., & Davis, P. K. (2004). *Challenges in Virtual Collaboration: Videoconferencing, Audio conferencing, and Computer-Mediated Communications.* Santa Monica: RAND National Defense Research Institute.

Wales, A. (2005). Managing knowledge to support the patient journey in NHS Scotland: strategic vision and practical reality. *Health Information and Libraries Journal, 22*(2), 83–95. doi:10.1111/j.1471-1842.2005.00572.x

Wales, A. (2008). A National Health Knowledge Network to support the patient journey. *Health Information and Libraries Journal, 25*(Suppl 1), 99–102. doi:10.1111/j.1471-1842.2008.00818.x

Walker, R. D., & Hurt, C. D. (1990). *Scientific And Technical Literature: An Introduction To Forms Of Communication*. Amer Library Assn.

Walker, C., & Millen, N. (2003). Stigma as social process: The role of stigma in chronic illness in C. Walker, C. Peterson, N. Millen and C. Martin (eds), *Chronic Illness: New Perspectives and New Directions*, Croydon, Tertiary Press, 82-93.

Wallerstein, N. (2006). *What is the evidence on effectiveness of empowerment to improve health? Health Evidence Network report*. Copenhagen: WHO Regional Office for Europe.

Walther, J. (1992). Interpersonal effects in computer-mediated interaction: A relational perspective. *Communication Research*, *19*(1), 52–90. doi:10.1177/009365092019001003

Wang, W. D., & Lue, B. H. (2003). National Taiwan University College of medicine: the design of medical humanities courses for clerkships. *Academic Medicine*, *78*, 1073–1074. doi:10.1097/00001888-200310000-00046

Ware, N. C. (1992). Suffering and the Social Construction of Illness: The Delegitimation of Illness Experience in Chronic Fatigue Syndrome. *Medical Anthropology Quarterly*, *6*(4), 347–361. doi:10.1525/maq.1992.6.4.02a00030

Ware, N. C., & Kleinman, A. (1992). Culture and somatic experience: the social course of illness in neurasthenia and chronic fatigue syndrome. *Psychosomatic Medicine*, *54*(5), 546–560.

Watanabe, M. (2007). Conflict and intolerance in a web community: Effects of a system integrating dialogues and monologues. *Journal of Computer-Mediated Communication*, *12*(3), 1020–1042. doi:10.1111/j.1083-6101.2007.00361.x

Waterloo Public Library. (2009). *Waterloo Public Library*. Retrieved from http://www.wplbookclub.blogspot.com uses blog as a book club

Watson, A. J. (2008). Brave New Worlds: How Virtual Environments Can Augment Traditional Care in the Management of Diabetes. *Journal of Diabetes Science and Technology*, *2*, 697–702.

Wear, D. (2003). The medical humanities at the northeastern Ohio Universities College of medicine: historical, theoretical, and curricular perspectives. *Academic Medicine*, *78*, 997–1000. doi:10.1097/00001888-200310000-00011

Weightman, A. L., & Williamson, J. (2005). The value and impact of information provided through library services for patient care: a systematic review. *Health Information and Libraries Journal*, *22*(1), 4–25. doi:10.1111/j.1471-1842.2005.00549.x

Weingarten, K. (2000). Witnessing, wonder and hope. *Family Process*, *39*(4), 389–402. doi:10.1111/j.1545-5300.2000.39401.x

Weingarten, K. (2001). Making sense of illness narratives: Braiding theory, practice and the embodied life. In *Dulwich Centre Publication Working with stories of women's lives*. Adelaide, Australia: Dulwich Centre.

Weingarten, K. (2003). *Common shock, witnessing violence every day: How we are harmed, how we can heal*. New York: Dutton.

Weingarten, K. (1995). Radical listening: Challenging cultural belief for and about mothers. In Weingarten, K. (Ed.), *Cultural resistance: Challenging belief about men, women and therapy*. New York: Haworth.

Weingarten, K. (2009, September). *Hope: In a time of global despair*. Keynote address presented at the New Zealand Association of Counsellors, Hamilton, New Zealand.

Weisz, G. (2005). From Medical Counting to Evidence-Based Medicine. In *Body Counts: Medical Quantification in Historical and Sociological Perspectives // La Quantification médicale, perspectives historiques et sociologiques*, (eds), Gérard Jorland, Annick Opinel and George Weisz, McGill-Queens Press, 2005, 377-393.

Weitzner, D. J., Abelson, H., Berners-Lee, T., Feigenbaum, J., Hendler, J., & Sussman, G. J. (2008). Information accountability. *Communications of the ACM*, *51*(6), 82–87. doi:10.1145/1349026.1349043

Wellbery, C., & Gooch, R. (2005). A web-based multimedia medical humanities curriculum. *Family Medicine*, *37*, 165–167.

Wenger, E. (1998). *Communities of practice: Learning, meaning and identity*. Cambridge, UK: Cambridge University Press.

Wenger, E., & Snyder, W. (2000). Communities of practice: The organizational frontier. *Harvard Business Review*, *78*(1), 139–145.

Werner, A., Isaksen, L. W., & Malterud, K. (2004). I am not the kind of woman who complains of everything': Illness stories on self and shame in women with chronic pain. *Social Science & Medicine*, *59*, 1035–1045. doi:10.1016/j.socscimed.2003.12.001

Westley, F., Zimmerman, B., & Patton, M. (2006). *Getting to maybe: How the world is changed*. Toronto, ON: Random House Canada.

White, D. L., & Hughes, T. P. (2009, April). Predicting the response of CML patients to tyrosine kinase inhibitor therapy. *Current Hematologic Malignancy Reports*, *4*(2), 59–65. doi:10.1007/s11899-009-0009-2

Whitehead, S. M. (2002). *Men and Masculinities*. Cambridge, MA: Polity.

Whitehead, L. C. (2006). Quest, status and restitution: Living with chronic fatigue syndrome/myalgic encephalomyelitis. *Social Science & Medicine*, *62*, 2236–2245. doi:10.1016/j.socscimed.2005.09.008

Whitworth, B., Gallupe, B., & McQueen, R. (2000). A cognitive three-process model of computer-mediated group interaction. *Group Decision and Negotiation*, *9*, 431–456. doi:10.1023/A:1008780324737

WHO (World Health Organization). (2009). *World report on child injury prevention*. Retrieved from http://www.who.int/violence_injury_prevention/child/injury/world_report/en/index.html

WHO. (2005). Priorities to take forward the health equity policy agenda WHO Task Force on Research priorities for equity in health. *Bulletin of the World Health Organization*, 12.

WHO Commission on Social Determinants of Health. *(2008)*. Closing the gap in a generation: health equity through action on the social determinants of health. Final report of the Commission on Social Determinants of Health. *Geneva*.

WHO (World Health Organization). (2003). *Influenza fact sheet*. Retrieved from http://www.who.int/mediacentre/factsheets/2003/fs211/en/

WHO. (2002). *Core Health Indicators for Papua New Guinea*. Retrieved from http://www3.who.int/whosis/country/compare.cfm?country=PNG&indicator=strMortChildMale2002,strMortChildFemale2002&language=english

WHO. (2004). *Roll Mack Malaria Partnership*. Retrieved from http://www.rbm.who.int/cgi-bin/rbm/rbmportal/custom/rbm/home.do

Whyte, W. F. (1991). *Participatory action research*. Newbury Park, CA: Sage.

Wiberg, M. (2007). Netlearning and Learning through Networks. *Journal of Educational Technology & Society*, *10*(4), 49–61.

Wiki Thing. (2009). *Wiki Thing or Library Things*. Visited February 2009. Retrieved from http://www.librarything.com/wiki/index.php/WikiThing:About

Wikipedia (2009). *Knowledge Engineering*. Retrieved from http://en.wikipedia.org/wiki/Knowledge_engineering#cite_note-3

Wikipedia (2009). *Online learning community*. Retrieved September 14th from http://en.wikipedia.org/wiki/Online_learning_community.

Wikipedia (2010, January 28). *Warfarin*. Retrieved February 11, 2010, from http://en/wikipedia.org/wiki/Warfarin

Wikipedia (n.d.). *List of open source healthcare software*. Retrieved July 24, 2009 from http://en.wikipedia.org/wiki/List_of_open_source_healthcare_software.

Williams, L., & Zipperer, L. (2003). Improving Access to Information: Librarians and Nurses Team Up for Patient Safety. *Nursing Economics, 21*(4), 199–201.

Williams, C. (1998) Mysticism Medicine Papua New Guinea. *Wellbeing magazine, 71,* 50-57

Williams, D. (2007). *Blog Glossary; Bloging Terms: Popular Products and Services.* Retrieved from http://www.webdesignseo.com/blogging-terms/web-20-terms.php)

Williams, S. J. (2006). Medical sociology and the biological body: Where are we now and where do we go from here? *Health (London) 10*(5).

Willis, E., Miller, R., & Wyn, J. (2001). Gendered embodiment and survival for young people with cystic fibrosis. *Social Science & Medicine, 53*(9), 1163–1174. doi:10.1016/S0277-9536(00)00416-0

Wilson, D., Chiroro, P., Lavelle, S., & Mutero, C. (1989). Sex worker, client sex behaviour and condom use in Harare, Zimbabwe. *AIDS Care, 1*(3), 269–280. doi:10.1080/09540128908253032

Wing, L., & Gould, J. (1979). Severe impairments of social interaction and associated abnormalities in children: epidemiology & classification. *Journal of Autism and Developmental Disorders, 9*(1), 11–29. doi:10.1007/BF01531288

Wingo, A. P., Harvey, P. D., & Baldessarini, R. J. (2009). Neurocognitive impairment in bipolar disorder patients: functional implications. *Bipolar Disorders, 11,* 113–125. doi:10.1111/j.1399-5618.2009.00665.x

Winkelman, W. J., Leonard, K. J., & Rossos, P. G. (2005). Patient-Perceived Usefulness of Online Electronic Medical Records: Employing Grounded Theory in the Development of Information and Communication Technologies for Use by Patients Living with Chronic Illness. *Journal of the American Medical Informatics Association, 12*(3), 306–314. doi:10.1197/jamia.M1712

Winograd, T., & Flores, R. (1987). *Understanding computers and cognition.* Reading, MA: Addison-Wesley.

Wolf, G., & Hegde, B. M. (1976). Syphilitic Aortic Regurgitation. An appraisal of surgical treatment. *The British Journal of Venereal Diseases, 52,* 366–369.

World Health Organisation (WHO). (2001). *International Classification of Functioning, Disability and Health (ICF)*. Geneva: Williams, G. C., Frankel, R. M., Campbell, T. L., & Deci, E. L. (2000). Research on relationship-centered care and healthcare outcomes from the Rochester biopsychosocial program: A self-determination theory integration. *Families, Systems & Health, 18*(1), 79–90.

Wray, J., & Maynard, L. (2008). Specialist cardiac services: what do young people want? *Cardiology in the Young, 18*(6), 569–574. doi:10.1017/S104795110800317X

Yates, S. (2001). Gender, language and CMC for education. *Learning and Instruction, 11,* 21–34. doi:10.1016/S0959-4752(00)00012-8

Yin, R. (1989). *Case study research.* Newbury Park, CA: SAGE.

Yoshida, K. K. (1993). Reshaping of self: a pendular reconstruction of self and identity among adults with traumatic spinal cord injury'. *Sociology of Health & Illness, 15*(2), 217–245. doi:10.1111/1467-9566.ep11346888

Young, J. (1997). *ITP personal stories: Success story. Platelet disorder support association.* Retrieved April 7, 2010 from http://www.pdsa.org/join-the-community/personal-stories/item/129-success-story.html.

Youngson, R. (2008). *Disabled doctoring – how can we rehabilitate the medical profession?* Paper presented at the Australian and New Zealand Spinal Cord Society Conference, Christchurch, New Zealand.

Zeng, Q. T., Crowell, J., Plovnick, R. M., Kim, E., Ngo, L., & Dibble, E. (2006). Assisting Consumer Health Information Retrieval with Query Recommendations. *Journal of the American Medical Informatics Association, 13*(1), 80–90. doi:10.1197/jamia.M1820

Zhang, B., Shen, L., Jeng, M., Jones, C., Wong, W., Engleman, E., & Zehnder, J. (2009). Increased VNN1/PPARG Gene Expression Ratio Is Correlated with Developing Chronic ITP and Oxidative Stress Exposure to PBMC in Vitro. *Blood, 114*(22), 368.

Zimmerman, P. (2001). *Summary and comment to "Complementary Methodology in Clinical Research - Cognition-based Medicine" - a new book by Helmut Kiene*. New York: Springer Publishers.

Zwick, D., & Dholakia, N. (2004). Consumer subjectivity in the age of internet: The radical concept of marketing control through customer relationship management. *Information and Organization, 14*(3), 211–236. doi:10.1016/j.infoandorg.2004.01.002

About the Contributors

Rakesh Biswas is a professor of Medicine in the Center for Scientific Research and Development, PCMS Campus, Bhopal, India. His interests include clinical problem solving applied to patient centered health care and health education. He has extensively published his experiences in clinical problem solving in global academic journals and books. He is presently a deputy editor for BMJ Case reports, UK, chief editor for the International Journal of User Driven Healthcare, US and a regional editor for the Journal of Evaluation in Clinical Practice, UK. He is an academic co-investigator in funded programs of research on "User Driven Healthcare" in India and Ireland.

Carmel M. Martin is an Associate Professor of Family Medicine at the Northern Ontario School of Medicine and Visiting Professor, University of Buckingham, UK and Visiting Research Fellow Department of Public Health and Primary Care, Trinity College, Dublin. She is active in clinical general practice with a particular interest in chronic disease and illness, patient centered care and complex systems. Carmel has a large volume of publications around this area and she also edits a journal section on Complexity in the Health Sciences for the Journal of Evaluation in Clinical Practice, UK. Carmel is a lead Clinical Principal Investigator on the Patient Journey Record Program in user driven healthcare at the National Digital Research Center NDRC, an independent organization formed by a consortium of members comprising different academic institutes in Dublin.

* * *

Nicole R. Agostinelli, MD, New York Presbyterian/Columbia-Cornell. Dr Agostinelli will be entering her final year of residency at New York Presbyterian Hospital. She graduated from Howard University College of Medicine and completed a year of Surgical internship at Mount Sinai Hospital in New York, NY. Upon completion of her residency, she will continue along her path of providing care to under-served populations world-wide.

Willie Ako is a Commonwealth Professional Scholar. He originates from the Batri community of the Southern Highlands Province of Papua New Guinea (PNG). His recent work focuses on participatory research approaches, combining education and health initiatives for the prevention of Malaria in the Batri community. This work has directly contributed to a decrease in the incidence of deaths through child and maternal malaria in the community. Dr. Ako has contributed to the launch of the 2009 Global Monitoring Report on Education for the Commonwealth Secretariat in London and consulted with UNESCO/International Institute of Educational Planning (IIEP), in Paris in identifying key issues affecting the development of effective educational strategies to address global poverty. Currently, Dr. Ako is working with the Minister of Higher Education in developing cross sectoral educational programs that will enhance strategies for poverty alleviation in PNG.

Mary Allan is a researcher at the School of Social and Political Sciences University of Canterbury, Christchurch, New Zealand and her research interests are led by her key passion for studying relationships. One strand of her work focuses on the study of electronically mediated interactions and their potential for supporting collaboration across work, research, and study environments. In studying this field, Mary focuses on the socio technical relationships emerging against the backdrop of today's Knowledge Economy.The other strand of Mary's work is the study of complex systems and the relationships at play in systems and subsystems. Working in this area Mary developed an innovative model for the implementation and support of change in complex situations. Mary is fascinated by the tensions between individuals and social structures in the context of a society and economy driven by information and the technologies enabling its transfer.

Tom Axtell obtained a M.A. in Education from Bishop's and a Bachelor's Degree in Communication Arts from Concordia University. His main interest is in health education using new media. Tom Axtell worked during the 80's in the Canadian Arctic to establish Inuit language radio and television services. In the 90's he managed the award winning Atii Training Inc. an Inuit management development training program in the years leading to the creation of the Nunavut Territory. He developed Internet services in Nunavik, Quebec, and K-NET in Northern Ontario, including teaching in the first one-room Internet High School in the North. He is the Project Coordinator for the Naasautit: Inuit Health Statistics project with the National Aboriginal Health Organization in Ottawa. (119)

Ayesha Aziz. A medical doctor from Pakistan who acquired a Master in Public Health from the University of Pittsburgh. She has strong interest in health systems and policies. Ayesha had been engaged with different projects in Pakistan that have ranged from infectious diseases to reproductive health issues. She helped in development of the health policy and management component of supercourse and hopes to link health research, advocacy and policy making through it.

Arindam Basu is a medical doctor and an epidemiologist-health services researcher. In addition to teaching courses on research methods, he works as a senior researcher at the Health Services Assessment Collaboration (HSAC) at the University of Canterbury at Christchurch, New Zealand. Before joining Canterbury, he was working as the Associate Director of the Fogarty International Training Program in Environmental and Occupational Health at Kolkata, India.Arin's primary research interests are in systematic reviews and meta analyses in the context of health services and outcomes research. His area of interest in inter-disciplinary linkage between health services research and environmental epidemiology. He has published on health impacts and determinants of Arsenic toxicity in the India, and currently edits a systematic review on middle ear pain in airplane travellers for "Clinical Evidence" – a secondary evidence based journal.

Paramartha Bhattacharya graduated in medicine in 1992 from Kolkata National Medical College, Kolkata in 1992 and id his post graduate diploma in Tropical Medicine from School of Tropical Medicine, Kolkata in 1995-97 when he worked with HIV pts with secondary infections such as Kaalazar and multi dermatomal HZ.Presently working as senior meical officer, Institute of Cadiovascular Sciences, SSKM hosp and IPGMER Kolkata, India ,interested in echocardiography of foetus.Happily married it Moonmoon and having a small family with two little sons he practices medicine esp, cardiology and diabetes in Kolkata and downtown at Serampore and Chanditala, Hooghly.

Kresten Bjerg. Born 1935 in Copenhagen. Married since 1955 with Beth Bjerg, speech therapist, with whom I have 3 daughters and 5 grandchildren. Studied Theater & Drama, Sorbonne, Paris 1953-54. Ph.d. in Psychology, University of Copenhagen, 1961. Research fellow, Harvard University (under professor Henry A. Murray) 1962."The Suicide Prevention Center, Los Angeles (under Dr Edwin Shneidman),1963. Research & teaching at Department of Psychology, University of Copenhagen, 1964-99. Interpersonal communication, Altered states of consciousness, Home-oriented Informatics & Telematics, Qualitative Research Methods in Psychology and "In and out of Theories of Personality". Developed & maintained an "Experimental Home" in the Department of Psychology, for user-oriented empirical research on domestic information-technology & domestic information dynamics 1974 -98. Development and testing of a cross-platform tool for maintaining electronic diary, 1995- 2010. Retired 1999.

Paul Bradley MRCPsych is a Specialty Registrar in Psychiatry working in the UK's National Health Service based in Hertfordshire, England. He is specialising in the support of people with learning disabilities and intellectual impairment.

Anirban Chaudhuri, originally a resident of Calcutta, India, graduated from Calcutta National Medical College in 1993.From 1996 to 1998,he worked and trained in the capacity of Honorary Clinical Attachee in the departments of Intensive Care Medicine and Traumatology in Scunthorpe General Hospital in North Lincolnshire, United Kingdom.He also was a member of the first Mobile Cardiac Care Unit of Goole Hospital, North Lincolnshire and worked there for 8 months in 1999, after which he came back to India, and shifted base to Mumbai in 2000.He worked in the capacity of the Clinical Assistant in the Emergency ICU in Hinduja Hospital for 5 years. Since 2007, he is attached to Mangalmurti Group of Hospitals, North Mumbai, as a Consultant Physician, with special interest in Cardiology and Intensive Care Medicine. Apart from Medicine, he does extensive reading in anthropology, history, theoretical physics and philosophy. He is an avid sports fan of cricket and Formula One Motor Racing. He is married and is a doting father of a one year old daughter.

Cassandra Chaulk, a Health Data Analyst with the Nunatsiavut Government in Labrador, was hired through the Naasautit Inuit Health Information Project and has worked on various projects such as the National Aboriginal Youth Suicide Prevention Strategy (NAYSPS) Evaluation along with a mentorship on an internal Seniors Survey from start to finish; and assisted with the regional component of the Inuit Health Survey with McGill University. She has travelled throughout Nunatsiavut teaching Microsoft Word and Excel to Department of Health and Social Development employees. She has completed a vast amount of training which includes: Public Health of Canada online Epidemiology courses: "Basic Epidemiological Concepts"; "Measurement of Health Status" and "Epidemiologic Methods"; Statistics Canada: "Surveys from Start to Finish" and "Aboriginal Statistical Training"; Canada's Evaluation Society, Newfoundland and Labrador Chapter: "Essentials Skills Series I- IV." Cassandra also provides on an ongoing basis statistical support to various departments within the Nunatsiavut Government.

Ronán Conroy is associate professor of biostatistics in the Royal College of Surgeons in Ireland, an independent medical school. He graduated in psychology and, later, in music. He teaches evidence based health in the undergraduate curriculum, a module which includes a significant ethics component, and research methods at postgraduate level. His research includes work on on health in developing countries, including the use of solar disinfection, health psychology, psychiatric epidemiology, and cardiovascular risk assessment. He is surprised as anyone by all of this, having more or less expected to be a music teacher.

Anjan Kumar Das was born in Calcutta and educated in the Medical College, Calcutta and at the Institute of Postgraduate Medical Education and Research, Calcutta. He trained first in general surgery and then as a cardiothoracic surgeon and spent 25 years as a medical teacher and consultant In Cardiothoracic Surgery first in Calcutta, then at Pokhara, Nepal and Gangtok, Sikkim, India where he headed the Department of Surgery at the Sikkim Manipal Institute of Medical Sciences.. At present he is working in clinical research in the field of stem cells and is based in Kuala Lumpur, Malaysia. Dr Das has had a long standing interest in the fields of basic research and low cost health care. He spends his holidays trekking in the Himalayas.

Brenda Dervin is Full Professor of Communication and Joan N. Huber Fellow in Social and Behavioral Sciences, Ohio State University. She received her bachelor's degree from Cornell University and master's and doctoral degrees from Michigan State, all in communication. She holds an honorary doctorate in social sciences from the University of Helsinki. Her Sense-Making Methodology, in development for some 35 years, has been applied as approach to research, dialogue, and design in multiple fields -- e.g., library and information science, health communication, telecommunication policy, audience reception, participatory pedagogy, organizational communication, and media uses. She is past president and fellow of the International Communication Association (ICA) and one of few North Americans to serve the European-based International Association of Media and Communication Research board. She has been recipient of research excellence awards from ICA and from the American Society for Information Science and Technology (ASIST). She is a fellow in the ASIST Special Interest Group focusing on information needs, seeking and use.

Binod Dhakal, MD was born in a small suburb in Kathmandu City in Nepal. After finishing his high school from the city he did his medical school in Manipal College of Medical Sciences in Pokhara, Nepal. He did his Internal medicine residency at Saint Francis Hospital at Evanston Illinois, USA.He is currently working as Assistant Professor in Internal Medicine in Medical College of Wisconsin in Milwaukee USA from July 2010 after completing his residency. His hobbies include reading science books, listening to music and travelling. He has also published few articles on narrative medicine in international journals focusing on the multidimensional aspects of health care. His areas of interest include basic science research and non linear approach to health care.

Rachel H. Ellaway is an Assistant Dean Informatics in the Northern Ontario School of Medicine-Sudbury, Ontario, CANADA and some of her resesarch interests include, Cultural Informatics, Narrative Medicine, Simulation in health-care and creation of Virtual Patient Banks.

Jane Fitzpatrick is a senior lecturer at the University of the West of England, Bristol. She has a keen interest in the development of collaborative learning cultures and draws on research approaches which focus on empowerment and capacity building as change agents. This interest combined with her clinical perspective as a public health nurse led to an innovative project with a disadvantaged, urban community in Papua New Guinea. This was extended to a malaria prevention initiative in the Batri Villages in the Southern Highlands. This has enabled the people of the villages to develop an effective strategy which demonstrates effective use and deployment of resources in the use of WHO approved ITN bed nets and thus enhance their health experiences. The people of the villages report that they have had no deaths from Malaria since the introduction of the nets and that generally 'people are walking straighter and feeling better

J.M. Garg is a passionate naturalist & a wildlife photographer. He has been trekking a lot since last 15 years. He is creating awareness about our Trees & Plants, winged friends (Birds), Butterflies, etc. in particular & nature around us in general. He has published a book called 'A Photo guide to the birds of Kolkata & Common birds of India'. He has held few Exhibitions mainly focusing on Bird Photography. He is the owner of 'Efloraofindia' - a Google group http://groups.google.co.in/group/indiantreepix?hl=en (around 1400 members on 10/10/10), the largest e-group in India (more than 50,000 messages so far in last three years & four months). Efloraofindia is the largest Google e-group in the world in this field & largest nature related e-group (and the most constructive) in India devoted to creating awareness, helping in identification etc. along with discussion on & documentation of Indian Flora. 'Efloraofindia' Database of around 4100 species can be downloaded from home page at http://groups.google.co.in/group/indiantreepix?hl=en

Vahideh Zarea Gavgani, PhD. LIS. Is a Researcher, Assistant Professor in LIS and healthcare, Member of Center for EBM in Tabriz University of Medical Science (Iran). She has published many research papers and books, worked on research projects and lectured for medical student, residents Library science student thorough formal academic courses and workshops. Her topic of interests are: EBM, EBLIP, Information Therapy (Ix), Healthcare, Consumer Health Information (CHI), Web 2.0, Digital Repositories, Digital libraries, LIS education.

Sheila Glenn is Professor of Applied Developmental Psychology at Liverpool John Moores University. She has previously held posts at the Universities of London, Southampton, Manchester and Central Lancashire and has published widely in the field of developmental disability.

Rishi K Goyal, MD, M.Phil New York Presbyterian/Columbia-Cornell Dr. Goyal is currently a Chief Resident at New York Presbyterian and will be an Assistant Professor of Emergency Medicine in June at the University of Arizona where he will also lead the Humanism education for the University of Arizona Medical School. He graduated from Columbia College of Physicians and Surgeons following which he enrolled in a Ph.D. program in English Literature at Columbia University. Dr. Goyal will be defending his dissertation on the Invention of Old Age in April, 2010. Dr. Goyal is actively involved in initiatives to bridge the concerns of evidence based medicine and narrative medicine.

Daz Greenop is Senior Lecturer at Liverpool John Moores University Centre for Social Work. He has worked in a variety of settings providing group therapy, one-to-one counselling and care management for a range of service user groups. Prior to his current academic post, Daz worked as a medical social worker at Liverpool Heart & Chest Hospital. He has particular interest in qualitative and participatory research methods, health psychology and medical sociology.

Ann Griffin is the mother of four sons, two with a diagnosis of Asperger syndrome/ADHD and one with ADHD. Ann works full time at a local college and helps with a local support group for families who live with autism. Ann's aim is to raise awareness of autism and to campaign to change how people view autism.

Peter Griffin is 29 years old with a diagnosis of Asperger syndrome/ADHD. Peter was diagnosed at the age of 19 having spent many years trying to find the answers about who he was. Peter was relieved to be diagnosed as he had thought he was going mad. Since then he has made it a focus to tell his story to ensure people understand autism.

BM Hegde was Professor, Director and Dean of Kasturba Medical College, Manipal, India and later the Vice Chancellor of Manipal University, India. He has more than 250 research articles and thousands of lay articles to educate the common man about health and wellness concepts. He has 35 books both for doctors and lay people in English and Kannada. Govt. of India has recently honored him with the prestigious Padma Bhushan award (akin to Knighthood in the UK). He is still active in spreading his Healing philosophy and Wellness Concept all over the world.

Richard James was born in Palmerton PA USA in 1920, He received an M.D. from the University of Pennsylvania in 1943. He served as a Flight Surgeon with the US Army Air Corps at Hickam Field Hawaii. After WWII, he received additional training in internal medicine at Cornell University, New York, The University of Pennsylvania, and completed a 2-year residency at Emory University, Atlanta, GA. He practiced primary care internal medicine in Charlotte, NC for many years. On retirement in 1985, he embarked on an effort to help busy clinicians keep up with the current literature and currently edits the "Practical Pointers for Primary Care Medicine" that is now accessed through the internet by over 12 000 individuals monthly.

Ankur Joshi perused his graduation in Medicine and a Masters in Community Medicine from Gandhi Medical College, Bhopal, respectively, in 2004 and 2008. His area of interest is infectious disease epidemiology (more specifically TB, HIV and related issues) and health policy analysis. He has been involved in some community oriented studies during his residency period. Several of which were funded by reputed internal organizations and the Government of India. He has presented several papers at national and international conferences. His thesis topic in post graduation was addressing the issue of non adherence in Tuberculosis. He believes that User Driven Healthcare may be an appropriate, acceptable and affordable as well as a sustainable response to meager resources in a developing country set up.

Edward Kim, MD, MBA, has over 15 years of experience in mental health as a provider, teacher, and researcher. A board-certified psychiatrist, he was vice chair of clinical programs at the Robert Wood Johnson Medical School, where he is a Clinical Associate Professor of Psychiatry. He received his bachelor's degree from Harvard University and his MD from Jefferson Medical College in Philadelphia, completing his psychiatric residency at Thomas Jefferson University Hospital. While Medical Director of Adult Services at the University of Medicine and Dentistry of New Jersey – University Behavioral HealthCare, a statewide integrated behavioral delivery system, he led quality improvement initiatives to reduce barriers to patient transfers across levels of care, and increase integration of physical health with mental health services. He earned an MBA from the University of Massachusetts at Amherst.

Dianne Kinnon is the Director of Inuit Tuttarvingat (the Inuit-specific centre) of the National Aboriginal Health Organization in Ottawa. She grew up in the countryside in Saskatchewan, attended university in Regina and then moved to Ontario where she worked in community health services. After getting a Master of Arts degree in public administration from Carleton University, Dianne worked for many years as an independent consultant in social and health issues and travelled throughout the country. She has worked continuously for and with Inuit, Métis and First Nations organizations over the last 17 years, on topics such as recruitment and retention of Aboriginal students in medical schools, Indigenous research capacity, community health capacity, national strategies for violence prevention and for residential schools healing, and sexual/reproductive health.

Monica Kochar has been in teaching profession for over 15 years teaching middle and senior classes. She started from Mothers International School and Mirambika in New Delhi in the year of 1993, to The Blue Mountain School in Ooty and then The Valley School in Bangalore. Apart from excellent capability in teaching skills and techniques, Monica comes with strengths in Specialist support to SEN children in Mathematics & Creating individualized programs for SEN children. She has also given/attended many workshops and written articles on new/alternate methods of teaching mathematics. Monica is qualified with Level 2 certificate course in IGCSE, she has been trained by IBO for MYP level 1 Mathematics, apart from Inclusive Education – teaching children with learning disability in the classroom Bangalore (2005-2006). Apart from this she has done B. Ed. From CIE and M. Sc. (Maths) and B. Sc (Honors) in Maths from Delhi University.

Elmarie Kotzé is an educational psychologist and senior lecturer at the Department of Human Development and Counselling at the University of Waikato, New Zealand. Her professional life has taken her through various disciplines. What has remained constant throughout her journey is a passionate search for ways that counselling practice and theory can come together to sustain and enrich the hopes and dreams that people hold for themselves, their families, and communities. As a teacher she has committed herself to students' interests and professional development. The papers students have published and their grateful support for what has been most precious to them stands as a testimony to her commitment. Susan Sliedrecht has a Masters degree in counselling and in social work. She works as a counsellor at the Auckland Spinal Rehabilitation Unit in New Zealand. She is committed to working collaboratively alongside patients and their families at both an individual and a community level to support them to achieve what is important to them.

Ronald LaPorte is a Cognitive Psychologist turned epidemiologist. His primary interest is the application of Internet Technology to the prevention of disease. His team has helped create the Supercourse which has over 65,000 faculties world-wide. He has published over 462 papers, and is a Director for Disease Monitoring and Telecommunications at the WHO Collaborating center.

Martin Ledson is Consultant Respiratory Physician at Liverpool Heart and Chest Hospital. He has published widely in his specialist areas of cystic fibrosis and lung cancer.

Richard Lehman is a Senior Research Fellow in the Department of Primary Care at Oxford University. He is perhaps best known for his individual weekly reviews of the principal general medical journals, maintained for the last 12 years and posted worldwide by the Centre for Evidence Based Medicine and on the BMJ website. His clinical interests are wide and in 2006 he was responsible for the first book on Palliative Care for Heart Failure. Following retirement this year from clinical practice R has been acting as medical adviser to the Health Experiences Research Group at Oxford and their groundbreaking website of patient interviews covering 70 clinical areas on www.healthtalkonline.org. His current main interest is in combining qualitative and quantitative research methods to identify patient-important outcome measures, especially in chronic illnesses as exemplified by type 2 diabetes.

Faina Linkov is a Research Assistant Professor of Medicine at the University of Pittsburgh School of Medicine, Department of Medicine, Division of Hematology and Oncology. Dr. Linkov holds PhD in Epidemiology, MPH in the Community and Behavioral Health Sciences, and Certificate of Advanced Studies in Global Health from the University of Pittsburgh. Her current research activities concentrate on the use of biological tumor markers to detect malignancies at early stages and on the link between obesity and cancer. Dr. Linkov served as a peer reviewer for the British Medical Journal (BMJ), Journal of Medical Internet Research, and others. Dr. Linkov participated in several Peer Review Congresses and has keen interest in peer review methods, publication planning, and authorship concerns. In the past ten years, Dr. Linkov has been working with Professor Ronald LaPorte in the Global Health Network Supercourse Project, supported by NASA and NIH www.pitt.edu/~super1. Supercourse is an open access Internet based library of lectures on public health and prevention hosted at the University of Pittsburgh server. With over 48,000 participants in 174 countries Supercourse is one of the largest efforts in the area of Public Health. One of the main goals of the Supercourse developers is to close the digital divide and deliver public health education materials to faculty members in the developing world. As a part of the Supercourse effort, Dr. Linkov was exploring the issues associated with open access publication, peer review, and alternatives to peer review. Exploration of peer review mechanisms has been the focus of Dr. Linkov's dissertation research. Several publications came out of this research, including one on the utility of Amazon.com type 5-star evaluation system for online lectures.

Mita Lovalekar is an Assistant Professor in the Department of Sports Medicine and Nutrition within the School of Health and Rehabilitation Sciences at the University of Pittsburgh. She is a physician trained in India, and completed both her Master's and Doctoral degrees in Epidemiology at the University of Pittsburgh. Her research interests include injury epidemiology and prevention, application of the Internet to dissemination of health information, and chronic disease epidemiology.

J. Huw C. Morgan was an inner-city General Practitioner and GP Educator in the United Kingdom for over two decades. For the last ten years has worked internationally in medical education in Eastern Europe, South Asia and Africa. He continues to work part time in General Practice and undergraduate medical education in the UK, as well as being a GP Educator on a post-graduate training programme for General Practice in South West England. He has published numerous papers on aspects of medical education and has always been interested in the interface of the humanities with medicine as a means of encouraging the development of compassion and other positive professional attributes in doctors.

Kamalika Mukherji M.R.C.Psych is a Consultant Psychiatrist in the National Health Service, U.K. and provides clinical leadership to a variety of community based services for adults with Learning Disabilities. She integrates her clinical work with academic activities in London and Cambridge.

Cameron Norman is an Assistant Professor in the Dalla Lana School of Public Health at the University of Toronto and the Director of Evaluation for the Peter A. Silverman Global eHealth Program. His research looks at the intersection of systems and design thinking and information technology and how they combine to facilitate diverse groups in collaborating to solve complex health problems. Through the use of social media, Dr. Norman seeks to understand how to leverage networks more effectively to promote knowledge translation for health and support social innovation on issues of public health and health promotion with professionals and the community alike. His research focuses on eHealth, transdisciplinary collaboration, communities of practice, knowledge integration in public health, systems thinking and complexity science, and health behaviour change. He lives in Toronto, Canada.

Matthew T. O'Neill, MD New York Presbyterian Hospital, Columbia-Cornell Dr. O'Neill is currently a Chief Resident of Emergency Medicine at New York Presbyterian, and in July will be an Instructor of Emergency Medicine at the New York Presbyterian Weill Cornell Medical Center. He graduated from the University of Illinois College of Medicine in Chicago and received his undergraduate degree from the University of Chicago. Dr. O'Neill's interests in Medicine are broad and range from the basic sciences to the medical humanities.

Brendan O' Shea practices medicine in Ireland, qualifying from TCD (1986), and is on The Specialist Regsiter of The Irish Medical Council for General Practice and Occupational Medicine. In 2005 he achieved Fellowship of The RCGP by assessment, the only GP to do so practicing outside of the UK. His current committements include GP Principal at The Bridge Medical Centre in Co. Kildare. He is an Assistant Director at the TCD HSE GP Training Scheme, and Medical Director at K Doc, a GP Co Operative including 104 GP Members. He also holds a part time academic post of Lecturer at Trinity Collge Dublin, Department of Primary Care and Public Health. He is presently writing an MD Thesis on Multimorbidity and Chronic Disease Management. His extra professional interests include intermittent bad golf, occassional dodgy boating, the odd decent photograph, and he considers himself very fortunate indeed to be taken for a walk most days by his best friend and two dogs. He is married to Corinna, and they have three boys.

Billy O' Steen is a researcher at the School of Educational Studies and Human Development, University of Canterbury, NZ. His research focuses on innovative curriculum design and professional development with a particular emphasis on experiential education and service-learning.

Max Overton was educated in New Zealand and Australia. He attended Victoria University in Wellington, New Zealand, where he majored in botany and zoology before getting his master's degree in plant physiology. He spent many years working for the New Zealand Government and private industry as a tissue culture researcher, before returning to academic studies at Massey University. Here he studied butterfly genetics and bumblebee ecology. Moving to Australia, Max worked as a lecturer at James Cook University in Townsville, and undertook doctoral research on butterfly ecology. He also entered the field of science education, working with Aboriginal communities in Queensland. Max is currently working for a microscopy supply house in Townsville, and writing fiction. He has nine published novels.

Chris Peterson works in the School of Social Sciences at La Trobe University and conducts research in the Youth Research Centre, University of Melbourne. He previously worked in the School of Public Health at La Trobe, and together with his work at the National Centre for Epidemiology and Population Health at the Australian National University has developed an epidemiological focus to his sociological research into health and illness and particularly chronic diseases. He has a jointly edited book on chronic illness and has published widely in local and international journals on chronic disease. He has also focussed on chronic disease as an occupational health and safety concern. He works on chronic illness projects both in Australia and as part of some international groups of researchers.

Asanga (Amar Puri) has traveled extensively throughout India, following many spiritual masters and for the past 20 years has dedicated his life to the study of Hatha Yoga and Ayurvedic principles. For many years, Asanga was disciple of Yogi Vikashanand at the Ananda Yoga Centre, Kathmandu, where he specialized in Yogic Cleansing, asanas and spiritual healing, and was the principal yoga teacher. He then went on to study Naturopathy and Yoga Therapy with the Indian Board of Alternative Medicines in Calcutta, India and gained a Bachelor Certificate on 2001. In 2002, Asanga married his wife Durga. Asanga also has 2 sons, and runs a yoga centre in Pokhara, Nepal

Susan D. Ross, MD, FRCPC, is a practicing internist in the Boston area, and an independent consultant in Evidence-based Medicine (EBM). She was a co-founder of MetaWorks, an AHRQ Evidence-based Practice Center, in Boston, where for many years she led MetaWorks' technical teams performing literature-based systematic reviews and meta-analyses. Prior to MetaWorks, Dr. Ross served as a Vice President of Clinical Research at a biotech company in Boston, as well as a clinical research consultant to industry. Her previous clinical practice experience includes a stint in outpatient Internal Medicine at a Boston-area HMO, and a hospital-based practice in Toronto. She is an honors graduate of the University of Toronto Faculty of Medicine, and completed an advanced course in Biomedical Research Management at the Harvard School of Public Health The unifying theme of her career to date has been the development and utilization of better ways to harness the power of data for healthcare. To this end, she has over 60 scientific publications and 90 abstracts presented at professional meetings, and she has authored/delivered numerous online and in-person seminars and workshops in EBM. She is presently intrigued with the challenge of how best to marry EBM and User-Driven Healthcare.

Suptendra Nath Sarbadhikari, MBBS, PhD A physician and a biomedical engineer, is currently the Founding Director of CAL2CAL Institute. He has written a book "A Short Introduction to Biomedical Engineering" and has edited another book "Depression and Dementia: Progress in Brain Research, Clinical Applications and Future Trends". He is a Faculty and Fellow of PSG FAIMER Regional Institute. He is the Editor-in-Chief of the Indian Journal of Medical Informatics (2007-2011). He is the Chair of the Education Committee, HL7 India (2009-2011) and the Chair-Elect, HL7 India (2010-2011). He has numerous publications and awards for medical informatics and education. He is a member of the Expert

Committee on Standards for Electronic Medical Records, Working Groups on Indian Health Information Network Development (i-HIND) and Health Literacy and Portal, of the Ministry of Health and Family Welfare, Government of India. Globally he is an emissary of health informatics standards in the form of being an HL7 Ambassador – a select representative of the global standards HL7 for healthcare information exchange and also as the India representative for the international Vital Records Functional Profile, being developed by the Center for Diseases Control, Atlanta and HL7 International.

Francois Sauer, MD, University of Mexico, UNAM; MBA, Harvard Business School program in Mexico City and MS Systems Analysis, Spanish-American University, Mexico City. CEO Trans Am Group. Trustee of the Baker University Board. Board member of the International Relations Council. Prior to this, he was the CEO of Cerner International, which produces IT products for health industry applications including presence in Australia, Singapore, Malaysia, Saudi Arabia, and Europe. At Transquest, Inc., he participated in an expansion strategy for the AT&T joint venture with Delta Airlines. Before that, he was at AT&T's Global Information Solution (old NCR) 1994 Developer, Global Health Network. Author of numerous publications on health care, IT, telecom, and the options for their collaborative application.

David J. Schaefer (Ph.D., The Ohio State University) is Professor and Chair in the Department of Communication Arts at Franciscan University of Steubenville in Ohio. His research interests include digital media literacy and dialogic theory, global/intercultural communication, South Asian cinema, and broadcast production. He has presented numerous conference papers and published journal articles and book chapters on these topics. His paper "Rethinking Electronic Public Spheres: Beyond Consensus/ Dissensus" won the Millennium Outstanding Paper Award at the 2000 Rochester Institute of Technology intercultural communication conference. He is a member of the Phi Kappa Phi National Honor Society, the International Communication Association, the Communication Institute for Online Scholarship, the Asian Media Information and Communication Centre, and serves on the Board of Directors for Urban Mission Ministries. In 2004-2005, he was awarded the Fulbright lecturing-research senior fellowship at the Wee Kim Wee School of Communication and Information, Nanyang Technological University, Singapore; in 2008 and 2009, he returned to NTU as a visiting research fellow.

P. Ravi Shankar is a Professor in Clinical Pharmacology and in Medical Education at KIST Medical College, a new medical school in Kathmandu valley, Nepal. He had started a Medical Humanities module at Manipal College of Medical Sciences, Pokhara as a curriculum innovation project as part of a FAIMER fellowship. He has conducted modules for faculty members and students at KIST Medical College. Dr. Shankar is a creative writer and a keen trekker and photographer.

Eugene Shubnikov, MD, is research scientist of the Laboratory of clinical, population and prevention studies of therapeutic and endocrine diseases, Institute of Internal Medicine, Novosibirsk, Russia from 1986. He graduated from Novosibirsk Medical Institute, Novosibirsk in 1985. Member of the European Association for the study of Diabetes from 1992. Fellowship under Freedom Support Act at University of Pittsburgh, Graduated School of Public Health, Department of Epidemiology. Moderator of Internet prevention program for Former Soviet Union countries in the frame of Supercourse Global Library Project in Public Health, Epidemiology and Internet, Developer of the Global Free Library of Lectures at Internet - Supercourse project from 2000. www.pitt.edu/~super1/index.htm

Susan Sliedrecht has a Masters degree in counselling and in social work. She works as a counsellor at the Auckland Spinal Rehabilitation Unit in New Zealand. She is committed to working collaboratively alongside patients and their families at both an individual and a community level to support them to achieve what is important to them.

Kevin Smith is a translational research leader with the National Digital Research Centre, Ireland and a scientific advisor on collaborative medical education to the Northern Ontario School of Medicine. In 1977 he received an MPhil in pure mathematics from Murdoch University in Western Australia and then spent 10 years at the University of London working on the application of massively parallel computing to a wide range of applications from lattice gauge simulations to medical image processing. He returned to Australia in 1990 and joined CSIRO - the Australian Government's main R&D agency. There he set up the joint Australian National University - CSIRO Virtual Environments Laboratory that pioneered the development and application of collaborative hapto-visual environments to surgical training. In 2001, he was the founding Director of the Western Australian Interactive Virtual Environments Centre before moving to Canada in 2003 to be a Strategic Advisor to the National Institute for Nanotechnology.

Joachim P. Sturmberg is an Associate Professor of General Practice at Monash University Melbourne and the University of Newcastle, Australia. He has a longstanding involvement in under- and post-graduate teaching in General Practice. His main research interest relates to the complex adaptive nature of health service structures and their impact on patient care.

Maartje Swennen graduated Medical School at the University Medical Centre Utrecht in 2002 and to date has been working here as a staff member for the Executive Board. In 2004 she obtained an MSc in Healthcare Management at the Erasmus Medical Centre in Rotterdam. Her Master Thesis concerned the barriers for the implementation of Evidence-based Medicine (EBM). This Thesis has gradually evolved into a PhD-fellowship that started late 2008 within the PhD Programme Epidemiology of the division Julius Centre for Health Sciences and Primary Care. Her aim is to triage doctors to their specific characteristics and behaviour in order to match the implementation strategy with the actual needs and wishes of diverse types of doctors. Her supervisors are Professor Yolanda van der Graaf and Professor Cor Kalkman. Her co-supervisor is Associate Professor Geert van der Heijden.

Dinesh Vigneshwar Valke, is into software testing with IBM India Pvt. Ltd in its Websphere division of India Software Lab.He had graduated as a Mechanical Engineer from Manipal Institute of Technology in 1986. For a decade, he worked in Engineering industry related to pumps. It was at Voltas Ltd. that the computer-shy Dinesh got hands-on experience with user-friendly inventory and purchase applications. Fine Arts, his basic interest moved him towards Computer Graphics - IT industry, since 1998.

Handan Vicdan is an Assistant Professor of Marketing at Eastern Kentucky University. Her research stream includes studies of social, cultural, and technological transformations in how consumers (re) organize their lives and become producers of their experiences in actual/virtual theaters of consumption; specifically issues of consumer freedom, body, power, resistance, the effects of online media technologies on consumer literacy and consumer-marketer collaboration, and implications of social networking in healthcare. She has published in numerous journals such as Journal of Customer Behaviour, Journal of

MacroMarketing, and Journal of Virtual Worlds Research, and in conference proceedings such as Association for Consumer Research, Academy of Marketing Science, and American Marketing Association.

Martin Walshaw is Consultant Respiratory Physician at Liverpool Heart and Chest Hospital and Director of the Regional Adult Cystic Fibrosis Unit. He has published widely and carried out pioneering work looking at infection in CF patients, much of which has been incorporated into the national recommendations for managing CF patients.

Evan Willis is Professor of Sociology and Associate Dean (Regions) at La Trobe University. Over a long career primarily as a medical sociologist he has worked on a variety of topics including the division of labour in health care, occupational health and safety, complementary and alternative health care, RSI, evidence based health care, genomics, the social relations of medical technology, and most recently the health impacts of Climate Change. His 1989 book Medical Dominance, was in 2003 voted by peers one of the 10 most influential books in Australian Sociology. He has served on a number of both federal and state inquiries at various times, including a national inquiry into Medicare, the Australia Health Technology Advisory Committee of the NHMRC, and the future of Chinese Medicine in Victoria

Michele Wood has been the Researcher/Evaluator for the Nunatsiavut Government, Department of Health and Social Development since 2007. She is a beneficiary of the Labrador Inuit Land Claims Agreement and was born in North West River, Labrador. Michele is currently working on the completion of a Masters of Information Management through Dalhousie University with an undergraduate degree obtained from Acadia University. Prior to working with the Nunatsiavut Government, Michele worked with the Government of Newfoundland and Labrador for 12 years with her most recent position being as a Senior Analyst with the Department of Labrador and Aboriginal Affairs. Recent work includes: coordinating regional participation in national and international research projects (such as the Inuit Health Survey); participating in national forums and committees on ethics, protocol development and health research. She also coordinates projects specific to the Aboriginal Health Transition Fund for the Nunatsiavut region.

Peter C. Wyer, MD Columbia University, NY Dr. Wyer is Associate Clinical Professor of Medicine, Columbia University College of Physicians & Surgeons. He is a recognized author and educator in the area of EBM. He is a member of the Evidence-Based Medicine Working Group and a substantial contributor to the JAMA Users' Guides to the Medical Literature series. He originated and edited innovative educational series on EBM in the CMAJ, Journal of General Internal Medicine and Annals of Emergency Medicine. He is the founder and chair of the SEBHC of NYAM, is a Fellow of the Academy and has overseen EBM educational initiatives in that venue since 1996, as well as at McMaster University and other international EBM workshops. He was principal investigator of a project to develop and validate assessment tools for EBM within the ACGME practice-based learning and improvement model funded by the Stemmler Fund of the National Board of Medical Examiners, and was principal investigator of a 2007 Consensus Conference on "Knowledge Translation and Emergency Medicine" funded by AHRQ, NIH and the Canadian Institutes for Healthcare Research.

Joan Young is the founder of the Platelet Disorder Support Association (PDSA) and author of the book, Wish by Spirit: A journey of recovery and healing from an autoimmune blood disease. Ms. Young has a BS in Education from Kutztown University and an MBA from Lehigh University. Prior to her involvement with PDSA she was a teacher and later led system implementation projects, including work for a hospital consortia and several pharmaceutical companies. Ms. Young has been a consultant and invited speaker at the National Institutes of Health, an author of three journal articles, and a member of an international coalition that published a consensus report on the treatment of ITP.

Index